IMMUNOLOGY OF INFLAMMATION

Handbook of inflammation

Volume 4

Series Editors

L.E. Glynn, John C. Houck and
Gerald Weissmann

1983
ELSEVIER
AMSTERDAM · NEW YORK · OXFORD

Immunology of inflammation

Editor

Peter A. Ward
Department of Pathology, University of Michigan Medical School,
Ann Arbor, Michigan, USA

1983
ELSEVIER
AMSTERDAM · NEW YORK · OXFORD

ISBN Vol. 4: 0-444-90286-4
ISBN Series: 0-444-80118-9

Published by:
Elsevier Science Publishers B.V.
P.O. Box 1126
1000 BC Amsterdam

Sole distributors for the U.S.A. and Canada:
Elsevier Science Publishing Co., Inc.
52 Vanderbilt Avenue
New York, N.Y. 10017

Printed in the Netherlands by Casparie Amsterdam

Preface

The editors propose to publish, over the course of the next few years, a series of at least five volumes entitled 'The Handbook of Inflammation', each volume focussing on a major element of the inflammatory process. Insofar as possible the editors have endeavored to select authors who were both knowledgeable and willing to review in detail the voluminous literature of their particular view of the field of inflammation in an interdisciplinary fashion. Each of the various editors are solely responsible for the selection of authors and subject of each volume, while all of the editors collectively are responsible for the volume topic.

The purpose of the series is to provide detailed and definitive reports of many of the multiplex components which go into the inflammatory process and to do this on an interdigitated and integrated basis. Because of the multidisciplinary aspects of inflammation, this is both necessary and difficult. In this field investigators must be capable of both 'looking down the tube' as well as 'pouring things into it'. To some workers the expression 'broken cell' means biological and membrane disaster, whereas to others it means that the ultracentrifuge is broken. Over the past decade, however, biologists have learned biochemistry to some degree and biochemists have had to learn some biology. Because of a shared vocabulary which has been developing as a consequence of this understanding of another discipline, a greater dialogue is now possible about inflammation than ever before. It is the conclusion of the editors that the compilation of interdisciplinary reviews side-by-side in the same volume will contribute to the further development of this colloquy.

L.E.G.
J.C.H.
G.W.

Volume 1–Chemical messengers of the inflammatory process
Volume 2–The cell biology of inflammation
Volume 3–Tissue repair and regeneration
Volume 4–Immunology of inflammation
Volume 5–The molecular basis for anti-inflammatory therapy

Introduction to Volume 4

The first three volumes of the *Handbook of Inflammation* have dealt with a wide variety of topics related to the inflammatory system. In Volume 4 we have tried to incorporate both basic and clinical investigative approaches in the broad context of Immunopathology. Some of the contributions deal with fundamentals of the inflammatory system, such as consideration of the toxic oxygen products from activated phagocytic cells, determinants of the fibrotic response, phlogistic derivatives of arachidonic acid metabolites, chemotactic mechanisms, inflammatory mediators of the complement and the coagulation systems, and related topics. It is interesting to note how the chapters in this volume differ in their content from similar chapters contained within the first three volumes, even though Volume 1 was published only rather recently (1979). For instance, in the newest volume's chapter dealing with chemotaxis, even though it has been preceded by two earlier and similar chapters, we now see an emphasis on how much is now known about chemotactic responses of nonphagocytic cells such as fibroblasts, platelets, and even tumor cells. In addition, the rapid growth of understanding about the relationship of the chemotactic responses and increases in adherence properties of responding cells is emphasized. In Volume 4 there are several contributions on the role of arachidonate metabolites in inflammation and the cell-damaging effects of H_2O_2 and oxygen-derived free radicals. With the rapid and expansive growth of knowledge, it is now possible to present more definitive information on the role of these factors in the inflammatory reaction in ways that were unimagined only two or three years ago.

Interspersed in this current volume are also contributions that emphasize our recent understanding of how immunopathologic mechanisms participate in disease processes affecting specific organs. In each instance, an attempt has been made to focus on new concepts. For instance, the chapter dealing with renal diseases describes the role of macrophage-like as well as unique stromal cells of the glomerular mesangium, the response of these cells to phlogistic stimuli, and the ultimate outcome. In the chapter dealing with mechanisms of lung diseases, we can begin to see the accumulating evidence that toxic oxygen products from activated leukocytes and alveolar macrophages have important determining effects that may result in both acute and chronic lung damage.

It is obvious that we are on the verge of a new era in our understanding of the inflammatory system. The information will transform clinical approaches to anti-inflammatory therapy. It can be predicted that there will soon be new classes of anti-inflammatory drugs quite unlike we have seen since the advent of the corticosteroids. This optimistic note should not hide the fact that we still understand very little about the immunopathologic basis for human diseases. On the other hand, the progress over the past 20 years in the field of inflammation has been nothing short of spectacular. We can confidently look forward to a new era of exciting developments. This being the case, I am quite unable to predict the contents of succeeding volumes of the *Handbook of Inflammation*, but they will surely be interesting.

Peter A. Ward

List of contributors

Charles G. Cochrane 361
Department of Immunopathology, Scripps Clinic and Research Foundation, La Jolla, CA 92037

Joseph C. Fantone 89
Department of Pathology, University of Michigan Medical School, Ann Arbor, MI 48109

Edward J. Goetzl 163
Department of Medicine, University of California Medical Center, San Francisco, CA 94143

Daniel W. Goldman 163
Department of Medicine, Harvard Medical School, Boston, MA 02115

Gerald D. Iliffe 279
Department of Internal Medicine, University of Manitoba, Winnipeg, Canada

Kent J. Johnson 1
Department of Pathology, University of Michigan Medical School, Ann Arbor, MI 48109

David F. Keren 337
Department of Pathology, University of Michigan Medical School, Ann Arbor, MI 48109

Paul Killen 1
Department of Pathology, University of Washington, Seattle, WA

Steven L. Kunkel 245
Department of Pathology, University of Michigan Medical School, Ann Arbor, MI 48109

Cynthia L. Marcelo 189
Department of Dermatology, University of Michigan Medical School, Ann Arbor, MI 48109

F. William Orr 211, 279
Department of Pathology, University of Manitoba School of Medicine, Winnipeg, Manitoba, Canada

Sem H. Phan 121
Department of Pathology, University of Michigan Medical School, Ann Arbor, MI 48109

Gary Striker 1
Department of Pathology, University of Washington, Seattle, WA

Alan Sugar 245
Department of Ophthalmology, University of Michigan Medical School, Ann Arbor, MI 48109

Gerd O. Till 373
Department of Pathology, University of Michigan Medical School, Ann Arbor, MI 48109

James Varani 211
Department of Pathology, University of Michigan Medical School, Ann Arbor, MI 48109

John J. Voorhees 189
Department of Dermatology, University of Michigan Medical School, Ann Arbor, MI 48109

Peter A. Ward 89, 373
Department of Pathology, University of Michigan Medical School, Ann Arbor, MI 48109

Stephen J. Weiss 37
Department of Internal Medicine, Simpson Research Institute, University of Michigan, Ann Arbor, MI 48109

Contents

1. Immunopathology of glomerular disease **1**
Kent J. Johnson, Gary Striker and Paul Killen
1.1. Introduction 1
1.2. Glomerular components 5
1.2.1. Cells 5
1.2.2. Extracellular matrix 7
1.3. Glomerular localization of immune reactants 10
1.3.1. Antigen–antibody deposition 11
1.3.2. Local formation of immune complexes 12
1.3.3. The role of charge 12
1.3.4. Non-immune materials 13
1.3.5. Renal localization of antiglomerular antibody 13
1.4. Removal of glomerular immune deposits 14
1.4.1. Cellular uptake 14
1.4.2. Mesangial cells 14
1.4.3. Endothelial cells 15
1.4.4. Visceral epithelial cells 15
1.4.5. Extracellular routes of disappearance 15
1.5. Mediator systems implicated in glomerulonephritis 16
1.5.1. Complement and glomerulonephritis 16
1.5.2. Prostaglandins 19
1.5.3. Bradykinins 20
1.6. Regulatory role of cell-mediated immunity in glomerulonephritis 20
1.7. Resolution of glomerular injuries 22
1.7.1. Cell and matrix changes associated with acute injury 22
1.7.2. Changes associated with chronic injury 27

2. Oxygen as a weapon in the phagocyte armamentarium **37**
Stephen J. Weiss
2.1. Introduction 37

2.2. Oxygen metabolites generated by phagocytes and their characteristics 37
2.2.1. Superoxide 38
2.2.2. Hydrogen peroxide 40
2.2.3. Hydrogen peroxide-peroxidase-halide derived oxidants 40
2.2.4. Hydroxyl radical 42
2.3. Role of oxygen metabolites in phagocyte–target cell interactions 44
2.3.1. Common methods used to identify responsible oxygen metabolites 45
2.3.1.1. Oxygen 45
2.3.1.2. Superoxide 46
2.3.1.3. Hydrogen peroxide 47
2.3.1.4. Hydrogen peroxide-peroxidase-halide system 47
2.3.1.5. Hydroxyl radical 48
2.3.2. Innocent bystander-type interactions mediated by phagocytes 49
2.3.2.1. Superoxide 49
2.3.2.2. Hydrogen peroxide 51
– H_2O_2 and erythrocytes 52
– H_2O_2 and platelets 54
– H_2O_2 and leukocytes 54
– H_2O_2 and endothelial cells 55
– H_2O_2 and tumor cells 56
2.3.2.3. Hydrogen peroxide-peroxidase-halide system 59
– Peroxidases and phagocytes 59
– Peroxidases and release reactions 60
– Peroxidases and tumor cells 61
2.3.2.4. The hydroxyl radical 63
2.3.3. Oxygen and antibody-dependent cellular cytotoxicity 64
2.3.3.1. Are oxygen metabolites generated by phagocytes bound to antibody-coated targets? 65
2.3.3.2. Are oxygen metabolites involved in phagocyte-mediated ADCC against erythroid targets? Yes, No, Maybe? 66
2.3.3.3. Role of oxidative metabolism in phagocyte-mediated ADCC against nucleated mammalian cells 67
2.4. Oxygen metabolites and the transformation of soluble inflammatory mediators 70
2.4.1. Oxygen metabolites and arachidonic acid 70
2.4.2. Oxygen metabolites and methionine-containing compounds 71
2.4.2.1. Chemotactic factors 71
2.4.2.2. α_1-Proteinase inhibitor 72
2.4.2.3. Methionine-enkephalin 73
2.4.3. Peroxidases and arachidonic acid metabolites 73
2.5. Summary 75

3. Mechanisms of neutrophil-dependent lung injury **89**
Joseph C. Fantone and Peter A. Ward
3.1. Introduction 89
3.2. Chemotactic factors of the lung: origin and regulation 93
3.2.1. Complement-derived chemotactic factors 93
3.2.2. Oxygen-metabolite-derived chemotactic factors 96
3.2.3. Cell-derived chemotactic factors 97
3.2.4. Bacterial- and viral-derived chemotactic factors 99
3.3. Leukocytic proteases in lung injury 100
3.4. Role of oxygen radicals and lung injury 100
3.5. Chemotactic-factor-mediated lung injury 103
3.5.1. Intravascular effects of chemotactic factors 103
3.5.2. Intra-alveolar chemotactic factors 105
3.6. Experimental models of immune-complex lung injury 106
3.7. Clinical examples of neutrophil-dependent lung injury 109

4. Fibrotic mechanisms in lung diseases **121**
Sem H. Phan
4.1. Introduction 121
4.2. Causes of pulmonary fibrosis 122
4.3. Review of connective tissue metabolism 124
4.3.1. Collagen 125
4.3.2. Elastin 128
4.3.3. Glycosaminoglycans and proteoglycans 130
4.4. Abnormalities in lung connective tissue composition and metabolism in pulmonary fibrosis 131
4.5. Abnormalities of regulation of connective tissue metabolism in pulmonary fibrosis 139
4.5.1. Non-immune mechanisms 140
4.5.2. Immune mechanisms 143
4.6. Conclusion 147

5. Mediation and modulation of immediate hypersensitivity and inflammation by products of the oxygenation of arachidonic acid **163**
Daniel W. Goldman and Edward J. Goetzl
5.1. Introduction 163
5.2. Products of arachidonic acid metabolism 164
5.3. Control of arachidonic acid release and metabolism 166
5.4. Pharmacologic modulation of arachidonic acid metabolism 169
5.5. Lipid mediators in hypersensitivity 171
5.6. Lipid mediators of the cellular elements of hypersensitivity and inflammation 174
5.7. Conclusions 180

6. Cyclic nucleotides and arachidonate metabolites in psoriasis **189**
Cynthia L. Marcelo and John J. Voorhees
6.1. Introduction 189

6.2. The cyclic nucleotide system 190
6.2.1. Cyclic AMP 190
6.2.2. Cyclic GMP 191
6.2.3. Cyclic AMP and cyclic GMP in psoriasis 191
6.2.4. The function of cyclic nucleotides in in-vitro and in-situ systems 193
6.3. Inflammation 193
6.3.1. Arachidonic acid metabolism 194
6.3.2. Cyclic nucleotides in leukocytes 195
6.3.3. Arachidonic acid metabolism in the skin 198
6.3.4. Arachidonic acid metabolites in psoriasis 199
6.4. Summary 200

7. Chemotaxis in non-leukocytic cells **211**
James Varani and F. William Orr
7.1 Introduction 211
7.2. Cell motility in vitro 212
7.3. Chemotactic responses in biological systems 218
7.3.1. Fertilization 218
7.3.2. Embryologic development of dorsal root ganglia 219
7.3.3. Tissue repair 221
7.3.3.1. Fibroblasts 222
7.3.3.2. Platelets 224
7.3.3.3. Endothelial cells and smooth muscle cells 226
7.3.4. Tumor cell invasion and metastasis 227
7.4. Biological basis of the chemotactic response 231
7.5. Adherence, motility and chemotaxis 235
7.6. Summary and conclusions 236

8. Inflammatory mechanisms in the eye **245**
Steven L. Kunkel and Alan Sugar
8.1. Introduction 245
8.2. Mediators derived from inflammatory cells and immune reactions 247
8.2.1. Complement and its split products 247
8.2.2. Cyclo-oxygenase and lipoxygenase products 253
8.2.3. Toxic products from oxygen metabolism 255
8.2.4. Products of lysosomal enzyme release from inflammatory cells 256
8.3. Experimental models of eye disease 257
8.3.1. Ocular inflammation due to infectious microorganisms 258
8.3.2. Experimental immune complex ocular vasculitis 260
8.3.3. Ocular inflammation due to alkali burns 261
8.3.4. Ocular inflammation due to endotoxemia 262
8.4. Autoimmune processes of the eye 263
8.4.1. Sympathetic ophthalmia 263
8.4.2. Vogt-Koyanagi-Harada syndrome 264
8.4.3. Reiter's syndrome 265

8.4.4. Behçet's syndrome 266
8.4.5. Cicatricial pemphigoid 266
8.5. Allergic keratitis 267
8.5.1. Atopic keratoconjunctivitis 267
8.5.2. Vernal catarrh 267
8.5.3. Staphylococcal marginal corneal ulceration 267
8.6. Ocular transplantation immunity 268
8.7. Other inflammatory eye diseases 269
8.7.1. Infections 269
8.7.1.1. Viral conjunctivitis 270
8.7.1.2. Chlamydial conjunctivitis 270
8.7.1.3. Bacterial corneal ulcers 270
8.7.1.4. Fungal keratitis 271
8.7.1.5. Herpes simplex keratitis 271
8.7.1.6. Scleritis 271

9. Inflammatory diseases of the liver 279
F. William Orr and Gerald D. Iliffe
9.1. Introduction 279
9.2. Hepatitis B 279
9.2.1. Hepatitis B virus (HBV) 279
9.2.2. Hepatitis B antigens 280
9.2.2.1. Hepatitis B surface antigen (HBsAg) 280
9.2.2.2. Hepatitis B core antigen (HBcAg) 282
9.2.2.3. Hepatitis B e-antigen (HBeAg) 283
9.2.2.4. Hepatitis B delta-antigen (HBδAg) 283
9.2.3. Antibodies to hepatitis B virus-associated antigens 285
9.2.3.1. Anti-HBs 285
9.2.3.2. Anti-HBc 285
9.2.3.3. Anti-HBe 287
9.2.4. HBV-related immune complex disease 287
9.2.4.1. Hepatocellular injury 287
9.2.4.2. Circulating immune complexes 288
9.2.4.3. Glomerulonephritis 289
9.2.4.4. Polyarteritis nodosa 290
9.2.4.5. Arthritis 290
9.2.4.6. Other diseases associated with HBV-related immune complexes 290
9.2.5. Anti-HBs-mediated cytotoxic reactions 291
9.2.6. Cell-mediated responses to HBV-related antigens 291
9.2.7. Relationships between antigenic expression, immune responses, and clinical presentation of HBV infection 292
9.2.7.1. Acute viral hepatitis 292
9.2.7.2. Chronic persistent hepatitis 295
9.2.7.3. Healthy carrier state 295
9.2.7.4. Chronic active liver diseases (CALD) 296
9.2.7.5. Additional clinical observations 298

9.2.7.6. Hepatocellular carcinoma (HCC) 298
9.3. Hepatitis A virus infection 299
9.3.1. General characteristics of the virus 299
9.3.2. Virus replication 299
9.3.3. Clinical features of human disease 300
9.3.4. Immunologic responses 300
9.3.5. Pathogenesis 301
9.4. Hepatocellular antigens 301
9.4.1. Liver-specific protein 301
9.4.2. Liver membrane antigen (LMA) 302
9.4.3. Biliary tract antigens 302
9.4.4. Humoral immune responses to hepatocelluar antigens 303
9.4.4.1. Antibodies to liver-specific protein and liver membrane antigen 303
9.4.4.2. Non-organ, non-species-specific antibodies 303
9.4.5. Cell-mediated responses to liver-specific protein 304
9.4.6. Experimental hepatitis induced by LSP 304
9.5. Chronic active liver disease (CALD) 304
9.5.1. Viral-related chronic active liver disease 305
9.5.1.1. Chronic active liver disease related to non-A,non-B hepatitis 305
9.5.2. Autoimmune-associated chronic liver disease 305
9.5.3. Drug-induced chronic active liver disease 307
9.5.4. Miscellaneous group 307
9.6. Alcohol-induced liver disease 308
9.6.1. Direct toxicity of alcohol 308
9.6.2. Humoral responses 310
9.6.2.1. Mallory bodies (alcoholic hyaline) and anti-Mallory-body antibodies 310
9.6.2.2. Other antibodies 310
9.6.3. Cell-mediated immunity 311
9.6.4. Genetic factors 312
9.7. Primary biliary cirrhosis 312
9.7.1. Humoral immune responses 314
9.7.1.1. Hypergammaglobulinemia 314
9.7.1.2. Antimitochondrial antibody 314
9.7.1.3. Anti-LSP 314
9.7.1.4. Other antibody responses 315
9.7.2. Immune complexes 315
9.7.3. Cell-mediated immunity 315
9.8. Summary 317

10. Mechanisms of immunologic injury in inflammatory bowel injury: ulcerative colitis and Crohn's disease 337
David F. Keren
10.1. Etiology of inflammatory bowel disease (IBD) 337
10.2. Humoral immunity in IBD 339

10.2.1. Local antibody production 339
10.2.2. Serum antibody levels 345
10.3. Role of inflammatory mediators: complement and prostaglandins 345
10.4. Immune complexes and inflammatory bowel disease 347
10.5. Antibody-dependent cell-mediated cytotoxicity (ADCC) 348
10.6. Cell-mediated immunity in inflammatory bowel disease 351
10.7. Mucosal immunocytes and inflammatory bowel disease 352

11. The contact system of plasma in inflammation **361**
Charles G. Cochrane
11.1. Introduction 361
11.2. Activation of proteins of the contact system by cellular enzymes 364
11.3. Pathophysiologic actions of the components of the contact system 366
11.3.1. Hageman factor and PF/dil 366
11.4. Leukocyte accumulation in blood vessels and tissues 367
11.5. High-MW kininogen 367
11.6. Bradykinin 367
11.7. Contact activation system and the plasma renin–angiotensin system 368
11.8. Summary 369

12. Altered inflammatory mechanisms in thermal injury **373**
Gerd O. Till and Peter A. Ward
12.1. Introduction 373
12.2. Serum complement in thermal injury 374
12.2.1. Activity of individual complement components 375
12.2.2. Alternative pathway of complement activation 376
12.2.3. Experimental studies on complement changes 377
12.2.4. Overview of clinical and experimental studies 378
12.3. Altered neutrophil functions in thermal injury 379
12.3.1. Chemotactic response 379
12.3.2. Chemotactic activity 383
12.3.3. Opsonization and phagocytosis 384
12.3.4. Bactericidal activity 385
12.4. Lung injury subsequent to thermal trauma 387
12.5. Immunological aberrations 390
12.6. Concluding remarks 392

Subject Index 401

CHAPTER 1

Immunopathology of glomerular disease

KENT J. JOHNSON
Department of Pathology, University of Michigan Medical School, Ann Arbor, Michigan 48109

and

GARY STRIKER and PAUL KILLEN
Department of Pathology, University of Washington, Seattle, Washington

1.1. INTRODUCTION

Great strides have been made in the study and treatment of renal diseases in the last few years. For example, in the United States an estimated 35,000 people per year die of various renal diseases, the mortality rate being far lower in number than in past decades. However, this statistic is somewhat misleading in that renal diseases, including the various glomerulonephrites, are still the source of a considerable degree of morbidity. For example, bacterial infections of the kidney and urinary system are the second most common site of infection in clinical medicine (Robbins and Cotran 1979). More specifically, if one turns attention to glomerulonephritis, the facts are also sobering. For, even though we have made great strides in the last two decades in understanding the immunopathogenesis of glomerulonephritis, this understanding has not progressed to a point where we have developed effective prevention and treatment of many of these diseases. There are today an estimated 50,000 people in the United States who are being treated with chronic hemodialysis, most cases the result of some type of glomerulonephritis, and the estimated total medical costs per year for these individuals exceeds one billion dollars (Kalata 1980). So, even though we have succeeded in decreasing mortality, we certainly have not effected a "cure" in terms of decreasing morbidity for these individuals, to say nothing of the tremendous social and economic costs involved.

The study of the etiology of glomerulonephritis has for many years centered on the apparent immunological mechanisms involved. This concept historically started with two sets of clinical observations made within the last 30 years. Firstly, it was observed that many cases of human glomerulonephritis were associated with a drop in serum complement levels (Lange and Treser 1973; Arroyave 1979). The second set of observations occurred with the development of immunofluorescence microscopy which revealed the presence of immune complexes and complement in the glomeruli of patients with certain types of glomerulonephritis (McCluskey and Leher 1974).

Further immunofluorescence studies on human renal biopsies with glomerulonephritis disclosed two main patterns of immunoglobulin and complement deposition. The predominant pattern is one of a granular ("lumpy-bumpy") pattern which was thought originally to represent the exclusive deposition of preformed circulating immune complexes. The second recognized immunofluorescence pattern was that of a linear deposit, usually of IgG, along the glomerular capillary wall.

With these important clinical observations, the next logical step was the development of experimental models that simulated human renal glomerular diseases. Major breakthroughs were made in this area with the development of two experimental models which appeared to closely mimic the histological and immunological appearances of the human glomerulonephritis.

The first major experimental model developed which simulated a type of human nephritis was anti-basement-membrane-induced nephritis. Recently reviewed by Wilson (1979), the model was originally extensively studied by Masugi who developed a crude anti-kidney antibody which upon injection into experimental animals caused a crescentic type of glomerulonephritis. Further studies revealed that this nephritis model had a biphasic pattern, with the first (heterologous) phase occurring with the binding of antibody to glomerular basement membrane (GBM) and the second (autologous) phase occurring with the development of an antibody against the foreign immunoglobulin. The hallmark of this model is the presence of a linear fluorescence pattern as well as detectable circulating anti-GBM antibodies. This model appears to be mediated in part by neutrophils and complement as described originally by Cochrane (1968). The model appears to correlate quite well with a few human renal diseases, most specifically those patients with Goodpasture syndrome as well as some patients with rapidly progressive glomerulonephritis (Wilson 1979).

The second major experimental model developed was that of acute ("one shot") serum sickness. Serum sickness is an acute self-limiting illness occurring 4–6 days after the injection of a foreign protein that is characterized by fever, arthralgias and edema, with an acute glomerulonephritis characterized by a drop in serum complement levels. Observations by Germuth and his colleagues (Germuth 1953; Germuth and McKinnon 1957) revealed that the lesions of serum sickness developed at the time when detectable antigen–antibody complexes were in the circulation. These observations were extended by Dixon et al. (1958, 1959) who found that coincidental with the presence of antigen—antibody complexes in the circulation there was a fall in serum complement levels and the appearance of a vasculitis and an acute glomerulonephritis which histologically resembled human acute glomerulonephritis. Evidence for deposition of the immune complexes in vessels and glomeruli was obtained by immunofluorescence which had a classical granular pattern. Further studies by Benacerraf and McCluskey (McCluskey et al. 1960; Benacerraf et al. 1960) using preformed immune complexes further strengthened the concept of the phlogistic potential of immune complexes deposited in glomeruli and vessel walls.

In view of the fact that the histological and immunofluorescence appearance of this experimental model of renal injury resembled that seen in many cases of human glomerulonephritis, it has been assumed that the deposition of preformed circulating immune complexes is responsible for most (70–80%) types of human glomerulonephritis (Wilson 1977). Indeed, further evidence including identification of specific antigens in the immune complexes has led to a whole group of human glomerular diseases which are widely accepted as being initiated by deposition of preformed, circulating immune complexes (Table 1).

For many years, our understanding of the immunological mechanisms of renal

TABLE 1.
Human glomerular diseases presumed to be mediated by immune complexes

Type of glomerulonephritis	Antigens identified in glomeruli
I. Secondary to bacterial infections	streptococcal treponemal ?other bacterial Ag (staphylococcal, listeria, enterococcus, coliforms)
II. Secondary to parasitic infections	malarial schistosomal filariasis
III. Secondary to viral infections	hepatitis (surface antigen)
IV. Secondary to malignancies	carcinoembryonic antigen ?oat-cell carcinoma ?renal-cell carcinoma (brush border Ag)
V. Secondary to collagen vascular diseases	DNA, IgG, thyroglobulin
VI. Primary glomerular diseases	
a) idiopathic membranous	none
b) membranoproliferative	none
c) IgA-mediated glomerulonephritis	none
d) some focal glomerulonephritis	none
e) some types of rapidly progressive glomerulonephritis	none

disease has not progressed much beyond this point. Lately, however, a number of observations have suggested that the serum sickness model of immune complex nephritis does not explain the findings seen in some types of human glomerular disease. For example, certain types of glomerular diseases do not show evidence of immune complex deposition. Secondly, in some types of human nephritis felt to be mediated by immune complexes, there is often no evidence of circulating immune complexes (CIC) even though immune complexes are present in renal glomeruli (Tung et al. 1978; Pussell et al. 1978). Some of this negative correlation might be explained on the basis of the known fluctuating levels of CIC in diseases such as lupus erythematosus. However, this explanation is probably not sufficient to explain the consistent lack of CIC in some types of nephritis such as membranous glomerulonephritis. Conversely, many conditions such as lipoid nephrosis, cancer and liver disease are commonly associated with CIC, but no deposition is seen in the kidney (McCluskey et al. 1978). This led to the concept of *in-situ immune complex formation* of which more will be said later. Doubts have also been raised about the specificity of immunofluorescence findings of deposits of immunoglobulins or complement. It is known, for example, that glomeruli contain Fc and C receptors and this may account for the occasional observation of faint mesangial IgM and C3 deposits in the absence of any known glomerular disease (McCluskey et al. 1978). Also, it has been known for many years that patients with diabetes mellitus often have a linear fluorescence pattern without evidence of circulating antibodies to glomerular basement membrane (Gallo 1970). Falsely positive linear fluorescence patterns have also been described in apparently normal kidneys obtained at the time of autopsy and in kidneys that have been subjected to perfusion preparatory to transplantation. Even normal kidney biopsies occasionally are positive for this fluorescence (Wilson 1979).

Finally, there is the almost complete lack of understanding of the mediator systems involved in the pathogenesis of glomerular disease. Outside of evidence implicating the complement system in the heterologous phase of anti-GBM nephritis, no conclusive evidence of involvement of other mediator systems has been obtained.

With these uncertainties in mind, we have chosen to look at glomerular injury in a sequential fashion starting with the normal, steady-state glomerulus and its resident cells. The next step will be to examine what is known about the type of immune complexes which deposit in renal glomeruli as well as the latest evidence implicating in-situ immune complex formation in some types of glomerulonephritis. This will then be followed by a description of the chronology of the inflammatory response, with particular emphasis placed on examining the possible role of various types of inflammatory cells with their subsequent elaboration of inflammatory mediators. Finally, the eventual outcome of the inflammatory response is discussed in terms of factors predisposing to glomerular fibrosis. By this, we hope to avoid the traditional approach of trying to match human nephritis with the experimental models and, instead, concentrate on the more recent experimental findings with a special emphasis on the possible mediator systems involved.

1.2. GLOMERULAR COMPONENTS

The glomerulus consists of three cell types and two distinct extracellular matrix regions.

1.2.1. Cells

The vascular loops are covered by the interdigitating pedicles of the visceral epithelial cells (Fig. 1). These cells have a thick glycocalyx which contains sialoglycoproteins (Mohos and Skoza 1969). In humans, C3b receptors have been demonstrated on the surfaces of these epithelial cells present in tissue sections (Gelfand et al. 1975). These cells have been isolated and maintained in vitro. They retain C3b receptors on their surface but lack Fc receptors. These cells synthesize in-vitro fibronectin, Type IV collagen (Killen and Striker 1979) and heparin-sulfate-containing proteoglycans (Striker et al. 1980b; Farin et al. 1982).

The endothelial cells are highly fenestrated over areas of the vascular wall which

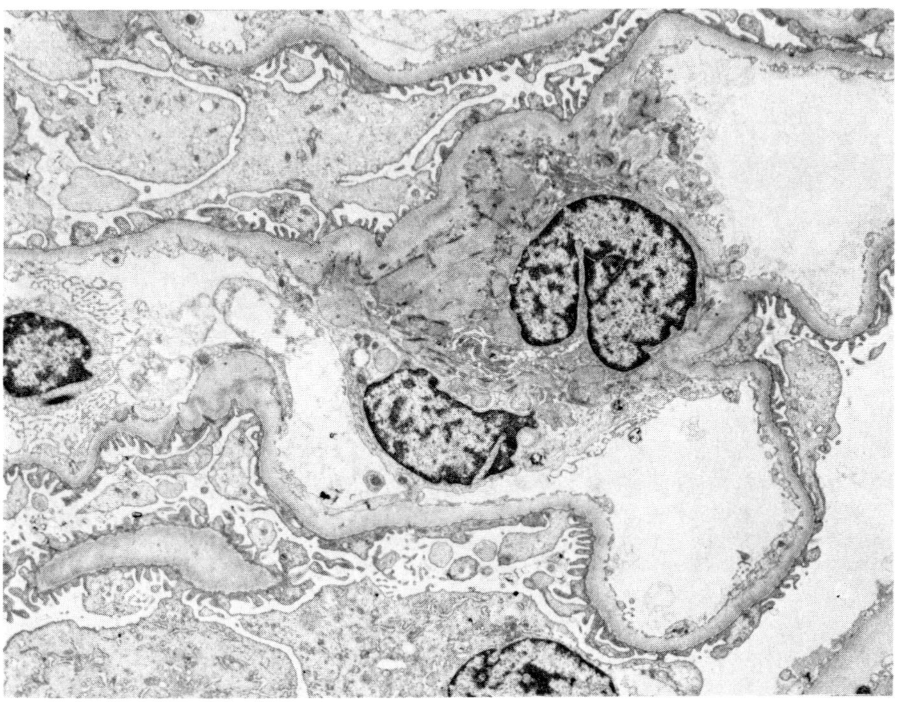

Fig. 1. Electron micrograph of a human glomerulus. The normal human glomerulus is composed of visceral epithelial cells, endothelial cells and at least 2 different populations of mesangial cells. The latter are difficult to distinguish on morphological grounds.

are not adjacent to the mesangium. The majority of the organelles and nucleus abut the mesangial region. Endothelial cells from several species and vascular beds have been propagated in vitro. Endothelial cells from umbilical cord vein retain cytoplasmic Factor VIII antigen. When quiescent, these cells lack Fc and C3b receptors, but following injury with white blood cell lysates (Ryan et al. 1981) or viral infection (Ryan et al. 1981; Cines et al. 1982), Fc and C3b receptors can be demonstrated on their surfaces. Endothelial cells from umbilical vein synthesize Factor VIII antigen in vitro (Jaffe et al. 1973). In addition, these cells synthesize elements of extracellular matrix, including Type IV collagen, fibronectin (Striker et al. 1980a) and proteoglycans (Buonassissi and Root 1975). Cells isolated from bovine aorta have a more complex biosynthetic profile (Sage et al. 1980). Preliminary evidence using capillary endothelial cells from the mouse brain suggest

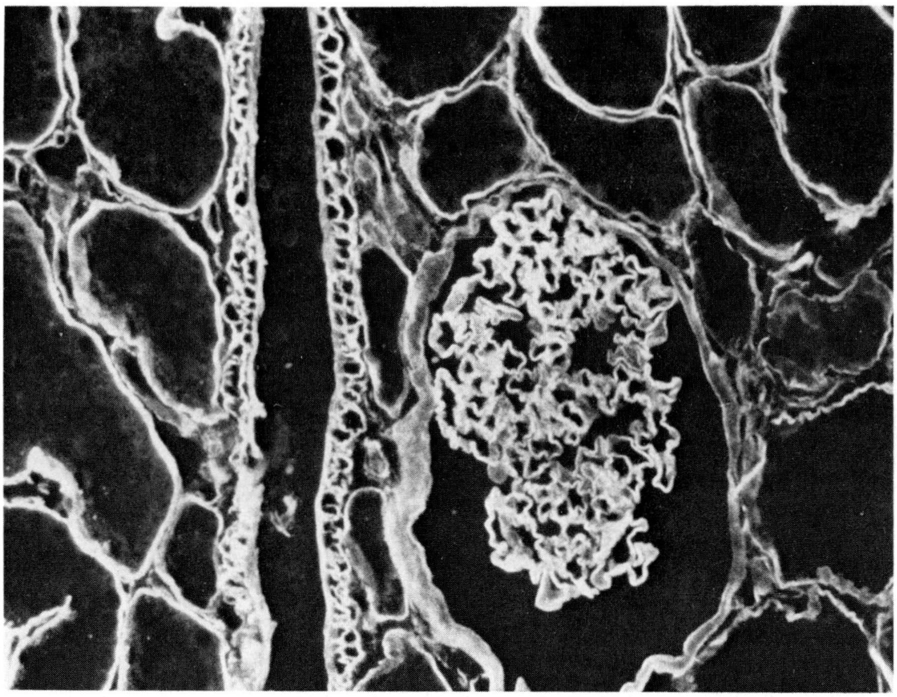

Fig. 2. Affinity purified antibody to Type IV collagen was applied to sections of normal human kidney tissue which had been fixed with Carnoy's solution and embedded in paraffin. The sections were partially digested with trypsin prior to application of the antibody. The distribution is similar for antibodies specific for laminin. In rats and mice a similar distribution is also noted for a proteoglycan containing heparin sulfate. The mesangium is difficult to detect. This may be due to the small amount of matrix normally found in the mesangium.

that biosynthetic profiles of endothelial cells from small blood vessels differ from the aorta.

At least two types of cells reside in the mesangium. One resembles smooth muscle cells and has been shown to contract in vitro when stimulated with angiotensin-II (Ausiello et al. 1980). This cell lacks Fc and C3b receptors and is not phagocytic. Collagen Types I, III and IV, as well as proteoglycans and glycoproteins, are synthesized by these cells in vitro (Striker et al. 1980b). This biosynthetic profile is similar to other vascular wall cells in vitro. The second cell type thus far identified in the mesangium resembles a macrophage. It expresses Ia antigen and processes antigen for lymphocytes. It has surface C3b and Fc receptors and is phagocytic (Schreiner et al. 1981).

1.2.2. Extracellular matrix

The extracellular matrix of the glomerulus consists of a basal lamina and a matrix in the centrolobular region, the mesangial matrix. The mesangial region appears to be

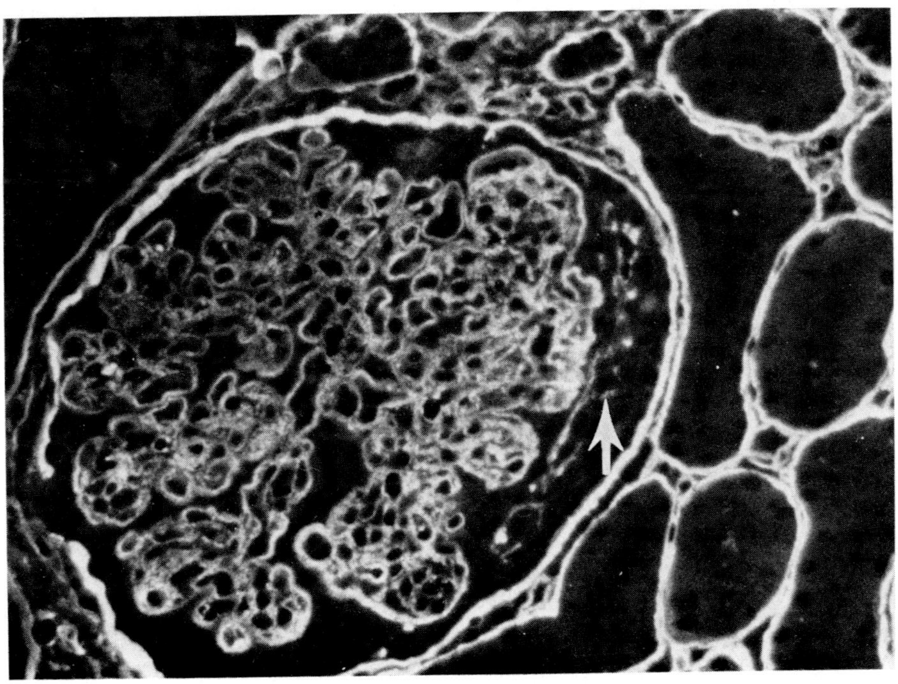

Fig. 3. The distribution of Type IV collagen in a diffuse proliferative glomerulonephritis due to systemic lupus erythematosus. Note synthesis of Type IV collagen by cells proliferating in the urinary space (arrow). There is also marked increase in Type IV collagen in the mesangium.

more permeable than the peripheral basal lamina, based on studies utilizing various sizes of tracers (Michael et al. 1976, 1980). The structural and biochemical basis for the observed differences in permeability are unknown. Huang (1979) has shown that there are differences in the composition of the mature mesangial matrix and the basal lamina by subjecting tissue to dissociating agents (guanidine-HCl). The basal lamina lying under the epithelial cell (GBL) has 3 laminae when adjacent to the fenestrated parts of the endothelium: the lamina rara externa, the lamina densa and the lamina rara interna. The lamina rara interna is no longer visible in areas adjacent to the mesangium. The antigenic composition of the basal lamina includes laminin in addition to the components known to be synthesized by visceral epithelial or endothelial cells in vitro. Immunocytochemical studies of the mesangial matrix reveal Type IV collagen and glycoproteins (Linder et al. 1980) (Fig. 2). In certain diseases (systemic lupus erythematosus), there appears to be an abundance of Type IV collagen (Figs 3 and 4). In contrast, Type III collagen is not found in normal

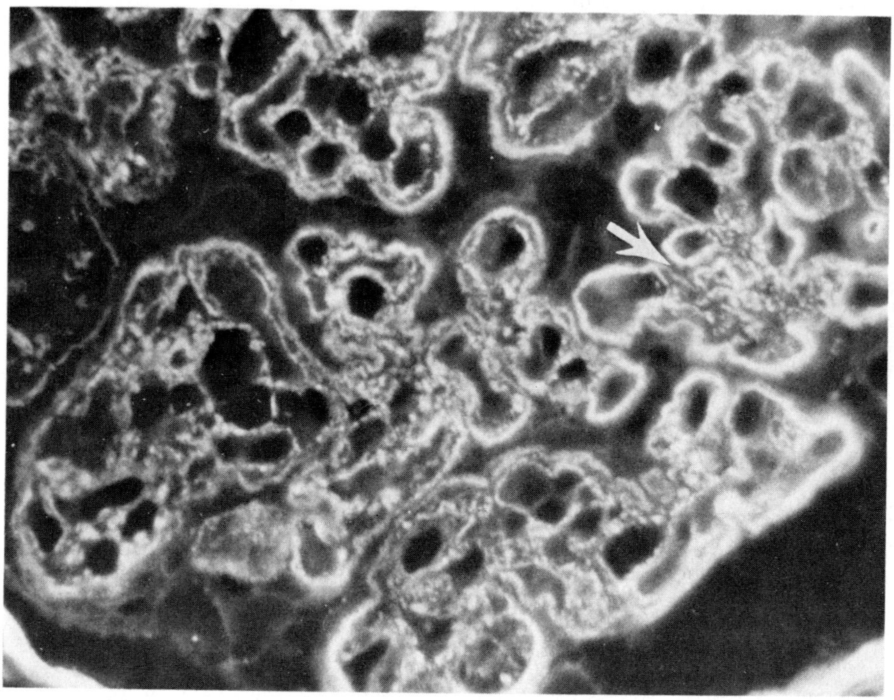

Fig. 4. A fluorescence photomicrograph of the glomerulus shown in Fig. 3. Note the obvious bilaminar distribution of Type IV collagen in the peripheral vascular loop. This would suggest that the endothelium in injury states may synthesize this collagen. The role of the endothelium in the synthesis of the normal glomerular basal lamina is unknown. Note the accumulation of Type IV collagen antigen in the mesangium (arrow).

glomeruli (Fig. 5), although it can be detected in diseased glomeruli (Fig. 6). It is not clear why there is a discrepancy between the in-vitro and in-vivo data with respect to the presence of Types I and III collagen. While each of 3 cell types synthesizes one or more of the individual components when studied in vitro, their relative contribution to the in-vivo structure remains conjectural (Cohen and Vogt 1975; Kanwar and Farquhar 1979b; Grant et al. 1975; Killen and Striker 1979). One approach to this question was to use the in-vivo labeling of basement membranes induced by adding silver nitrate to the drinking water of rats for a period of 6 weeks (Kurtz and Feldman 1962). Initially, there was diffuse stippling of the peripheral matrix with electron-dense granules. The silver nitrate was stopped and several weeks later examination of the glomeruli revealed an electron-lucent zone adjacent to the epithelial cells. The conclusion from this study was that visceral epithelial cells synthesized the glomerular basement membrane. However, it was subsequently found that, even if the animals were continuously exposed to silver nitrate in the

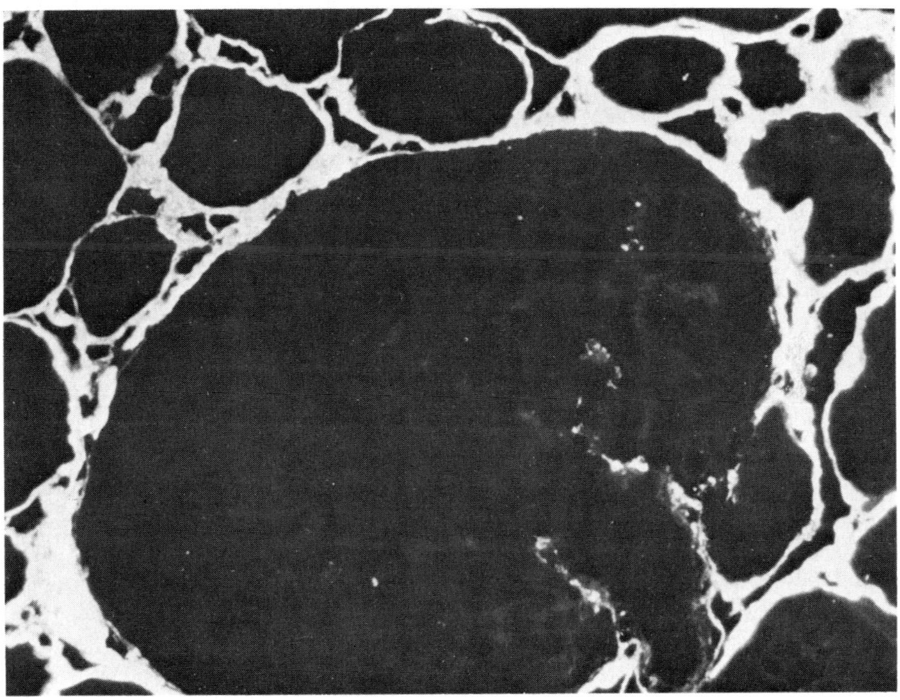

Fig. 5. The distribution of Type III collagen antigen studied in tissues prepared as in Fig. 3. Type III collagen antigens are present in the interstitium surrounding Bowman's capsule and in the adventitia of blood vessels. The only glomerular localization visible in normals is at the vascular pole.

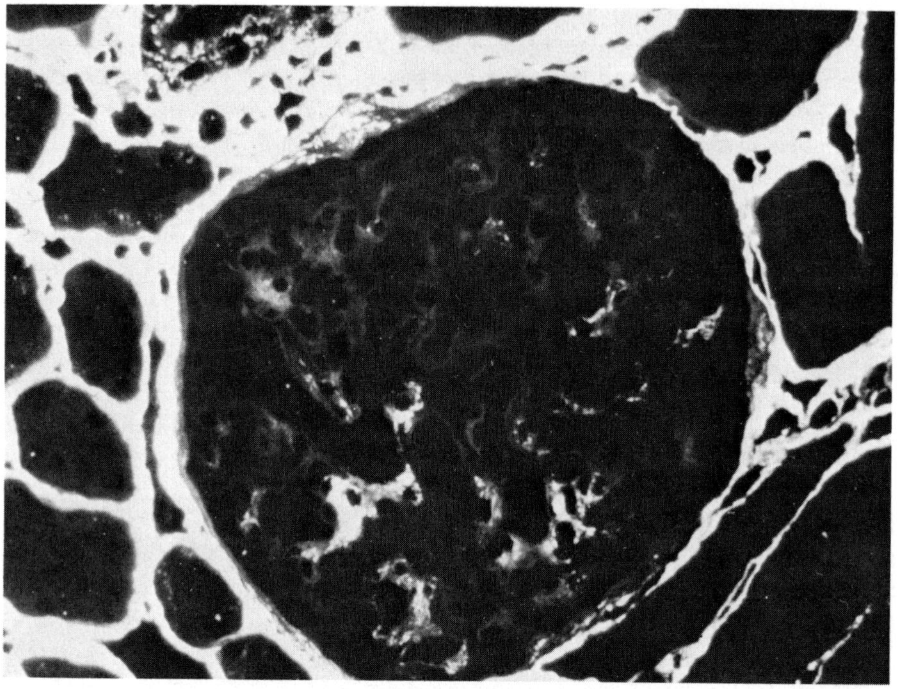

Fig. 6. In contrast to the normal glomerulus (see Fig. 4), Type III collagen is found in the mesangium of glomeruli in areas of marked sclerosis. These data suggest that there is abnormal expression of the gene product in pathological states.

drinking water, a subepithelial zone free of granules appeared (Striker and Smuckler 1970). Thus, this new zone was not identical to the initial basement membrane. Therefore, some doubts must be raised about the nature of this new material and the exact contribution of the visceral epithelial cells to the glomerular basement membrane in this model. In summary, there are morphological and biochemical differences between the matrix associated with mesangial and epithelial cells, which may relate to the observed differences in permeability and could be important to other aspects of the localization of material to these regions. Finally, the site(s) of the synthesis of the matrix components in vivo is still incompletely understood — a critical defect for future studies on the pathogenesis of glomerulosclerosis.

1.3. GLOMERULAR LOCALIZATION OF IMMUNE REACTANTS

There has recently been renewed interest in the initiation of glomerular injury by circulating immune materials. Based on extensive studies in experimental animals, two types of immunological injury were recognized: that directed against glomerular antigens (anti-GBL) and that secondary to deposition of circulating antigen—antibody complexes. While these two mechanisms are clearly valid, they fail to explain many of the glomerulonephrites which progress to end-stage renal disease. This is supported by 3 lines of evidence. Firstly, there is a rarity of patients with circulating antiglomerular antibodies (Wilson and Dixon 1979a). Secondly, it has become increasingly difficult to provide convincing evidence that patients with disease induced by circulating antigen—antibody complexes develop a progressive disease (Ooi et al. 1977; Van de Run et al. 1978). Finally, most patients with renal deposition of immunoglobulins do not have levels of circulating antigen—antibody complexes which differ from the control population (Dixon et al. 1971). These data have led to the search for additional means by which immunological materials might localize to the kidney. The following discussion will center on a brief summary of the localization and removal of soluble immune reactants in the kidney.

1.3.1. Antigen—antibody deposition

Renal deposition of circulating antigen—antibody complexes has been found to occur only when large-latticed complexes (greater than Ag_2Ab_2) are present in the circulation (Haakenstad et al. 1976). The deposits were found in the mesangial regions and, even though these latticed complexes persisted for 96 hours, no subepithelial deposits were found. Furthermore, glomerular deposits have not been identified if only small-latticed complexes are injected (Mannik and Haakenstad 1977). The in-vivo clearance of antigen—antibody complexes without bound C3 is not altered by depletion of C3 by cobra venom (Bockow and Mannik 1981).

The mechanism by which deposits appear in the mesangial regions is not clear. It has been postulated that circulating materials might first deposit in endothelial fenestrae, gain access to the lamina rara interna, and then be swept from the periphery of glomerular loops to the mesangium (Farquhar and Palade 1962). This may be true for certain large foreign particles such as ferritin and carbon. However, for immune materials it appears that there is localization of electron-dense material first in endothelial caveoli and then in the mesangial matrix (Haakenstad et al. 1976). In fact, Keane and Rai (1981) found that the number of endothelial fenestrae do not correlate with mesangial localization of aggregated immunoglobulins. These data suggest that endothelial cells may actively participate in the sequestration of material in the mesangium. It has recently been shown that endothelial cells may develop Fc receptors following injury (Ryan et al. 1981).

However, receptor-mediated endocytosis usually results in localization of the material in cell cytosomes rather than in transcellular transport. Thus, the role of endothelial cells in mesangial localization of materials requires clarification. Based on the observation that "blebs" of mesangial cytoplasm may be seen protruding between endothelial cells so that they are exposed to the circulation, it has been proposed that mesangial cells are actively involved in the local deposition of circulating materials. However, two factors bring this conclusion into question. Firstly, the frequency of mesangial "blebs" seems to correlate more closely with poor fixation than with other variables. Secondly, receptors for C3 or Fc have only been found on a small subset of mesangial cells which express Ia antigen in vitro (Schreiner et al. 1981).

1.3.2. Local formation of immune complexes

As noted in the previous section, it has not been possible to produce subepithelial deposits by the injection of the usual species of preformed antigen–antibody complexes. However, Germuth et al. (1979) found that subepithelial deposits could develop when low-avidity complexes were injected. These could be expected to dissociate in vivo, raising the possibility that free antigen and antibody might localize independently, to combine at an extravascular site. This possibility was nearly simultaneously described by Couser et al. (1978b) and Van Damme et al. (1978). They found that when antigen–antibody complexes were perfused into an isolated kidney, only mesangial deposits were formed, whereas alternate perfusion with antigen and antibody resulted in the appearance of subepithelial deposits. These observations provide strong evidence that the deposits were formed by the aggregation of antigen and antibody molecules which arrived independently in the subepithelial zone. This is not entirely without precedent since the tissue localization of one component of immune complexes with subsequent delivery of the other reactant is a well-established concept, as in the Arthus phenomenon. Further support for this postulate is provided by studies of the development of membranous (uniform, subepithelial) deposits in Heyman's nephritis. In this model, it has been shown that circulating antibody localizes in proximity to an antigen residing in the subepithelial region to form local complexes (Fleuren et al. 1980b). It is unclear how frequently this mechanism applies, but Globus and Wilson (1979) were able to induce a glomerulonephritis in animals that have been first injected with an antigen which localizes in the peripheral glomerular matrix (Con-A), followed by vascular infusion of antibody to Con-A, raising the possibility that a wide variety of antigenic moieties might localize in the basement membrane for various reasons, including size, charge and lectin-like binding. It seems likely that the local formation of antigen–antibody complexes is an important mechanism of immune injury since the resulting renal disease closely resembles the clinical and histological features of glomerulonephritis (Couser and Salant 1980).

1.3.3. The role of charge

As noted above, the glomerular vascular wall has a high, net-negative charge due, in part, to both sialoglycoproteins and proteoglycans (Kanwar and Farquhar 1979a; Mohos and Skoza 1969). There is recent evidence that the charge on immune complexes and/or the individual components may be important. Antibody eluted from kidneys of murine models of systemic lupus erythematosus was found to have a higher isoelectric point than those present within the circulation (Ebling and Hahn 1980). Similar observations were made in Heyman's nephritis when antibodies of different isoelectric points were isolated. Cationic antibody preferentially localizes in the glomerulus (Madaio et al. 1981a). In addition, the conclusion of the studies of Gallo and co-workers (Gallo 1970; Gallo et al. 1981) was that the positive charge on antigens was an important factor for glomerular deposition of immune deposits. This is a relatively new area of investigation and requires further study to place it in proper perspective.

1.3.4. Non-immune materials

The uptake of materials by the renal glomerulus has been studied utilizing a variety of markers. Studies using immunofluorescence as the major analytical tool have largely concentrated on aggregated serum proteins (Michael et al. 1976, 1980). These studies have demonstrated that the mesangial region is the principal renal site of the recognizable accumulation of these materials. Studies using the transmission electron-microscope have made use of many probes which share the property of being large and electron-dense (carbon, imposil and ferritin). Thus, these particles can be readily identified, often by light microscopy. These probes have a common disadvantage, mainly that they do not resemble substances for which they are supposed to serve as models, i.e. immune reactants. Some of the more obvious differences include size, charge, conformation and surface ligand activity. All of these features are known to be critical in the localization and subsequent fate of these materials. It is interesting that there is a distinct difference in the disposition of particles (such as carbon) when compared to the fate of endogenous proteins (Grond and Elema 1981). Therefore, it cannot be assumed that these two types of materials will be handled in the same way with respect to uptake in tissues, interaction with extracellular matrix and cells, and activation of the inflammatory system. Thus, use of particulates may not serve as reasonable models for tissue localization and processing of immune products (complexes etc.). Therefore, conclusions about deposition of immune reactants based on the use of particulates must be reviewed with considerable reservation at the present time.

1.3.5. Renal localization of antiglomerular antibody

As noted above, the composition of the glomerular wall is quite complex, consisting of collagenous and non-collagenous proteins and proteoglycans. Most likely, there are additional constituents associated with each of the several cell types. Heterologous anti-GBL antibodies localize to both the lamina rara interna and externa (Druet et al. 1973; Fresen and Vogt 1973; McCausland et al. 1976b). Depending on the purity and type of the immunizing agent, the resulting antibodies react with a few or several of the known glomerular antigens. Antibodies from sera of patients with Goodpasture's syndrome react principally with antigens in the lamina rara interna (Fish et al. 1979). They also react with the residue of isolated glomerular matrix following its digestion with collagenase (Wilson and Dixon 1979b; Golbus and Wilson 1979). While matrix residue includes non-collagenous glycoproteins, proteoglycans, the telopeptide portions of the associated collagens, and entrapped serum proteins, isolation of the glomerular basal lamina may result in the partial loss of antigen (Kanwar and Farquhar 1979b).

1.4. REMOVAL OF GLOMERULAR IMMUNE DEPOSITS

The elimination of deposited immune complexes has been shown to occur by two separate mechanisms: one which involves uptake by cells and another which appears to be independent of direct cellular interactions.

1.4.1. Cellular uptake

The cells responsible for removal of immune deposits could be either residential or they could be derived from infiltrating circulating cells. As noted above, there are several populations of glomerular cells: two resident cell types in the mesangium (smooth muscle and macrophage-like), endothelial cells and the visceral epithelial cells.

1.4.2. Mesangial cells

There are at least two cell types present in the mesangium under basal conditions. One is a contractile cell resembling smooth muscle. The other consists of cells closely resembling macrophages (Schreiner et al. 1981). A frequent observation has been that, in both human and experimental glomerulonephritis, immune deposits often persist in the mesangial matrix and are seldom visualized in the lysosomes of contractile cells, and macrophage-like cells are often present (Haakenstad et al. 1976). This has led to the question of whether mesangial cells are the principal cells responsible for the removal of immune complexes (Striker et al. 1979). It had previously been shown that non-immune tracers such as ferritin (Farquhar and Palade 1962), silver-associated materials (Striker and Smuckler 1970) and carbon particles (Elema et al. 1976) are taken up by cells in the mesangium. However, these particles have been shown to be endocytosed by many interstitial cells, including fibroblasts and may therefore not be relevant to studies of the fate of immune products. Using bone marrow transplantation in the Chediak-Higashi mouse model where phagocytic cells develop giant lysosomes, it has been shown that the increase in glomerular cells following administration of soluble, exogenous immune complexes is derived from the bone marrow (Striker et al. 1979). Furthermore, the contractile mesangial cells do not develop large lysosomes, suggesting that they are not actively engaged in the phagocytosis of immune deposits. Since the identification of immune complexes was limited to morphological appearances, endocytosis or extracellular degradation of the complexes by contractile mesangial cells could have been overlooked. However, it is clear that the major cell involved in bulk removal of immune complexes, in this model, is derived from the bone marrow. These experiments leave open the question of the contribution of marrow-derived cells which are resident in the glomerulus. A curious observation with regard to removal of glomerular aggregates has been made in animals chronically exposed to silver nitrate following removal of the chemical from the drinking water. Initially, the dense granules are distributed randomly on the endothelial aspect of the GBL and in the mesangial matrix. Later, the peripheral aspects of the GBL remain heavily labeled. However, the density of granules markedly decreases in both the mesangial matrix and that part of the GBL covering the mesangial region. This suggests that the mesangial matrix and the basal lamina covering the mesangium are more rapidly cleared of foreign deposits than are deposits in the central (mesangial) areas of GBL.

1.4.3. Endothelial cells

Electron microscopic studies have suggested that immune complexes first localize the endothelial cell caveoli in the juxtamesangial region (Haakenstad et al. 1976). However, the role of endothelial cells in removal of deposited complexes remains unknown.

1.4.4. Visceral epithelial cells

These cells encircle deposits in the subepithelial space; lysosomes are often present in their cytoplasm. While C3b receptors have been identified on the surfaces of these cells in humans (Gelfand et al. 1975), it has not been clearly shown whether these cells are involved in ingesting immune complexes deposited in the subepithelial space.

1.4.5. Extracellular routes of disappearance

Elema et al. (1976), using carbon particle injection, concluded that materials in the mesangial matrix can exit this region via the vascular stalk. This postulate was confirmed using aggregated proteins (Michael et al. 1980). Since these data have been obtained with particulates, it is unclear whether immune complexes residing in the extracellular mesangial matrix are handled in a similar manner. Recently, it was found that administration of excess antigen to animals with glomerular *mesangial* immune complex deposits causes disappearance of detectable complexes (Mannik and Striker 1980). In these studies, large latticed complexes were administered intravenously, resulting in mesangial localization. Then, large amounts of antigen were injected. A 40-fold excess of antigen removed all complexes when given 12 hours after administration of the immune complexes. If a longer time elapsed between the administration of complexes and the antigen, disappearance of the complexes was incomplete. In this case, immunofluorescence and electron-microscopic analysis suggested that the complexes which could not be removed were intracellular and that all of the extracellular deposits were gone. The route of disappearance is unknown. The possibilities include catabolism by the local cells, return to the glomerular circulation, loss into the filtrate, or egress through the stalk regions.

The mechanisms by which *subendothelial* deposits are removed are not known, but they are conceivably much more accessible to both circulating cells and antigen than immune reactants deposited in the mesangium.

Subepithelial deposits may be incorporated into the substance of the glomerular basement membrane in chronic glomerulonephritis. The exact mechanism by which these deposits disappear is, again, not known. However, we have recently obtained preliminary evidence that excess antigen may also remove subepithelial deposits in animals that have been repeatedly immunized (Haakenstad et al., unpublished data).

1.5. MEDIATOR SYSTEMS IMPLICATED IN GLOMERULONEPHRITIS

1.5.1. Complement and glomerulonephritis

It is somewhat sobering to realize that, even though over 20 years have passed since the basic pathological mechanisms of anti-GBM nephritis and serum sickness were described, only one mediator system — complement — has been incriminated, and only for some of these reactions. Pioneering studies in the 1960's by Cochrane et al. (1965) revealed that certain forms of experimental anti-GBM disease require complement for the development of the full-blown glomerulonephritis characterized histologically by the accumulation of neutrophils. It has been assumed that the complement activation is required primarily to attract neutrophils into the glomeruli mainly through the formation of C5a. Complement does not appear to be required in immune complex (serum sickness) models of glomerulonephritis and in some models of nephrotoxic nephritis (Cochrane 1979).

There are suggestions for participation of complement in many of the human glomerulonephrites, but it must be stressed that this evidence is inferential rather than direct. The evidence is based upon two major findings. The first is that there are many human glomerulonephrites associated with low total serum hemolytic complement (CH_{50}) (see Table 2). This low serum complement appears to be due to increased consumption rather than decreased synthesis of complement (Müller-Eberhard 1974). The other major evidence suggesting a role for complement is in the widespread use of the immunofluorescence technique which has revealed that many types of human glomerulonephritis are associated with immunoglobulin and complement deposits in the glomeruli (see Table 3). Thus, some types of human glomerulonephritis, particularly systemic lupus erythematosus, are associated with

TABLE 2.
Glomerulonephritis according to the complement systems (CH_{50})

I. Normocomplementemic

a) Henoch-Schönlein purpura
b) periarteritis nodosa
c) rapidly-progressive (idiopathic) glomerulonephritis
d) Goodpasture syndrome
e) lipoid nephrosis
f) idiopathic membranous glomerulonephritis
g) focal glomerular sclerosis

II. Hypocomplementemic

a) acute poststreptococcal glomerulonephritis
b) lupus erythematosus nephritis
c) membranoproliferative glomerulonephritis
d) post-transplant glomerulonephritis
e) sickle-cell disease
f) subacute bacterial endocarditis
g) postinfectious rapidly progressive
h) mixed cryoglobulinemia

From Arroyave (1979).

glomerular deposits of the early complement components such as C1q, C4 and C2, suggesting activation of the classical pathway of complement. Other types of glomerulonephritis such as IgA nephropathy and membranoproliferative glomerulonephritis are often associated with glomerular deposits of C3 and properdin, suggesting alternative pathway activation. These patients also often have a circulating antibody to C3 convertase, the so-called C3 nephritic factor. Finally, there are some types of glomerulonephritis (such as in patients with subacute bacterial endocarditis and membranoproliferative glomerulonephritis) where C3 deposits are found in the absence of immunoglobulins. The significance of finding C3 alone is not known. A final word of caution must be given in terms of the significance of complement and immunoglobulin deposition in glomeruli. IgM and C3 deposits have been reported in a variety of renal diseases which appear to have no immunological basis, such as Alport's syndrome, nephronophthisis cystinosis and oligomeganephronia (Berger et al. 1974). Also, IgM and C3 deposits have been described in glomeruli which do not show any evidence of glomerular disease.

TABLE 3.
Immune deposits in human glomerulonephritis as assessed by immunofluorescence

Type of glomerular disease	Pattern	Glomerular deposition						
		IgG	IgM	IgA	C3	C4	C1q	properdin
I. Immune complex disease								
Poststreptococcal glomerulonephritis	nodular	+	+	0	+	0	0	+
Systemic lupus erythematosus	granular	+	+	+	+	+	+	+
Subacute bacterial endocarditis	granular/nodular	+	+	0	+	+	+	0
Membranoproliferative glomerulonephritis								
Type I	granular/nodular	+/0	+	0	+	+/0	+	+
Type II	nodular	0	0	0	+	0	0	0
Membranous glomerulopathy	granular/nodular	+	+	0	+	+/0	+/0	+/0
IgG-IgM cryoglobulinemia	granular/nodular	+	+	0	+	+	+	+/0
Henoch-Schönlein purpura	granular	+	+	+	+	0	+/0	+/0
IgA nephropathy	granular	+	+/0	+	+	0	0	+/0
II. Anti-basement-membrane disease								
Goodpasture	linear	+	+/0	0	+	0	0	0
III. Idiopathic nephrotic syndrome								
Lipoid nephrosis	none	0	0	0	0	0	0	0
Mesangial proliferative glomerulonephritis	nodular/granular	+/0	+	0	+	0	0	0
Focal sclerosis	nodular/granular	+/0	+	0	+	0	0	0

Adapted from Fish and Michael (1979).

Finally, partially sclerotic glomeruli often contain IgM and C3, but whether these represent specific immune complexes or entrapped aggregated gamma-globulin remains unclear (McCluskey et al. 1978).

In summary, clinical evidence supports a role for complement in some types of human glomerulonephritis based upon determinations of total hemolytic complement levels, as well as immunofluorescence evidence of complement deposits in glomeruli. However, the exact role of the complement system in these entities remains to be determined.

1.5.2. Prostaglandins

Prostaglandins are a family of fatty acids synthesized from two unsaturated fatty acids: arachidonic acid and dihomo-γ-linolenic acid. These substances are essentially ubiquitous and seem to occur naturally in almost every animal species and tissues or cells studied (Horton 1979). It is not surprising, therefore, that prostaglandins are present in high levels in renal tissue. Precise identification of cells in the kidney synthesizing prostaglandins remains unclear, but there is evidence of synthesis in cortical and medullary collecting tubules, arterial endothelial cells and interstitial cells of the renal medulla. Recent preliminary evidence also reveals prostaglandin synthesis in isolated glomeruli grown in culture, although the exact cell of origin has not been determined (Sraer et al. 1981).

The biological effects of the prostaglandins appear at first glance as ubiquitous as their distribution. A main area of interest has revolved around their involvement in inflammation, with multiple studies relating prostaglandins to the production of pain, fever, vasodilatation and increased vascular permeability (Lewis 1977; Williams 1977). Other areas of study in which prostaglandins are becoming increasingly implicated are reproductive biology, gastric secretion, hypertension, congenital heart disease and platelet aggregation and thrombosis (Horton 1979).

In the kidney, the best understood regions implicating prostaglandin involvement are those areas that can be geographically related to control of water and electrolyte excretion, renal blood flow and blood pressure. There is surprisingly little information relating to the role of prostaglandins in renal inflammation, particularly glomerulonephritis. The one series of studies addressing this question relates to the study of NZB/W mice. These mice develop an autoimmune disease resembling lupus erythematosus, characterized by anti-DNA antibody formation and early death from immune-complex-induced glomerulonephritis (Dixon et al. 1971). Studies by Krakauer et al. (1978) revealed that treatment of female mice with prostaglandin E_1 (PGE_1) delays the appearance of the antinuclear antibodies and largely prevents the development of nephritis. The exact mechanism of action is unknown, but it may relate to evidence suggesting a direct effect of PGE_1 on lymphocytes with enhancement of T-cell and suppression of B-cell activity (Krakauer et al. 1978).

1.5.3. Bradykinins

Bradykinins are small peptides which are formed in the circulation by the cleavage of plasma kininogens by proteinases (kallikreins) (Wiggins and Cochrane 1982). These small peptides have a diverse array of biological activities including smooth muscle contraction or relaxation, production of pain, stimulation of cellular proliferation and potentiating activity for vasoactive amines and arachidonic acid metabolites. However, the main effects of bradykinin appear to be increased vascular permeability, arteriolar dilatation, and venular constriction (Wiggins and Cochrane 1982). Kinins promote the movement of fluid out of the vascular compartment into the extravascular space at the level of the postcapillary venule. Although kinins can themselves cause changes associated with inflammation (heat, pain, redness and swelling), there is no direct evidence that they are directly involved as mediators of inflammation. Nonetheless, there is indirect evidence to suggest that kinins may be important mediators in hereditary angioedema, gout, septic shock and acute pancreatitis (Curd et al. 1980; Kellermeyer and Breckenridge 1965; Hirsch et al. 1974; Toki et al. 1981). With the exception of acute pancreatitis, the postulated role of kinins in these reactions is related to Hageman factor activation with subsequent kinin formation (due to activation of prekallikrein). There is no evidence implicating a direct role for kinins in the pathogenesis of glomerulonephritis. However, the potential of kinins to reproduce the events seen in inflammatory processes could apply to the kidney. Some authors have suggested a role for activated Hageman factor in the nephrotic syndrome, but this remains to be determined (Wiggins and Cochrane 1982).

1.6. REGULATORY ROLE OF CELL-MEDIATED IMMUNITY IN GLOMERULONEPHRITIS

There is accumulating evidence that the cellular immune system may be indirectly involved in the development of glomerulonephritis. A variety of regulatory defects has been described in which there is an association with several types of glomerular diseases. It should be stressed that there is very little evidence to support the contention that cellular immune mechanisms play a direct role in glomerulonephritis. Classically, the experimental models of glomerulonephritis, as well as most types of human glomerulonephritis, appear to be caused by humoral immune mechanisms with the involvement of antigen—antibody reactions serving as triggering agents for the release of various mediators. Thus, glomerulonephritis is classically thought to represent Type III (immune-complex-mediated) hypersensitivity reaction. The cardinal feature of delayed-type hypersensitivity reactions is the presence of a small number of specifically sensitized lymphocytes interacting with antigen locally to elaborate various lymphokines that mediate the inflammatory response. Therefore, classical cell-mediated hypersensitivity depends on locally activated lymphocytes rather than on antibody. In none of the experimental or human types of glomerulonephritis has a direct role for the lymphocyte been shown.

On the other hand, there is indirect evidence that cell-mediated immunity may be incriminated in antibody-mediated glomerular injury. Some reports in humans with glomerulonephritis have suggested that blood lymphocytes from a few of these patients exhibit cellular hypersensitivity to purified glomerular basement membrane as measured by blastogenic reactions and production of lymphokines (Fillit et al. 1978).

In one form of human glomerular disease (lipoid nephrosis) cell-mediated immune mechanisms are thought to be important. Although there is no proof of an immune complex etiology for this disease, abnormalities of lymphocytic function have been noted. These patients appear to have a circulating inhibitor which suppresses lymphocyte transformation (Moarthy et al. 1976; Iitaka and West 1979). These patients also appear to have increased lymphocyte-mediated cytotoxicity in vitro for target cells (Eyres et al. 1976) as well as evidence of diminished levels of suppressor-cell activity (Taube et al. 1981). Finally, there is the well-known linkage between Hodgkin's disease and lipoid nephrosis. Hodgkin's disease is characterized by abnormalities of lymphocyte function and the nephrotic syndrome. This complication usually remits with radiation treatment of the Hodgkin's disease (Williams 1981).

Experimentally, two strains of mice have provided further evidence for a possible role for cellular immunity. The NZB/W mice spontaneously develop an autoimmune disease with an immune-complex-induced nephritis. Attempts have been made in these animals to ascertain proportions of the various lymphocyte subclasses (such as B-cells and helper and suppressor T-cells). There is general agreement that the proportion and number of B-cells increases, while there is a decreased proportion of T-cells and a specific decrease in the number of T-suppressor cells (Krakauer et al. 1976). It has been suggested that it is this decrease of T-suppressor-cell activity that accounts for the apparent activation of the B-cell system.

Another strain of mouse used is the athymic, or nude, mouse. These mice have little or no thymus and appear to have an almost total immunological defect of the T-cell system. Studies by Balton et al. (1978) using nude mice have revealed an inability to develop an autoimmune type of glomerulonephritis. However, criticism has been leveled at using nude mice, because there are suggestions that nude mice have abnormally distributed and functioning B-lymphocytes. Studies with neonatally thymectomized rats appear to corroborate the results in nude mice by revealing that an immune complex glomerulonephritis developed only with an intact T-cell system, in this case T-helper-cell activity (Palestro et al. 1980).

The finding that circulating (Ia-positive) mononuclear cells are present in the glomeruli in some types of experimental glomerular disease has renewed interest in the possible role of cell-mediated immune mechanisms, since the macrophage is the main infiltrating cell type found in typical delayed-type hypersensitivity reactions. To test this hypothesis, Bhan et al. (1978) used the model of anti-GBM nephritis which is known to be associated with large numbers of mononuclear cells in renal glomeruli. By using subnephritogenic doses of anti-GBM antisera, they were able to show that only animals receiving lymph node cells or enriched T-cell populations from previously sensitized animals together with the anti-GBM antibody develop histological evidence of glomerulonephritis. By using this complex model, the authors contend that specifically sensitized T-cells are responsible for the accumulation of macrophages in the glomeruli. However, no attempt was made to perform various in vitro assays on the sensitized T-cells in terms of measuring lymphokine activity such as the macrophage chemotactic factor (MCF) that has been described in extracts of delayed-hypersensitivity skin reaction sites (Cohen et al. 1973).

In summary, there is experimental evidence to suggest an indirect role for cell-mediated immune mechanisms in modulating antibody-mediated glomerular injury. The best evidence comes from studies in mice where levels of T-helper and T-suppressor cell activity appear important in modulating the B-cell response. There is also evidence, albeit indirect, that sensitized T-cells may contribute to monocyte deposition in glomeruli in certain types of experimental glomerulonephritis. There is no evidence, to date, implicating a direct role for lymphokines in the initiation of glomerular injury, which is the case for most reactions involving cell-mediated immunity.

1.7. RESOLUTION OF GLOMERULAR INJURIES

Consideration of the effect of growth factors on the various glomerular cell types is beyond the scope of this chapter. The degree and type of glomerular cell injury depends on the nature and severity of the inflammatory response. The focus has been on the glomerular reaction rather than on the nature of the injury. Glomerular cells have often been considered to be innocent bystanders, injured as a result of an inflammatory response directed at the deposited materials. The demonstration of circulating antibody to glomerular cells following the injection of mercury chloride raises the possibility that a direct response to antigens synthesized by glomerular cells may be a more important mechanism than previously realized (Bariety et al. 1971). The glomerulus may thus be the target of a direct immunological attack involving cellular and/or humoral immunity.

1.7.1 Cell and matrix changes associated with acute injury

In acute postinfectious glomerulonephritis, it has been noted that the mesangial region is difficult to define by electron microscopy (Strunk et al. 1964), suggesting that there are changes in both the cells and their surrounding matrix. Similar changes are noted following Habu snake venom injection, i.e. mesangiolysis (Sakaguchi and Kawamura 1963). Similarly, if glomerular injury is induced chemically, as by aminonucleosides, there is evidence of cellular injury and matrix alterations, since there is a reduction of immune complex deposition in damaged glomeruli (Mauer et al. 1972; Couser et al. 1978a; Salant et al. 1979). The exact alteration of the matrix associated with these lesions is not clear. Common to most is proteinuria and loss of colloidal iron staining and Fx1a antigen (Blau and Haas 1973; Couser et al. 1978a). The Fx1a antigen is located in the lamina rara externa region, as is one of the components of the charge barrier. Other components of this region include proteoglycans containing heparan sulfate. Thus, it has been thought that the loss of these components and the onset of proteinuria might be linked. Recent preliminary observations that adriamycin also induces podocyte changes and proteinuria without observable changes in either colloidal iron staining or the presence of glomerular Fx1a antigens suggest that some caution must be exercised in the correlation of these variables. In summary, the composition of the extracellular matrix of the glomerulus is still unclear. Therefore, it is premature for detailed analysis of alterations following acute injury. Similarly, the net biological effect of matrix changes is highly speculative since the importance of individual molecules in overall glomerular function or their interaction with immune reactants is largely unknown. This topic remains an important field of inquiry.

The cellular changes following acute injury have been mainly investigated by morphological means. The role of the neutrophils has been recently reviewed (Couser and Salant 1982). There is strong experimental evidence that, in certain types of immune-complex-mediated tissue injury, neutrophils are required for the injury to occur. The two experimental models in which this is true are the Arthus reaction, which is an immune complex vasculitis, and nephrotoxic nephritis or glomerulonephritis caused by antibody against glomerular basement membranes. In both of these models, ablation of the circulating neutrophils by either nitrogen mustard or specific anti-neutrophil antibody results in a marked protection from tissue injury (Cochrane et al. 1959). In the nephrotoxic nephritis model, the proteinuria is reduced or eliminated and there is evidence that the cellular proliferative reaction (see above) is reduced in these instances.

The neutrophil requirement in these experimental models parallels the requirement for an intact complement system. Ablation of complement by treating the animals with cobra venom factor prevents the accumulation of neutrophils at the inflammatory sites. The exact reason why complement is required is uncertain, but it is felt to relate to the generation of chemotactic factors for neutrophils derived from the complement system, presumably C5a. The constituents of neutrophils which cause the tissue injury are currently under active study. The neutrophil is capable of releasing many biologically active substances into the circulation (see Table 4). Traditionally, the various proteases have been felt to be exclusively responsible, since neutrophilic lysates or lysates from cytoplasmic granules from rabbit neutrophils hydrolyse, in vitro, various substrates including glomerular basement membrane. The proteases responsible were found to be cathepsins D and E (Cochrane 1968).

If proteases are in fact responsible for the tissue injury, one would expect that the use of various protease inhibitors would block the tissue injury. However, using the

Arthus reaction as a model, we have been unable to inhibit the reaction using the protease inhibitors α_2-macroglobulin, soybean trypsin inhibitor and α_1-antitrypsin (Johnson and Ward 1981). Other studies in which isolated granule extracts were used also have failed, for the most part, to inflict tissue damage (Cochrane and Janoff 1974). This is not to say that proteases do not play a role in inflammation. Proteases certainly can act to amplify the inflammatory response with their ability to generate leukotactic peptides for C3 and C5 (Ward and Hill 1970). Therefore, evidence to date suggests that leukocytic proteases act in the amplification of acute inflammatory reactions. It should also be pointed out that in some experimental models, such as nephrotoxic nephritis, there is evidence for proteolysis of glomerular basement membrane (Cochrane 1968), perhaps related to the intimate contact between neutrophils and the basement membrane. It seems likely that the ultimate effects of acute inflammatory reactions mediated by complement and neutrophils will be due to a combination of oxygen-derived free radical generation and the release of lysosomal proteases.

It has been known for many years that neutrophils undergoing activation during the "respiratory burst" produce large quantities of highly reactive oxygen products such as the superoxide anion (O_2^-), hydrogen peroxide (H_2O_2) etc. These products are released in considerable amounts into the extracellular space during phagocytosis and other conditions of surface activation (chemotactic factors, Fc and C3b receptor binding). Many in-vitro studies have shown a role for these oxygen free radicals in the antimicrobial activity of leukocytes (Klebanoff 1980). More recent in-vitro studies have shown that various oxygen free radicals are capable of inflicting cytotoxic injury on isolated cells (Clark and Klebanoff 1975; Nathan et al. 1979).

TABLE 4.
Biologically active constituents of neutrophils

Constituent	Activity
proteases	hydrolysis of basement membrane, histone, proteoglycan
fibrinolysis	degradation of fibrin
collagenase	hydrolysis of collagen basement membrane
elastase	hydrolysis of internal elastic lamina
basic proteins	
bands 1, 3, 4	increase in vascular permeability
band 2	activation of mast cells
thrombin-activating material	thromboplastin
slow-reacting substance	vascular permeability and smooth muscle contraction
kininogenase	release of kinin from kininogen
free radicals of oxygen	in-vitro cytotoxicity, acute tissue injury
surface protease	kinin release from plasma alpha-globulin

With this background information, we assessed the role of oxygen-derived free radicals and other toxic oxygen products (H_2O_2) from neutrophils on immune-complex-mediated tissue injury in vivo. Using inhibitors such as superoxide dismutase (SOD) and catalase, the tissue injury occurring in the Arthus reaction can be largely prevented (Johnson and Ward 1981). These studies suggest that a major mechanism responsible for the tissue damage occurring in these neutrophil-dependent reactions is the production of H_2O_2 or its derivatives by the neutrophil.

There are, however, some types of experimental glomerulonephritis that do not appear to require complement or neutrophils. The best-known example is acute serum sickness. While the vasculitis associated with acute serum sickness is complement- and neutrophil-dependent, the accompanying glomerulonephritis does not appear to be. In the absence of a requirement for complement and neutrophils, the mediators involved in this type of glomerulonephritis have not been identified. Recently, however, studies have suggested a critical role for macrophages in this as well as other types of experimental glomerulonephritis. This finding could also support the concept of free-radical-induced tissue injury, since it is well known that the monocytes and macrophages produce large amounts of oxygen free radicals under appropriate stimulation.

Recently, increasing attention has been focused on monocytes and macrophages, both as inflammatory cells with principally a phagocytic function and as an effector cell in cell-mediated immunity. Macrophages were postulated to be the principal cell responsible for phagocytosis of mesangial immune deposits following injection of preformed immune complexes (Haakenstad et al. 1976; Striker et al. 1979) (Fig. 7). In Masugi nephritis, macrophages have been identified at the light- and electron-microscopic levels as the main inflammatory cell at the onset of the lesion and remain identifiable up to 124 days (Morita et al. 1976). These cells have also been identified in a rabbit model of acute serum sickness as a major contributor to the early glomerular hypercellularity (Sano 1976). Subsequently, it has been estimated that 76% of the cells in rabbit glomerulonephritis induced by nephrotoxic antibody are monocytes (Akikusa et al. 1979). Similar findings have been reported in immune-complex-mediated diseases using a combination of histochemical and cell culture techniques (Holdsworth et al. 1980). Finally, there is abundant evidence in both human and experimental crescentic glomerulonephritis that macrophages contribute significantly to the increased number of cells in the crescents (Atkins et al. 1976; Thomson et al. 1979). In the case of non-crescentic glomerulonephritis, the contribution of macrophages to the hypercellularity has been recently questioned (Monga et al. 1981).

A direct contribution of the macrophage to glomerular injury has been shown by depletion experiments in a model of accelerated glomerulonephritis in which rats are preimmunized with rabbit IgG and subsequently injected with amounts of rabbit anti-rat kidney serum that are subnephrotoxic (Schreiner et al. 1978). The late proteinuria (48–96 hours) was abrogated when macrophages were eliminated by irradiation. Mononuclear cell preparations containing T-cells sensitized to

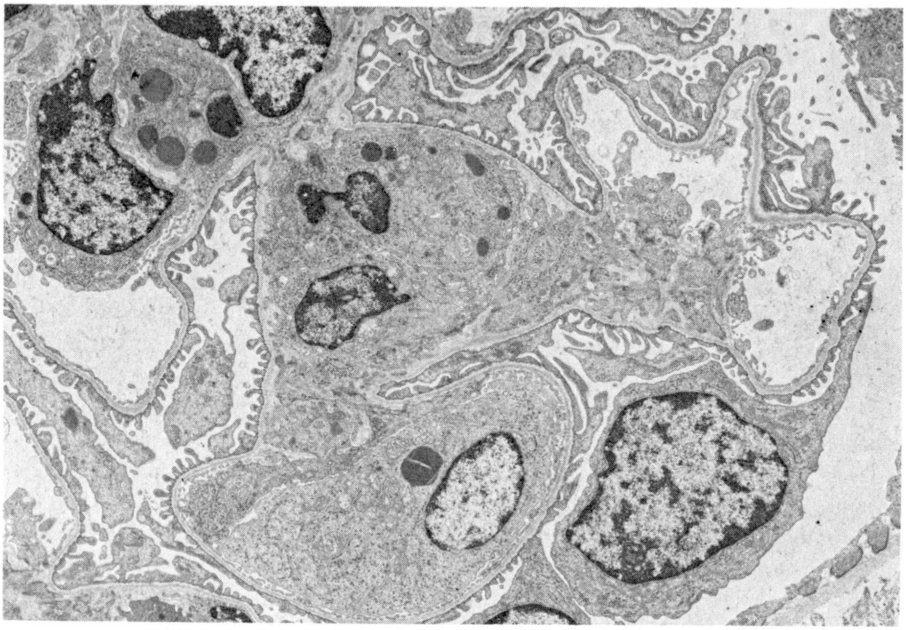

Fig. 7. Electron micrograph of glomerulus following administration of 5 mg of immune complexes. The mouse was a stable bone marrow chimera following engraftment with Chediak-Higashi marrow. The mesangial hypercellularity was due to infiltration of bone-marrow-derived cells with giant lysosomes characteristic of Chediak-Higashi syndrome.

glomerular antigens were shown after infusion into rabbits to induce focal glomerular hypercellularity and necrosis (Bhan et al. 1978). The hypercellularity was apparently due both to infiltrating monocytes and to locally proliferating endothelial cells.

Proliferation of endogenous glomerular cells following acute glomerular injury has been difficult to distinguish from infiltration of blood-derived cells. Most authors have relied on the presence of mitotic figures in cells which have anatomic features consistent with resident glomerular cells. Endothelial proliferation has been documented in anti-GBL and immune complex nephritis (Jennings and Haber 1961; Shigematsu 1970; Bradfield and Cattell 1977; Hawn and Janeway 1947). Mesangial cell proliferation has been shown in human and experimental animals (Shigematsu et al. 1976; Shigematsu and Kobayashi 1976; Johnston and Latta 1972; Bradfield and Cattell 1977; Cattell and Bradfield 1977). The cause of the proliferation is not clear, but it has been noted that glomerular hypercellularity is interrupted if immune deposits are removed by a large excess of antigen infusion prior to the onset of macrophage infiltration (Mannik and Striker 1980). Similarly, if macrophages are eliminated by irradiation, no local increase in glomerular cells is seen (Schreiner et al. 1978). In addition, supernatant fluids from cultured macrophages have been shown to stimulate proliferation of mesangial cells in vitro (Striker et al. 1980b). However, glomerular visceral epithelial cells and endothelial cells do not respond to this stimulus (Striker et al. 1979).

The role of platelets in the causation of an acute proliferative response is less clear. Following the report of Vassali et al. (1963) there was considerable interest in the role of coagulation factors in clinical and experimental renal diseases. The results from clinical trials to inhibit acute renal disease characterized by fibrin deposition have been inconsistent. Experimental studies also are difficult to interpret at this time. Using a model of mesangiolysis induced by Habu venom, it has been found that the injection of anti-platelet serum does not alter the early glomerular damage, whereas the late mesangial cell proliferation is blocked (Cattell 1979). In the same model, acetylsalicylic acid greatly increases the early glomerular damage; prostacyclin has been found to inhibit this change, suggesting that products of platelets and endothelial cells may play an important role in determining the outcome of glomerular injury subsequent to intravascular coagulation (Cattel and Mehotra 1980). In two other models of immune-mediated renal injury (Lavelle and Moseman, 1978; Sindrey et al. 1979), the role of platelets has been less clear. Platelets were depleted with anti-platelet serum during the autologous phase of glomerular immune injury induced in rabbits with BSA (Lavelle and Moseman 1978). There was no effect noted on the glomerulonephritis when hypotension was controlled. In an accelerated model of nephrotoxic nephritis, anti-platelet sera did not affect fibrin deposition or evidence of glomerular damage, although proteinuria was initially reduced (Sindrey et al. 1979). When nephrotoxic antibody injections were followed by antiserum to the heterologous IgG, platelet depletion resulted in the localization of fewer neutrophils in glomeruli, but fibrin deposition was not altered. Thus, the contribution of platelets to glomerular injury awaits further study. These data suggest that caution should be exercised in generalizations about the role of coagulation between the various experimental models and the different species.

1.7.2 Changes associated with chronic injury

Glomerulosclerosis has recently been described following administration of aminonucleoside of puromycin (Glasser et al. 1977) and N,N^1-diacetylbenzidine (Zimmerman 1979). These observations raise the possibility that other chemicals may be implicated in the genesis of glomerular scarring. The progression of injury to glomerulosclerosis may depend on the age and genetic background of the animal. "Spontaneous" glomerulosclerosis has been noted in Sprague-Dawley rats (Bolton and Sturgell 1980) and in the fawn-hooded rat (Kreisberg et al. 1979). These changes can be accentuated through increasing the functional load following unilateral nephrectomy (Striker et al. 1969). Recently, it has been shown that glomerular changes in spontaneously hypertensive rats whose blood pressure is controlled by drugs are rather similar to untreated controls except for a delayed appearance (Feld et al. 1981).

Strain differences in the susceptibility of mice to virally induced glomerular lesions have also been documented (Gresser et al. 1978; Morel-Maroger et al. 1979). Rats also demonstrate interstrain differences following immunization with human glomerular basement membrane preparation (McCausland et al. 1976). These data provide evidence that the genetic constitution as well as potential initiators of glomerular damage must be considered in the interpretations of glomerular injury.

REFERENCES

Akikusa, B., Shigematsu, H. and Kondo, Y. (1979) Cellular aspects of rabbit Masugi nephritis. IV. Cell quantitation of proliferative glomerulonephritis. *Acta Pathol. 29,* 509–522.

Arend, W.P. and Mannik, M. (1979) Studies on antigen–antibody complexes. II. Quantification of tissue uptake of soluble complexes in normal and complement-depleted rabbits. *Immunology 107,* 63–75.

Arroyave, C.M. (1979) The complement system in pediatric renal disease. *Paediatrician 8,* 349–363.

Atkins, R.C., Holdsworth, S.R., Glasgow, E.F. and Matthews, F. (1976) The macrophage in human rapidly progressive glomerulonephritis. *Lancet 2,* 830–832.

Ausiello, D.A., Kreisberg, J.I., Roy, C. and Karnovsky, M.J. (1980) Contraction of cultured rat glomerular cells of apparent mesangial origin after stimulation with angiotensin II and arginine vasopressin. *J. Clin. Invest. 65,* 754–760.

Balton, W.K., Benton, F.R. and Tobo, P.I. (1978) Requirement of functional T-cells in the production of autoimmune glomerulotubular nephropathy in man. *Clin. Exp. Immunol. 33,* 474–477.

Bariety, J., Druet, P., Saliberte, F. and Sapin, C. (1971) Glomerulonephritis with aα- and β-globulin deposits induced in rats by mercuric chloride. *Am. J. Pathol. 65,* 292–302.

Benacerraf, B., Patter, J.L., McCluskey, R.T. and Miller, F. (1960) The pathologic effects of IV administered soluble antigen–antibody complexes. II. Acute glomerulonephritis in rats. *J. Exp. Med. 111,* 195–200.

Berger, J., Nael, L.H. and Yaneria, H. (1974) Complement deposition in the kidney. In: J. Hamburger, J. Crasnier and M.H. Maxwell (Eds), *Advances in Nephrology,* Year Book Medical Publishers, Chicago, pp. 37–48.

Bhan, A.K., Schneeberger, E.E., Collins A.B. and McCluskey, R.T. (1978) Evidence for a pathogenic role of a cell-mediated immune mechanism in experimental glomerulonephritis. *J. Exp. Med. 148,* 246–260.

Blau, E.B. and Haas, J.E. (1973) Glomerular sialic acid and proteinuria in human renal disease. *Lab. Invest. 28,* 477–481.

Bockow, B.I. and Mannik, M. (1981) Clearance and tissue uptake of immune complexes in complement-depleted and control mice. *Immunology 42,* 497–504.

Bolton, W.K. and Sturgell, B.C. (1980) Spontaneous glomerulosclerosis in aging rats. II. Ultrastructural studies. *Am. J. Pathol. 98,* 399–356.

Border, W.A., Ward, H.J., Kamil, E.S. and Cohen, A.H. (1982) Induction of membranous nephropathy in rabbits by administration of an exogenous cationic antigen:

demonstration of a pathogenic role for electrical charge. *J. Clin. Invest.,* in press.

Bradfield, J.W.B. and Cattell, V. (1977) The mesangial cell in glomerulonephritis I. Mechanism of hypercellularity in experimental immune complex glomerulonephritis. *Lab. Invest. 36,* 481.

Brenner, B.M., Hostetter, T.H. and Humes, H.D. (1978) Molecular bases of proteinuria of glomerular origin. *N. Engl. J. Med. 298,* 826–833.

Buonassissi, V. and Root, M. (1975) Enzymatic degradation of heparin-related mucopolysaccharides from the surface of endothelial cell cultures. *Biochim. Biophys. Acta 385,* 1–10.

Cattell, V. (1979) Focal mesangial proliferative glomerulonephritis in the rat caused by Habu snake venom: the role of platelets. *Br. J. Exp. Pathol. 60,* 201–208.

Cattell, V. and Bradfield, J.W. (1977) Focal mesangial proliferative glomerulonephritis in rat caused by Habu snake venom. *Am. J. Pathol. 87,* 511.

Cattell, V. and Mehotra, A. (1980) Focal mesangial proliferative glomerulonephritis in the rat caused by Habu venom: the effect of antiplatelet agents. *Br. J. Exp. Pathol. 61,* 310–314.

Chang, R.L.S., Deen, W.M., Robertson, C.R., Bennett, C.M., Glassock, R.J. and Brenner B.M. (1976) Permselectivity of the glomerular capillary wall: studies of experimental glomerulonephritis in the rat using neutral dextran. *J. Clin. Invest. 57,* 1272–1286.

Cines, D.B., Lyss, A.P., Bina, M., Corkey, R., Kefalides, N.A. and Friedman, H.M. (1982) Fc and C3b receptors induced by herpes simplex virus on cultured human endothelial cells. *J. Clin. Invest. 69,* 123–128.

Clark, R.A. and Klebanoff, S.J. (1975) Neutrophil-mediated tumor cell cytotoxicity: role of the peroxidase system. *J. Exp. Med. 141,* 1442–1447.

Cochrane, C.G. (1968) Immunologic tissue injury mediated by neutrophilic leukocytes. *Adv. Immunol. 9,* 97–162.

Cochrane, C.G. (1979) Immune complex mediated tissue injury. In: S. Cohen, P.A. Ward and R.T. McCluskey (Eds), *Mechanisms of Immunopathology,* John Wiley and Sons, New York, pp. 29–48.

Cochrane, C.G. and Janoff, A. (1974) The Arthus reaction: a model of neutrophil complement-mediated injury. In: B. Zweifach, L. Grant and R.T. McCluskey (Eds), *The Inflammatory Process, Vol. 3,* 2nd edn., Academic Press, New York.

Cochrane, C.G., Weigle, W.O. and Dixon, F.J. (1959) The role of polymorphonuclear leukocytes in the imitation and cessation of the Arthus vasculitis. *J. Exp. Med. 110,* 481.

Cochrane, C.G., Unanue, E.R. and Dixon, F.G. (1965) A role of polymorphonuclear leukocytes and complement in nephrotoxic nephritis. *J. Exp. Med. 122,* 99–116.

Cohen, M.P. and Vogt, C.A. (1975) Collagen synthesis and secretion by isolated rat renal glomeruli. *Biochim. Biophys. Acta 393,* 78–87.

Cohen S., Ward, P.A., Yashida, T. and Burek, C.L. (1973) Biologic activity of extracts of delayed hypersensitivity skin reaction sites. *Cell. Immunol. 9,* 363–376.

Couser, W.G. (1981) What are circulating immune complexes doing in glomerulonephritis? (Editorial) *N. Engl. J. Med. 304,* 1230–1232.

Couser, W.G. (1982) Idiopathic rapidly progressive glomerulonephritis (Editorial Review) *Am. J. Nephrol.,* in press.

Couser, W.G. and Salant, D.J. (1980) In situ immune complex formation and glomerular injury. *Kidney Int. 17,* 1–13.

Couser, W.G. and Salant D.J. (1982) Immunopathogenesis of glomerular capillary wall injury in nephrotic states. In: *Contemporary Issues in Nephrology,* in press.

Couser, W.G., Spargo, B.H., Stilmant, M.M. and Lewis, E.J. (1975) Experimental glomerulonephritis in the guinea pig. II. Ultrastructural lesions of the basement membrane associated with proteinuria. *Lab. Invest. 32,* 46–55.

Couser, W.G., Jermanovich, N.B., Belok, S., Stilmant, M.M. and Hoyer, J.R. (1978a) The effect of aminonucleoside nephrosis on immune complex localization in autologous immune complex nephropathy in rats. *J. Clin. Invest. 61,* 561–572.

Couser, W.G., Steinmuller, D.R., Stilmant, M.M., Salant, D.J. and Lowenstein, L.M. (1978b) Experimental glomerulonephritis in the isolated perfused rat kidney. *J. Clin. Invest. 62,* 1275–1287.

Curd, J.G., Prograis, L.J. and Cochrane, C.G. (1980) Detection of active kallikrein in induced blister fluids of hereditary angioedema patients. *J. Exp. Med. 152,* 742–747.

Dixon, F.J., Vasquez, J.T., Weigle, W.O. and Cochrane, C. (1958) Pathogenesis of serum sickness. *Arch. Pathol. 65,* 18–28.

Dixon, F.J., Vasquez, J.T., Weigle, W.O. and Cochrane, C.G. (1959) In: H.S. Lawrence (Ed.), *Proceedings, Symposium on Cellular and Humoral Aspects of the Hypersensitive States,* Hoeber Division, Harper and Row, New York.

Dixon, F.J., Oldstone, M.D.A. and Tometti, B. (1971) Pathogenesis of immune complex glomerulonephritis of New Zealand mice. *J. Exp. Med. 134,* 655–715.

Druet, P., Letontur, P., Contet, A. and Mandet, C. (1973) Cryoglobulinemia in human renal diseases: study of 76 cases. *Clin. Exp. Immunol. 15,* 483–496.

Ebling, F. and Hahn, B.H. (1980) Restricted sub-populations of DNA antibodies in kidneys of mice with systemic lupus: comparison of antibodies in serum and renal eluates. *Arthritis Rheum. 23,* 392–403.

Editorial (1981) Prostaglandins and the kidney. *Lancet 2,* 343–345.

Edgington, T.F., Glassock, R.J. and Dixon, F.J. (1968) Autologous immune complex nephritis induced with renal tubular antigen. I. Identification and isolation of the pathogenetic antigen. *J. Exp. Med. 127,* 555–572.

Elema, J.D., Hoyer, J.R. and Vernier, R.L. (1976) Glomerular mesangium uptake and transport of intravenously injected colloidal carbon in rats. *Kidney Int. 9,* 395–406.

Eyres, K., Mallick, N.P. and Taylor, G. (1976) Evidence for cell-mediated immunity to renal antigens in minimal change nephrotic syndrome. *Lancet 1,* 1158–1159.

Farin, F.M., Killen, P.D. and Striker, G.E. (1982) Human glomerular epithelial cells in vitro, proteoglycan synthesis. *Physiology,* in press.

Farquhar, M.G. and Palade, G.E. (1962) Functional evidence of a third cell type in the renal glomerulus: phagocytosis of filtration residues by a distinctive third cell. *J. Cell Biol. 13,* 55–87.

Feld, L.G., Van Liew, J.B., Brentjiens, J.R. and Boylan, W. (1981) Renal lesions and proteinuria in the spontaneously hypertensive rat made normotensive by treatment. *Kidney Int. 20,* 606–614.

Fillit, H.M., Reed, S.E., Sherman, R.L., Zabriskie, J.B. and Rijn, I. (1978) Cellular reactivity to altered basement membranes in glomerulonephritis. *N. Engl. J. Med. 298,* 861–868.

Fish, A.J. and Michael, A.F. (1979) Immunopathogenesis of renal disease. In: L.E. Early and C.W. Gottschalke (Eds), *Diseases of the Kidney,* Ch. 15, Little, Brown and Co., Boston.

Fish, A.J., Carmody, K.M. and Michael, A.F. (1979) Spatial orientation and distribution of antigens with human glomerular basement membrane. *J. Lab. Clin. Med. 94,* 447–457.

Fleuren, G., Grond, J. and Hoedemaeker, Ph. J. (1980a) In situ formation of subepithelial glomerular immune complexes in passive serum sickness. *Kidney Int. 17,* 613–637.

Fleuren, G., Grond, J. and Hoedemaeker, Ph.J. (1980b) The pathogenetic role of free circulating antibody in autologous immune complex glomerulonephritis. *Clin. Exp. Immunol., 41,* 205–217.

Fresen, K.O. and Vogt, A. (1973) Ultrastructural localization of peroxidase-labelled nephrotoxic antibodies after intravenous application. *Exp. Pathol. 8,* 276–282.

Gallo, G.R. (1970) Elution studies in kidneys with linear deposition of immunoglobulin in glomeruli. *Am. J. Pathol. 61,* 377–394.

Gallo, G.R., Caulin-Glaser, T. and Lamm, M.E. (1981) Charge of circulating immune complexes as a factor in glomerular basement membrane localization in mice. *J. Clin. Invest. 67,* 1305–1313.

Gelfand, M.C., Frank, M.M. and Green, I. (1957) A receptor for the third component of complement in the human renal glomerulus. *J. Exp. Med. 142,* 1029–1034.

Germuth, F.G. (1953) A comparative histologic and immunologic study in rabbits of induced hypersensitivity of the serum sickness type. *J. Exp. Med. 97,* 257–282.

Germuth, F.G. and McKinnon, G.E. (1957) Studies on the biological properties of antigen–antibody complex. I. Anaphylactic shock induced by antigen–antibody complex in unsensitized normal guinea pigs. *Bull. Johns Hopk. Hosp. 101,* 13–14.

Germuth, F.G., Jr., Rodriguez, E., Lorelle, C.A., Trump. E.I., Milano, L.L. and Wise, O. (1979) Passive immune complex glomerulonephritis in mice: models for various lesions found in human disease. II. Low avidity complexes and diffuse proliferative glomerulonephritis with subepithelial deposits. *Lab. Invest. 41,* 366–271.

Glasser, R.J., Velosa, J.A. and Michael, A.F. (1977) Experimental model of focal sclerosis. I. Relationship to protein excretion in aminonucleoside nephrosis. *Lab. Invest. 36,* 519–526.

Golbus, S. and Wilson, C.B. (1979) Experimental glomerulonephritis induced by in situ formation of immune complexes in glomerular capillary wall. *Kidney Int. 16,* 148–157.

Grant, M.E., Harwood, R. and Williams, I.F. (1975) The biosynthesis of basement membrane collagen by isolated rat glomeruli. *Eur. J. Biochem. 54,* 531–540.

Gresser, I., Maury, C., Tovey, M., Morel-Maroger, L. and Pontillon, F. (1978) Progressive glomerulonephritis in mice treated with interferon preparations at birth. *Nature (London) 263,* 420–422.

Grond, J. and Elema, J.D. (1981) Glomerular mesangium: analysis of the increased activity observed in experimental acute aminonucleoside nephrosis in the rat. *Lab. Invest. 45,* 400–409.

Haakenstad, A.O., Striker, G.E. and Mannik, M. (1976) The glomerular deposition of soluble immune complexes prepared with reduced and alkylated antibodies and with intact antibodies in mice. *Lab. Invest. 35,* 293–301.

Hawn, C.V. and Janeway, C.A. (1947) Histological and serological sequences in experimental hypersensitivity. *J. Exp. Med. 85,* 571.

Hirsch, E.F., Nakajima, T., Oshima, G., Erdas, F.G. and Herman, C.M. (1974) Kinin system responses in sepsis after trauma in man. *J. Surg. Res. 17,* 147–153.

Holdsworth, S.R., Thomson, N.R., Glasgow, E.F., Dowling, J.P. and Atkins, R.C. (1978) Tissue culture of isolated glomeruli in experimental crescentic glomerulonephritis. *J. Exp. Med. 147,* 98–109.

Holdsworth, S.R., Neale, T.J. and Wilson, C.B. (1980) The participation of macrophages and monocytes in experimental immune complex glomerulonephritis. *Clin. Immunol. Immunopathol. 15,* 510–524.

Holdsworth, S.R., Neale, T.J. and Wilson, C.B. (1981) Abrogation of macrophage-dependent injury in experimental glomerulonephritis in the rabbit. Use of an antimacrophage serum. *J. Clin. Invest. 68,* 686–698.

Horton. E.W. (1979) Prostonoids in health and disease. In: S.M. Roberts and F. Schneinmann (Eds), *Biochemistry and Pharmacological Activity of Prostonoids,* Pergamon Press, New York.

Huang, T.W. (1979) Basal lamina heterogeneity in the glomerular capillary tufts of human kidneys. *J. Exp. Med. 149,* 1450–1459.

Iitaka, K. and West, C.D. (1979) A serum inhibitor of blastogenesis in idiopathic nephrotic syndrome transferred by lymphocytes. *Clin. Immunol. Immunopathol. 12,* 62–71.

Jaffe, E.A., Hoyer, L.W. and Nachman, R.L. (1973) Synthesis of antihemophilic factor antigen by cultured human endothelial cells. *J. Clin. Invest. 52,* 2757–2764.

Jennings, R.B. and Haber, M.H. (1961) Intraglomerular mitosis in rat nephritis: experimental antikidney serum nephritis in the rat. *Arch. Pathol. (Chicago) 71,* 330–335.

Johnson, K.J. and Ward, P.A. (1981) Role of oxygen metabolites in immune complex injury of lung. *J. Immunol. 126,* 2365–2369.

Johnston, W.H. and Latta, H. (1972) Acute focal glomerulonephritis in the rabbit induced by infection of Saccharomyces cerevisiae: an electron microscopic study. *Lab. Invest. 26,* 741.

Kalata, G.B. (1980) Dialysis after nearly a decade. *Science 208,* 473–476.

Kanwar, Y.S. and Farquhar, M. (1979a) Presence of heparin sulfate in the glomerular basement membrane. *Proc. Natl. Acad. Sci. USA 76,* 1303–1307.

Kanwar, Y.S. and Farquhar, M.G. (1979b) Isolation of glycosaminoglycans (heparin sulfate) from glomerular basement membranes. *Proc. Natl. Acad. Sci. USA 76,* 4493–4497.

Keane, W.F. and Rai, L. (1981) Determinants of glomerular mesangial localization of immune complexes: role of endothelial fenestrae. *Lab. Invest. 45,* 366.

Kellermeyer, R.W. and Breckenridge, R.T. (1965) The inflammatory process in gouty arthritis. I. Activation of Hageman factor by sodium urate crystals. *J. Lab. Clin. Med. 65,* 307–315.

Killen, P.D. and Striker, G.E. (1979) Human glomerular visceral epithelial cells synthesize a basal lamina collagen in vitro. *Proc. Natl. Acad. Sci. USA 76,* 3518–3522.

Klebanoff, S.J. (1980) Oxygen metabolism and the toxic properties of phagocytes. *Am. J. Intern. Med. 93,* 480.

Krakauer, R.S., Waldmann, T.A. and Strober, W. (1976) Loss of suppressor T cells in adult NZB/NZW mice. *J. Exp. Med. 144,* 662–673.

Krakauer, K.A., Taney, S.B. and Zurier, R.D. (1978) Prostaglandin E_1 treatment of NZB/W mice. *Clin. Immunol. Immunopathol. 11,* 256–266.

Kreisberg, J.I., Wayne, D.B. and Karnovsky, M.J. (1979) Rapid and focal loss of negative charge associated with mononuclear cell infiltration early in nephrotoxic serum nephritis. *Kidney Int. 16,* 290–300.

Kurtz, S.M. and Feldman, J.D. (1962) Experimental studies on the formation of the glomerular basement membrane. *J. Ultrastruct. Res. 6,* 19–27.

Lange, K. and Treser, G. (1973) Acute poststreptococcal glomerulonephritis, mechanism and sequelae: attempts at a unifying concept. *Clin. Nephrol. 1,* 55–60.

Lavelle, K.J. and Moseman, A.M. (1978) Influence of selective thrombocytopenia on immune-complex glomerulonephritis. *J. Lab. Clin. Med. 92,* 737–749.

Lewis, J.P. (1977) Prostaglandins in inflammation. *J.Reticuloendothel. Soc. 22,* 389–402.

Linder, E., Miettinen, A. and Tornroth, T. (1980) Fibronectin as a marker for the glomerular mesangium in immunohistology of renal biopsies. *Lab. Invest. 42,* 70–75.

Madaio, M.P., Salant, D.J., Couser, W.G., Darby, C. and Capparell, N. (1981a) Influence of antibody charge and concentration on sub-epithelial immune deposit formation (Abstract). *Kidney Int. 19,* 186.

Madaio, M.P., Salant, D.J., Stilmant, M.M., Darby, C., Capparell, N. and Couser, W.G. (1981b) A comparative study of subepithelial immune deposit (SID) formation in active (AICN) and passive (PHN) Heymann nephritis (Abstract). *Kidney Int. 19,* 186.

Mannik, M. and Haakenstad, A.O. (1980) Circulation and glomerular deposits of immune complexes. *Arthritis Rheum. 20,* S148–S157.

Mannik, M. and Striker, G.E. (1980) Removal of glomerular deposits of immune complexes in mice by administration of excess antigen. *Lab. Invest. 42,* 483–489.

Matre, R., Tonder, O. and Wesenberg, F. (1980) Human renal glomeruli possess no Fcγ receptors. *Clin. Immunol. Immunopathol. 17,* 157–162.

Mauer, S.M., Fish, A.J., Blau, E.B. and Michael, A.F. (1972) The glomerular mesangium. I. Kinetic studies of macromolecular uptake in normal and nephrotic rats. *J. Clin. Invest. 51,* 1092–1101.

McCausland, I.P., Herdson, P.B. and Gavin, J.B. (1976a) Experimental autoimmune glomerulonephritis in the rat. I. Factors influencing induction. *Pathology. 8,* 109–115.

McCausland, I.P., Seelye, R.M., Gavin, J.B. and Herdson, P.B. (1976b) The electron microscopic localization of nephrotoxic antibodies in isolated glomeruli. *Pathology 8,* 73–80.

McCluskey, R.T. and Leher, P.D. (1974) An evaluation of immunologic mechanisms. In: F. Ingelfinger, R.V. Ebert, M. Finland and A.S. Relman (Eds), *Controversy in Internal Medicine, Vol. 2,* W.B. Saunders Co., Philadelphia.

McCluskey, R.T., Benacerraf, B., Patter, J.L. and Miller, F. (1960) The pathologic effects of intravenously administered soluble antigen–antibody complexes. I. Passive serum sickness in mice. *J. Exp. Med. 111,* 181–194.

McCluskey, R.T., Hall, C.L. and Calvin, R.B. (1978) Immune complex mediated diseases. *Hum. Pathol. 9,* 71–84.

McLeish, K.R., Gohara, A.F., Gunning, W.T. and Senitezer, D. (1980) Prostaglandin E_1 therapy of murine chronic serum sickness. *J. Lab. Clin. Med. 96,* 470–479.

Melcion, C., Killen, P.D., Morel-Maroger, L., Farin, F.M. and Striker, G.S. (1982) Synthesis of matrix constituents by cells derived from the renal interstitium (in preparation).

Michael, A.F., Fish, A.J. and Good, R.A. (1976) Glomerular localization and transport of aggregated protein in mice. *Lab. Invest. 17,* 14–29.

Michael, A.F., Keane, W.F., Raiz, L., Vernier, R.L. and Mauer, S.M. (1980) The glomerular mesangium. *Kidney Int. 17,* 141–154.

Moarthy, A.V., Zimmerman, S.W. and Burkholder, P.M. (1976) Inhibition of lymphocyte blastogenesis by plasma of patients with minimal change nephrotic syndrome. *Lancet 1,* 1160–1162.

Mohos, S.C. and Skoza, L. (1969) Glomerular sialoprotein. *Science 164,* 1519–1521.

Monga, G., Mazzucco, G., De Belgiojoso, G.B. and Bosnach, G. (1981) Monocyte infiltration and glomerular hypercellularity in human acute and persistent glomerulonephritis. *Lab. Invest. 44,* 381–387.

Morel-Maroger, L., Sloper, J.C., Vinter, J., Woodrow, D. and Bresser, I. (1979) An ultrastructural study of the development of nephritis in mice treated with interferon in the neonatal period. *Lab. Invest. 39,* 513–522.

Morita, T., Kihara, I., Oite, T. and Yamaoto, T. (1976) Participation of blood borne cells in rat Masugi nephritis. *Acta Pathol. Jpn. 26,* 409–422.

Müller-Eberhard, H.J. (1974) The complement system and nephritis. In: *Advances in Nephrology, Vol. 4,* Year Book Medical Publishers, The Hague, pp. 3–15.

Nathan, C.F., Brukner, L., Silverstein, S.C. and Cohn, Z.A. (1979) Extracellular cytolysis of activated macrophages and granulocytes. *J. Exp. Med. 149,* 100–113.

Ooi, Y.M., Ooi, B.S. and Pollak, V.E. (1977) Relationship of levels of circulating immune complexes to histologic patterns of nephritis: a comparative study of membranous glomerulonephropathy and diffuse proliferative glomerulonephritis. *J. Lab. Clin. Med. 90,* 891–898.

Palestro, G., Mazzucco, G., Navone, R., Canese, M.G., Coda, R., Navero, D., Micra, F.B. and Leonardo, E. (1980) Role of the T-cell system in glomerulonephritis induced in rats by human serum albumin (HSA). *Virchows Arch. B 35,* 19–32.

Pussell, B.A., Lockwood, C.M., Scott, D.M., Pinching, A.J. and Peters, D.K. (1978) Value of immune-complex assays in diagnosis and management. *Lancet 2,* 359–364.

Robbins, S.L. and Cotran, R.S. (1979) *Pathologic Basis of Disease, 2nd edn.,* pp. 1115–1185. W.B. Saunders Company, Philadelphia.

Rudofsky, U.H. (1981) Murine lupus nephritis is accelerated by anti-glomerular basement membrane autoantibodies. *Clin. Exp. Immunol. 44,* 18–23.

Ryan, U.S., Schultz, D.R. and Ryan, J.W. (1981) Fc and C3b receptors on pulmonary endothelial cells: induction by injury. *Science 214,* 557–558.

Sage, H., Pritzl, P. and Bornstein, P. (1980) A unique, pepsin-sensitive collagen synthesized by aortic endothelial cells in culture. *Biochemistry 19,* 5747–5755.

Sakaguchi, H. and Kawamura, S. (1963) Electron microscopic observations of the mesangiolysis — the toxic effects of the "Habu Snake" venom on the renal glomerulus. *Keio J. Med. 12,* 99–112.

Salant, D.J., Belok, S., Stilmant, M.M., Darby, C. and Couser, W.G. (1979) Determinants of glomerular localization of subepithelial immune deposits: effects of altered antigen:antibody ratio, steroids, vasoactive amine antagonists and aminonucleoside of puromycin on passive Heymann nephritis in rats. *Lab. Invest. 41,* 89–99.

Salant, D.J., Belok, S., Madaio, M.P. and Couser, W.G. (1980a) A new role for complement in experimental membranous nephropathy in rats. *J. Clin. Invest. 66,* 1339–1350.

Salant, D.J., Darby, C. and Couser, W.G. (1980b) Experimental membranous glomerulonephritis in rats: quantitative studies of glomerular immune deposit formation in isolated glomeruli and whole animals. *J. Clin. Invest. 66,* 71–81.

Sano, M. (1976) Participation of monocytes in glomerulonephritis in acute serum sickness of rabbit. *Acta Pathol. Jpn. 26,* 423–433.

Schreiner, G.F., Cotran, R.S., Pardo, V. and Unanue E.R. (1978) A mononuclear cell component in experimental immunologic glomerulonephritis. *J. Exp. Med. 147,* 369–384.

Schreiner, G.F., Kiely, J.M., Cotran, R.S. and Unanue, E.R. (1981) Characterization of resident glomerular cells in the rat expressing Ia determinants and manifesting genetically restricted interactions with lymphocytes. *J. Clin. Invest. 68,* 920–931.

Shigematsu, H. (1970) Glomerular events during the initial phase of rat Masugi nephritis. *Virchows. Arch. B 5,* 187–200.

Shigematsu, H. and Kobayashi, Y. (1976) Accelerated serum sickness in the rabbit. II. Glomerular ultrastructural lesions in transient proliferative and progressive disorganizing glomerulonephritis. *Virchows Arch. Pathol. Anat. Physiol. 369,* 269–282.

Shigematsu, H., Dikman, S.H., Churg, J., Grishman, E. and Duffy, J.L. (1976) Mesangial involvement in hemolytic-uremic syndrome. *Am. J. Pathol. 85,* 349.

Sindrey, M., Marshall, T.L. and Naish, P. (1979) Quantitative assessment of the effects of platelet depletion in the autologous phase of nephrotoxic serum nephritis. *Clin. Exp. Immunol. 36,* 90–96.

Sraer, J., Sraer, J.D., Momlonguet, L., Siess, W. and Ardaillou, R. (1981) Prostaglandins: synthesis by glomeruli isolated from rats with glycerol-induced acute renal failure (Abstract). *Kidney Int. 19,* 215.

Striker, G.E. and Smuckler, E.A. (1970) An ultrastructural study of glomerular basement membrane (GBM) synthesis. *Am. J. Pathol. 58,* 531–555.

Striker, G.E., Nagle, R., Kohnen, P. and Smuckler, E.A. (1969) Response to unilateral nephrectomy in old rats. *Arch. Pathol. 87,* 439–442.

Striker, G.E., Mannik, M. and Tung, M.Y. (1979) Role of marrow derived monocytes and mesangial cells in removal of immune complexes from renal glomeruli. *J. Exp. Med. 149,* 127–136.

Striker, G.E., Harlan, J.M. and Schwartz, S.M. (1980a) Human endothelial cells in vitro. *Methods Cell Biol. 21,* 135–151.

Striker, G.E., Killen, P.D. and Farin, F.M. (1980b) Human glomerular cells in vitro, isolation and characterization. *Transplant. Proc. 12,* 88–99.

Strunk, S.E., Hammond, W.S. and Benditt, E.P. (1964) The resolution of acute glomerulonephritis: an electron microscopic study of four sequential biopsies. *Lab. Invest. 13,* 401.

Taube, D., Brawn, Z. and Williams, D.G. (1981) Long-term impairment of suppressor–cell function by cyclophosphamide in minimal change nephropathy and its association with therapeutic response. *Lancet 1,* 235–238.

Thomson, N.M., Holdsworth, S.R., Glasgow, E.F. and Atkins, R.C. (1979) The macrophage in the development of experimental crescentic glomerulonephritis: studies using tissue culture and electron microscopy. *Am. J. Pathol. 94,* 223–240.

Toki, N., Sumi, H. and Takasugi, S. (1981) Purification and characterization of kallikrein from plasma of patients with acute pancreatitis. *Clin. Sci. 60,* 199–205.

Tung, K.S.K., Woodroffe, A.J., Ahlin, T.D., William, R.C., Jr. and Wilson, C.B. (1978))

Application of the solid phase CIQ and Raji cell radioimmune assays for the detection of circulating immune complexes in glomerulonephritis. *J. Clin. Invest. 62,* 61–72.

Unanue, E.R., Schreiner, G.F. and Cotran, R.S. (1978) The role of mononuclear phagocytes in immunologically induced glomerulonephritis. In: A. Michael and N. Cummings (Eds), *Immune Mechanisms in Renal Disease,* Plenum Press, New York, in press.

Van Damme, B.J.C., Fleuren, G.J., Bakker, W.W., Vernier, R.L. and Hoedemaeker, P.J. (1978) Experimental glomerulonephritis in the rat induced by antibodies directed against tubular antigens. V. Fixed glomerular antigens in the pathogenesis of heterologous immune complex glomerulonephritis. *Lab. Invest. 38,* 502–510.

Van de Run, I., Fillh, H., Brandeis, W.E., Reid, H., Poon-King, T., McCarthy, M., Day, N.K. and Zabriskie, J.B. (1978) Serial studies on circulating immune complexes in post-streptococcal sequelae. *Clin. Exp. Immunol. 34,* 318–325.

Van Es, L.A., Blok, A.P.R., Schoenfeld and Glassock, R.J. (1977) Chronic nephritis induced by antibodies reacting with glomerular bound immune complexes. *Kidney Int. 11,* 106–115.

Vassali, P., Simon, G. and Roullier, G. (1963) Electron microscopic study of glomerular lesions resulting from intravascular fibrin formation. *Am. J. Pathol. 43,* 579.

Ward, P.A. and Hill, J.H. (1970) C5 chemotactic fragments produced by an enzyme in lysosomal granules of neutrophils. *J. Immunol. 104,* 535–543.

Wiggins, R.C. and Cochrane, C.G. (1982) Kinins and kinin-forming systems. In: M.M. Dale and J.C. Fareman (Eds), *Immunopharmacology, A Basic Course on the Pharmacology of Inflammation and the Immune Response,* Blackwell Scientific Publications, in press.

Williams, D.G. (1981) New ideas in the pathogenesis of nephritis. *J. Clin. Pathol. 34,* 1223–1227.

William, T.J. (1977) Edema and vasodilatation in inflammation: the relevance of prostaglandins. *Postgrad. Med. J. 53,* 660.

Wilson, C.B. (1977) Recent advances in the immunological aspects of renal disease. *Fed. Proc. 36,* 2171–2175.

Wilson, C.B. (1979) Immunopathology of anti-basement membrane antibodies. In: S. Cohen, P.A. Ward and R.T. McCluskey (Eds), *Mechanisms of Immunopathology,* John Wiley and Sons, New York.

Wilson, C.B. and Dixon, F.J. (1979a) Renal injury from immune reaction involving antigens in or of the kidney. In: C.B. Wilson, B.M. Brenner and J.H. Stein (Eds), *Contemporary Issues in Nephrology, Vol. 3,* Churchill-Livingston, New York, pp. 35–66.

Wilson, C.B. and Dixon, F.J. (1979b) Immunological mechanisms in nephritogenesis. *Hosp. Pract. 14,* 54–69.

Zager, R.A., Couser, W.G., Andrews, B.S., Bolton, W.K. and Pohl, M.A. (1979) Membranous nephropathy: a radioimmunologic search for antirenal tubular epithelial antibodies and circulating immune complexes. *Nephron 24,* 10–16.

Zimmerman, S.W. (1979) Characterization of chronic N,N^{1}-diacetylbenzidine-induced nephropathy. *Am. J. Pathol. 94,* 285–300.

CHAPTER 2

Oxygen as a weapon in the phagocyte armamentarium

STEPHEN J. WEISS
University of Michigan, Simpson Research Institute, Ann Arbor, Michigan 48109

2.1. INTRODUCTION

Phagocytic leukocytes are mobile arsenals capable of seeking and destroying a wide variety of biological targets. Recent insights into the mechanisms of phagocyte-mediated destruction have derived from the observation that these cells can consume and metabolize oxygen to generate an impressive array of reactive oxygen intermediates. The role of oxygen metabolites in antimicrobial defense mechanisms has been the subject of intensive study but only recently has attention focused on the potential import of oxygen in phagocyte—mammalian cell interactions. In this review we will examine evidence obtained in a variety of in-vitro model systems demonstrating the ability of intact phagocytes to generate oxygen metabolites capable of destroying normal or neoplastic tissue, altering cellular function and modulating inflammation. A basic understanding of the biochemistry of phagocyte-mediated oxygen dependent events should allow us to elucidate and potentially modulate immunologic defenses against neoplastic invasion, the destruction of normal tissue in pathogenic states and the course of the inflammatory response. The role of phagocyte-derived oxygen metabolites in microbicidal activity will not be the subject of this report and the reader is directed to several comprehensive reviews (Klebanoff and Clark 1978; Babior 1978; Johnston 1978; Root and Cohen 1981).

2.2. OXYGEN METABOLITES GENERATED BY PHAGOCYTES AND THEIR CHARACTERISTICS

Following specific membrane perturbation by either soluble or particulate stimuli, phagocytic leukocytes begin to discharge lysosomal components and exhibit a burst in oxygen consumption (termed the respiratory burst) coincident with the generation of reactive oxygen metabolites (for recent reviews see Roos 1980; Badwey and Karnovsky 1980). The primary species generated are the univalent and divalent reduction products of oxygen, superoxide and hydrogen peroxide. These species can then play a role in the generation of additional and more reactive oxidants including the hydroxyl radical and halide oxidation products. In this section we will briefly discuss only those oxygen metabolites implicated in the injury or modulation of cell function and inflammation. Due to the extensive literature in this area the reader will be referred to general reviews whenever possible.

2.2.1. *Superoxide*

After the phagocyte has been exposed to the appropriate stimulus, a reduced pyridine nucleotide oxidase capable of utilizing NADH or NADPH is activated and begins to shuttle electrons from the appropriate electron donor to oxygen (Roos 1980; Badwey and Karnovsky 1980). Although the characteristics and localization of the oxidase are controversial, it appears that the enzyme is membrane-bound and comprises a mini-electron transport chain with a flavoprotein, a b-cytochrome and perhaps a quinone. The reduced pyridine nucleotides can donate two electrons via the oxidase to two molecules of oxygen to form two molecules of superoxide ($O_2^{\cdot -}$).

$$2O_2 + \text{NAD(P)H} \xrightarrow[\text{oxidase}]{\text{NAD(P)H}} 2O_2^{-} + \text{NADP}^+ + H^+$$

Thus, $O_2^{\cdot -}$ is an oxygen molecule that contains one extra, unpaired electron. This extra electron gives $O_2^{\cdot -}$ a net negative charge (12 protons, 13 electrons) and the fact that the extra electron is unpaired characterizes the species as a free radical. $O_2^{\cdot -}$ can be protonated to form $HO_2^{\cdot}$, the perhydroxyl radical (13 protons, 13 electrons), but the pK_a is 4.8 and only $\sim$1% will exist in this form at neutral pH (for an introduction to the biology of oxygen and its products see Fridovich 1976, 1978).

Although there are a number of comprehensive reviews dealing with the chemistry of superoxide (Fee and Valentine 1977; Valentine 1979; Sawyer and Gibian 1979), some of its biological characteristics should be noted. Based on the general reactivity of free radicals, $O_2^{\cdot -}$ was initially considered a likely mediator of phagocyte-dependent cytotoxicity but it is now clear that its reactivity in aqueous media is restricted. $O_2^{\cdot -}$ may act as a reducing agent, an oxidizing agent, a ligand, base or nucleophile but its ability to participate in these reactions is strongly solvent-dependent (see reviews). In an aqueous medium the reactivity of $O_2^{\cdot -}$ is in part dictated by its rapid dismutation reaction wherein:

$$O_2^{\cdot -} + O_2^{\cdot -} + 2H^+ \longrightarrow H_2O_2 + O_2$$

Thus, in order for $O_2^{\cdot -}$ to react with a given material, the rate of this reaction must be competitive with the rate of dismutation. The rate of interaction between two $O_2^{\cdot -}$ molecules to form H_2O_2 is a function of the availability of protons, i.e., pH. The fastest rate of spontaneous dismutation occurs at a pH of 4.8 where the $O_2^{\cdot -}$ and $HO_2^{\cdot}$ concentrations are equal.

$$O_2^{\cdot -} + HO_2^{\cdot} \longrightarrow H_2O_2 + O_2 \qquad k = 8.5 \times 10^7 \text{ mol l}^{-1} \text{ s}^{-1}$$

At neutral pH, the rate constant is decreased by a factor of 200 ($k = 4.5 \times 10^5$ mol l^{-1} s^{-1}) which might allow $O_2^{\cdot -}$ to diffuse considerable distances away from its site of generation. At very high pH's, or in an aprotic solvent, the rate constant is < 0.5 mol l^{-1} s^{-1} and solutions containing $O_2^{\cdot -}$ can be stored for weeks.

The dismutation of $O_2^{\cdot -}$ can also be enzymatically catalyzed by superoxide dismutases, a family of metallo-enzymes that may contain copper-zinc, iron or manganese (Fridovich 1976). The rate constant for the copper-zinc enzyme catalyzed reactions is 1.9×10^9 mol l^{-1} s^{-1} over a wide pH range (5.0−9.5) and seems to be limited by rates of diffusion alone. Thus, superoxide dismutase would be particularly effective in lowering the steady-state concentrations of $O_2^{\cdot -}$ at neutral or alkaline pH's.

In aqueous systems the predominant reactivity of $O_2^{\cdot -}$ capable of competing with the dismutation reaction is that of a reductant or a ligand and, in a few circumstances, as an oxidant (Fee and Valentine 1977; Valentine 1979). $O_2^{\cdot -}$ can donate an electron to a variety of organic compounds and inorganic transition metal ions. Nitroblue tetrazolium and cytochrome c are examples of electron acceptors employed in quantitating $O_2^{\cdot -}$ generation by phagocytes. As a ligand, $O_2^{\cdot -}$ can form complexes with metal ions that are not easily reduced such as Ca^{2+}, Zn^{2+} or Ba^{2+}. The reactivity of these complexes in biological systems remains to be established. $O_2^{\cdot -}$-mediated oxidations are energetically favorable only when protons are available. In the absence of a proton the addition of one electron to $O_2^{\cdot -}$ would result in the formation of a highly unstable peroxide dianion (O_2^{-2}). Apparently a proton requirement would stabilize the dianion as HO_2^- (hydrogen peroxide anion). Despite the oxidizing potential of $O_2^{\cdot -}$ there are few well-documented examples of $O_2^{\cdot -}$ acting as an oxidant. $O_2^{\cdot -}$ can directly oxidize ascorbate, hydroquinones, transition metal complexes (Fee and Valentine 1977; Valentine 1979), and possibly tocopherol (Nishikimi et al. 1980), pamoate (Hassan et al. 1980), the 1,2-dihydroxy-ethylthiamine pyrophosphate intermediate of the transketolase reaction (Takabe et al. 1980), and tetrapyrroles (Robertson and Fridovich 1982). In an interesting example of the influence of the microenvironment in determining rates of reactivity, Bielski and Chan (1976) demonstrated that $O_2^{\cdot -}$ did not react at significant rates with free NADH but rapidly oxidized NADH bound to lactate dehydrogenase. It should be noted that the perhydroxyl radical ($HO_2^{\cdot}$, the protonated form of $O_2^{\cdot -}$) is a much stronger oxidant than $O_2^{\cdot -}$ (Sawyer and Gibian 1979; Bielski and Shiue 1979) and may be found in substantial concentrations within the acidic environment of the phagocytic vacuole. Thus, despite the limited reactivity of $O_2^{\cdot -}$, its ability to reduce or oxidize transition metal ion complexes, to form ligands with metals, to oxidize organic substrates and to be protonated to $HO_2^{\cdot}$, could allow this species to play an important role in phagocyte-mediated cytotoxicity.

2.2.2. *Hydrogen peroxide*

Stoichiometric analysis of $O_2^{\cdot -}$ and H_2O_2 generation by human neutrophils ingesting opsonized bacteria revealed that ~80% of the H_2O_2 generated arises from the dismutation of $O_2^{\cdot -}$ (Root and Metcalf 1977). Similar results have been obtained with cells exposed to other ingestable (Weening et al. 1975) as well as soluble stimuli (Cohen et al. 1980). However, the ability of a cell to generate $O_2^{\cdot -}$ may not indicate its ability to form H_2O_2. Nathan et al. (1979a) have reported that the macrophage cell line J774 did not generate detectable quantities of H_2O_2 despite its ability to form $O_2^{\cdot -}$. In this system the fate of the generated $O_2^{\cdot -}$ is unknown.

Although phagocytes may generate H_2O_2 via the dismutation of $O_2^{\cdot -}$, the ability of cell's oxidase to release H_2O_2 directly remains undetermined. Certain enzymes (e.g., glucose oxidase) can apparently reduce oxygen to H_2O_2 by a two-electron pathway (see Fridovich 1976). It is conceivable that under the appropriate conditions phagocytes could generate H_2O_2 without a demonstrable $O_2^{\cdot -}$ intermediate.

H_2O_2 can exist as an anion (HO_2^-) but the pK_a is high so that almost all of the molecule exists as H_2O_2 under physiological conditions. H_2O_2 is a strong oxidant but its reactions with organic substances are slow (Fee and Valentine 1977). In contrast, H_2O_2 reacts with transition metal ions and their complexes at rapid rates to form highly reactive oxygen metabolites (Fee and Valentine 1977; and see Section 2.2.4.). Many H_2O_2-mediated reactions may be dependent on the formation of reactive oxygen intermediates initiated by homolytic cleavage of the O—O bond by transition metals.

2.2.3. *Hydrogen peroxide-peroxidase-halide derived oxidants*

Neutrophils and monocytes from a variety of species contain a heme-enzyme in the primary lysosomal granules known as myeloperoxidase (for recent reviews and specific references for this section see Klebanoff and Clark 1978; Root and Cohen 1981; Roos 1980; Klebanoff 1980a). Phagocytes exposed to a variety of stimuli discharge granules containing myeloperoxidase into the phagocytic vacuole or into the extracellular millieu. In the presence of H_2O_2, myeloperoxidase can catalyze the oxidation of the halides, chloride (Cl^-), iodide (I^-) or bromide (Br^-) but not fluoride. In this reaction, myeloperoxidase effectively transfers two electrons from the halide (the electron donor) to H_2O_2 (the electron acceptor) to generate an oxidized halide.

$$H_2O_2 + \underset{(Cl^-,\ I^-,\ Br^-)}{X^-} \xrightarrow[H^+]{\text{myeloperoxidase}} HOX + H_2O$$

The pH optimum of the myeloperoxidase system is approximately 4.5–5.0 but can be regulated by both the H_2O_2 and halide concentrations. Thus, under the appropriate experimental conditions, the enzyme may function over a much wider pH range. The halide employed by the myeloperoxidase system in vivo is unknown, however Cl^- is present at much higher concentrations than either I^- or Br^-. It should be noted that phagocytes can deiodinate thyroid hormones and may be able to concentrate I^-. In addition, Br^- is found in the blood at concentrations that may be sufficient for utilization by the peroxidase (Ramsey et al. 1982). Thus, the phagocyte could have a pool of halides for its use, depending on the characteristics of the particular environment.

Eosinophils also contain a granule associated peroxidase that functions similarly to myeloperoxidase but the eosinophil peroxidase has a different primary structure and heme group. In addition, its ability to oxidize the various halides, particularly Cl^-, may differ from that of myeloperoxidase. Recently, a peroxidase has been described associated with mast cell granules and appears functionally similar to the eosinophil peroxidase (Henderson and Kaliner 1979).

Although most phagocytes do contain granule-associated peroxidases, there are several noteworthy exceptions, e.g., normal chicken neutrophils (Penniall and Spitznagel 1975) as well as rabbit monocytes (Nichols et al. 1971) lack a granule peroxidase. In addition, human neutrophils and monocytes from individuals with myeloperoxidase deficiency are peroxidase negative while eosinophils remain peroxidase positive. Finally, as blood monocytes mature into macrophages, the granule-associated peroxidase disappears while peroxidase-positive material may appear in the rough endoplasmic reticulum, nuclear envelope and Golgi complex (reviewed in Klebanoff 1980b). This peroxidase does not seem to be discharged following membrane perturbation and its role in cytotoxic reactions is unknown.

Phagocytes ingesting particles or responding to soluble stimuli release sufficient amounts of H_2O_2 and peroxidase to catalyze the halogenation of susceptible target molecules. In vitro, the halide oxidation product generated by a model system consisting of H_2O_2, purified myeloperoxidase and Cl^- has been identified as the powerful oxidant hypochlorous acid (HOCl) (Harrison and Schultz 1976). Although the products of I^- and Br^- oxidations by myelo- or eosinophil peroxidase have not been identified, hypoiodous acid (HOI) and hypobromous acid (HOBr) seem likely candidates.

The hypohalous acids, HOCl, HOI, and HOBr, are weak acids with pK_a's of approximately 7.4, 11.0 and 8.3 (for review see Downs and Adams 1973). Thus, substantial quantities of these species will exist in the unionized form at physiologic pH. These acids and their salts (hypochlorite, hypoiodite, hypobromite) are potent oxidants and can react with a wide variety of biologically important molecules. Indeed, hypochlorite salts are the active ingredients in household cleansing powders and bleach. However, hypohalites are weaker oxidants than their respective acids. Although HOCl is the strongest hypohalous oxidant from a thermodynamic consideration, HOCl and HOBr react with susceptible molecules at much faster rates. From a biological standpoint, the reactivity of the hypohalous acids has been most carefully examined with HOCl. This oxidant reacts rapidly with amines, amino acids, sulfhydryl compounds, thioethers, aromatics and other unsaturated carbon groups (Klebanoff and Clark 1978; Downs and Adams 1973; Held and Hurst 1978; Harrison et al. 1978; Albrich et al. 1981). HOCl may also be able to react with other oxygen metabolites generated by the phagocyte to produce new reactive intermediates. Of potential interest is the ability of $O_2^{\cdot -}$ to react with HOCl to form an extremely powerful oxidant, the hydroxyl radical (OH·) (Long and Bielski 1980).

$$O_2^{\cdot -} + HOCl \longrightarrow OH\cdot + Cl^- + O_2$$

Although OCl^- can react with H_2O_2 to form singlet oxygen ($^1O_2$), an activated form of oxygen with increased chemical reactivity, there is no clear evidence supporting the formation of this product by the phagocyte (Foote 1979).

2.2.4. Hydroxyl radical

The ability of phagocytes to generate the hydroxyl radical (OH·) and the mechanisms involved remain unclear. The OH· is an extremely powerful oxidant capable of interacting with a host of organic and inorganic molecules at diffusion controlled rates (Willson 1979). Interest in the ability of phagocytes to generate this species stemmed from the observation that xanthine and xanthine oxidase, an enzyme capable of generating $O_2^{\cdot -}$ and H_2O_2, could oxidize the thioether methional with ethylene gas as a quantitatable end product (Beauchamp and Fridovich 1970; Diguiseppi and Fridovich 1980). Beauchamp and Fridovich (1970) demonstrated that neither $O_2^{\cdot -}$ nor H_2O_2 alone could oxidize the thioether and suggested that the two species interacted via the Haber-Weiss reaction to form OH·.

$$O_2^{\cdot -} + H_2O_2 \longrightarrow OH\cdot + OH^- + O_2 \qquad \text{Haber-Weiss reaction}$$

A role for OH· was based on the ability of OH· scavengers, compounds known to react rapidly with OH·, to inhibit ethylene generation. This observation unleashed a flood of reports describing the formation of the OH· or an OH·-like oxidant in cell-free systems generating both $O_2^{\cdot -}$ and H_2O_2 (for review see Willson 1979; Cohen 1977; Halliwell 1981). Subsequently, it became clear that the Haber-Weiss reaction, although energetically favorable, occurred at very slow rates. In order to resolve this apparent conflict it was postulated and demonstrated that iron salts and their complexes could effectively catalyze an interaction between $O_2^{\cdot -}$ and H_2O_2 (see Halliwell 1981).

$$O_2^{\cdot -} + M^{n+} \longrightarrow O_2 + M^{(n-1)+}$$

$$M^{(n-1)+} + H_2O_2 \longrightarrow Mn^{+} + OH\cdot + OH^{-}$$

Thus, $O_2^{\cdot -}$ acts to reduce the transition metal ion and H_2O_2 then interacts with the reduced metal ions in a Fenton reaction to form the OH· or a species with similar reactivity. Because $O_2^{\cdot -}$ is acting only as a reducing agent it may be replaced by other compounds capable of reducing the metal, e.g., ascorbic acid (see review by Halliwell 1981). Nonetheless, there are numerous examples of $O_2^{\cdot -}$, H_2O_2 and various transition metal chelates interacting to form an oxidant with OH·-like characteristics. Attempts to identify a potential biological metal chelator capable of catalyzing a similar reaction in vivo have yielded conflicting results. In almost all systems iron plus EDTA is an effective catalyst while iron chelated to other small molecular weight compounds or large proteins (e.g., transferrin, lactoferrin, etc.) may or may not function effectively depending on assay conditions employed (see reviews and for recent studies with extensive bibliographies Diguiseppi and Fridovich 1980; Ambruso and Johnston 1981; Rosen and Klebanoff 1981; Samuni et al. 1981). Despite these contradictions, it seems clear that in the presence of $O_2^{\cdot -}$, H_2O_2 and a properly coordinated transition metal a powerful oxidant with characteristics similar to, if not identical with, OH· is generated.

Attempts to chemically detect OH· generation by intact phagocytes have primarily depended on quantitating the ability of the cell to oxidize a variety of exogenous compounds including thioethers (Weiss et al. 1977; Tauber and Babior 1977; Weiss et al. 1978), dimethylsulfoxide (Repine et al. 1979), and benzoate (Sagone et al. 1980). The formation of the oxidized product should be quantitable, insensitive to $O_2^{\cdot -}$ or H_2O_2 alone, and inhibitable by compounds known to scavenge OH·. Polymorphonuclear leukocytes (primarily neutrophils and eosinophils) and monocytes appear to be able to oxidize thioethers but the mechanism is complicated by a potential requirement for myeloperoxidase. Klebanoff and Rosen (1978) demonstrated that a model H_2O_2-myeloperoxidase-Cl^- system could oxidize thioethers but EDTA-stimulated activity and the reaction mechanism seemed to be dependent on both H_2O_2 and $O_2^{\cdot -}$. A myeloperoxidase-mediated reaction dependent on EDTA and $O_2^{\cdot -}$ is unusual and serves to highlight the complex mechanisms involved in phagocyte-mediated thioether oxidations. In a similar light the role of OH· in the oxidation of dimethysulfoxide or benzoate by polymorphonuclear leukocytes must be interpreted cautiously since myeloperoxidase inhibitors blocked these reactions (Repine et al. 1979; Sagone et al. 1980). It should be noted, however, that peroxidase-negative, animal (Drath et al. 1979), and human macrophages (Hoidal et al. 1979) can oxidize thioethers or dimethylsulfoxide by a mechanism dependent on $O_2^{\cdot -}$ and H_2O_2 and inhibitable by OH· scavengers.

An additional and potentially more specific technique to detect OH· generation by phagocytes utilized the ability of OH· to react with 5,5'-dimethyl-1-pyrroline-N-oxide (DMPO) to form a semi-stable free radical adduct (Green et al. 1979; Rosen and Klebanoff 1979). The product can then accumulate and be identified by its characteristic electron spin resonance spectrum. Stimulated neutrophils generated the OH· adduct of DMPO by a mechanism dependent on $O_2^{\cdot -}$ and independent of myeloperoxidase. Interestingly, attempts to demonstrate a role for H_2O_2 were unsuccessful in both studies. The addition of the OH· scavenger mannitol decreased the formation of the DMPO adduct (Green et al. 1979; Rosen and Klebanoff 1979), however, another OH· scavenger ethanol had no effect (Green et al. 1979). Indeed, the addition of ethanol to a OH·-forming system should result in the formation of an α-hydroxyethyl radical ($CH_3\mathring{C}HOH$) which can then react with DMPO to form a new spectrum (Finkelstein et al. 1980). Although the ability of the phagocyte to generate OH· requires further study, it is clear from these experiments that the cell can generate a powerful oxidant(s) by a myeloperoxidase-independent mechanism.

In summary, the phagocyte can engage in combat by unleashing an almost bewildering array of oxygen-derived metabolites. Target molecules can be exposed to $O_2^{\cdot -}$, $HO_2^{\cdot}$, H_2O_2 and the products of their various interactions, including HOCl, HOI, HOBr and OH·. These species can in turn react with certain target molecules (e.g., unsaturated fatty acids) to initiate the propagation of additional oxidants in complex, interconnected reaction schemes (see, e.g., Mead 1976). In the remainder of this review we will focus on studies designed to demonstrate the ability of the phagocyte to utilize these oxygen metabolites in host defense, host tissue destruction and the modulation of the inflammatory response.

2.3. ROLE OF OXYGEN METABOLITES IN PHAGOCYTE–TARGET CELL INTERACTIONS

The biological reactivity of phagocyte-derived oxygen metabolites has been partially dissected in a number of simple model systems wherein phagocytes (i.e., the effector cell) are coincubated with target cells in the presence of an appropriate stimulus. A variety of stimuli have been used in these model systems but for the purposes of this discussion will be divided into two groups. The first group includes those agents that stimulate the phagocyte in an undirected manner such that all adjacent targets are non-specifically exposed to the released toxins. These innocent bystander-type reactions are triggered by a variety of stimuli including opsonized zymosan particles, latex spherules, plant lectins, the croton oil derivative phorbol myristate acetate (PMA), the activated complement component C5a and endotoxin (Goldstein 1979). In the second group the phagocyte directs its attack specifically against antibody-coated target cells (Henney 1977). Evidence is accumulating demonstrating the ability of phagocyte-derived oxygen metabolites to alter or destroy cellular function with either class of stimulating agent.

2.3.1. Common methods used to identify responsible oxygen metabolites

In order to identify the oxygen metabolites involved in phagocyte–target cells interactions a variety of environmental manipulations, enzymes, inhibitors, oxygen metabolite scavengers and cell populations are employed. Some of the more common techniques used to demonstrate a requirement for O_2, $O_2^{\cdot -}$, H_2O_2, the H_2O_2-peroxidase-halide system and OH· will be discussed along with their potential pitfalls. Again, whenever applicable, the reader is directed to existing comprehensive reviews for further details.

2.3.1.1. Oxygen

A requirement for oxygen in a phagocyte-mediated event can be tested by observing the effect of anaerobic conditions. In the absence of oxygen, phagocytes cannot generate oxygen metabolites but the conditions must be strictly anaerobic since phagocytes are quite effective in extracting small amounts of oxygen from their environment (Gabig et al. 1979). The cells should be directly tested for their ability to generate oxygen metabolites under these conditions and be able to function normally after re-exposure to air. In addition, the effector cells' dependence on aerobic metabolism for maintenance of its energy charge should be established and potential effects of the conditions on the target cell considered. Based on a reported synergistic relationship between oxygen metabolites and prostaglandins (Metzger et al. 1980; and see Section 2.3.2.2. under "H_2O_2 and endothelial cells"), a requirement for oxygen in syntheses catalyzed by cyclo-oxygenase and lipoxygenase cannot be overlooked.

Phagocytes obtained from individuals with classic chronic granulomatous disease (CGD), a rare genetic disorder, are incapable of generating any oxygen metabolites but can release lysosomal components (Klebanoff and Clark 1978; Babior 1978, Root and Cohen 1981; Roos 1980). Thus, CGD cells may provide specific data regarding requirements for intact oxidative metabolism. However, these individuals must be carefully identified because there exist a number of variants of this disease. Phagocytes have been isolated from patients with CGD-like disorders where the cells fail to respond to some but not all stimuli (Weening et al. 1976; Harvath and

Andersen 1979). In other variants the cells generate reduced but potentially significant quantities of the oxygen metabolites (Dilworth and Mandell 1977; Lew et al. 1981). In addition, CGD neutrophils do release myeloperoxidase and if small amounts of H_2O_2 are present, either from auto-oxidizable material in the suspending medium or from the target cell, oxygen-dependent activity may be expressed. Finally, recent data indicate that changes in the vacuolar pH normally associated with phagosome formation may be altered in CGD neutrophils (Van Zwieten et al. 1981; Segal et al. 1981*). Thus, results obtained with CGD phagocytes should be cautiously interpreted.

2.3.1.2. Superoxide

The steady-state concentration of $O_2^{\cdot-}$ can be dramatically lowered by catalyzing its dismutation to H_2O_2 with superoxide dismutase (Fridovich 1976, 1978). Thus, in the presence of superoxide dismutase, the concentration of $O_2^{\cdot-}$ is lowered without decreasing the H_2O_2 concentration. At present, the enzyme is considered specific for $O_2^{\cdot-}$ but other factors bear consideration. Copper-zinc superoxide dismutase can slowly react with H_2O_2 (Hodgson and Fridovich 1975a), can function as a non-specific peroxidase (Hodgson and Fridovich 1975b), is inhibitable by cyanide (Fridovich 1976), and may be inactivated by H_2O_2 (Hodgson and Fridovich 1975a) or a combination of $O_2^{\cdot-}$ and H_2O_2 (Sinet and Garber 1981). If these difficulties are suspected, the manganic form of superoxide dismutase does not catalyze peroxidations (Hodgson and Fridovich 1975b), is insensitive to cyanide (Ravindranath and Fridovich 1975), and is not inactivated by H_2O_2 (Hodgson and Fridovich 1975b; Sinet and Garber 1981). Recent evidence indicates that certain types of reactions may be indirectly inhibited by superoxide dismutase where $O_2^{\cdot-}$ is not a major or significant product. Winterbourn demonstrated that high concentrations of superoxide dismutase inhibited a reaction dependent on semiquinone radicals by displacing its equilibrium with O_2 far to the right (Winterbourn 1981).

$$\text{Semiquinone} + O_2 \rightleftharpoons \text{quinone} + O_2^{\cdot-} \xrightarrow[\text{dismutase}]{\text{Superoxide}}$$

Thus, despite the specificity of superoxide dismutase for $O_2^{\cdot-}$, its effects in complex systems should be interpreted cautiously.

---

*Although Segal et al. (1981) examined possible complicating effects of oxygen metabolites on their pH probes with a hypoxanthine–xanthine oxidase system, the ability of myeloperoxidase to interfere was not tested. For an example of a myeloperoxidase-dependent oxidation of a fluorescent probe, see Whitin et al. 1981.

2.3.1.3. *Hydrogen peroxide*

Catalase is a heme-enzyme that can reduce the H_2O_2 concentration by catalyzing a rapid dismutation reaction (Fridovich 1976). It should be noted that at low H_2O_2 concentrations this enzyme can catalyze a variety of interesting peroxidative reactions.

$$H_2O_2 + H_2O_2 \xrightarrow{\text{catalase}} 2H_2O + O_2$$

For example, although azide is normally considered an inhibitor of catalase, the enzyme can use H_2O_2 to oxidize azide to nitrous oxide, nitric oxide and nitrogen with an associated reduction of the heme iron (Keilin and Hartree 1945, 1955). In addition, Klebanoff has demonstrated that under acidic conditions and, in the presence of low concentrations of H_2O_2, catalase can oxidize I^- to a bactericidal or fungicidal compound (Klebanoff 1969). Catalase is also sensitive to inactivation by $O_2^{\cdot -}$ via the formation of an oxyheme derivative (Odajima and Yamazaki 1972). Again, this information does not preclude the use of catalase in complex systems but rather cautions the interpretation of anomalous results.

H_2O_2 as well as alkyl hydroperoxides can also be reduced by the seleno-enzyme glutathione peroxidase (Fridovich 1976). This enzyme has a much lower K_m for H_2O_2 but requires glutathione as an electron donor and is difficult to purify.

Finally, if H_2O_2 is produced via an $O_2^{\cdot -}$ intermediate, the addition of an agent capable of oxidizing the $O_2^{\cdot -}$ should also block the subsequent production of H_2O_2. Cytochrome c (cyt c) can interact with $O_2^{\cdot -}$ to form the reduced cytochrome and O_2.

$$\underset{Fe^{+++}}{\text{cyt c}} + O_2^{\cdot -} \longrightarrow \underset{Fe^{++}}{\text{cyt c}} + O_2$$

However, the ability of H_2O_2 to react with reduced cyt c does not render this intervention palatable (Roos et al. 1977).

2.3.1.4. *Hydrogen peroxide-peroxidase-halide system*

Effects mediated by this system can be blocked by reducing the H_2O_2 concentration, inhibiting the peroxidase or removing the required halide (Klebanoff and Clark 1978; Klebanoff 1980a). As discussed, the H_2O_2 concentration can be reduced with catalase but sufficient enzyme must be present to compete with the peroxidase. Myeloperoxidase is sensitive to heme-enzyme inhibitors such as azide, cyanide or aminotriazole while eosinophil and mast cell peroxidase seem somewhat more resistant to inhibition by cyanide (Klebanoff 1980a). Finally, if experiments are performed under halide-free conditions, the peroxidase system will not be able to form the respective hypohalous acid. Important considerations regarding these manipulations include the specificity of the peroxidase inhibitors and the effects of halide-free conditions on cell function. For example, azide or cyanide can block oxidative phosphorylation and endogenous catalase in both effector and target cell populations. Inhibition of myeloperoxidase and catalase can also allow the generated H_2O_2 to accumulate to significant concentrations. Halide-free conditions, although commonly used to inhibit peroxidase-mediated reactions, may alter the discharge of lysosomal components (Weissman et al. 1980).

Perhaps the most direct means of demonstrating a myeloperoxidase requirement in a given system is the use of phagocytes isolated from patients with hereditary myeloperoxidase deficiency (Klebanoff and Clark 1978; Roos 1980). Originally considered a rare disorder it appears that the frequency of this deficiency is quite high (Parry et al. 1981). Neutrophils and monocytes from these individuals can generate $O_2^{\cdot -}$ and H_2O_2 but are peroxidase-negative. It should be noted that these cells appear to generate increased amounts of $O_2^{\cdot -}$, H_2O_2 and possibly $OH\cdot$ (Rosen and Klebanoff 1979). Finally, the eosinophil peroxidase content in myeloperoxidase deficiency is normal and contamination of cell preparations with eosinophils could complicate results.

Peroxidase-mediated reactions may also be blocked by attempting to scavenge the end product of the halide oxidation, i.e., the hypohalous acid. The scavenger must react with the oxidant rapidly, the scavenger cannot non-specifically inhibit cellular metabolism, and the product of the interaction should not be a reactive or toxic species. The reactivity and potential toxicity of the products formed when HOCl is scavenged with amines or amino acids is especially relevant. HOCl can react with amines to form chloramines (if the chloramine reacts with a second HOCl a dichloramine is formed) which are also strong oxidizing agents (Downs and Adams 1973). Amino acids and HOCl can also interact to generate chloramines which may oxidize a potential electron donor or undergo oxidative decarboxylation to an aldehyde, carbon dioxide and ammonia (for references see Klebanoff and Clark 1978 or Roos 1980). Thus, the inability of a known scavenger to block a HOCl-mediated reaction does not necessarily rule out a role for HOCl. Perhaps the most important limitation of these scavengers is their lack of specificity for a given oxidant. Any species with an oxidizing potential similar to the hypohalous acid would also be scavenged. Indeed, all compounds used to scavenge $^1O_2$ react rapidly with HOCl (Held and Hurst 1978; Harrison et al. 1978). Therefore, in the remainder of this review $^1O_2$ scavengers will be referred to as $HOCl/^1O_2$ scavengers.

2.3.1.5. Hydroxyl radical

Based on questions concerning the ability of intact phagocytes to generate $OH\cdot$ and the specific reaction mechanisms involved, the criteria for implicating $OH\cdot$ in cell-mediated events are not clear. $OH\cdot$ generation by phagocytes may be inhibitable by superoxide dismutase alone or by either superoxide dismutase and catalase (see

Section 2.2.4.). Unfortunately, a great deal of evidence relies on the effects of non-specific OH· scavengers. As with the hypohalous acid scavengers, the OH· scavengers must react rapidly with OH·, cannot non-specifically depress cellular metabolism, and should not form a powerful oxidant as a result of their interaction with OH·. In addition, special care must be employed in choosing OH· scavengers that do not react with hypohalous acids. To further complicate matters, it is clear that in a variety of model systems where the OH· is the probable final mediator, high concentrations of OH· scavengers remain ineffective (e.g., see Willson 1979; Samuni et al. 1981; Hodgson and Fridovich 1975a; Sinet and Garber 1981; Van Hemmen and Meuling 1977). This seems to be especially true when H_2O_2 reacts with a protein-bound transition metal. Apparently, the formation of OH· in the immediate vicinity of its biological target precludes scavenging. This is an extremely important point not only for the OH· but for all the species discussed. In the presence of a tightly coupled effector—target cell interface, the ability to intercept a given oxygen metabolite, especially with large enzymes, may be severely restricted.

Thus, a brief overview of the techniques and limitations commonly employed to identify the oxygen metabolites involved in cell-mediated events has been provided. Although it would appear that these considerations would impede any effort to dissect oxygen-dependent mechanisms, considerable progress has been made. In the next section we will present evidence supporting roles for $O_2^{\cdot-}$, H_2O_2, the H_2O_2-peroxidase-halide systems and OH· in phagocyte-mediated, innocent bystander-type reactions.

2.3.2. Innocent bystander-type interactions mediated by phagocytes

Phagocytes incubated with either particulate or soluble stimuli will discharge their lysosomal content and generate oxygen metabolites. If a target cells lies adjacent to the stimulated phagocyte it will be non-specifically exposed to all those species that can diffuse from the effector cells to the target cell. Although several of the stimuli used in these studies are not physiological (i.e., would not be encountered in vivo), they provide a convenient technique to trigger the phagocyte. These studies allow us to examine and dissect the cytotoxic potential of the phagocytes' armamentarium. Target cells that have been tested in these models include erythrocytes, platelets, phagocytes, lymphocytes, endothelial cells and tumor cells. In this section the ability of phagocyte-derived oxygen metabolites to alter or destroy target cell function will be examined.

2.3.2.1. Superoxide

A potential role of $O_2^{\cdot-}$ alone in phagocyte-mediated cytotoxicity was first described in a system that examined the ability of lectin-stimulated human neutrophils to destroy chicken erythrocytes. Simchowitz and Schur demonstrated that neutrophils incubated with the lectins, PHA or Con A, rapidly destroyed chicken erythrocyte targets (although sheep and human erythrocytes were considerably more resistant)

(Simchowitz and Schur 1976a, b). In their system cytolysis required cell—cell contact, correlated with agglutination, did not involve erythrophagocytosis and was dependent on anaerobic glycolysis but independent of oxidative phosphorylation. Based on the ability of lectin to stimulate the phagocyte to generate oxygen metabolites, Simchowitz and Spilberg (1979) postulated a potential role for oxygen, $O_2^{\cdot -}$ and/or H_2O_2 in cytolysis. Lectin-stimulated neutrophils incubated under anaerobic conditions failed to generate $O_2^{\cdot -}$ or mediate hemolysis suggesting a critical requirement for oxygen metabolites. In order to determine the role of $O_2^{\cdot -}$ or H_2O_2 in cytotoxicity, experiments were performed in the presence of superoxide dismutase or catalase. At an effector to target cell ratio of 10:1 (10 neutrophils vs 1 erythrocyte), superoxide dismutase partially inhibited cytotoxicity. In contrast, catalase had no protective effect and the authors concluded that H_2O_2 did not play a strong role in their systems. Although the inability of catalase to inhibit hemolysis may be related to its difficulty in gaining access to the neutrophil—erythrocyte interface in the agglutinated mixture, the data suggested that $O_2^{\cdot -}$ might play an important role in their system.

Stronger evidence for $O_2^{\cdot -}$ in phagocyte-mediated destruction was provided by a series of studies (Weiss and LoBuglio 1980; Weiss 1980). Human neutrophils were stimulated with PMA and examined for their ability to destroy erythrocyte targets in a model system similar to that first described by Nathan et al. (1979a) (see Section 2.3.2.2. under "H_2O_2 and tumor cells"). Neutrophils were able to mediate a powerful cytotoxic effect and under optimal conditions each neutrophil could destroy more than 10 erythrocyte targets. Additional studies demonstrated that purified suspensions of human monocytes were able to mediate comparable cytotoxicity (Weiss et al. 1980). Early attempts to determine the mechanism of cytotoxicity revealed that either superoxide dismutase or catalase could inhibit hemolysis (Weiss and LoBuglio 1980; Weiss et al. 1980) but additional studies performed with highly purified catalase or glutathione peroxidase demonstrated that only superoxide dismutase was protective (Weiss 1980). The ability of superoxide dismutase to almost completely protect the erythrocytes indicated that $O_2^{\cdot -}$ played an important role in cytolysis while the product of its dismutation, H_2O_2, did not appear to participate in target cell destruction. A role for $OH\cdot$ or HOCl could not be demonstrated since compounds known to scavenge these oxidants failed to inhibit cytolysis. In confirmatory studies, neutrophils isolated from patients with chronic granulomatous disease did not destroy erythrocyte targets while myeloperoxidase deficient neutrophils lysed erythrocytes comparably to normal cells by a $O_2^{\cdot -}$ dependent mechanism (S.J. Weiss, unpublished observations). Because all these data indicated that $O_2^{\cdot -}$, a chemically unreactive species, was responsible for cytotoxicity, a cooperative interaction between $O_2^{\cdot -}$ and oxyhemoglobin was considered as a potential prerequisite for hemolysis. $O_2^{\cdot -}$ can react with oxyhemoglobin to form methemoglobin and H_2O_2 (Lynch et al. 1976; Sutton et al. 1976) which can then combine to form a peroxide—methemoglobin complex (for references see Weiss 1980) with a strong oxidizing potential. Thus, the following reaction sequence was proposed to occur within the erythrocyte targets:

$$O_2^{\cdot -} + \text{Hgb-Fe}^{++} \cdots O_2 \xrightarrow{2H^+} H_2O_2 + \text{Hgb-Fe}^{+++} + O_2$$

oxyhemoglobin methemoglobin

$$H_2O_2 + \text{Hgb-Fe}^{+++} \longrightarrow \left[\text{Hgb-Fe}^{+++} \cdots H_2O_2\right] \longrightarrow \text{lysis}$$

peroxidative complex

This scheme was supported by 1) the inability of PMA-stimulated neutrophils to destroy erythrocytes after the oxyhemoglobin was derivatized to carbon monoxyhemoglobin, 2) the ability of neutrophils to destroy methemoglobin-rich erythrocytes by a mechanism independent of $O_2^{\cdot -}$ but dependent on H_2O_2, and 3) the marked sensitivity of methemoglobin-rich erythrocytes to hemolysis by H_2O_2 (Weiss 1980). Additional studies demonstrated that $O_2^{\cdot -}$ could traverse the erythrocyte plasma membrane via the anion channels to oxidize intracellular hemoglobin to methemoglobin (Lynch and Fridovich 1978b; Weiss 1982). It appears that $O_2^{\cdot -}$ generated by human neutrophils can mediate cytotoxicity by interacting with a hemoprotein activator within the target cell. It is interesting to note that in the electron spin resonance studies of Rosen and Klebanoff (1979), an oxidant was generated by a mechanism also dependent on $O_2^{\cdot -}$ but not H_2O_2. They postulated that $O_2^{\cdot -}$ might interact with a source of iron to generate an oxidant with characteristics similar to OH· (see Section 2.2.4.). In the erythrocyte model the source of the iron may be hemoglobin but other hemoproteins (in the erythrocyte or phagocyte) cannot be ruled out.

Are there any other examples of $O_2^{\cdot -}$ dependent phagocyte-mediated cytotoxicity? At present we are unaware of any additional reports although erythrocytes have been exposed to oxidant fluxes generated by cell-free model systems. Despite a number of different mechanisms, in two reports erythrocyte (Bartosz et al. 1977) or erythrocyte vesicles (Lynch and Fridovich 1978a) exposed to $O_2^{\cdot -}$ and H_2O_2 were lysed by a mechanism inhibitable by superoxide dismutase but not catalase. In addition, Kellogg et al. (1979) recently demonstrated that bacteria could be destroyed by a negative air ion identified as $O_2^{\cdot -}$. These data support the concept that $O_2^{\cdot -}$ (and possibly $HO_2\cdot$) may be sufficiently reactive to play an important role in phagocyte-mediated extracellular cytotoxicity.

2.3.2.2. Hydrogen peroxide

A large number of studies have implicated H_2O_2 alone as an effective oxidant capable of injuring or altering cell function. Potentially susceptible targets studied include erythrocytes, platelets, phagocytes, lymphocytes, endothelial cells and tumor cells. Much of the early evidence supporting a role for H_2O_2 alone is questionable, i.e., other reactive species dependent on H_2O_2 for their generation were not suspected or considered. These early studies focused on H_2O_2 as a potent oxidant but, with the discovery that phagocytes could generate more reactive species, the toxicity of H_2O_2 was questioned or assumed negligible. Recently, Nathan and co-workers convincingly demonstrated the cytotoxic potential of H_2O_2 alone (see section 2.3.2.2. under "H_2O_2 and tumor cells"), once again resurrecting interest in this oxidant. In this section we will review evidence supporting or demonstrating a role for H_2O_2 phagocyte-mediated events.

H_2O_2 and erythrocytes Perhaps the earliest report demonstrating a role for oxygen metabolites in phagocyte—target cell interactions was a study describing the ability of human polymorphonuclear leukocytes to alter glutathione levels in glucose-6-phosphate dehydrogenase (G6PD)-deficient erythrocytes (Baehner et al. 1971). Normal erythrocytes (along with almost all mammalian cells) are armed with two enzyme systems capable of degrading H_2O_2, catalase and the glutathione peroxidase-reductase system (Aebi and Wyss 1978). Catalase can directly degrade H_2O_2 (H_2O_2 is both the electron donor and electron acceptor) while glutathione peroxidase catalyzes the reduction of H_2O_2 by glutathione (GSH, α-glutamyl-cysteinylglycine):

$$H_2O_2 + H_2O_2 \xrightarrow{\text{catalase}} 2H_2O + O_2$$

$$H_2C_2 + 2GSH \xrightarrow[\text{peroxidase}]{\text{GSH}} 2H_2O + GSSG$$

The oxidized gluthathione (GSSG) is reduced back to GSH by NADPH and glutathione reductase.

$$GSSG + NADPH + H^+ \xrightarrow[\text{reductase}]{\text{GSH}} 2\ GSH + NADP^+$$

Finally, the NADPH is regenerated by the first two enzymatic steps (G6PD and 6-phosphogluconate dehydrogenase) in the hexose monophosphate shunt. Both catalase and the GSH reductase system are important in protecting erythrocytes from oxidant stress; however, the GSH system seems to preferentially reduce low concentrations of H_2O_2 (Cohen and Hochstein 1963; Jacob et al. 1965). In G6PD-deficient erythrocytes insufficient NADPH is available to reduce GSSG. Patients with this disorder may suffer from a hemolytic anemia during infection and Baehner et al. (1971) hypothesized that H_2O_2 generated by phagocytosing leukocytes might injure G6PD-deficient erythrocytes. Indeed, phagocytes ingesting latex spherules generated sufficient H_2O_2 to mediate GSH oxidation in G6PD-deficient but not normal erythrocytes. Although GSH was oxidized there was no methemoglobin or Heinz body (hemoglobin precipitates) formation observed. GSH oxidation in G6PD-deficient erythrocytes was accelerated in the presence of cyanide possibly due to increased H_2O_2 release from the phagocyte (cyanide would inhibit myeloperoxidase and catalase) and/or a further decline in the ability of the erythrocyte to degrade the H_2O_2 (cyanide would also block catalase in the erythrocyte). As expected, chronic granulomatous disease phagocytes did not oxidize GSH in the G6PD-deficient erythrocytes. Finally, G6PD-deficient erythrocytes exposed to a flux of enzymatically generated H_2O_2 had a decreased survival in vivo. The authors concluded that H_2O_2 could oxidize GSH in G6PD-deficient erythrocytes and may alter the cell such that in vivo survival is shortened. Recent studies have demonstrated that human neutrophils stimulated with PMA (a stronger stimulus for oxygen metabolite generation than latex) can oxidize hemoglobin to methemoglobin in intact, normal erythrocytes by a mechanism dependent on H_2O_2 (Weiss 1982; Winterbourn et al. 1981). These studies did not measure possible changes in the GSH concentration but they reinforce the concept that H_2O_2 can play an important role in oxidizing susceptible intracellular targets.

Although there are no specific studies demonstrating the ability of H_2O_2 alone to destroy erythrocytes, it has been implicated in cytolysis in several reports. Nathan et al. (1979a) demonstrated that murine phagocytes stimulated to generate large amounts of H_2O_2 could efficiently destroy mouse erythrocytes. However, the mechanism of cytolysis was not examined with this target cell population. In addition, Keisari and Pick (1981) reported that guinea pig macrophages stimulated with PMA or its methylated derivative (4-O-methyl PMA), wheat germ agglutinin or Con A could lyse guinea pig erythrocytes. The addition of catalase inhibited cytotoxicity mediated by PMA or 4-O-methyl PMA-stimulated macrophages but was ineffective in either lectin-stimulated systems. Finally, Greene et al. (1980) examined the role of oxygen in Con A-dependent neutrophil-mediated cytotoxicity against chicken erythrocytes (similar to the system of Simchowitz and Schur, see Section 2.3.2.1.). They demonstrated that at an effector to target cell ratio of 12.5:1, Con A-stimulated human neutrophils could destroy ~25−75% of the chicken erythrocytes. Neutrophils isolated from patients with CGD were incapable of mediating lysis while myeloperoxidase-deficient neutrophils could destroy the erythrocyte comparably to control cells. Thus, destruction was mediated by an oxygen-dependent, myeloperoxidase-independent mechanism. Either superoxide dismutase or catalase could partially reduce cytotoxicity while in the presence of both enzymes their effects were additive. The addition of OH· or $HOCl/{}^1O_2$ scavengers had no effect on hemolysis and the authors concluded that although both $O_2^{\cdot -}$ and H_2O_2 were involved, the final mediator could not be identified. Whether these results indicate that $O_2^{\cdot-}$ and H_2O_2 together form an oxidant that is difficult to scavenge, or indicate that the erythrocytes are lysed by either $O_2^{\cdot-}$ alone or H_2O_2 alone, remains to be determined.

H_2O_2 and platelets Platelets and neutrophils are commonly seen together in thrombi, and Levine et al. (1976) examined a potential interaction between these two cell populations. In an interesting model, human neutrophils stimulated with latex spherules were placed in dialysis bags and then suspended in solutions containing washed platelets. They found that neutrophils generated a product that could diffuse across the dialysis membrane and inhibit the ability of the platelets to aggregate. The addition of catalase to this system significantly protected the platelets. In addition, the neutrophil could be replaced by either reagent H_2O_2 or enzymatically generated H_2O_2 with similar results. Thus, it appeared that neutrophils generated sufficient H_2O_2 to impair platelet function. Although the effect of other oxygen metabolites generated by the phagocyte were not examined, it seems unlikely that the more reactive intermediates could diffuse across the dialysis membrane before reacting with other substrates.

A number of additional studies have examined the effects of oxygen metabolites generated by model systems on platelet function (for a recent study with complete bibliography see Levine et al. 1981). Handin et al. (1977) demonstrated that $O_2^{\cdot-}$ generated by the xanthine-xanthine oxidase system could aggregate platelets but this observation is complicated by reports that commercial xanthine oxidase may be contaminated with a heat-labile component capable of aggregating platelets (Levine et al. 1981; Patscheke et al. 1978). In contrast, it appears that H_2O_2 generated by a variety of cell-free systems can alter platelet function possibly by altering intracellular levels of ATP (Holmsen and Robkin 1977).

H_2O_2 and leukocytes Although phagocytes can generate appreciable amounts of H_2O_2, they do not appear to be invulnerable to this oxidant. Baehner et al. (1977) demonstrated that human neutrophils were hyperphagocytic under anaerobic conditions relative to aerobic controls. Phagocytosis or chemotaxis in the presence of oxygen could be enhanced by catalase but not by superoxide dismutase, OH· or $HOCl/^1O_2$ scavengers. Neutrophils exposed to enzymatically generated or reagent H_2O_2 had depressed phagocytic function, decreased C3b receptor activity and could be protected by catalase (Baehner et al. 1977; Boxer et al. 1978). -Tocopherol, a fat-soluble, membrane-associated, antioxidant also played a protective role in this system (Baehner et al. 1977; Harris et al. 1980). In contrast, Casciato et al. (1978) demonstrated that neutrophil chemotaxis induced by bacterial factors was actually depressed under anaerobic conditions, but the mechanism remains unclear. Other reports have suggested that phagocyte-derived H_2O_2 may be important in chemotactic deactivation (Nelson et al. 1979), time-dependent loss of chemotactic responsiveness of isolated phagocytes (Ferrante et al. 1980) and phagocytosis-induced injury (McGee and Myrvik 1979), but the precise identity of the responsible oxidant(s) require further clarification.

Additional evidence supporting a potential role for H_2O_2 in phagocyte injury has been uncovered in studies of neutrophils isolated from patients with glutathionine synthetase deficiency, glutathione reductase deficiency and acatalasemia (for review see Roos 1980 and Roos et al. 1980). Phagocytosing leukocytes with either genetic deficiency in the glutathione redox system are easily damaged by their own oxidants while both glutathione reductase deficient or acatalasemic cells can also be damaged by extracellular fluxes of H_2O_2. At present, it appears that both the glutathione system and catalase are required for the preservation of phagocyte function in the face of high concentrations of H_2O_2.

H_2O_2 generated by model systems can impair a number of lymphocyte functions (see Kraut and Sagone 1981), but few studies have examined the role of oxygen in phagocyte—lymphocyte interactions. Metzger et al. (1980) recently demonstrated the ability of *Corynebacterium parvum* or thioglycolate induced macrophages to suppress Con A-induced proliferation of murine splenic lymphocytes. Analysis of the macrophages' inhibitory effect revealed that catalase and indomethacin synergistically protected the lymphocytes. Apparently both H_2O_2 and prostaglandins play an important role in controlling lymphocyte proliferation in this model.

H_2O_2 and endothelial cells Studies by Craddock et al. (1979) indicated that activation of the alternative complement cascade occurs in patients undergoing hemodialysis with cellophane membrane equipment. Animals treated in a similar manner develop pulmonary leukostasis, pulmonary artery hypertension, pulmonary edema and an associated protein-rich pulmonary lymph fluid. The authors hypothesized that granulocytes exposed to activated complement components damaged the endothelial cell barrier and permitted a protein leak. Hence, Sacks et al. (1978) examined the ability of human granulocytes incubated with activated complement to induce endothelial cell damage in an in-vitro system. Granulocytes incubated with serum fractions enriched with C5a damaged endothelial cells by a mechanism inhibitable by catalase but only inconsistently blocked with superoxide dismutase. Similar results were obtained if the phagocyte was replaced with the xanthine-xanthine oxidase system. C5a stimulated cells released little myeloperoxidase and cells isolated from a patient with chronic granulomatous disease mediated half as much damage as control granulocytes. The authors concluded that C5a stimulated granulocytes could injure endothelial cells by generating an uncharacterized oxygen metabolite. Additional studies revealed that endotoxin-stimulated granulocytes could also damage endothelial cells by a similar mechanism (Yamado et al. 1981).

Weiss et al. (1981) attempted to identify those oxygen metabolites capable of damaging endothelial cells in a model similar to that used by Sacks et al. (1978) but in which C5a was replaced with PMA. Human neutrophils could destroy endothelial cells when stimulated with PMA while chronic granulomatous disease cells were ineffective. Damage was inhibited by catalase but not by superoxide dismutase, suggesting a critical role for H_2O_2. Neither OH· nor HOCl scavengers protected the endothelial cells and myelo-peroxidase-deficient neutrophils effectively mediated cytotoxicity by a H_2O_2-dependent mechanism. Although PMA is not a strong stimulus for the release of myeloperoxidase (see Goldstein 1979), the addition of purified enzyme failed to stimulate cytolysis by either the normal or myeloperoxidase-deficient cells. Because these data indicated that H_2O_2 might be the cytotoxic effector, the neutrophil was replaced with an enzyme system capable of generating H_2O_2 at a rate similar to that of the intact cell. As expected, glucose-glucose oxidase, an enzyme system that generates H_2O_2 directly, effectively destroyed the endothelial cell targets. Thus, it appeared that neutrophils could destroy endothelial cells by generating toxic quantities of H_2O_2.

In contrast, Harlan et al. (1981) demonstrated that human neutrophils stimulated with opsonized zymosan particles did not lyse endothelial cells but could mediate their detachment from a monolayer. Although reagent H_2O_2 could induce both lysis and detachment, neither catalase nor superoxide dismutase inhibited zymosan-stimulated neutrophils from detaching the endothelial cells. Chronic granulomatous disease neutrophils were also able to cause detachment, suggesting a role for an oxygen-independent mechanism. Cell-free postsecretory media from zymosan-stimulated cells or partially purified granule fractions could mediate detachment and their effects could be blocked by neutral protease inhibitors. The authors concluded that neutrophils could damage endothelial cell monolayers by releasing a lysosomal enzyme(s) with characteristics similar to elastase. Although these conclusions differ from the other reports, the results are not necessarily contradictory. First, both C5a and PMA are weak stimuli for the release of the elastase-rich, primary granules from the neutrophil. Second, serum was present in the H_2O_2-dependent models whereas enzyme-mediated detachment was serum-inhibitable. Third, it should be noted that the ability of PMA-stimulated neutrophils to damage endothelial cells was blocked in the presence of unopsonized zymosan particles by an uncharacterized mechanism (Weiss et al. 1981). Indeed, levels of H_2O_2 reported by Harlan et al. to cause both extensive detachment and lysis are similar to those generated by PMA-stimulated neutrophils in the study by Weiss et al. Nonetheless, it appears that neutrophils have the capacity to injure endothelial cells by both H_2O_2-dependent and oxygen-independent mechanisms.

H_2O_2 and tumor cells Nathan et al. (1979a, b) provided the first evidence indicating that H_2O_2 alone, generated by intact phagocytes, could clearly mediate cytotoxicity. Bacillus Calmette-Guérin (BCG), *C. parvum* or casein-activated murine macrophages or thioglycolate-elicited granulocytes could rapidly destroy a variety of malignant and non-malignant target cells when triggered with PMA. Cytolysis was complete within 4.5 hours and could be demonstrated in the presence of serum. The ability of various effector cell populations to mediate cytotoxicity closely correlated with their ability to generate H_2O_2. However, both thioglycolate-elicited macrophages and the macrophage-like tumor cell J774 failed to mediate cytotoxicity

or generate detectable quantities of H_2O_2 despite their ability to release substantial amounts of $O_2^{\cdot -}$. An analysis of the susceptibility of the target cells to lysis by PMA-stimulated phagocytes revealed a close correlation with their sensitivity to reagent H_2O_2. Based on these observations, a direct role for H_2O_2 in macrophage and granulocyte-mediated cytolysis of one of the tumor cell lines (P388 lymphoma) was examined (Nathan et al. 1979b). Under anaerobic conditions, BCG-activated macrophages stimulated with PMA did not destroy the tumor cell target. H_2O_2 generation and cytolysis by the PMA-triggered macrophages or thioglycolate-elicited granulocytes were similarly inhibited if glucose was omitted from the incubation mixture. Tumor cell lysis by the PMA-stimulated phagocytes was also blocked in the presence of catalase while superoxide dismutase had no protective effect. Neither $OH\cdot$ nor $HOCl/^1O_2$ scavengers inhibited cytolysis and peroxidase inhibitors augmented cytotoxicity. Thus, despite the presence of myeloperoxidase in the granulocytes, it did not appear to play a cytotoxic role in this system. Finally, phagocyte-mediated killing could be mimicked by particle-bound glucose oxidase generating H_2O_2 at rates similar to those of the effector cells. It seems clear that PMA could trigger either BCG-activated macrophages or thioglycolate-elicited granulocytes to generate sufficient quantities of H_2O_2 to destroy the lymphoma target*.

Because target cells varied widely in their susceptibility to H_2O_2-mediated lysis, Nathan et al. (1980) examined potential antioxidant defenses in six murine tumors that varied over 50-fold in their sensitivity to enzymatically generated H_2O_2. Intracellular concentrations of catalase, GSH peroxidase or GSH reductase did not correlate with the resistance of the tumors to H_2O_2. In contrast, the intracellular concentrations of GSH correlated with the logarithm of the flux of H_2O_2 causing 50% lysis. It should be noted, however, that cells that varied in their sensitivity to H_2O_2 by a factor of 4 had essentially identical GSH contents. In a much smaller sample, Bozzi et al. (1979) reported that the sensitivity of four different strains of ascites tumors to H_2O_2 also seemed to correlate with the intracellular glutathione content. Blockade of tumor cell glutathione reductase with 1,3-bis(2-chloroethyl)-1-nitrosourea (BCNU) or the reduction of glutathione peroxidase levels by passing the tumor cells in selenium-deficient mice markedly increased their sensitivity to enzymatically generated H_2O_2 or PMA-stimulated phagocytes (Nathan et al. 1980). In contrast, inhibition of catalase with aminotriazole failed to enhance the tumor cells' sensitivity to enzyme- or phagocyte-generated H_2O_2. In a complementary

*It is puzzling that dihydrocytochalasin B, an agent that did not inhibit glucose transport in the macrophage and had minimal effects on PMA-triggered H_2O_2 generation, markedly inhibited cytotoxicity mediated by PMA-stimulated BCG macrophages (Nathan and Cohn 1980). These findings may indicate an added requirement for an intact macrophage contractile network in PMA-triggered cytolysis.

study, Arrick et al. (1982) examined the effect of GSH depletion on lysis of tumor cells by H_2O_2. GSH levels were depleted by either blocking γ-glutamylcysteine synthetase with buthionine sulfoximine or by treating the cells with 1-chloro-2,4-dinitrobenzene which covalently binds GSH via catalysis by GSH S-transferase. Tumor cells with depleted GSH levels demonstrated increased sensitivity to a constant flux of H_2O_2 generated enzymatically or by PMA-stimulated phagocytes but not to a bolus of H_2O_2. In contrast, the susceptibility of catalase-inhibited targets to a flux or bolus of H_2O_2 was unaltered. However, target cells were sensitive to a bolus of H_2O_2 if both the catalase activity was inhibited and GSH levels depleted. Thus, tumor cells seem to utilize only the GSH redox system for protection when exposed to a steady flux of H_2O_2 while either the GSH system or catalase was effective when the target was suddenly exposed to large quantities of H_2O_2.

In summary, phagocytes can generate sufficient quantities of H_2O_2 to oxidize intracellular components in erythrocyte targets, damage or modulate leukocyte function, injure endothelial cells and destroy tumor cells. The ability of H_2O_2 to mediate these effects is regulated, in part, by antioxidant defenses in the target cell population. The GSH redox system is a critical component in determining the susceptibility of the erythrocyte, phagocyte and tumor cells to H_2O_2-induced damage. Whether the GSH system plays this protective role by effectively handling low concentrations of H_2O_2, reducing lipid hydroperoxides or repairing oxidant damage is unknown. Catalase may also act as an antioxidant defense in the phagocyte or tumor cell but apparently only in the face of high concentrations of H_2O_2. The role of other protective enzymes or compounds, e.g., GSH transferase, cysteine, ascorbic acid, α-tocopherol, etc., remains to be determined.

Although all of these studies implicate H_2O_2 as a toxic intermediate, it is intriguing to note that fat cells can also generate substantial quantities of H_2O_2. Mukherjee and Lynn (1977) demonstrated that fat cells contain a membrane-bound NADPH oxidase that can be activated with insulin to produce H_2O_2. Though the amounts of H_2O_2 released extracellularly versus intracellularly are unclear, this oxidant actually mimics many of insulin's effects on the fat cell (May and DeHaen 1979). Apparently the quantities of H_2O_2 released, its site of production, and the cell population responsible for generation, all play an important role in defining its biological effects.

How does H_2O_2 mediate cell injury? At present, few studies have addressed this problem but, based on the slow reaction rates of H_2O_2 with most organic substrates, catalysis by transition metal ions or their chelates, is an attractive hypothesis. Repine et al. (1981) recently demonstrated that H_2O_2 can react with iron incorporated into *Staphylococcus aureus* to generate a staphylocidal species with characteristics similar, if not identical, with OH·. Thus, the sensitivity of a target cell to H_2O_2 may be determined by both its antioxidant defenses and the presence or location of metal-containing target molecules. In addition, Adams et al. (1981) have shown that H_2O_2 can interact synergistically with a macrophage-secretory product known as cytolytic factor to effect tumor cell destruction. It appears that H_2O_2 (like $O_2^{\cdot -}$; Section

2.3.2.1.) may evade target cell defense mechanisms and react with intracellular (or membrane-associated) targets in order to generate highly reactive oxidants. The final damage resulting from this oxidant attack may then be amplified by other phagocyte-derived products.

2.3.2.3. Hydrogen peroxide-peroxidase-halide system

Model systems consisting of H_2O_2, purified peroxidases and halides have been extensively studied (for reviews see Klebanoff and Clark 1978; Klebanoff 1980a) and it is clear that the oxidants generated can both modify cell function and mediate cytotoxicity. Clark and Klebanoff (1975) were the first to demonstrate the ability of intact phagocytes to destroy an extracellular target cell by a peroxidase-dependent mechanism. Subsequently, it has been demonstrated that neutrophils, eosinophils, monocytes and mast cells may utilize their peroxidases to modulate their own function, mediate platelet or mast cell release reactions and destroy neoplastic cells.

Peroxidases and phagocytes During ingestion neutrophils release myeloperoxidase into both the phagocyte vacuole and the extracellular milieu. Thus, in the presence of H_2O_2 and a halide, the phagocyte is exposed to myeloperoxidase-generated oxidants at multiple sites. Evidence currently indicates that the myeloperoxidase system is an important component in the termination of the respiratory burst, the inactivation of lysosomal enzymes and autotoxicity.

The earliest evidence suggesting a role for the myeloperoxidase system in the termination of the respiratory burst was provided by metabolic studies of myeloperoxidase-deficient neutrophils. When stimulated, these cells had increased rates of oxygen consumption, $O_2^{\cdot -}$ generation and H_2O_2 production as compared to normal controls (Rosen and Klebanoff 1976). A kinetic study of $O_2^{\cdot -}$ production by normal and myeloperoxidase-deficient neutrophils revealed that the initial rates of generation by the stimulated cells were comparable. However $O_2^{\cdot -}$ production by normal cells ceased after ~60 minutes while it continued for at least 2 hours with the myeloperoxidase-deficient neutrophils. These results indicated that the respiratory burst was significantly prolonged in the absence of myeloperoxidase. Subsequently, Jandl et al. (1978) examined the various factors regulating the $O_2^{\cdot -}$-forming activity in the 27,000 x *g* particulate fraction from neutrophils stimulated with zymosan. Activity began to rapidly decline in particles prepared from neutrophils that were exposed to zymosan for more than 3 minutes. After a 60-minute incubation, the $O_2^{\cdot -}$-forming activity was almost completely gone. However, in the presence of myeloperoxidase inhibitors, the $O_2^{\cdot -}$-forming activity was preserved for approximately 10 minutes before subsequently declining. Inhibition of the myeloperoxidase system might allow other oxygen metabolites (e.g. $O_2^{\cdot -}$, H_2O_2, $OH^{\cdot}$) to play a role in the loss of activity but anaerobic conditions did not protect the $O_2^{\cdot -}$-forming activity beyond the first 10 minutes. Apparently the $O_2^{\cdot -}$-forming activity of intact neutrophils declines after stimulation by an early myeloperoxidase-dependent mechanism and a later oxygen-independent scheme.

The myeloperoxidase system also plays a role in the inactivation of the phagocytes' own lysosomal enzymes. Skosey et al. (1981) reported that lysosomal enzyme release from phagocytosing neutrophils was stimulated as the oxygen concentration was decreased. In addition, enzyme release under aerobic conditions was apparently increased in the presence of catalase, azide and a number of scavengers most of which react with HOCl. They concluded that oxygen metabolites generated by the neutrophil during phagocytosis inhibited lysosomal enzyme release. Voetman et al. (1981) made a similar observation when they noted that stimulated CGD neutrophils released more lysosomal enzyme activity (β-glucuronidase, lysozyme or α-glucosidase) than normal cells. An analysis of the amount of enzyme activity released into the extracellular medium and remaining in the cell pellet of the CGD cells revealed that all of the activity could be recovered. However, approximately 20% of the total enzyme activity was lost from the incubation mixtures with normal neutrophils. Thus, the smaller amount of lysosomal enzyme activity found in the supernate from the normal cells was due to enzyme inactivation. The inactivation process was inhibited under anaerobic conditions indicating a central role for oxygen. Lysosomal enzyme inactivation was enhanced in the presence of the myeloperoxidase inhibitor, azide, but, paradoxically, myeloperoxidase-deficient cells did not inactivate their own lysosomal enzymes. Apparently phagocytes require H_2O_2 and myeloperoxidase to inactivate their enzymes but the addition of azide allows the H_2O_2 to reach a concentration sufficient to directly inactivate the enzymes independently of myeloperoxidase. Enzyme inactivation took place in the phagolysosome and could not be inhibited by exogenous superoxide dismutase, catalase or albumin illustrating the inability of large molecules to gain entrance into the vacuolar space. Although the results illustrate the sensitivity of lysosomal enzymes to myeloperoxidase-derived oxidants, it should be noted that myeloperoxidase itself may be susceptible to its own products. HOCl can reversibly or irreversibly inactivate myeloperoxidase, suggesting that the enzyme may self-deactivate in the absence of oxidizable substrates (Harrison and Schultz 1976; Naskalski 1977).

The neutrophils' $O_2^{\cdot -}$-forming activity and lysosomal enzymes may be sensitive to myeloperoxidase-derived oxidants but in addition the phagocytes' own viability may be at stake. Clark and Klebanoff (1977a) demonstrated that a model H_2O_2-myeloperoxidase-Cl^- system could destroy leukocytes, while Tsan and Denison (Tsan 1980; Tsan and Denison 1980) later examined the ability of PMA-stimulated neutrophils to mediate autotoxicity. Injury was blocked by catalase and by histidine or methionine; compounds known to react with HOCl. However, azide did not inhibit autotoxicity. These results may indicate that the H_2O_2-myeloperoxidase-Cl^- system is involved in autotoxicity but, in the presence of azide, the H_2O_2 concentration reaches toxic levels and destroys the neutrophil by a myeloperoxidase-independent mechanism.

Peroxidases and release reactions Clark and Klebanoff (1979a) demonstrated that platelets labeled with adenine (a cytoplasmic marker) and serotonin (a granule component) released serotonin in excess of adenine if exposed to a model H_2O_2—myeloperoxidase—Cl^- system. In addition, serotonin release also required intact platelet metabolism, which suggested that this myeloperoxidase-dependent effect was non-lytic and analogous to the platelet release reaction. In a similar system, platelets incubated with neutrophils and opsonized zymosan released equal amounts of adenine and serotonin by a mechanism dependent on H_2O_2 and a halide (Clark and Klebanoff 1980). Whether these results reflect platelet lysis, the release reaction or a combination of the two processes, is unclear. Neither CGD- nor myeloperoxidase-deficient neutrophils could mediate this release. However, the addition of myeloperoxidase inhibitors (azide, cyanide) to normal or myeloperoxidase-deficient neutrophils significantly enhanced release. These results suggested that H_2O_2 alone, in the presence of heme-enzyme inhibitors, could enhance the release reaction. Indeed, either reagent or enzymatically generated H_2O_2 could initiate a release reaction that was stimulated by the addition of azide, cyanide or aminotriazole probably as a consequence of the inhibition of the platelet's catalase. Thus, in several models (see Section 2.3.2.3. under "Peroxidases and phagocytes"), H_2O_2 alone can mediate effects similar to those observed with the intact myeloperoxidase system, but only if conditions allow high concentrations of H_2O_2 to accumulate.

Recent evidence indicates that the ability of the peroxidase system to initiate a release reaction may not be limited to neutrophils and platelets. Eosinophils and mast cells are commonly associated in areas of immediate hypersensitivity and Henderson et al. (1980a) postulated that activated eosinophils might alter mast cell activity. In a model system, H_2O_2, eosinophil peroxidase and a halide could either induce the specific secretion of granules from intact mast cells or mediate mast cell destruction depending on the eosinophil peroxidase concentration. In addition, eosinophil peroxidase could also bind to the matrix of the mast cell granule in a manner that potentiated its secretory activity on mast cells (Henderson et al. 1980a, b). Thus, the eosinophil peroxidase has the opportunity to amplify its own activity by inducing mast cell granule exocytosis and binding to the released matrix.

Peroxidases and tumor cells Human neutrophils can be stimulated to release sufficient H_2O_2 and myeloperoxidase into the extracellular milieu to destroy adjacent tumor cell targets. Clark and Klebanoff (1975) first described the ability of neutrophils stimulated with opsonized zymosan to destroy extracellular tumor cells by a mechanism depending on H_2O_2, myeloperoxidase and Cl^- or I^-. On a molar basis, I^- was more effective than Cl^- in this system with equivalent cytotoxicity being obtained with 10^{-4} mol l^{-1} I^- or 10^{-1} mol l^{-1} Cl^-. Cytolysis was also observed if a combination of I^- and Cl^- was used at concentrations where either halide alone showed minimal activity. Neither CGD- nor myeloperoxidase-deficient neutrophils could destroy tumor cells unless supplemented with exogenous H_2O_2 or myeloperoxidase, respectively. Subsequent studies have demonstrated that Con A or PMA-stimulated neutrophils can also destroy either murine or human tumor cells by an essentially identical myeloperoxidase system (Clark and Klebanoff 1979c; Slivka et al. 1980; Jong and Klebanoff 1980; Clark and Szot 1981). All three halides (I^-, Cl^- or Br^-) are effective and cytotoxicity can be demonstrated in the presence of serum (Clark and Szot 1981).

Can other cells utilize their peroxidases to mediate tumor cell destruction? In comparisons with human neutrophils, monocytes contain about one-third the myeloperoxidase concentration (Bos et al. 1978) and appear to generate less H_2O_2 (Reiss and Roos 1978), but they can effectively mediate tumor cell cytotoxicity. Weiss and Slivka (1982) demonstrated that purified monocytes stimulated with PMA could destroy tumor cells comparably to neutrophils by a mechanism dependent on the H_2O_2-myeloperoxidase-Cl^- system.

Mast cells and eosinophils may be observed associated together in certain types of neoplasms and their potential to mediate peroxidase-dependent cytotoxicity has been examined. Jong and Klebanoff (1980) demonstrated that a model H_2O_2—eosinophil peroxidase—halide system could destroy tumor cell targets. Unlike myeloperoxidase, eosinophil peroxidase could only utilize I^- to mediate cytotoxicity at pH 7.0. However, Cl^- could significantly increase cytolytic activity at ineffective I^- concentrations. In contrast, at pH 6.0, the halide requirement of the model system could be filled with either Cl^-, I^- or Br^-. Intact guinea pig eosinophils stimulated with PMA or opsonized zymosan could also kill tumor cells but required I^- supplementation for their maximal cytotoxic effect.

Mast cells also contain small amounts of a granule-associated peroxidase that can effectively mediate cytotoxicity. Henderson et al. (1981) demonstrated that mast cells incubated with H_2O_2 could discharge their granules and, in the presence of I^-, mediate tumor cell cytolysis. As discussed, eosinophil peroxidase alone can destroy tumor cell targets (Jong and Klebanoff 1980) but its cytotoxic potential is clearly enhanced if bound to the mast cell granule (Henderson et al. 1981). Thus, eosinophils and mast cells have the potential to cooperate and amplify their tumoricidal potential.

At present, there is no evidence supporting a role for macrophage-mediated, peroxidase-dependent cytotoxicity but it is important to note that macrophages may utilize endocytosed or phagocytosed peroxidases from neutrophils, eosinophils, monocytes or mast cells in cytotoxic reactions (Heifets et al. 1980). In addition, the cationic properties of myeloperoxidase and eosinophil peroxidase may allow these enzymes to bind to target cell membranes and thus enhance the cytotoxic potential of the H_2O_2 generated by the macrophage (Ramsey et al. 1982).

Although the final mediator of myeloperoxidase-dependent cytotoxicity has not been directly identified, evidence supports a role for the hypohalous acids. HOCl is indeed tumoricidal (Slivka et al. 1980) and tumor cell cytotoxicity mediated by reagent HOCl, a model H_2O_2—myeloperoxidase—Cl^- system, PMA-stimulated neutrophils or monocytes can all be blocked by HOCl scavengers (Weiss and Slikva 1982). The precise mechanisms by which HOCl administers the death blow is unknown but, based on its microbicidal properties, the oxidant could attack both membrane and intracellular components (Thomas 1979a, b; Selvaraj et al. 1980; Albrich et al. 1981). Membrane sulfhydryl groups, proteins, and lipids may be at risk while intracellular nucleotides and components of the respiratory redox chain are particularly reactive with HOCl. Based on their pK_a's, the hypohalous acids would primarily exist in their uncharged form at neutral or acidic pH and could rapidly diffuse into the intracellular compartment. Cellular defense mechanisms against HOCl have not been defined but it seems unlikely that an enzyme could directly catalyze its reduction. However, target cells could indirectly limit the HOCl concentration by degrading extracellular H_2O_2 before it is utilized by the peroxidases. In addition, the oxidizing equivalents of HOCl (or HOI, HOBr) could be shuttled into the GSH system via GSSG formation ($HOCl + 2\,GSH — GSSH + H_2O + Cl^- + H^+$). Finally, the GSH redox system's ability to repair hypohalous acid-mediated damage is unknown. Despite these potential protective mechanisms, in the face of large concentrations of the hypohalous acids, cell death would seem to be an inevitable consequence.

In summary, myeloperoxidase, eosinophil peroxidase and mast cell peroxidase are all members of a specialized class of peroxidases that can generate free hypohalous acids. Phagocytes can utilize these species to either modulate cell function, enhance or attenuate the generation of oxidants or mediate cytotoxicity. Based on the reactivity of the hypohalous acids, requirements for transition-metal activation or evasion of antioxidant defenses (re: $O_2^{\cdot -}$ or H_2O_2) are probably unnecessary. Thus, these oxidants are self-contained and independently acting toxins capable of attacking target cells at multiple sites. Nevertheless, the importance and cytotoxic potential of the phagocyte-associated peroxidases has been questioned. Normal macrophages and phagocytes from individuals with myeloperoxidase deficiency effectively mediate oxygen-dependent but peroxidase-independent cytotoxic effects. Rather than invalidating the important role of the H_2O_2−peroxidase−halide system, these findings serve to highlight the effectiveness and redundancy of the phagocytes' arsenal of oxygen metabolites.

2.3.2.4. The hydroxyl radical

The $OH^{\cdot}$ has been implicated in phagocyte-mediated antimicrobial activity (Johnston et al. 1975; Murray et al. 1979) but few studies have demonstrated the ability of leukocytes to utilize $OH^{\cdot}$ to destroy mammalian cell targets. Indeed, reports suggesting a role for $OH^{\cdot}$ in cytotoxic events are limited to phagocyte autoinjury. Salin and McCord (1975) first demonstrated the ability of superoxide dismutase, catalase or the $OH^{\cdot}$ scavenger mannitol to protect phagocytosing leukocytes from self-inflicted damage. High concentrations of bovine superoxide dismutase were required for protection, possibly owing to an electrostatic repulsion between the negatively charged enzyme and plasma membrane. In support of this explanation, positively charged superoxide dismutase (a polylysyl derivative) protected the leukocytes at much lower concentrations than the native system (Salin and McCord 1977). Thus, $O_2^{\cdot -}$ and H_2O_2 were involved in the generation of a species with $OH^{\cdot}$-

like characteristics that was capable of damaging the phagocytes. In an additional report implicating OH·, Klock and Stossel (1977) demonstrated that normal granulocytes adhering to nylon wool fibers damaged themselves but only under aerobic conditions. CGD granulocytes did not injure themselves in this system, suggesting that the damage was dependent on oxygen metabolite generation. The addition of superoxide dismutase prevented damage as did the OH· scavengers mannitol and benzoate, but catalase was ineffective. Although the authors questioned the ability of catalase to degrade small amounts of H_2O_2 at the fiber-cell interface, it appeared that $O_2^{\cdot -}$ might be involved in the generation of an OH·-like species independently of H_2O_2.

Both of these studies implicated an oxygen intermediate with characteristics similar to OH· but it is interesting to note that they detected damage in the presence of a variety of OH· scavengers. Salin and McCord demonstrated phagocyte autotoxicity in a medium containing 5% serum and 55 mM glucose while Klock and Stossel reported injury in the presence of plasma. Although these conditions did not impair OH·-mediated attack, the further addition of exogenous scavengers in 1−2 mM concentration completely protected the phagocytes from damage. How the OH· evaded the endogenous scavengers (serum, glucose, plasma) to mediate cell injury and yet was intercepted by low concentrations of the exogenous traps, is unclear. It is possible that the interaction of OH· with oxidizable compounds found in the control systems could result in the formation of secondary radicals that are less reactive but more selective in their action (for interesting examples of this phenomenon in radiobiology, see Willson 1979).

Do these two reports constitute the only "proof" for OH·-mediated cellular injury? Clearly, our early requirements for establishing the role of OH·, i.e., inhibition by superoxide dismutase, catalase and OH· scavengers are too restrictive. As discussed earlier, $O_2^{\cdot -}$ alone or H_2O_2 alone may react with transition-metal chelates to form OH·-like oxidants. Indeed, $O_2^{\cdot -}$, H_2O_2, myeloperoxidase and a halide could all be involved in OH· generation via an interaction between $O_2^{\cdot -}$ and a hypohalous acid. Finally, attempts to trap OH· are dependent on the ability of the scavengers to gain access to the site of reaction and the reactivity of the resultant product. It should be emphasized that there is still no proof for OH· generation by phagocytes and the possibility of an OH·-like species with characteristics similar, but not identical with OH·, cannot be overlooked (Bors et al. 1979). It may well be that the ability of an OH· scavenger to inhibit phagocyte-mediated, "OH·"-dependent events is the exception rather than the rule.

2.3.3. Oxygen and antibody-dependent cellular cytotoxicity (ADCC)

Non-immune leukocytes bearing Fc receptors can bind and destroy antibody-coated target cells by a process known as antibody-dependent cellular cytotoxicity or ADCC (for review see Henney 1977; Pearson 1978). Unlike the innocent bystander-type reactions discussed in the previous sections, the phagocytes' cytotoxic arsenal is specifically directed against a sensitized target. Thus, adjacent, but unbound targets, are not damaged during this process. Apparently the tight coupling between the effector and target cell membranes (e.g., see micrographs in LoBuglio et al. 1967) assures a closed environment for the generated toxins. However, the efficiency of this process also impedes our attempts to manipulate events at this interface. Enzymes that might be able to inhibit ADCC, e.g., superoxide dismutase or catalase, may not gain access to these sites in sufficient quantities to effectively lower the $O_2^{\cdot -}$ or H_2O_2 concentrations (see discussion in Clark and Klebanoff 1977b, Hafeman and Lucas 1979, or Nathan and Cohn 1980). Indeed, if an oxygen metabolite and its biological target are in close proximity, even small molecular weight scavengers might be unable to inhibit cytotoxicity (see Section 2.3.2.4.). Thus, the failure to block a localized event in ADCC (or similar immune processes) with these techniques must be cautiously interpreted before a role for oxygen is excluded.

In 1977, Clark and Klebanoff provided the first evidence supporting a role for oxygen metabolites in phagocyte-mediated ADCC. Since that time a number of studies have attempted to define the processes involved in ADCC but most of the information regarding the importance of oxidative metabolism is indirect. The most common approaches include 1) the detection of oxygen metabolites generated during ADCC, 2) the effects of anaerobiosis on ADCC and 3) the (in)ability of CGD- or myeloperoxidase-deficient phagocytes to mediate ADCC. Despite the "deficiencies" in our investigative tools, evidence continues to accumulate implicating oxygen metabolites in phagocyte-mediated ADCC against both erythroid and nonerythroid mammalian targets.

2.3.3.1. Are oxygen metabolites generated by phagocytes bound to antibody-coated targets?

For the phagocyte to mediate ADCC, it first must bind to the target cell. This is a complex mechanism regulated by the type of effector cell, the distribution of its Fc receptors, the immunoglobulin type, subtype and concentration, the density and distribution of antigen-binding sites on the target cell, and a variety of other factors which are beyond the scope of this review (see Henney 1977; Pearson 1978). However, even if the phagocyte is bound to the target cell, oxygen metabolites will not play a role in the cytotoxic event unless the antibody provides a suitable stimulus for the respiratory burst. Perhaps the earliest reports demonstrating the ability of antibody-coated targets to stimulate phagocyte oxidative metabolism were the studies of Handin and Stossel (1974) and Boxer and Stossel (1974). Human neutrophils or rabbit alveolar macrophages incubated with antibody-coated platelets or neutrophils, respectively, ingested the sensitized cells and reduced the redox dye nitroblue tetrazolium. (It was later demonstrated that phagocytes reduce the dye by generating $O_2^{\cdot -}$; Baehner et al. 1976.) Subsequent studies revealed that aggregated immunoglobulins in solution (Henson and Oades 1975; Goldstein et al. 1975) or surface-bound (Johnston and Lehmeyer 1976; Johnston et al. 1976), and IgG bound to beads (Goldstein et al. 1976) or erythrocytes (Newman and Johnston 1979) could all stimulate phagocyte oxidative metabolism in a concentration-dependent manner. Recent evidence indicates that the physical properties of the antibody-coated target are an additional important consideration. In a series of studies, Hafeman et al. (1979, 1980, 1981) and Lewis et al. (1980) examined antibody-dependent interactions between phagocytes and haptenated lipid vesicles or monolayers. The stimulation of macrophage oxidative metabolism was strongly dependent upon both the density of the antibodies on the vesicle surface and the "fluidity" of the lipid membrane. The kinetics of antibody-dependent binding to macrophages were enhanced with fluid vesicles when compared to solid vesicles but, in contrast, the solid vesicles were far more effective in stimulating the respiratory burst. Indeed, at antibody concentrations where 50% of either type vesicle was bound and internalized, only the solid vesicles stimulated oxidative metabolism. Although neutrophils did not recognize differences in the fluidity of vesicles coated with this specific antibody, these findings illustrate the complexity of the factors regulating oxygen metabolite generation by the target-bound phagocyte.

Is there any evidence that phagocytes actually generate oxygen metabolites while mediating ADCC? The respiratory burst is normally associated with the "four increases"; an increase in O_2 consumption, $O_2^{\cdot -}$ generation, H_2O_2 production and hexose monophosphate shunt activity (Babior 1978). Hafeman and Lucas (1979) were the first to demonstrate an associated increase in O_2 consumption, $O_2^{\cdot -}$ generation and shunt activity (measured as the release of labeled carbon dioxide from [1-^{14}C]glucose) during granulocyte-mediated ADCC against a tumor cell target. In addition, other reports have demonstrated enhanced rates of [1-^{14}C]glucose oxidation during neutrophil or monocyte-mediated ADCC against erythrocyte targets (Borregaard and Kragballe 1980; Klassen and Sagone 1980; Sagone et al. 1981). Fc-bearing lymphocytes can also mediate cytotoxicity but there was no evidence for activation of a respiratory burst (Hafeman et al. 1981; Sagone et al. 1981). There is, however, a report by Thorne et al. (1980) which suggests that T-lymphocytes can generate H_2O_2 during their interaction with a mastocytoma cell line.

These studies demonstrate that phagocyte oxidative metabolism can be stimulated during ADCC but it should be noted that these increases are extremely small when compared to phagocytosing cells. Nonetheless, the local concentrations of the oxidants generated at the effector cell—target cell interface may be sufficient to mediate damage.

2.3.3.2. *Are oxygen metabolites involved in phagocyte-mediated ADCC against erythroid targets? Yes, No, Maybe?*

In a number of reports normal human neutrophils or monocytes could mediate ADCC against erythrocytes by a process that was inhibitable under anaerobic conditions (Table 1). The degree of inhibition was variable (40—80%) but the absolute differences in cytotoxicity between aerobic and anaerobic conditions were small. CGD phagocytes had an impaired cytotoxic potential in some studies but mediated ADCC comparably to controls in others (Table 1). Although these results appear contradictory, they may be partially reconciled by the findings of Katz et al. (1980). In suspension, normal neutrophils or monocytes rapidly phagocytosed and destroyed antibody-coated erythrocytes while CGD phagocytes ingested the targets but were unable to mediate effective hemolysis. However, if ingestion was prevented by using a monolayer of target cells, both normal and CGD phagocytes mediated comparable cytotoxicity. Similarly, the ability of CGD cells to mediate hemolysis while in suspension could be normalized by blocking phagocytosis with colchicine. Apparently, extracellular cytolysis, unlike intracellular destruction, did not require an intact system for generating oxygen metabolites. The biochemical basis for this phenomenon is unknown.

As expected, in almost all of these systems superoxide dismutase, catalase and a variety of oxygen metabolite scavengers failed to inhibit ADCC (Fleer et al. 1979; Klassen and Sagone 1980; Koller and LoBuglio 1981) but there are two noteworthy exceptions. In a preliminary report, Capsoni et al. (1979) reported that superoxide dismutase could inhibit neutrophil-mediated ADCC against chicken erythrocytes but we are unaware whether this observation has been confirmed. Borregaard and Kragballe (1980) demonstrated that neutrophil- or monocyte-mediated ADCC could be stimulated by azide or cyanide and modestly inhibited by high concentrations of mannitol (e.g., mannitol inhibited neutrophil or monocyte ADCC from 22 to 16% and 17 to 11%, respectively). Azide and mannitol did not inhibit CGD cells from mediating hemolysis. The authors concluded that normal phagocytes could mediate ADCC by generating $OH\cdot$ via a mechanism similar to that proposed by Green et al. (1979) and Rosen and Klebanoff (1979).

2.3.3.3. Role of oxidative metabolism in phagocyte-mediated ADCC against nucleated mammalian cells

As in the erythrocyte models, the requirement for oxidative metabolism in phagocyte-mediated ADCC against nucleated mammalian cells is variable (Table 1). Anaerobic conditions could inhibit neutrophil- or macrophage-mediated cytolysis but in one study hypoxia had no effect on monocyte-mediated ADCC (Klassen and Sagone 1980). In this model, monocytes destroyed erythrocytes by an oxygen-dependent process but lysed tumor cells by a mechanism that did not stimulate the hexose monophosphate shunt, did not require oxygen and could be mediated normally by CGD cells. Of all the systems described (Table 1), this is apparently the only example of normal phagocytes mediating cytotoxicity by an oxygen-independent process alone.

Extracellular cytolysis is the predominant mode of destruction with nucleated, non-erythroid mammalian cell targets (Pearson 1978) and one might predict that CGD phagocytes should destroy these cells normally (see Katz et al. 1980). However, Clark and Klebanoff (1977b) demonstrated that both normal and myeloperoxidase-deficient neutrophils could destroy antibody-coated tumor cells

TABLE 1.
A role for oxidative metabolism in phagocyte-mediated ADCC?

Reference	Effector*	Target	Oxidative metabolism stimulated?	Effect of anaerobiosis on ADCC	CGD-phagocyte toxicity?
Fleer et al. 1979	MN	HRBC	Not done	Not done	Normal
Katz et al. 1980**	PMN, MN	HRBC	Not done	Not done	Decreased
Borregaard and Kragballe 1980	PMN, MN	HRBC	Yes	Decreased	Decreased
Klassen and Sagone 1980	MN	HRBC	Yes	Decreased	Decreased
Sagone et al. 1981	MN	HRBC	Yes	Decreased	Decreased
Koller and LoBuglio 1981	MN	HRBC	Not done	Decreased	Normal
Clark and Klebanoff 1977	PMN	Lymphoma	Not done	Not done	Decreased
Hafeman and Lucas 1979	PMN	Adenocarcinoma	Yes	Decreased	Not done
Siebens et al. 1979	PMN	Herpes-infected CEM	Not done	Not done	Normal
Katz et al. 1980	PMN	Lymphoid	Not done	Not done	Normal
Nathan and Cohn 1980	Macrophage	Lymphoma	Not done	Decreased	Not done
Klassen and Sagone 1980	MN	Lymphoblast	No	No effect	Normal

* MN = monocyte; PMN = polymorphonuclear leukocyte; HRBC = human red blood cell.
** Results of assays performed in suspension.

while CGD cells were only minimally active. Cytotoxicity was blocked by inhibitors of glycolysis or anti-microtubule agents and it was concluded that ADCC required a burst in oxidative metabolism, glycolysis and intact microtubular function.

Phagocyte-mediated ADCC against nucleated targets could not be inhibited by superoxide dismutase, catalase or oxygen metabolite scavengers in any of these systems (Clark and Klebanoff 1977b; Hafeman and Lucas 1979; Nathan and Cohn 1980; Klassen and Sagone 1980) and further attempts to implicate oxygen are indirect. Nathan and Cohn (1980) demonstrated that anaerobiosis, glucose deprivation or the addition of thioglycolate broth could inhibit H_2O_2 release from PMA-stimulated macrophages and similarly depress macrophage-mediated ADCC. Further evidence implicating H_2O_2 in the cytotoxic process was based on the increased susceptibility of BCNU-treated tumor cells (GSH reductase inhibited) to macrophage-mediated cytolysis (Nathan et al. 1980). However, macrophage-mediated ADCC was not enhanced against GSH depleted (buthionine sulfoximine treated) tumor cell targets (Arrick et al. 1982). At present, there is no evidence to support the role of other oxygen metabolites in macrophage, neutrophil or monocyte mediated, antibody-dependent destruction.

In summary, the precise role of oxygen metabolites in phagocyte-mediated ADCC remains unclear. A requirement for oxygen in this model is partially dependent on the effector cell, sensitizing antibody, target cell and assay conditions. Clearly, the inability to effectively utilize superoxide dismutase, catalase and oxygen metabolite scavengers hampers our analysis of this system. These same problems may account for a reported lack of dependence upon oxygen in other "physiological" models of phagocyte-mediated cytotoxicity (Weinberg and Hibbs 1977; Sorrel et al. 1978; Rinehart et al. 1978). However, preliminary results indicate that, in at least one model, immunologically activated macrophages can recognize and destroy tumor cells via a catalase-inhibitable process (personal communication M. L. Karnovsky; see Badwey and Karnovsky 1980, pp. 713–714).

At present, evidence implicating oxygen metabolites in phagocyte-mediated ADCC is indirect; however, the data are remarkably similar to those obtained in studies of phagocyte-dependent microbicidal mechanisms. First, depending on the particular micro-organism, normal phagocytes can destroy bacteria and fungi by either oxygen-dependent or oxygen-independent processes (for review see Root and Cohen 1981). Second, CGD phagocytes can also kill a variety of micro-organisms by oxygen-independent mechanisms (Root and Cohen 1981). Third, normal phagocytes can exert a microbicidal effect that is normally resistant to exogenous superoxide dismutase, catalase or oxygen metabolite scavengers (Root and Cohen 1981). These findings do not diminish the importance of oxygen metabolites in the microbicidal process nor should they in phagocyte-mediated ADCC. Rather, these data highlight the multiplicity of cytotoxic processes operable within the phagocyte.

Are there alternate schemes that might explain an oxygen requirement in ADCC or the inability of CGD phagocytes to mediate cytolysis that do not directly involve oxygen metabolites? Based on recent evidence associating the respiratory burst with extracellular (Van Zwieten et al. 1981) and phagosomal pH changes (Segal et al. 1981), one should not overlook the possibility of an altered pH (and possibly altered lysosomal enzyme activity) in the microenvironment at the effector cell—target cell interface. Nevertheless, oxygen metabolites can be generated during phagocyte-mediated ADCC and these species clearly possess a strong cytotoxic potential. The identification of sensitized targets that clearly stimulate the phagocytes' oxidative metabolism and the utilization of new techniques designed to insert exogenous enzymes between the activated effector cell and its target (enzymes coupled to the antibody or directly to the target cell membrane?) may provide new insights into the cytotoxic processes involved.

2.4. OXYGEN METABOLITES AND THE TRANSFORMATION OF SOLUBLE INFLAMMATORY MEDIATORS

As phagocytes migrate into an inflammatory focus they find themselves immersed in a complex milieu containing a variety of soluble, bioactive materials including enzymes, proteins, peptides, lipids and lipid oxidation products. The biological activity of this environment is in constant flux as mediators are generated, transformed or inactivated. Although the phagocyte can modulate the activity of a number of these components by processes independent of oxygen metabolites (see Chapters 3 and 5), the leukocytes may utilize products of the respiratory burst to modify the inflammatory response. In this section we will examine interactions between oxygen metabolites and 1) arachidonic acid, 2) methionine-containing peptides and proteins and 3) prostaglandin and leukotriene products.

2.4.1. Oxygen metabolites and arachidonic acid

Arachidonic acid oxidation products generated after auto-oxidation (Turner et al. 1975) or exposure to a $O_2^{\cdot -}$-H_2O_2 generating system (Perez et al. 1980) possess either chemokinetic and/or chemotactic activity for human neutrophils. The chemotactic factor produced by an acetaldehyde-xanthine oxidase system (generates $O_2^{\cdot -}$, H_2O_2 and secondary oxidants) required both $O_2^{\cdot -}$ and H_2O_2 for its generation (Perez et al. 1980). In a similar model, one of the major products formed after exposure of purified arachidonic acid to an acetaldehyde-xanthine oxidase system was 5-hydroperoxy-eicosatetraenoic acid, the initial metabolite of the arachidonic acid-lipoxygenase pathway (Fridovich and Porter 1981). Although chemotactic factor generation and arachidonic acid oxidation were dependent on the formation of a secondary oxygen metabolite, Petrone et al. (1980) demonstrated that xanthine-xanthine oxidase could transform serum albumin into a potent chemotactic factor by a mechanism dependent on $O_2^{\cdot -}$ alone. Apparently, $O_2^{\cdot -}$ reacted with a fatty acid—albumin complex to generate the chemotactic factor. The ability of intact phagocytes to mediate this reaction has not been reported but leukocyte infiltration into sites of induced inflammation was inhibited in superoxide dismutase-treated animals (Petrone et al. 1980). It appears that $O_2^{\cdot -}$ generated by stimulated phagocytes may react with plasma precursors to regulate chemotactic activity at inflammatory site.

2.4.2. Oxygen metabolites and methionine-containing compounds

A variety of methionine-containing compounds may be found at inflammatory sites and several of these mediators are sensitive to phagocyte-mediated oxidative reactions. Methionine has a highly nucleophilic thioether bond (RSR) that can be readily oxidized to its sulfoxide ($R-\overset{\displaystyle O}{\overset{\|}{S}}-R$; see below). If the thioether group is integral to the compound's activity and is accessible to the attacking oxidant, then loss of function will occur. At present, three groups of methionine-containing compounds sensitive to phagocyte-derived oxidants have been identified: 1) chemotactic factors, 2) peroxidase inhibitors, and 3) enkephalins.

2.4.2.1. Chemotactic factors

Phagocytes will migrate into an inflammatory focus as a direct response to the formation of chemotactic factors (see Chapter 3). The complement-derived agent, C5a (Clark and Klebanoff 1979a), and the oligopeptides, F-Met-Leu-Phe (Clark and Klebanoff 1979) or F-Met-Leu-Phe-Lys (Clark et al. 1980) are chemotactic factors that each contain a single methionine and can be inactivated by a model, H_2O_2—myeloperoxidase—halide system. Synthetic chemoattractants that do not contain methionine were not inactivated by this system (Clark et al. 1980). Additional studies have demonstrated that F-Met-Leu-Phe will also lose its chemotactic activity following exposure to a H_2O_2-horseradish peroxidase-I^- system (Anderson and Grabow 1980). These results suggested that methionine may be an important factor in determining the sensitivity of these compounds to peroxidase-mediated attack. Clark et al. (1980) examined the chromatographic characteristics of myeloperoxidase-treated F-Met-Leu-Phe and found that the product had an R_f value corresponding to a methionine-oxidized derivative. Subsequently, Tsan and co-workers demonstrated that intact, stimulated neutrophils could oxidize either free methionine (Tsan and Chen 1980) or the methionyl moiety of F-Met-Leu-Phe (Tsan and Denison 1981) to the corresponding sulfoxide by a H_2O_2-myeloperoxidase-Cl^- dependent mechanism. The key role of the myeloperoxidase system in this process was underlined by the inability of either CGD or hereditary myeloperoxidase-deficient neutrophils to inactivate the oligopeptide unless H_2O_2 or purified myeloperoxidase, respectively, were added (Clark and Szot 1982). Thus, intact phagocytes can utilize the H_2O_2—myeloperoxidase—halide system to inactivate chemotactic factors containing critical (and accessible) methionine residues.

2.4.2.2. α_1-Proteinase inhibitor

After phagocytes migrate into an inflammatory site they may discharge proteinases capable of degrading the surrounding connective tissue (see Chapter 3). The steady-state activity of these lysosomal enzymes is determined by the amount of enzyme released and the quantities inactivated by endogenous antiproteinases. Based on the sensitivity of α_1-proteinase inhibitor, a powerful antiproteinase, to chemical oxidation, Carp and Janoff speculated that phagocytes might indirectly enhance proteinase-mediated tissue destruction by oxidizing and inactivating the inhibitor (Carp and Janoff 1979). Indeed, immune complex-stimulated phagocytes could suppress the activity of α_1-proteinase inhibitor by a process that could be partially blocked by either superoxide dismutase, catalase, azide or mannitol. Similar results were obtained with PMA-stimulated phagocytes; however, OH· scavengers were not protective in this system (Carp and Janoff 1980).

Although the precise mechanisms involved in the phagocyte-mediated inactivation of α_1-proteinase inhibitor were unclear, Johnson and Travis (1979) demonstrated that the protein could be inhibited by chemical oxidation of a single methionyl residue at the reactive center to its sulfoxide. Subsequently, the ability of a H_2O_2-myeloperoxidase—halide system to inactivate the antiproteinase has been reported (Matheson et al 1979; Carp and Janoff 1980; Matheson et al. 1981; and Clark et al. 1981). Matheson et al. (1979, 1981) clearly demonstrated that the myeloperoxidase-inactivated α_1-proteinase inhibitor was identical in size to the native protein. However, amino acid analysis revealed that two methionyl residues were oxidized to the sulfoxide form, one of which represented the reactive-site methionine. This is not a general characteristic of antiproteinases and both α_1-antichymotrypsin and $_2$-macroglobulin are insensitive to the myeloperoxidase system under similar conditions (Matheson et al. 1979, 1981 and Clark et al. 1981).

Earlier studies demonstrated the ability of intact phagocytes (neutrophils, mononuclear cells and alveolar macrophages) to inactivate α_1-proteinase inhibitor by a mechanism only partially dependent on the myeloperoxidase system (Carp and Janoff 1979, 1980). Based on the sensitivity of the inhibitor to the model myeloperoxidase system, Clark et al. (1981) re-examined the ability of stimulated neutrophils to inactivate α_1-proteinase inhibitor and described a process solely dependent on H_2O_2, myeloperoxidase and a halide. Although these reports are contradictory, it seems likely that the electron-rich thioether bond of methionine is sensitive to a number of oxidants. High concentrations of H_2O_2 alone can oxidize methionine to its sulfoxide (Tsan and Chen 1980) and Carp and Janoff (1980) demonstrated the ability of a xanthine-xanthine oxidase system to inactivate α_1-proteinase inhibitor*. Indeed, PMA-stimulated alveolar macrophages could inactivate the antiproteinase despite the absence of a granule-associated peroxidase

*It is interesting to note the similarities between the effects of superoxide dismutase, catalase, myeloperoxidase inhibitors and OH· scavengers on phagocyte-mediated α_1-proteinase inactivation and ethylene generation from thioether probes (Section 2.2.4.).

(see, however, Matheson et al. 1981 and Klebanoff 1980b). Apparently, a number of oxidants may inactivate the α_1-proteinase inhibitor and the responsible species is dictated in part by the effector cell, the stimulus and the assay conditions.

2.4.2.3. Methionine-enkephalin

Met-enkephalin is a bioactive, endogenous peptide with morphine agonist activity. Turkall et al. (1982) demonstrated the ability of resting neutrophils to degrade the pentapeptide by releasing a single amino acid residue. However, when the neutrophils were stimulated, the enkephalin was both degraded and the methionyl residue oxidized to its sulfoxide. As expected, sulfoxide generation was dependent on the H_2O_2–myeloperoxidase–halide system. Because both the degradation products and the sulfoxide derivative have reduced opiate agonist activity, it was suggested that the neutrophil may contribute to the development of pain at an inflammatory focus.

2.4.3. Peroxidases and arachidonic acid metabolites

The oxidation of arachidonic acid by the cyclooxygenase or lipoxygenase pathways leads to the formation of a series of potent lipid mediators (see Chapter 5). Leukotrienes, a complex family of lipoxygenase derived products, were the first group of lipid compounds that appeared sensitive to attack by the peroxidase system. Henderson and Kaliner (1979) demonstrated that slow-reacting substance of anaphylaxis (primarily leukotrienes C_4 and D_4) could be inactivated by H_2O_2 and mast cell granule peroxidase in a Cl^--containing buffer. Because eosinophils can generate leukotrienes (Jörg et al. 1982), secrete eosinophil peroxidase and generate oxygen metabolites (section 2.2.3.), a potential interaction between lipoxygenase and eosinophil peroxidase-derived products was examined in this cell population. Indeed, a model H_2O_2–eosinophil peroxidase–halide system could inactivate leukotrienes B_4, C_4 and D_4 while the recovery of endogenous leukotrienes from stimulated eosinophils was enhanced in the presence of catalase or myeloperoxidase inhibitors (Henderson et al. 1982). Apparently, stimulated eosinophils both generate leukotrienes and inactivate a portion of these lipids by an eosinophil peroxidase-dependent process.

In addition to leukotrienes, a variety of prostaglandins also seem susceptible to neutrophil-mediated transformation. Paredes and Weiss (1982) demonstrated that stimulated neutrophils could rapidly transform large quantities of exogenous 6-keto-$PGF_{1\alpha}$, PGE_2 or $PGF_{2\alpha}$ as assessed by thin layer radiochromatography. Identical products were formed by a model H_2O_2-myeloperoxidase-Cl^- system and stimulated neutrophils did not transform prostaglandins in the presence of catalase or myeloperoxidase inhibitors. These data indicate that phagocytes can alter or transform a variety of arachidonic acid oxidation products by a H_2O_2-peroxidase-halide dependent process. The site of oxidant attack on these molecules has not been identified but leukotrienes C_4 and D_4 are thioether-containing compounds. In addition, the remainder of the sensitive lipids have multiple unsaturated carbon groups that may be susceptible to halogenation (e.g., Boeynaems and Hubbard 1980).

In summary, phagocytes may utilize their oxygen metabolites to modulate the intensity of the inflammatory response by interacting with a number of soluble mediators. $O_2^{\cdot -}$ is involved in the generation of a chemotactic factor and the inactivation of $_1$-proteinase inhibitor but the majority of the effects described are directly mediated by the peroxidase systems. Intact phagocytes appear capable of utilizing the H_2O_2—peroxidase—halide system to attack either thioether bonds or alkenes. However, based on the reactivity of the peroxidase-derived oxidants, a wider spectrum of targets may be affected. The myeloperoxidase system can attack N-terminal amino acids (Stelmaszynska and Zgliczynski 1979) and intact phagocytes can decarboxylate and deaminate both free amino acids (Strauss et al. 1971; Tsan and Denison 1981b; see, however, Adeniyi-Jones and Karnovsky 1981). Indeed, Matheson et al. (1979) reported the ability of a model H_2O_2—myeloperoxidase—Cl^- system to inactivate neutrophil cathepsin G or pancreatic trypsin by oxidizing critical tryptophan residues. (For other examples of susceptible targets see Albrich et al. 1981.) Thus, the sensitivity of a given molecule is dictated by the susceptibility of the groups found at the reactive site and its accessibility to the generated oxidant.

At present, the peroxidase-derived oxidants responsible for those effects have not been directly identified but the hypohalous acids are the most likely candidates. Hypohalous acids can oxidize thioethers (Tsan and Chen 1980) and halogenate alkenes (Downs and Adams 1973). Although amino acids, compounds known to react rapidly with HOCl, failed to inhibit methionine oxidation in some systems (e.g., see Tsan and Denison 1981a or Turkall et al. 1982), it is important to note that the product of this interaction is a chloramine, a powerful oxidant that may proceed to oxidize the thioether. In a similar manner, the formation of chloramine may explain the ability of a peroxidase-derived oxidant to diffuse through serum to inactivate α_1-proteinase inhibitor (Carp and Janoff 1979, 1980 and Clark et al. 1981). Indeed, chloramines may be an excellent example of a "secondary" oxidant that is less reactive than the original species (i.e., HOCl) but is more selective in its action.

Finally, is there any in-vivo evidence to support a role for oxidative-control of the inflammatory response? As discussed by Clark et al. (1982), CGD patients frequently develop large and multiple abscesses and some myeloperoxidase-deficient patients may develop fungal abscesses or inflammatory skin lesions. It is especially intriguing to note that inactivated α_1-proteinase inhibitor recovered from either rheumatoid synovial fluid (Wong and Travis 1980) or the lungs of cigarette smokers (Carp et al. 1982) contains methionyl sulfoxide residues. Additional evidence indicates that these changes are reversible and that the biological activity of α_1-proteinase inhibitor can be restored by enzyme systems capable of reducing the sulfoxide (Abrams et al. 1982). These data suggest that the ultimate course of the inflammatory response may be regulated by a complex equilibrium between rates of activation, inactivation and reactivation of the soluble mediators.

2.5. SUMMARY

In summary, we have reviewed the ability of phagocytes to consume and metabolize oxygen to generate a diverse array of reactive intermediates. Evidence obtained from in-vitro model systems has demonstrated the ability of these oxygen metabolites to alter cell function, mediate cytotoxicity or transform inflammatory mediators. Currently, the data suggest that $O_2^{\cdot -}$, H_2O_2, hypohalous acids and the OH· may all be utilized either separately or in concert by the phagocyte to mediate oxygen-dependent inflammatory events. Depending on the particular set of in-vivo circumstances, phagocyte-derived oxygen metabolites could play a pivotal role in host defense, host tissue destruction and the modulation of the inflammatory response. Hopefully, an understanding of the biochemistry of these events will allow us to manipulate the phagocyte and the inflammatory response to augment host defense or attenuate tissue destruction in a variety of pathological states.

ACKNOWLEDGEMENTS

This study was supported in part by PHS grant No. R01 A1-16524-03, awarded by the National Institute of Allergy and Infectious Disease, and PHS grant No. HL-28024-01, awarded by the National Institute of Heart and Lung Disease.

REFERENCES

Abrams, W.R., Weinbaum, G., Weissbach, L., Weissbach, H. and Brot, N. (1981) Enzymatic reduction of oxidized α-1-proteinase inhibitor restores biological activity. *Proc. Natl. Acad. Sci. USA 78,* 7483–7486.

Adams, D.D., Johnson, W.J., Fiorito, E. and Nathan, C.F. (1981) Hydrogen peroxide and cytolytic factor can interact synergistically in effecting cytolysis of neoplastic targets. *J. Immunol. 127,* 1973–1977.

Adeniyi-Jones, S.K. and Karnovsky, M.L. (1981) Oxidative decarboxylation of free and peptide-linked amino acids in phagocytizing guinea pig granulocytes. *J. Clin. Invest. 68,* 365–373.

Aebi, H.E. and Wyss, S.R. (1978) Acatalasemia. In: J.B. Stanbury, J.B. Wyngaarden and D.S. Frederickson (Eds), *The Metabolic Basis of Inherited Disease,* 4th edn., McGraw-Hill Book Co., New York, pp. 1792–1807.

Albrich, J.M., McCarthy, C.A. and Hurst, J.K. (1981) Biological reactivity of hypochlorous acid: implications for microbicidal mechanisms of leukocyte myeloperoxidase. *Proc. Natl. Acad. Sci. USA 78,* 210–214.

Ambruso, D.R. and Johnston, R.B. (1981) Lactoferrin enhances hydroxyl radical production by human neutrophils, neutrophil particulate fractions, and an enzymatic generating system. *J. Clin. Invest. 67,* 352–360.

Anderson, R. and Grabow, G. (1980) In vitro stimulation of neutrophil motility by metoprolol and sotalol related to inhibition of both H_2O_2 production and peroxidase mediated iodination of the cell and leucoattractant. *Int. J. Immunopharmacol. 2,* 321–331.

Arrick, B.A., Nathan, C.F., Griffith, O.W. and Cohn, Z.A. (1982) Glutathionine depletion sensitizes tumor cells to oxidative cytolysis. *J. Biol. Chem. 257,* 1231–1237.

Babior, B.M. (1978) Oxygen-dependent microbial killing by phagocytes. *N. Engl. J. Med. 298,* 659–668, 721–725.

Badwey, J.A. and Karnovsky, M.L. (1980) Active oxygen species and the functions of phagocytic leukocytes. *Ann. Rev. Biochem. 49,* 695–726.

Baehner, R.L., Nathan, D.G. and Castle, W.B. (1971) Oxidant injury of caucasian glucose-6-phosphate dehydrogenase-deficient red blood cells by phagocytosing leukocytes during infection. *J. Clin. Invest. 50,* 2466–2473.

Baehner, R.L., Boxer, L.A. and Davis, J. (1976) The biochemical basis of nitroblue tetrazolium reduction in normal and chronic granulomatous disease polymorphonuclear leukocytes. *Blood 48,* 309–313.

Baehner, R.L., Boxer, L.A., Allen, J.M. and Davis, J. (1977) Autooxidation as a basis for altered function by polymorphonuclear leukocytes. *Blood 50,* 327–335.

Bartosz, G., Fried, R., Grzelinska, E. and Leyko, W. (1977) Effect of hyperoxide radicals on bovine-erythrocyte membrane. *Eur. J. Biochem. 73,* 261–264.

Beauchamp, C. and Fridovich, I. (1970) A mechanism for the production of ethylene from methional. *J. Biol. Chem. 245,* 4641–4646.

Bielski, B.H.J. and Chan, P.C. (1976) Re-evaluation of the kinetics of lactate dehydrogenase-catalyzed chain oxidation of nicotinamide adenine dinucleotide by superoxide radicals in the presence of ethylenediamine-tetraacetate. *J. Biol. Chem. 251,* 3841–3844.

Bielski, B.H.J. and Shiue, G.G. (1979) Reaction rates of superoxide radicals with the essential amino acids. In: *Oxygen Free Radicals and Tissue Damage,* Ciba Foundation Symposium 65, Excerpta Medica, Amsterdam, pp. 43–48.

Boeynaems, J.-M. and Hubbard, W.C. (1980) Transformation of arachidonic acid into an iodolactone by the rat thyroid. *J. Biol. Chem 255,* 9001–9004.

Borregaard, N. and Kragballe, K. (1980) Role of oxygen in antibody-dependent cytotoxicity mediated by monocytes and neutrophils. *J. Clin. Invest. 66,* 676–683.

Bors, W., Michel, C. and Saran, M. (1979) On the nature of biochemically generated hydroxyl radicals: Studies using bleaching of p-nitrosodimethylaniline as a direct assay method. *Eur. J. Biochem. 95,* 621–627.

Bos, A., Wever, R. and Roos, D. (1978) Characterization and quantification of the peroxidase in human monocytes. *Biochim. Biophys. Acta 525,* 37–44.

Boxer, L.A. and Stossel, T.P. (1974) Effects of anti-human neutrophil antibodies in vitro: quantitative studies. *J. Clin. Invest. 53,* 1543–1545.

Boxer, L.A., Richardson, S.B. and Baehner, R.L. (1978) Effects of surface-active agents in neutrophil receptors. *Infect. Immun. 21,* 28–33.

Bozzi, A., Mavelli, I., Mondovi, B., Strom, R. and Rotilio, G. (1979) Differential sensitivity of tumor cells to externally generated hydrogen peroxide: role of glutathione and related enzymes. *Cancer Biochem. Biophys. 3,* 135–141.

Capsoni, F., Meroni, P.L., Ciboddo, G.F. and Colombo, G. (1979) Cytotoxic mechanisms in white blood cells (Letter). *N. Engl. J. Med. 300,* 44.

Carp, H. and Janoff, A. (1979) In vitro suppression of serum elastase-inhibitory capacity by reactive oxygen species generated by phagocytosing polymorphonuclear leukocytes. *J. Clin. Invest. 63,* 793–797.

Carp, H. and Janoff, A. (1980) Potential mediator of inflammation: phagocyte-derived oxidants suppress the elastase-inhibitory capacity of α_1-proteinase inhibitor in vitro. *J. Clin. Invest. 66,* 987–995.

Carp, H., Miller, F., Hoidal, J. and Janoff, A. (1982) Potential mechanism of emphysema: α_1-proteinase inhibitor recovered from lungs of cigarette smokers contains oxidized methionine and has decreased elastase inhibitory capacity. *Proc. Natl. Acad. Sci. USA 79,* 2041–2045.

Casciato, D.A., Goldberg, L.S. and Bluestone, R. (1978) Polymorphonuclear neutrophil chemotaxis under aerobic and anaerobic conditions. *Infect. Immun. 21,* 381–386.

Clark, R.A. and Klebanoff, S.J. (1975) Neutrophil-mediated tumor cell cytotoxicity: role of the peroxidase system. *J. Exp. Med. 141,* 1442–1447.

Clark, R.A. and Klebanoff, S.J. (1977a) Myeloperoxidase–H_2O_2–halide systems: cytotoxic effect on human blood leukocytes. *Blood 50,* 65–70.

Clark, R.A. and Klebanoff, S.J. (1977b) Studies on the mechanism of antibody-dependent polymorphonuclear leukocyte-mediated cytotoxicity. *J. Immunol. 119,* 1413–1418.

Clark, R.A. and Klebanoff, S.J. (1979a) Chemotactic factor inactivation by the myeloperoxidase–hydrogen peroxide–halide system. *J. Clin. Invest. 64,* 913–920.

Clark, R.A. and Klebanoff, S.J. (1979b) Myeloperoxidase-mediated platelet release reaction. *J. Clin. Invest. 63,* 177–183.

Clark, R.A. and Klebanoff, S.J. (1979c) Role of the myeloperoxidase–H_2O_2–halide system in concanavalin A-induced tumor cell killing by human neutrophils. *J. Immunol. 122,* 2605–2610.

Clark, R.A. and Klebanoff, S.J. (1980) Neutrophil–platelet interaction mediated by myeloperoxidase and hydrogen peroxide. *J. Immunol. 124,* 399–405.

Clark, R.A. and Szot, S. (1981) The myeloperoxidase–hydrogen peroxide halide system as effector of neutrophil-mediated tumor cell cytotoxicity. *J. Immunol. 126,* 1295–1301.

Clark, R.A. and Szot, S. (1982) Chemotactic factor inactivation by stimulated human neutrophils mediated by myeloperoxidase-catalyzed methionine oxidation. *J. Immunol. 128,* 1507–1513.

Clark, R.A., Szot, S., Venkatasubramanian, K. and Schiffmann, E. (1980) Chemotactic factor inactivation by myeloperoxidase-mediated oxidation of methionine. *J. Immunol. 124,* 2020–2026.

Clark, R.A., Stone, P.J., El Hag, A., Calore, J.D. and Franzblau, C. (1981) Myeloperoxidase-catalyzed inactivation of α_1-protease inhibitor by human neutrophils. *J. Biol. Chem. 256,* 3348–3353.

Cohen, G. (1977) In defense of Haber-Weiss. In: A.M. Michelson, J.M. McCord and I. Fridovich (Eds), *Superoxide and Superoxide Dismutases,* Academic Press, New York, pp. 316–321.

Cohen, G. and Hochstein, P. (1963) Glutathione peroxidase: the primary agent for the elimination of hydrogen peroxide in erythrocytes. *Biochemistry 2,* 1420–1428.

Cohen, M.S., Metcalf, J.A. and Root, R.K. (1980) Regulation of oxygen metabolism in human granulocytes: relationship between stimulus binding and oxidative response using plant lectins as probes. *Blood 55,* 1003–1010.

Craddock, P.R., Hammerschmidt, D.E., Moldow, C.F., Yamado, D. and Jacob, H.S. (1979) Granulocyte aggregation as a manifestation of membrane interactions with complement: possible role of leukocyte margination, microvascular occlusion and endothelial damage. *Semin. Hematol. 16,* 140−147.

Diguiseppi, J. and Fridovich, I. (1980) Ethylene from 2-keto-4-thiomethyl butyric acid: the Haber-Weiss reaction. *Arch. Biochem. Biophys. 205,* 323−329.

Dilworth, J.A. and Mandell, G.L. (1977) Adults with chronic granulomatous disease of childhood. *Am. J. Med. 63,* 233−243.

Downs, A.J. and Adams, C.J. (1973) Hypohalous acids and hapohalites. In: J.C. Bailar, H.J. Emeleus, R. Nyholm and A.F. Trotman-Dickenson (Eds), *Comprehensive Inorganic Chemistry,* Pergamon Press, Ltd., Oxford, pp. 1399−1412.

Drath, D.B., Karnovsky, M.L. and Huber, G.L. (1979) Hydroxyl radical formation in phagocytic cells of the rat. *J. Appl. Physiol. 46,* 136−140.

Fee, J.A. and Valentine, J.S. (1977) Chemical and physical properties of superoxide. In: A.M. Michelson, J.M. McCord and I. Fridovich (Eds), *Superoxide and Superoxide Dismutases,* Academic Press, New York, pp. 19-60.

Ferrante, A., Beard, L.J. and Thong, Y.H. (1980) Early decay of human neutril chemotactic responsiveness following isolation from peripheral blood. *Clin. Exp. Immunol. 39,* 532−537.

Finkelstein, E., Rosen, G.M. and Rauckman, E.J. (1980) Spin trapping of superoxide and hydroxyl radical: practical aspects. *Arch. Biochem. Biophys. 200,* 1−16.

Fleer, A., Roos, D., Von Dem Borne, A.E.G.K. and Engelfriet, C.P. (1979) Cytotoxic activity of human monocyte towards sensitized red cells is not dependent on the generation of reactive oxygen species. *Blood 54,* 407−411.

Foote, C.S. (1979) Detection of singlet oxygen in complex systems: a critique. In: W.S. Caughey (Ed.), *Biochemical and Clinical Aspects of Oxygen,* Academic Press, Inc., New York, pp. 603−626.

Fridovich, I. (1976) Oxygen radicals, hydrogen peroxide and oxygen toxicity. In: W.A. Pryor (Ed.), *Free Radicals in Biology, Vol. 1,* Academic Press, New York, pp. 239−277.

Fridovich, I. (1978) The biology of oxygen radicals. *Science 201,* 875−880.

Fridovich, S.E. and Porter, N.A. (1981) Oxidation of arachidonic acid in micelles by superoxide and hydrogen peroxide. *J. Biol. Chem. 256,* 260−285.

Gabig, T.G., Bearman, S.I. and Babior, B.M. (1979) Effects of oxygen tension and pH on the respiratory burst of human neutrophils. *Blood 53,* 1133−1139.

Goldstein, I.M. (1979) Polymorphonuclear leukocyte functions: role of the plasma membrane. In: *Current Topics in Hematology Vol. 2,* Alan P. Liss, Inc., New York, pp. 145−202.

Goldstein, I.M., Roos, D., Kaplan, H.B. and Weissman, G. (1975) Complement and immunoglobulins stimulate superoxide production by human leukocytes independently of phagocytosis. *J. Clin. Invest. 56,* 1155−1163.

Goldstein, I.M., Kaplan, H.B., Radin, A. and Frosch, M. (1976) Independent effects of IgG and complement upon human polymorphonuclear leukocyte function. *J. Immunol. 117,* 1282−1287.

Green, M.R., Hill, A.D., Okolow-Zubkowska, M.J. and Segal, A.W. (1979) The production of hydroxyl and superoxide radicals by stimulated human neutrophils: measurements by EPR spectroscopy. *FEBS Lett. 100,* 23−26.

Greene, W.H., Colclough, L., Anton, A. and Root, R.K. (1980) Lectin-dependent neutrophil-mediated cytotoxicity against chicken erythrocytes: a model of non-myeloperoxidase-mediated oxygen-dependent killing by human neutrophils. *J. Immunol. 125,* 2727–2734.

Hafeman, D.G. and Lucas, Z.J. (1979) Polymorphonuclear leukocyte-mediated, antibody-dependent, cellular cytotoxicity against tumor cells: dependence on oxygen and the respiratory burst. *J. Immunol. 123,* 55–62.

Hafeman, D.G., Parce, J.W. and McConnel, H.M. (1979) Specific antibody dependent activation of neutrophils by liposomes containing spin-label lipid haptens. *Biochem. Biophys. Res. Commun. 86,* 522–528.

Hafeman, D.G., Lewis, J.T. and McConnel, H.M. (1980) Triggering of the macrophage and neutrophil respiratory burst by antibody bound to a spin-label phospholipid hapten in model lipid bilayer membranes. *Biochemistry 19,* 5287–5394.

Hafeman, D.G., Von Tscharner, V. and McConnel, H.M. (1981) Specific antibody-dependent interactions between macrophages and lipid haptens in planar lipid monolayers. *Proc. Natl. Acad. Sci. USA 78,* 4552–4556.

Halliwell, B. (1981) The biological effects of the superoxide radical and its products. *Bull. Eur. Physiopathol. Respir. 17 (Suppl.),* 21–28.

Handin, R.I., and Stossel, T.P. (1974) Phagocytosis of antibody coated platelets by human granulocytes. *N. Engl. J. Med. 290,* 989–993.

Handin, R.I., Karabin, R. and Boxer, G.J. (1977) Enhancement of platelet function by superoxide anion. *J. Clin. Invest. 59,* 959–965.

Harlan, J.M., Killen, P.D., Harker, L.A., Striker, G.E. and Wright, D.G. (1981) Neutrophil-mediated endothelial injury in vitro: mechanism of cell detachment. *J. Clin. Invest. 68,* 1394–1403.

Harris, R.E., Boxer, L.A. and Baehner, R.L. (1980) Consequences of vitamin-E deficiency on the phagocytic and oxidative functions of the rat polymorphonuclear leukocyte. *Blood 55,* 338–343.

Harrison, J.E. and Schultz, J. (1976) Studies on the chlorinating activity of myeloperoxidase. *J. Biol. Chem. 251,* 1371–1374.

Harrison, J.E., Watson, B.S. and Schultz, J. (1978) Myeloperoxidase and singlet oxygen: a reappraisal. *FEBS Lett. 92,* 327–332.

Harvath, L. and Andersen, B.R. (1979) Defective initiation of oxidative metabolism in polymorphonuclear leukocytes. *N. Engl. J. Med. 300,* 1130–1135.

Hassan, H.M., Dougherty, H. and Fridovich, I. (1980) Inhibitors of superoxide dismutases: a cautionary tale. *Arch. Biochem. Biophys. 199,* 349–354.

Heifets, L., Imai, K. and Goren, M.B. (1980) Expression of peroxidase-dependent iodination by macrophages ingesting neutrophil debris. *J. Reticuloendothel. Soc. 28,* 391–404.

Held, A.M. and Hurst, J.K. (1978) Ambiguity associated with the use of singlet oxygen trapping agents in myeloperoxidase catalyzed oxidations. *Biochem. Biophys. Res. Commun. 81,* 878–885.

Henderson, W.R. and Kaliner, M. (1979) Mast cell granule peroxidase: location, secretion and SRS-A inactivation. *J. Immunol. 122,* 1322–1328.

Henderson, W.R., Chi, E.Y. and Klebanoff, S.J. (1980a) Eosinophil peroxidase-induced mast cell secretion. *J. Exp. Med. 152,* 265–279.

Henderson, W.R., Jong, E.C. and Klebanoff, S.J. (1980b) Binding of eosinophil peroxidase to mast cell granules with retention of peroxidase activity. *J. Immunol. 124,* 1383−1388.

Henderson, W.R., Chi, E.Y., Jong, E.C. and Klebanoff, S.J. (1981) Mast cell-mediated tumor-cell cytotoxicity. *J. Exp. Med. 153,* 520−533.

Henderson, W.R., Jörg, A. and Klebanoff, S.J. (1982) Eosinophil peroxidase-mediated inactivation of leukotrienes B_4, C_4, D_4. *J. Immunol.* 126, 2609−2613.

Henney, C.S. (1977) Mechanisms of tumor cell destruction. In: I. Green, S. Cohen and R.T. McCluskey (Eds), *Mechanisms of Tumor Immunity,* John Wiley and Sons, New York, pp. 55−86.

Henson, P. and Oades, Z.G. (1975) Stimulation of human neutrophils by soluble and insoluble immunoglobulin aggregates: secretion of granule constituents and increased oxidation of glucose. *J. Clin. Invest. 56,* 1053−1061.

Hodgson, E.K. and Fridovich, I. (1975a) The interaction of bovine erythrocyte superoxide dismutase with hydrogen peroxide: inactivation of the enzyme. *Biochemistry 14,* 5294−5298.

Hodgson, E.K. and Fridovich, I. (1975b) The interaction of bovine erythrocyte superoxide dismutase with hydrogen peroxide: chemiluminescence and peroxidation. *Biochemistry 14,* 5299−5303.

Hoidal, J.R., Beall, G.D. and Repine, J.E. (1979) Production of hydroxyl radical by human alveolar macrophages. *Infect. Immun. 26,* 1088−1092.

Holmsen, H. and Robkin, L. (1977) Hydrogen peroxide lowers ATP levels in platelets without altering adenylate energy charge and platelet function. *J. Biol. Chem. 252,* 1752−1757.

Jacob, H.S., Ingbar, S.H. and Jandl, J.H. (1965) Oxidative hemolysis and erythrocyte metabolism in hereditary acatalasia. *J. Clin. Invest. 44,* 1187−1199.

Jandl, R.C., Andre-Schwartz, J., Borges-Dubois, L., Kipnes, R., McMurrich, B.J. and Babior, B.M. (1978) Termination of the respiratory burst in human neutrophils. *J. Clin. Invest. 61,* 1176−1185.

Johnson, D. and Travis, J. (1979) The oxidative inactivation of human α1-proteinase inhibitor. *J. Biol. Chem. 254,* 4022-4026.

Johnston, R.B. (1978) Oxygen metabolism and the microbicidal activity of macrophages. *Fed. Proc. 37,* 2759−2764.

Johnston, R.B., Keele, B.B., Misra, H.P., Lehmeyer, J.E., Webb, L.S., Baehner, R.L. and Rajagopolan, K.V. (1975) The role of superoxide anion generation in phagocytic bactericidal activity: studies with normal and chronic granulomatous disease leukocytes. *J. Clin. Invest. 55,* 1357−1372.

Johnston, R.B. and Lehmeyer, J.E. (1976) Elaboration of toxic oxygen by-products by neutrophils in a model of immune complex disease. *J. Clin. Invest. 57,* 836−841.

Johnston, R.B., Lehmeyer, J.E. and Guthrie, L.A. (1976) Generation of superoxide anion and chemiluminescence by human monocytes during phagocytosis and on contact with surface bound immunoglobulin G. *J. Exp. Med. 143,* 1551−1556.

Jong, E.C. and Klebanoff, S.J. (1980) Eosinophil-mediated mammalian tumor cell cytotoxicity: role of the peroxidase system. *J. Immunol. 124,* 1949−1953.

Jörg, A., Henderson, W.R., Murphy, R.C. and Klebanoff, S.J. (1982) Leukotriene generation by eosinophils. *J. Exp. Med. 155,* 390−402.

Katz, P., Simone, C.B., Henkart, P.A. and Fauci, A.S. (1980) Mechanisms of antibody-dependent cellular cytotoxicity: the use of effector cells from chronic granulomatous disease patients as investigative probes. *J. Clin. Invest. 65,* 55–63.

Keilin, D. and Hartree, E.F. (1945) Properties of azide-catalase. *Biochem. J. 39,* 148–157.

Keilin, D. and Hartree, E.F. (1955) Catalase, peroxidase and metmyoglobin as catalysts of coupled peroxidatic reactions. *Biochem. J. 60,* 310–325.

Keisari, Y. and Pick, E. (1981) Macrophage-mediated cytolysis of erythrocytes in the guinea pig: Activation by stimulators of the oxidative burst. *Cell. Immunol. 62,* 172–185.

Kellog, E.W., Yost, M.G., Barthakur, N. and Kreuger, A.P. (1979) Superoxide involvement in the bactericidal effects of negative air ions on Staphylococcus albus. *Nature (London) 281,* 400–401.

Klassen, D.K. and Sagone, A.L. (1980) Evidence for both oxygen and non-oxygen dependent mechanisms of antibody sensitized target cell lysis by human monocytes. *Blood 56,* 985–992.

Klebanoff, S.J. (1969) Anti-microbial activity of catalase at acid pH. *Proc. Soc. Exp. Biol. Med. 132,* 571–574.

Klebanoff, S.J. (1980a) Oxygen metabolism and the toxic properties of phagocytes. *Ann. Intern. Med. 93,* 480–490.

Klebanoff, S.J. (1980b) Oxygen intermediates and the microbicidal event. In: R. Van Furth (Ed.), *Mononuclear Phagocytes, Functional Aspects, Part II,* Martinus Nijhoff, The Hague, pp. 1105–1141.

Klebanoff, S.J. and Clark, R.A. (1978) *The Neutrophil: Function and Clinical Disorders,* Elsevier/North-Holland Publ. Co., Amsterdam.

Klebanoff, S.J. and Rosen, H. (1978) Ethylene formation by polymorphonuclear leukocytes: Role of myeloperoxidase. *J. Exp. Med. 148,* 490–506.

Klock, J.C. and Stossel, T.P. (1977) Detection, pathogenesis, and prevention of damage to human granulocytes caused by interaction with nylon wool fiber: implications for filtration leukapheresis. *J. Clin. Invest. 60,* 1183–1190.

Koller, C.A. and LoBuglio, A.F. (1981) Monocyte-mediated antibody-dependent cell-mediated cytotoxicity: the role of the metabolic burst. *Blood 58,* 293–299.

Kraut, E.H. and Sagone, A.L. (1981) The effect of oxidant injury on the lymphocyte membrane and functions. *J. Lab. Clin. Med. 98,* 697–703.

Levine, P.H., Weinger, R.S., Simon, J., Scoon, K.L. and Krinsky, N.I. (1976) Leukocyte–platelet interaction: Release of hydrogen peroxide by granulocytes as a modulator of platelet reactions. *J. Clin. Invest. 57,* 955–963.

Levine, P.H., Sladdin, D.G. and Krinsky, N.I. (1981) Superoxide, xanthine oxidase and platelet reactions: Further studies on mechanisms by which oxidants influence platelets. *Thrombos. Haemostas. 45,* 290–293.

Lew, P.D., Southwick, F.S., Stossel, T.P., Whitin, J.C., Simons, E. and Cohen, H.J. (1981) A variant of chronic granulomatous disease: deficient oxidative metabolism due to a low affinity NADPH oxidase. *N. Engl. J. Med. 305,* 1329–1333.

Lewis, J.T., Hafeman, D.G. and McConnel, H.M. (1980) Kinetics of antibody-dependent binding of haptenated phospholipid vesicles to a macrophage-related cell line. *Biochemistry 19,* 5376–5386.

LoBuglio, A.F., Cotran, R.S. and Jandl, J.H. (1967) Red cells coated with immunoglobulin G: binding and sphering by mononuclear cells in man. *Science 158,* 1582–1585.

Long, C.A. and Bielski, B.H.J. (1980) Rate of reaction of superoxide radical with chloride containing species. *J. Phys. Chem. 84,* 555–557.

Lynch, R.E. and Fridovich, I. (1978a) Effects of superoxide on the erythrocyte membrane. *J. Biol. Chem. 253,* 1838–1845.

Lynch, R.E. and Fridovich, I. (1978b) Permeation of the erythrocyte stroma by superoxide radical. *J. Biol. Chem. 253,* 4697–4699.

Lynch, R.E., Lee, G.R. and Cartwright, G.E. (1976) Inhibition by superoxide dismutase of methemoglobin formation from oxyhemoglobin. *J. Biol. Chem. 251,* 1015–1019.

Matheson, N.R., Wong, P.S. and Travis, J. (1979) Enzymatic inactivation of human α-1-proteinase inhibitor by neutrophil myeloperoxidase. *Biochem. Biophys. Res. Commun. 88,* 402–409.

Matheson, N.R., Wong, P.S., Schuyler, M. and Travis, J. (1981) Interaction of human α-1-proteinase inhibitor with neutrophil myeloperoxidase. *Biochemistry 20,* 331–336.

May, J.M. and deHaen, C. (1979) Insulin-stimulated intracellular hydrogen peroxide production in rat epididymal fat cells. *J. Biol. Chem. 254,* 2214–2220.

McGee, M.P. and Myrvik, Q.N. (1979) Phagocytosis-induced injury of normal and activated alveolar macrophages. *Infect. Immun. 26,* 910–915.

Mead, J.F. (1976) Free radical mechanisms of lipid damage and consequences for cellular membranes. In: W.A. Pryor (Ed.), *Free Radicals in Biology, Vol. 1,* Academic Press, New York, pp. 51–68.

Metzger, Z., Hoffeld, J.T. and Oppenheim, J.J. (1980) Macrophage-mediated suppression. I. Evidence for participation of both hydrogen peroxide and prostaglandins in suppression of murine lymphocyte proliferation. *J. Immunol. 124,* 983–988.

Mukherjee, S.P. and Lynn, W.S. (1977) Reduced nicotinamide adenine dinucleotide phosphate oxidase in adipocyte plasma membrane and its activation by insulin: possible role in the hormone's effects on adenylate cyclase and the hexose monophosphate shunt. *Arch. Biochem. Biophys. 184,* 69–76.

Murray, H.W., Juanghanich, C.W., Nathan, C.F. and Cohn, Z.A. (1979) Macrophage oxygen dependent antimicrobial activity. II. The role of oxygen intermediates. *J. Exp. Med. 150,* 950–964.

Naskalski, J.W. (1977) Myeloperoxidase inactivation in the course of catalysis of chlorination of taurine. *Biochim. Biophys. Acta 485,* 291–300.

Nathan, C. and Cohn, Z. (1980) Role of oxygen-dependent mechanisms in antibody-induced lysis of tumor cells by activated macrophages. *J. Exp. Med. 152,* 198–208.

Nathan, C.F., Brukner, L.H., Silverstein, S.C. and Cohn, Z.A. (1979a) Extracellular cytolysis by activated macrophages and granulocytes. I. Pharmacologic triggering of effector cells and the release of hydrogen peroxide. *J. Exp. Med. 149,* 84–99.

Nathan, C.F., Silverstein, S.C., Brukner, L.H. and Cohn, Z.A. (1979b) Extracellular cytolysis by activated macrophages and granulocytes. II. Hydrogen peroxide as a mediator of cytotoxicity. *J. Exp. Med. 149,* 100–113.

Nathan, C.F., Arrick, B.A., Murray, H.W., DeSantis, N.M. and Cohn, Z.A. (1980) Tumor cell anti-oxidant defenses: inhibition of the glutathionine redox cycle enhances macrophage-mediated cytolysis. *J. Exp. Med. 153,* 766–782.

Nelson, R.D., McCormack, R.T., Fiegel, V.D., Herron, M., Simmons, R.L. and Quie, P.G. (1979) Chemotactic deactivation of human neutrophils: Possible relationship to stimulation of oxidative metabolism. *Infect. Immun. 23,* 282–286.

Newman, S.L. and Johnston, R.B. (1979) Role of binding through C3b and IgG in polymorphonuclear neutrophil function: studies with trypsin-generated C3b. *J. Immunol. 123,* 1839–1846.

Nichols, B.A., Bainton, D.F. and Farquhar, M.G. (1971) Differentiation of monocytes, origin, nature and fate of their azurophil granules. *J. Cell Biol. 50,* 498–515.

Nishikimi, M., Yamada, H. and Yaki, K. (1980) Oxidation by superoxide of tocopherols dispersed in aqueous media with deoxycholate. *Biochim. Biophys. Acta 627,* 101–108.

Odajima, T. and Yamazaki, I. (1972) Myeloperoxidase of the leukocyte of normal blood. III. The reaction of ferric myeloperoxidase with superoxide anion. *Biochim. Biophys. Acta 284,* 355–359.

Paredes, J.-M. and Weiss, S.J. (1982) Human neutrophils transform prostaglandins by a myeloperoxidase-dependent mechanism. *J. Biol. Chem. 257,* 2738–2740.

Parry, M.F., Root, R.K., Metcalf, J.A., Delaney, K.K., Kaplow, L.S. and Richar, W.J. (1981) Myeloperoxidase deficiency: prevalence and clinical significance. *Ann. Intern. Med. 95,* 293–301.

Patscheke, H., Paschen, W. and Worner, P. (1978) Superoxide-independent platelet response to xanthine oxidase. *Hoppe-Seyler's Z. Physiol. Chem. 359,* 933–937.

Pearson, G.R. (1978) In vitro and in vivo investigations on antibody-dependent cellular cytotoxicity. *Curr. Top. Microbiol. Immunol. 80,* 65–90.

Penniall, R. and Spitznagel, J.K. (1975) Chicken neutrophils: oxidative metabolism in phagocytic cells devoid of myeloperoxidase. *Proc. Natl. Acad. Sci. USA 72,* 5012–5015.

Perez, H.D., Weksler, B.B. and Goldstein, I.M. (1980) Generation of a chemotactic lipid from arachidonic acid by exposure to a superoxide-generating system. *Inflammation 4,* 313–328.

Petrone, W.F., English, D.K., Wong, K. and McCord, J.M. (1980) Free radicals and inflammation: Superoxide-dependent activation of a neutrophil chemotactic factor in plasma. *Proc. Natl. Acad. Sci. USA 77,* 1159–1163.

Ramsey, P.G., Martin, T., Chi, E. and Klebanoff, S.J. (1982) Arming of mononuclear phagocytes by eosinophil peroxidase bound to Staphylococcus aureus. *J. Immunol. 128,* 415–420.

Ravindranath, S.D. and Fridovich, I. (1975) Isolation and characterization of a manganese-containing superoxide dismutase from yeast. *J. Biol. Chem. 250,* 6107–6112.

Reiss, M. and Roos, D. (1978) Differences in oxygen metabolism of phagocytosing monocytes and neutrophils. *J. Clin. Invest. 61,* 480–488.

Repine, J.E., Eaton, J.W., Anders, M.W., Hoidal, J.R. and Fox, R.B. (1979) Generation of hydroxyl radical by enzymes, chemicals and human phagocytes in vitro. *J. Clin. Invest. 64,* 1642–1651.

Repine, J.E., Fox, R.B. and Berger, E.M. (1981) Hydrogen peroxide kills Staphylococcus aureus by reacting with Staphylococcal iron to form hydroxyl radical. *J. Biol. Chem. 256,* 7094–7096.

Rinehart, J.J., Lange, P., Gormus, B.J. and Kaplan, M.E. (1978) Human monocyte-induced tumor cell cytotoxicity. *Blood 52,* 211–220.

Robertson, P. and Fridovich, I. (1982) A reaction of the superoxide radical with tetrapyrroles. *Arch. Biochem. Biophys. 213,* 353–357.

Roos, D. (1980) The metabolic response to phagocytosis. In: G. Weissman (Ed.), *Handbook of Inflammation, Vol. 2: The Cell Biology of Inflammation,* Elsevier/North-Holland, New York, pp. 337–385.

Roos, D., Van Schaik, M.L.J., Weening, R.S. and Wever, R. (1977) Superoxide generation in relation to other oxidative reactions in human polymorphonuclear leukocytes. In: A.M. Michelson, J.M. McCord, and I. Fridovich (Eds), *Superoxide and Superoxide Dismutases,* Academic Press, New York, pp. 307–316.

Roos, D., Weening, R.S. and Voetman, A.A. (1980) Protection of human neutrophils against oxidative damage. *Agents Actions 10,* 528–535.

Root, R.K. and Cohen, M.S. (1981) The microbicidal mechanisms of human neutrophils and eosinophils. *Rev. Inf. Dis. 3,* 565–598.

Root, R.K. and Metcalf, J.A. (1977) H_2O_2 release from human granulocytes during phagocytosis: relationship to superoxide anion formation and cellular catabolism of H_2O_2: studies with normal and cytochalasin B-treated cells. *J. Clin. Invest. 60,* 1266–1279.

Rosen, H. and Klebanoff, S.J. (1976) Chemiluminescence and superoxide production by myeloperoxidase-deficient leukocytes. *J. Clin. Invest. 58,* 50–60.

Rosen, H. and Klebanoff, S.J. (1979) Hydroxyl radical generation by polymorphonuclear leukocytes measured by electron spin resonance spectroscopy. *J. Clin. Invest. 64,* 1725–1729.

Rosen, H. and Klebanoff, S.J. (1981) Role of iron and ethylenediaminetetraacetic acid in the bactericidal activity of a superoxide anion-generating system. *Arch. Biochem. Biophys. 208,* 512–519.

Sacks, T., Moldow, C.F., Craddock, P.R., Bowers, T.K. and Jacob, H.S. (1978) Oxygen radicals mediate endothelial cell damage by complement-stimulated granulocytes: and in vitro model of immune vascular damage. *J. Clin. Invest. 61,* 1161–1167.

Sagone, A.L., Decker, M.A., Wells, R.M. and Democko, C. (1980) A new method for the detection of hydroxyl radical production by phagocytic cells. *Biochim. Biophys. Acta 628,* 90–97.

Sagone, A.L., Klassen, D., Decker, M.A., Clark, L. and Metz, E.N. (1981) Characteristics of the metabolic response of human monocytes to red cells sensitized with anti-D alloantibodies. *J. Lab. Clin. Med. 98,* 382–395.

Salin, M.L. and McCord, J.N. (1975) Free radicals and inflammation: protection of phagocytosing leukocytes by superoxide dismutase. *J. Clin. Invest. 56,* 1319–1323.

Salin, M.L. and McCord, J.M. (1977) Free radicals in leukocyte metabolism and inflammation. In: A.M. Michelson, J.M. McCord and I. Fridovich (Eds), *Superoxide and Superoxide Dismutases,* Academic Press, New York, pp. 257–270.

Samuni, A., Chevion, M. and Czapski, G. (1981) Unusual copper-induced sensitization of the biological damage due to superoxide radicals. *J. Biol.Chem. 256,* 12632–12635.

Sawyer, D.T. and Gibian, M.J. (1979) The chemistry of superoxide ion. *Tetrahedron 35,* 1471–1481.

Segal, A.W., Geisow, M., Garcia, R., Harper, A. and Miller, R. (1981) The respiratory burst of phagocytic cells is associated with a rise in vacuolar pH. *Nature (London) 290,* 406–409.

Selvaraj, R.J., Zgliczynski, J.M., Paul, B.B. and Sbarra, A.J. (1980) Chlorination of reduced nicotinamide adenine dinucleotides by myeloperoxidase: a novel bactericidal mechanism. *J. Reticuloendothel. Soc. 27,* 31–38.

Siebens, H., Tevethia, S.S. and Babior, B.M. (1979) Neutrophil-mediated antibody-dependent killing of herpes-simplex-virus-infected cells. *Blood 54,* 88–94.

Simchowitz, L. and Schur, P.H. (1976a) Lectin-dependent neutrophil-mediated cytotoxicity. I. Characteristics. *Immunology 31,* 303–311.

Simchowitz, L. and Schur, P.H. (1976b) Lectin-dependent neutrophil-mediated cytotoxicity. II. Possible mechanisms. *Immunology 31,* 313−322.

Simchowitz, L. and Spilberg, I. (1979) Evidence for the role of superoxide radicals in neutrophil-mediated cytotoxicity. *Immunology 37,* 301−309.

Sinet, P. - M. and Garber, P. (1981) Inactivation of CuZn superoxide dismutase during exposure to $O_2^{\cdot-}$ and H_2O_2. *Arch. Biochem. Biophys. 212,* 411−416.

Skosey, J.L., Chow, D.C., Nusinow, S., May, J., Gestautas, V. and Niwa, Y. (1981) Effect of oxygen tension on human peripheral blood leukocytes: lysosomal enzyme release and metabolic responses during phagocytosis. *J. Cell Biol. 88,* 358−363.

Slivka, A., LoBuglio, A.F. and Weiss, S.J. (1980) A potential role for hypochlorous acid in granulocyte-mediated tumor cell cytotoxicity. *Blood 55,* 347−350.

Sorrel, T.C., Lehrer, R.I. and Cline, M.J. (1978) Mechanism of nonspecific macrophage-mediated cytotoxicity: evidence for lack of dependence upon oxygen. *J. Immunol. 120,* 347−352.

Stelmaszynska, T. and Zgliczynski, J.M. (1978) N-(2-Oxoacyl)amino acids and nitriles as final products of dipeptide chlorination mediated by the myeloperoxidase/H_2O_2/Cl^- system. *Eur. J. Biochem. 92,* 301−308.

Strauss, R.R., Paul, B.B., Jacobs, A.A. and Sbarra, A.J. (1971) Role of the phagocyte in host-parasite interactions. XXVII. Myeloperoxidase−H_2O_2−Cl^- mediated aldehyde formation and its relationship to antimicrobial activity. *Infect. Immun. 3,* 595−602.

Sutton, H.C., Roberts, P.B. and Winterbourn, C.C. (1976) The rate of reaction of superoxide radical ion with oxyhaemoglobin and methaemoglobin. *Biochem. J. 155,* 503−510.

Takabe, T., Asami, S. and Akazawa, T. (1980) Glycolate formation catalyzed by spinach leaf transketolase utilizing the superoxide radical. *Biochemistry 19,* 3985−3989.

Tauber, A.I. and Babior, B.M. (1977) Evidence for hydroxyl radical formation by human neutrophils. *J. Clin. Invest. 60,* 374−379.

Thomas, E.L. (1979a) Myeloperoxidase, hydrogen peroxide, chloride antimicrobial system: nitrogen−chlorine derivatives of bacterial components in bactericidal activity against Escherichia coli. *Infect. Immun. 23,* 522−531.

Thomas, E.L. (1979b) Myeloperoxidase−hydrogen peroxide−chloride antimicrobial system: effect of exogenous amines on antibacterial action against Escherichia coli. *Infect. Immun. 25,* 110−116.

Thorne, K.J.I., Svvennsen, R.J. and Franks, D. (1980) Role of hydrogen peroxide in the cytotoxic reaction of T-lymphocytes. *Clin. Exp. Immunol. 39,* 486−495.

Tsan, M.F. (1980) Phorbol myristate acetate induced neutrophil autotoxicity. *J. Cell Physiol. 105,* 327−334.

Tsan, M. and Chen, J.W. (1980) Oxidation of methionine by human polymorphonuclear leukocytes. *J. Clin. Invest. 65,* 1041−1050.

Tsan, M.F. and Denison, R.C. (1980) Phorbol myristate acetate-induced neutrophil autotoxicity: a comparison with H_2O_2 toxicity. *Inflammation 4,* 371−380.

Tsan, M. and Denison, R.C. (1981a) Oxidation of amino acids by human neutrophils. *Inflammation 5,* 379−386.

Tsan, M. and Denison, R.C. (1981b) Oxidation of n-formyl methionyl chemotactic peptide by human neutrophils. *J. Immunol. 126,* 1387−1389.

Turkall, R.M., Denison, R.C. and Tsan, M. (1982) Degradation and oxidation of methionine enkephalin by human neutophils. *J. Lab. Clin. Med. 99,* 418−427.

Turner, S.R., Campbell, J.A. and Lynn, W.S. (1975) Polymorphonuclear leukocyte chemotaxis toward oxidized lipid components of cell membranes. *J. Exp. Med. 141,* 1437–1447.

Valentine, J.S. (1979) The chemical reactivity of superoxide anion in aprotic versus protic media: a review. In: W.S. Caughey (Ed.), *Biochemical and Clinical Aspects of Oxygen,* Academic Press, New York, pp. 659–677.

Van Hemmen, J.J. and Meuling, W.J.A. (1977) Inactivation of Escherichia coli by superoxide radicals and their dismutation products. *Arch. Biochem. Biophys. 182,* 743–748.

Van Zwieten, R., Wever, R., Hamers, M.N., Weening, R.S. and Roos, D. (1981) Extracellular proton release by stimulated neutrophils. *J. Clin. Invest. 68,* 310–313.

Voetman, A.A., Weening, R.S., Hamers, M.N., Meerhof, L.J., Bot, A.A.A.M. and Roos, D. (1981) Phagocytosing human neutrophils inactivate their own granular enzymes. *J. Clin. Invest. 67,* 1541–1549.

Weening, R.S., Wever, R. and Roos, D. (1975) Quantitative aspects of the production of superoxide radicals by phagocytizing human granulocytes. *J. Lab. Clin. Med. 85,* 245–252.

Weening, R.S., Roos, D., Weemaes, C.M.R., Homan-Muller, J.W.T. and Van Schaik, M.L.J. (1976) Defective initiation of the metabolic stimulation in phagocytizing granulocytes: a new congenital defect. *J. Lab. Clin. Med. 88,* 757–768.

Weinberg, J.B. and Hibbs, J.B. (1977) Endocytosis of red blood cells or haemoglobin by activated macrophages inhibits their tumoricidal effect. *Nature (London) 269,* 245–247.

Weiss, S.J. (1980) The role of superoxide in the destruction of erythrocyte targets by human neutrophils. *J. Biol. Chem. 255,* 9912–9917.

Weiss, S.J. (1982) Neutrophil-mediated methemoglobin formation in the erythrocyte: the role of superoxide and hydrogen peroxide. *J. Biol. Chem. 257,* 2947–2953.

Weiss, S.J. and LoBuglio, A.F. (1980) An oxygen dependent mechanism of neutrophil-mediated cytotoxicity. *Blood 55,* 1020–1024.

Weiss, S.J. and Slivka, A. (1982) Monocyte and granulocyte-mediated tumor cell destruction: a role for the hydrogen peroxide–myeloperoxidase–chloride system. *J. Clin. Invest. 69,* 255–262.

Weiss, S.J., King, G.W. and LoBuglio, A.F. (1977) Evidence for hydroxyl radical formation by human monocytes. *J. Clin. Invest. 60,* 370–373.

Weiss, S.J., Rustagi, P.K. and LoBuglio, A.F. (1978) Human granulocyte generation of hydroxyl radical. *J. Exp. Med. 147,* 316–323.

Weiss, S.J., LoBuglio, A.F. and Kessler, H.B. (1980) Oxidative mechanisms of monocyte-mediated cytotoxicity. *Proc. Natl. Acad. Sci. USA 77,* 584–587.

Weiss, S.J., Young, J., LoBuglio, A.F., Slivka, A. and Nimeh, N.F. (1981) Role of hydrogen peroxide in neutrophil-mediated destruction of cultured endothelial cells. *J. Clin. Invest. 68,* 714–721.

Weissman, G., Smolen, J.E. and Korchak, H.M. (1980) Release of inflammatory mediators from stimulated neutrophils. *N. Engl. J. Med. 303,* 27–34.

Whitin, J.C., Clark, R.A., Simons, E.R. and Cohen, H.J. (1981) Effects of the myeloperoxidase system on fluorescent probes of granulocyte membrane potential. *J. Biol. Chem. 256,* 8904–8906.

Willson, R.L. (1979) Hydroxyl radicals and biological damage in vitro: what relevance in vivo? In: *Oxygen Free Radicals and Tissue Damage, Ciba Foundation Symposium 65,*

Excerpta Medica, Amsterdam, pp. 19–42.

Winterbourn, C.C. (1981) Cytochrome c reduction by semiquinone radicals can be indirectly inhibited with superoxide dismutase. *Arch. Biochem. Biophys. 209,* 159–167.

Winterbourn, C.C., Williamson, D., Vissers, M.C.M. and Carrel, R.W. (1981) Unstable haemoglobin haemolytic crises: contributions of pyrexia and neutrophil oxidants. *Brit. J. Haematol. 49,* 111–116.

Wong, P.S. and Travis, J. (1980) Isolation and properties of oxidized alpha-1-proteinase inhibitor from human rheumatoid synovial fluid. *Biochem. Biophys. Res. Commun. 96,* 1449–1454.

Yamado. O., Moldow, C.F., Sacks, T., Craddock, P.R., Boogaerts, H.A. and Jacob, H.S. (1981) Deleterious effects of endotoxin on cultured endothelial cells: an in vitro model of vascular injury. *Inflammation 5,* 115–126.

CHAPTER 3

Mechanisms of neutrophil-dependent lung injury

JOSEPH C. FANTONE

and

PETER A. WARD

Department of Pathology, University of Michigan Medical School, Ann Arbor, Michigan 48109

3.1. INTRODUCTION

The lung is a critical organ whose primary physiological function is to maintain the homeostatic balance of oxygen and carbon dioxide within the body and the metabolism of a variety of biologically active substances including polypeptides, amines and prostaglandins. As a result, the lung is exposed to a variety of substances in the external environment, many of which are potentially pathogenic for the host. These include toxic gases and particles as well as a variety of infectious organisms and organic materials capable of initiating acute and/or chronic inflammatory responses within the lung. In recent years, a wealth of experimental evidence has accumulated, increasing our understanding of the pathogenesis of a variety of lung diseases. Specific examples of each of the classical categories of immunological tissue injury, as described by Gell and Coombs in 1969 (see Gell et al. 1975), have been observed. Examples of each of these reactions in the lung are noted in Table 1. However, rarely is a lung immunopathological reaction limited to a single mechanism. In most cases of immunological lung injury, one can find components of at least two of these mechanisms occurring, e.g. hypersensitivity pneumonitis in which cellular immune and immune complex mechanisms have been implicated. It is beyond the scope of this review to present adequately the experimental evidence describing both non-immunological and immunological inflammatory mechanisms in the lung. However, since the polymorphonuclear leukocyte is an important component of most acute inflammatory reactions and certain forms of chronic lung injury, the following chapter will focus on the mechanisms of neutrophil-mediated lung injury and its relevance to human disease.

TABLE 1.
Immunological mechanisms of lung injury

Type		Lung manifestation
I.	Immediate hypersensitivity reactions (anaphylaxis)	Asthma
II.	Cytotoxic antibody	Goodpasture's disease
III.	Antigen–antibody complexes	Polyarteritis nodosa
IV.	Delayed hypersensitivity (cell-mediated)	Tuberculosis Berryliosis Sarcoidosis

Metchnikoff first described in the late 1800's the presence of specific cells in tissues which are capable of ingesting a variety of pathogenic substances. The process of cellular recognition and internalization of a particular substance has been termed "phagocytosis" (for reviews see Roos 1980; Cline and Territo 1980). Three of the most extensively studied phagocytic cells are the polymorphonuclear leukocyte, the tissue macrophage, and the circulating monocyte. Each of these cells has been shown to be an important component in acute and chronic inflammatory reactions in the lung and in other tissues.

When pathogenic agents are formed and/or deposited in the lung, circulating neutrophils may be recruited from the intravascular compartment into the lung parenchyma by the local generation of a variety of soluble phlogistic mediators. These mediators are derived from numerous sources including resident alveolar macrophages and/or activation of plasma components including complement (see below). Directed cell migration – chemotaxis, is the process by which leukocytes, responding to a soluble chemical stimulus, migrate from the circulation to an inflammatory site (Ward 1980; Ward et al. 1979). When neutrophils are exposed to a chemotactic agent in vitro, the cell migrates in the direction of increasing concentration of chemical stimulus. Under certain conditions, particulate and soluble phlogistic mediators generated at sites of inflammation will bind to specific receptors on the neutrophil surface, leading to its activation. A recent review describes in detail the complex biochemical mechanisms involved in the process of neutrophil activation (Roos 1980). In summary, when a foreign particle is deposited in the host tissue, it may or may not be coated with specific host proteins, defined as opsonins. These include immunoglobulins and complement components. These phlogistic mediators have the ability to enhance recognition of foreign particles by neutrophils (and macrophages) by binding to specific receptors on the neutrophil cell surface (e.g. Fc receptor, C3b receptor). After recognition, the foreign particle is ingested by the

TABLE 2.
Lysosomal granule contents of neutrophils

Lysosomal enzyme	Primary substrate	Granule
Elastase	Elastin, collagen, proteoglycans	Azurophil
Collagenase	Collagen	Specific
Myeloperoxidase	H_2O_2, halide; microbicidal	Azurophil
Lysozyme	Bacterial murein	Azurophil and specific
α-Glucosaminidase	Proteoglycans	Azurophil
Hyaluronidase	Proteoglycans	Azurophil
β-Glucuronidase	Proteoglycans	Azurophil
N-Acetyl-β-glucosaminidase	Proteoglycans	Azurophil
β-Glycerophosphatase	Proteoglycans	Azurophil
β-Galactosidase	Proteoglycans	Azurophil
β-Xylosidase	Proteoglycans	Azurophil
β-L-Iduronidase	Proteoglycans	Azurophil
Heparin sulfatase	Proteoglycans	Azurophil
Cathepsin B	Proteoglycans	Azurophil
Cathepsin D	Proteoglycans	Azurophil
Cathepsin G	Proteoglycans, collagen	Azurophil
Cathepsin F	Proteoglycans	Azurophil
Alkaline phosphatase	Phosphoric acid esters	Specific
Lactoferrin	Iron-chelator	Specific

neutrophil and internalized within cytoplasmic vacuoles. These vacuoles fuse with lysosomal granules, forming phagolysosomes. Hydrolytic enzymes capable of degrading a wide variety of biological substances including collagen, elastin, mucopolysaccharides, and bacterial cell membranes (Table 2) are released into the phagolysosome by an active metabolic process known as "degranulation" (Fig. 1).

Neutrophils and other phagocytic cells experience a "respiratory burst" after recognition of either phagocytic or soluble stimuli (reviewed; Cline and Territo 1980; Roos 1980). An increase in oxygen consumption occurs with activation of the hexosemonophosphate shunt and the generation of superoxide anion (O_2^-) generated from molecular oxygen (O_2) by a cell-membrane-associated NADPH oxidase (Fig. 2). In-vitro studies have shown that during either the process of phagocytosis or stimulation by specific chemotactic factors (especially in the presence of cytocylasin

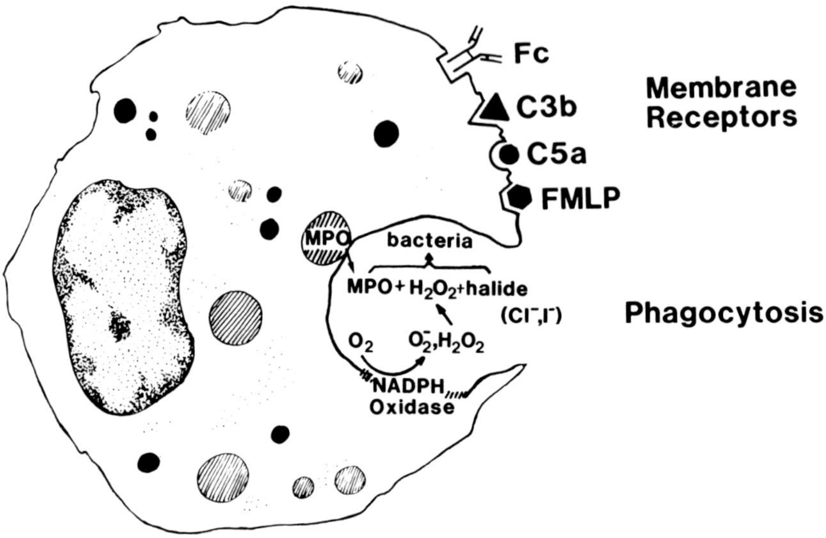

Fig. 1. Neutrophil activation and degranulation by chemotactic and phagocytic stimuli.

B, an inhibitor of microfilaments), neutrophils and other phagocytic cells release lysosomal enzymes and O_2^- into the external environment. O_2^- may be converted to hydrogen peroxide (H_2O_2) and other toxic metabolic products (such as the hydroxyl radical, OH·) via a modified Haber-Weiss reaction (in the presence of metallo-ion). In turn, the reaction of myeloperoxidase with H_2O_2 in the presence of a halide ion will generate additional toxic products (Becker et al. 1978; Curnette and Babior 1979; Root et al. 1975). Current evidence suggests that both lysosomal enzymes and oxygen-derived free radicals and their metabolites play important roles in neutrophil-mediated lung injury.

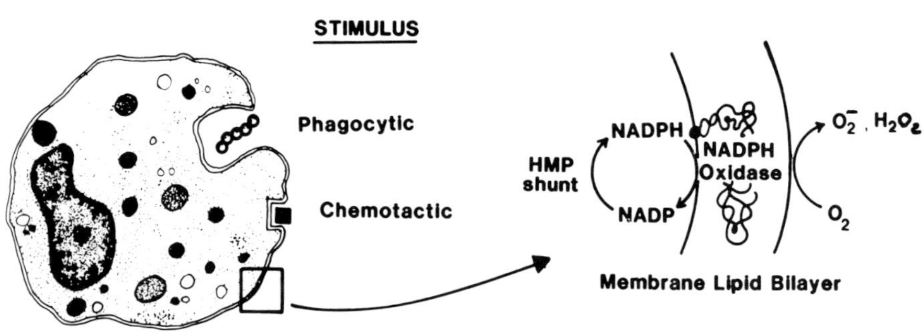

Fig. 2. Proposed mechanism(s) of membrane-associated NADPH oxidase activation.

3.2. CHEMOTACTIC FACTORS OF THE LUNG: ORIGIN AND REGULATION

3.2.1. Complement-derived chemotactic factors

The human complement system is the most extensively studied source of chemotactic factors. This enzymatic cascade may be activated through either the classical or alternative complement pathways with the generation of two potent anaphylatoxins C3a (Mr = 9,000) and C5a (Mr = 12,000) (Hugli and Muller-Eberhard 1978; Hugli 1978) (Fig. 3). These biologically active molecules are defined in vitro by their ability to cause contraction of smooth muscle and the release of vasoactive amines from mast cells and basophils (Table 3). In addition to its anaphylatoxin activity, C5a is a potent chemoattractant for neutrophils. Active in nanomole concentrations, C5a will cause unidirectional movement, not only of neutrophils, but also monocytes, basophils and eosinophils (Fernandez et al. 1978). Initial studies suggested that C3a may also be chemotactically active for neutrophils. However, recent studies using highly purified C3a at physiological concentrations have failed to demonstrate significant chemotactic activity (Hugli, 1978). One of the major regulatory proteins in serum for anaphylatoxins is carboxypeptidase-N (SCPN), which is capable of cleaving the C-terminal arginine residue from several inflammatory mediators including C3a, C5a, and bradykinin. Present in human plasma at concentrations of 30–40 ng/ml, SCPN cleaves a C-terminal arginine from

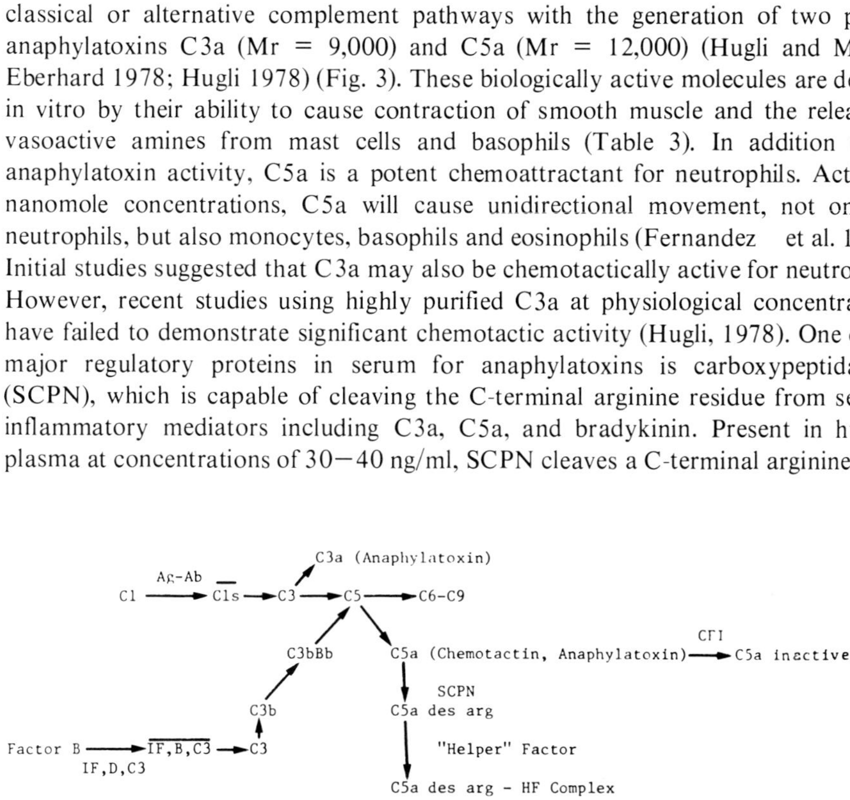

COMPLEMENT PRODUCTS

	Molecular Weight	Activity
C3a	9,000	Anaphylatoxin
C5a	12,500	Anaphylatoxin, Chemotactin Enzyme Release, Aggregation
C5a des arg	12,300	Chemotaxis, ± "Helper" Factor
"Helper" Factor	68,000	Binds to C5a des arg (Increases chemotactic activity)

Fig. 3. Complement-derived chemotactic factors.

TABLE 3.
Activators of the classical and alternative complement pathway

Classical complement pathway	Alternative complement pathway
1. Aggregated antibodies	1. Zymosan (yeast cell wall)
2. Protein A (staphylococcus)	2. Bacterial cell wall
3. IgM	3. Cobra venom factor
4. IgG	4. Endotoxin (lipopolysaccharide)
5. C-reactive protein	5. Aggregated antibody
6. Proteases	6. C3-nephritic factor (IgG against C3b-dependent convertase)

C5a, producing C5a-des-Arg (Chenoweth and Hugli 1980). The chemotactic activity of C5a-des-Arg is approximately 1/40 that of C5a. Recent studies have identified an acidic serum protein that has the capacity to interact with C5a-des-Arg to restore the majority of its chemotactic activity (Beebe et al. 1980; Perez et al. 1980). Since SCPN is present in serum in relatively large quantities, the evidence suggests that the C5a-des-Arg—"helper factor" complex, and not C5a per se, may be responsible for most of the chemotactic activity generated in vivo by complement activation.

A second group of regulatory substances present in serum are the chemotactic factor inactivators that irreversibly inactivate chemotactic factors derived from the complement system, bacteria and lymphocytes (Till and Ward 1975). Chemotactic factor inactivator (CFI) activity is distinct from SCPN and appears to inactivate both C5a and C5a-des-Arg (Kreutzer et al. 1979a). Although the precise physical and chemical parameters of the various CFI's present in serum have not been fully characterized, preliminary evidence suggests that the CFI that reacts with the C5a molecule has an approximate molecular weight of 150,000 and functions through the enzymatic cleavage of C5a. Recent in-vivo studies have shown that intratracheal instillation of CFI purified from human serum into animal lungs will inhibit immune-complex-induced lung injury (Johnson et al. 1977).

Recently, several studies have shown that soluble products derived from leukocyte granules are capable of generating chemotactically active substances from both serum and the structural components of the lung (Fig. 4). In-vitro experiments have shown that, when C3 and C5 are incubated in the presence of cathepsins or elastase (purified from human neutrophils), anaphylatoxin activity is generated from C3 and chemotactic activity from C5 (Orr et al. 1979; Verge and Olsson 1975). Using a model of immune-complex-induced vasculitis in the dermis of rats, greater than a 90% of the C5-derived chemotactic activity has been shown to be the result of lysozymal enzyme cleavage of C5 and not from in-situ activation of the complement system (Ward and Hill 1970). Additional studies have shown that local activation of

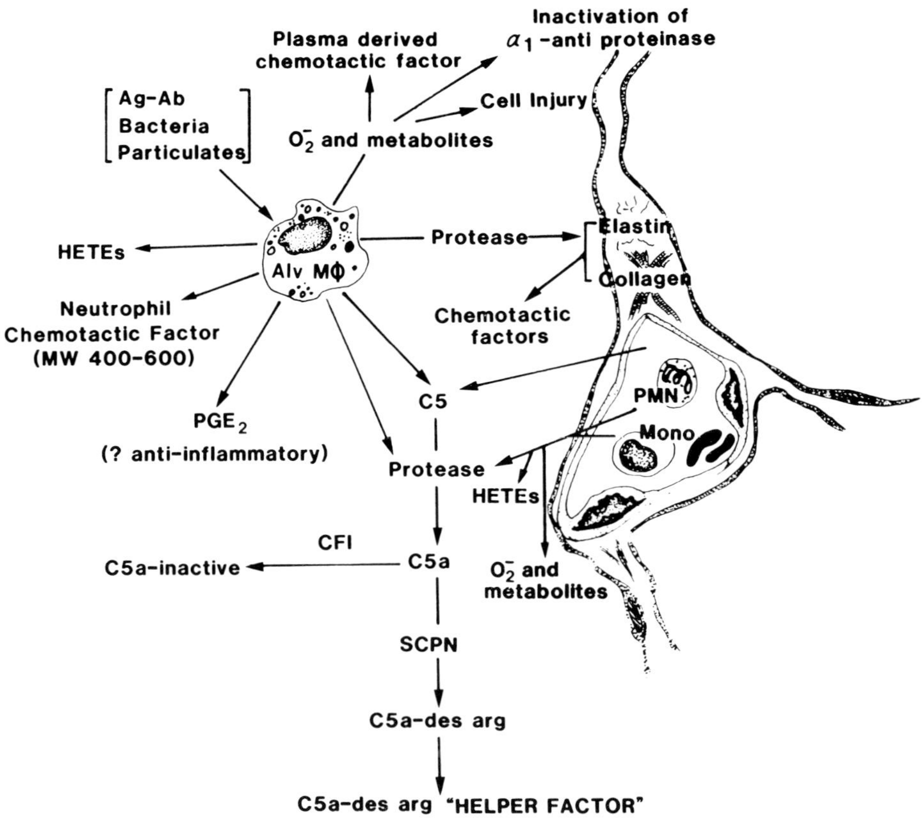

Fig. 4. Phagocyte-derived phlogistic factors in the lung.

either the coagulation or fibrinolytic system has the potential to generate chemotactic activity in serum (Taylor and Ward 1967). When plasminogen and streptokinase are incubated in the presence of serum, chemotactically active substances are generated as a result of enzymatic cleavage of C5 by plasmin. Since neutrophils (Granelli-Piperno et al. 1977) and macrophages (Unkeless et al. 1974) have been shown to secrete plasminogen activator in response to specific stimuli, the initiation of an inflammatory response may be amplified by the local activation of plasminogen to plasmin with the further production of chemotactic agents.

Several studies have shown that proteolytic enzymes released from activated neutrophils have the capacity to generate chemotactically active products from structural substrates in the lung. In-vitro experiments have demonstrated the generation of collagen-derived peptides chemotactic for both monocytes and fibroblasts after incubation of collagen with collagenase (Postlewaite and Kang

1976; Postlewaite and Snyderman 1975; Postlewaite et al. 1978). However, these fragments have not been fully characterized at this time. In addition, elastin, after incubation with human neutrophil elastase, is degraded into biologically active fragments that are chemotactic for monocytes, neutrophils and alveolar macrophages (Senior et al. 1980). These chemotactically active fragments are high in desmosine cross-links and have a molecular weight of approximately 14,000–20,000 daltons. Since recent studies have shown an increased secretion of elastase from macrophages isolated from smokers as compared to non-smokers (Rodriguez et al. 1977), these data described above suggest that the local generation of chemotactic factors as a result of neutrophil and/or macrophage elastase degradation of lung elastin may lead to an influx of inflammatory cells and play an important role in the structural injury present in the lungs of smokers. This provides an additional mechanism in which an inflammatory reaction may be initiated or amplified in vivo.

3.2.2. *Oxygen-metabolite-derived chemotactic factors*

Upon activation of neutrophils by phagocytic or chemotactic stimuli, the primary oxygen-derived products secreted into the extracellular environment are superoxide anion (O_2^-) and hydrogen peroxide H_2O_2 (reviewed, Fantone and Ward 1982a; Klebanoff 1980; Babior 1978). Further studies suggest that other potent oxygen metabolites may be generated by the modified Haber-Weiss (Fenton) reaction in which O_2^- and H_2O_2 are converted to O_2, OH^-, and hydroxyl radical ($OH\cdot$) in a metal-catalysed non-enzymatic reaction:

$$M^{(n+)} + O_2^- = O_2^- + M^{(n-1)}$$

$$\underline{M^{(n-1)} + H_2O_2 = OH^- + OH^{\cdot} + M^{(n+)}}$$

$$O_2^- + H_2O_2 = O_2 + OH^- + OH^{\cdot}$$

In addition, myeloperoxidase in the presence of H_2O_2 has been shown to oxidize various halide ions to hypohalite and, under certain conditions, also to generate singlet oxygen, $^1O_2$. Numerous in-vitro (Clark and Klebanoff 1975; Kellogg and Fridovich 1977; Nathan et al. 1979; Weiss et al. 1980) and in-vivo (Johnson et al. 1981; McCormick et al. 1981) studies have directly implicated products of oxygen metabolism in neutrophil-mediated cell and tissue injury (see Chapter 2). Reactive oxygen metabolites have also been implicated in tissue injury secondary to antineoplastic drugs (Doroshow et al. 1980), hyperoxia (Rister and Baehner 1976; Saltzman and Fridovich 1975), and toxic agents such as paraquat (Burls et al. 1980).

The possible role of oxygen metabolites in the generation of chemotactically active substances has recently been investigated. When human plasma is incubated with xanthine−xanthine oxidase (an O_2^- and H_2O_2 generating system), a biologically active lipid is produced that is chemotactic for neutrophils (Petrone et al. 1980). Its production is closely correlated with generation of O_2^-. This biologically active substance is heat-labile and binds to albumin in its active form. However, the precise characterization of the physical and structural properties of this lipid has not been determined. An additional study has demonstrated the generation of a chemotactic lipid in vitro after incubation of arachidonic acid with an O_2^- generating system (Perez and Goldstein 1980). This material is functionally active at a concentration of 3.0 ng/ml and is chromatographically distinct from arachidonic acid. These studies demonstrate the potential ability of potent oxidants derived from neutrophils to generate additional chemotactic factors at sites of inflammation. The data also suggest that oxidants derived from other sources, such as inhaled noxious gases and/or cigarette smoke, may also function to initiate or amplify local inflammatory responses in the lung. Whether similar chemotactically active lipids are generated in vivo awaits further study.

A second mechanism by which oxidants may augment the local generation of chemotactic factors in the lung is via the inactivation of normal serum inhibitors of leukocyte and monocyte proteases. In-vitro experiments have shown inhibition of α_1-antiprotease (the primary inhibitor of neutrophil elastase present in serum) by oxygen metabolites (Carp and Janoff 1979) and cigarette smoke (Carp and Janoff 1978). Hydroquinone and thymol, both phenolic antioxidants, block the effects of the smoke-derived inactivation of α_1-antiprotease. These data suggest that the local generation of potent oxidants or lung inhalation may lead to the inactivation of the natural inhibitors of neutrophil- and monocyte-derived proteases. This could result in increased destruction of the structural components of the lung (e.g. collagen and elastin) and may lead to the local increase in chemotactic factors derived from these structural substrate elements.

A recent report has complicated our interpretation of the role of oxygen metabolites in tissue injury. When C5a or the synthetic chemotactic peptide, N-formyl-methionyl-leucyl-phenylalanine (f-Met-Leu-Phe), is incubated with a myeloperoxidase−H_2O_2−halide system in vitro, there is a loss of chemotactic activity which appears to be the result of oxidation of methionine residues (Clark et al. 1980). A recent report has demonstrated inhibition of chemotactic activity of f-Met-Leu-Phe when incubated in the presence of activated neutrophils (Clark and Szot 1982). Therefore, clarification of the phlogistic role of oxidants and oxygen metabolites in the lung awaits further study.

3.2.3. Cell-derived chemotactic factors

Additional chemotactic factors in the lung may be derived directly from activated inflammatory cells. When neutrophils or other phagocytic cells are activated by either particulate or soluble stimuli, arachidonic acid is generated from membrane phospholipids and may be metabolized by specific lipoxygenases generating a class of biologically active hydroxyeicosatetranoic acids (HETES) and intermediate compounds. A detailed review of arachidonic acid metabolism in inflammatory cells is presented elsewhere (see Chapter 5). Several of the HETES and other intermediate compounds of arachidonic acid metabolism have been shown to be chemotactic for neutrophils in vitro, the most potent of which are 5-HETE, 5,12-di-HETE, and leukotrine B_4, the last having chemotactic activity in a dose range similar to that for C5a. Therefore local activation of inflammatory cells can result in activation of a membrane-associated phospholipase with the generation of arachidonic acid from membrane phospholipids. Further metabolism by activation of the lipoxygenase enzyme system may result in the generation of potent biologically active products, several of which have been shown to be chemotactic for neutrophils with a potential for amplifying the inflammatory response. Under certain conditions, these potent mediators may be the primary phlogistic agents of the inflammatory response.

Additional products of alveolar macrophages have also been suggested as potential sources of chemotactic activity in vivo. Recent studies have demonstrated the presence of hemolytically active C5 in bronchoalveolar lavage fluids. Although in-vitro studies suggest that mononuclear phagocytes may secrete several complement components (Schrieber et al. 1973), there is conflicting evidence suggesting that alveolar macrophages are the source of C5 in bronchoalveolar lavage fluids (Henson et al. 1979; Robertson et al. 1976). Therefore, without prior vascular injury and exudation of plasma, C5-derived chemotactic peptides could theoretically be generated in the alveolus following an insult to the alveolar area prior to the triggering of an inflammatory response. Alveolar macrophages have also been shown to secrete a low-molecular-weight chemotactic factor for neutrophils following stimulation by immune complexes, micro-organisms and particulate matter (Hunninghake et al. 1978b, 1980b; Kazmierowski et al. 1977; Merrill et al. 1980; Roos et al. 1977). The chemotactic factor derived from alveolar macrophages attracts neutrophils preferentially and has a molecular weight of between 400–600 daltons. Additional studies have shown that stimulated alveolar macrophages also secrete unsaturated fatty acids, primarily linoleic acid which stimulates macrophage motility (Lynn and Mukherjee 1979). Further in-vitro studies of macrophage chemotaxis have shown that both linoleic acid, which is found in elevated concentrations of certain inflammatory cells, and phosphatidic glycerol, which is present in bronchoalveolar lavage fluids, enhance macrophage migration. These studies suggest that the alveolar macrophage plays a potentially pivotal role in the initiation and modulation of lung inflammation.

Certain classes of lymphocytes when stimulated with either antigens or mitogens respond by the secretion of a class of soluble mediators defined as lymphokines. Although a large number of biological activities have been described for lymphokines in a number of species, precise structure definition and characterization of the biochemical behavior of these active materials is not complete. Of these various biologically active materials, several investigators have demonstrated chemotactic activity for a variety of inflammatory cells including neutrophil chemotactic factor

(NCF), macrophage chemotactic factor (MCF), basophil chemotactic factor (BCF), eosinophil chemotactic factor (ECF), lymphocyte (T-cell) chemotactic factor (LCF), eosinophil stimulation promotor (ESP), and fibroblast chemotactic factor (FCF) (reviewed, Altman 1978). Although the biological activities of lymphokines have been defined in vitro, it is believed that they play an important role in the mobilization of inflammatory cells in vivo.

A distinct group of cell-derived chemotactic factors for eosinophils has also been defined. Activated neutrophils have been shown to release small peptides that are chemotactic for eosinophils. These peptides are biochemically identical to the eosinophil chemotactic factor of anaphylaxis (ECF-A) which is released during IgE-mediated anaphylactic triggering of the mast cell. ECF-A has been identified as a tetrapeptide with one of two chemical structures Ala-Gly-Ser-Glu or Val-Gly-Ser-Glu (Goetzl and Austen 1975; Kay and Austen 1971). These peptides appear to react with a specific receptor on the cell membrane which triggers the locomotive response of the eosinophil. The activity of these peptides was originally thought to be specific for eosinophils; however, these peptides have also been shown to be chemotactic for neutrophils.

3.2.4. *Bacterial- and viral-derived chemotactic factors*

An additional source of neutrophil chemotactic factor production in the lung includes infectious agents. Several studies have shown the ability of bacteria to elaborate small peptides (Mr approx. 1,000) which are chemotactic for neutrophils (Schiffman et al. 1975; Ward et al. 1968). Current evidence suggests that these active peptides represent formylated signal peptides derived from the NH_2 terminus of newly synthesized proteins (Schiffman et al. 1975). Additional studies have shown a structure–function relationship between formylated peptides and neutrophil chemotactic activity with the subsequent identification of a specific receptor for formylated peptides on the neutrophil surface (Showell et al. 1976; Marasco et al. 1982; Marasco and Becker 1982). In the process of activating neutrophils, these low-molecular-weight compounds cause a respiratory burst, O_2^- and H_2O_2 generation, and lysosomal enzyme degranulation. Although the in-vitro activity of the formylated peptides has been well established, their relevance in vivo awaits further study.

A second mechanism in which bacteria have been shown capable of generating chemotactic agents is secondary to the release of enzymes which are capable of cleaving C5 into active fragments (Ward et al. 1973). Similarly, viruses have been shown to induce release of chemotactic factors which do not contain viral particles and are complement-independent. Virus-infected cells also produce C5-cleaving enzymes which are most likely derived from the host-cell lysosomal granules (Brier et al. 1970; Ward et al. 1972). This evidence indicates that specific infectious agents are capable of either directly or indirectly producing chemotactic activity in the lung and potentially initiating an inflammatory response.

3.3. LEUKOCYTIC PROTEASES IN LUNG INJURY

Human neutrophils as well as alveolar macrophages have been shown to contain numerous lysosomal enzymes including collagenase, elastase, chymotrypsin and cathepsins (Dewald et al. 1975). These enzymes are capable of degrading the structural elements of lung (collagen, elastin, basement membrane, and proteoglycans). Of these different proteases, the role of leukocyte elastase in the pathogenesis of lung injury has been the most extensively studied. Leukocytic elastase is thought to play a significant role in the pathogenesis of emphysema. This has been based on two observations. The first and most direct evidence is derived from humans with α_1-antitrypsin deficiency (Leiberman 1969; Kueppers and Black 1974). This protein is the primary protease inhibitor in serum for leukocyte elastase. Patients with homozygote (PiZZ) deficiency of serum α_1-antitrypsin show a high incidence of pulmonary emphysema. Additional evidence for the role of elastase in pulmonary emphysema comes from experiments in dogs and hamsters in which either lysosomal granule extracts or purified leukocyte elastase is instilled intratracheally. These animals show rapid development of pulmonary emphysema associated with a loss of elastin but not of collagen (Janoff et al. 1977; Senior et al. 1977).

Additional studies of leukocytic neutral proteases have shown that these enzymes are capable of cleaving both C3 and C5 with the production of biologically active fragments. Elastase and cathepsin purified from human neutrophils are capable in vitro of generating anaphylatoxin activity from C3 and chemotactic fragments from C5 (Ward and Hill 1970; Verge and Olsson 1975) (see previous section). Thus, the role of leukocytic proteases in lung injury appears to be twofold. Not only do the proteases have the ability to effect damage to the structural components of the lung, but they also have the capacity to amplify inflammatory reactions by generating chemotactic mediators and anaphylatoxins from complement.

3.4. ROLE OF OXYGEN RADICALS AND LUNG INJURY

Until recently, it was thought that the neutral proteases derived from neutrophils and macrophages were the primary agents responsible for the tissue injury occurring in many inflammatory responses. However, protease inhibitors failed to significantly decrease neutrophil-mediated tissue injury induced with immune complexes (Johnson and Ward 1981). In addition, beige mice whose leukocytes are deficient in neutral protease, do not show decreased neutrophil-mediated tissue injury (Johnson et al. 1978). These studies suggest that alternative mechanisms are responsible for neutrophil-mediated tissue injury.

During the last several years there has accumulated considerable evidence suggesting that oxygen metabolites derived from inflammatory cells may be responsible for acute injury of cells and tissue (reviewed; Fantone and Ward 1982a; Klebanoff 1980; Babior 1978). Since most bacteria are metabolized and degraded within intracellular phagolysosomes where relatively high concentrations of oxygen metabolites and myeloperoxidase occur, it would appear that injury to cells in the external environment by phagocytic cells would be unlikely. However, several investigators have reported in-vitro studies demonstrating that oxygen metabolites released from the surfaces of activated neutrophils and macrophages are cytotoxic to a wide variety of cells including erythrocytes (Kellogg and Fridovich 1977; Klebanoff and Clark 1975; Weiss et al. 1980), endothelial cells (Sachs et al. 1978; Weiss et al. 1981), fibroblasts (Simon et al. 1981), tumor cells (Clark et al. 1975; Nathan et al. 1979; Clark and Klebanoff 1975; Hafeman and Lucas 1979), leukocytes (Baehner et al. 1977; Roos et al. 1980), and platelets (Clark and Klebanoff 1979). It appears that the toxic effects on eukaryotic cells of oxygen metabolites derived from neutrophils and other phagocytes occur in a manner that is strikingly similar to their bactericidal system (see Chapter 2). Each of the various oxygen metabolites including O_2^-, H_2O_2, HOCl, OH^- and $^1O_2$ have been implicated in extracellular injury of host cells. Several in-vitro studies using scavengers of free radicals and specific enzymes — superoxide dismutase (SOD) and catalase — have implicated products of the interaction between H_2O_2 and O_2^- or products of the myeloperoxidase—H_2O_2—halide system as the most potent cytolytic agents.

Recent in-vivo studies have demonstrated the ability of SOD to suppress carrageenin-induced inflammation (Huber and Saifer 1977). When carrageenin is injected into the pleural cavity of normal and SOD-treated animals, the amount of pleural effusion is reduced by approximately 50% and the number of neutrophils decreased by 30% in the SOD-treated animals. These studies suggest that neutrophil-derived O_2^- or its metabolic product is necessary for the full expression of the inflammatory response. Systemic treatment with SOD has been shown to suppress carrageenin-induced footpad edema in the rat (Oyanagui 1976). SOD has also been shown to suppress several other forms of phagocyte-mediated tissue injury including kaolin-induced inflammation and chronic adjuvant arthritis in the rat (Huber and Saifer 1977).

A recent report has shown that the intratracheal instillation of specific enzyme—substrate systems known to generate oxygen metabolites will cause acute lung injury (Fig. 5) (Johnson et al. 1981). Intratracheal instillation of xanthine and xanthine oxidase into rats causes increased vascular permeability with only minor intra-alveolar edema formation and focal hemorrhage at 4 hours. These pathological changes are inhibited by the simultaneous instillation of SOD. When glucose and glucose oxidase (an H_2O_2-generating system) are instilled into the airways, there is a marked increase in vascular permeability, edema, hyaline membrane (fibrin) formation, hemorrhage and a marked neutrophil influx. These changes are consistent with the pathological changes that have been observed in humans and defined as "diffuse alveolar damage" and associated with adult respiratory distress syndrome (Katzenstein et al. 1976). These pathological alterations are inhibited with catalase,

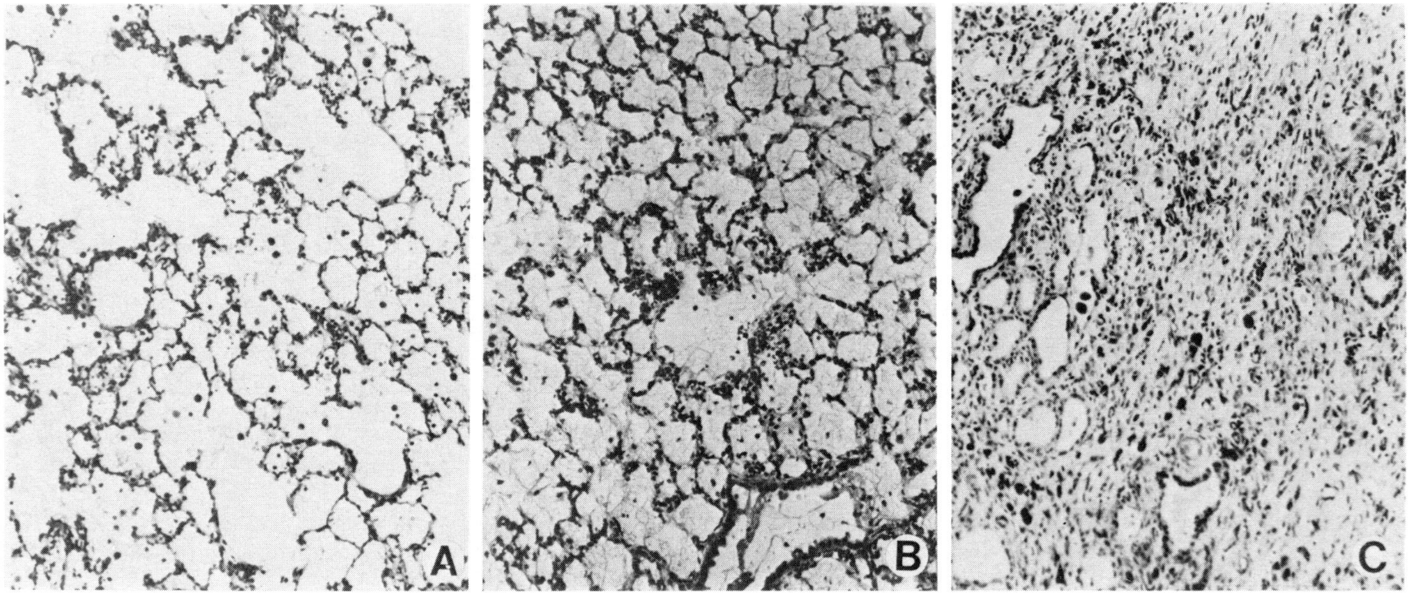

Fig. 5. In-vivo lung damage by enzymatically generated oxygen metabolites. (A) Section of lung from a rat 4 hr after intratracheal instillation of glucoseoxidase (70 U) and glucose (1 mg). There is smudging of alveolar walls with neutrophil infiltration, and early intra-alveolar hemorrhage with fibrin deposition (H and E; x 48). (B) Section of rat lung 4 hr after treatment with glucoseoxidase (28 U), glucose (1 mg) and lactoperoxidase (1.7 U). The pathological changes within the lung show increased neutrophils, increased accumulation of fibrin and minimal hemorrhage (H and E; x 48). (C) Section of rat lung from animals tested as in Fig. 5B, 14 days after instillation of enzymes. Sections of lung show collapse of lung tissue, loss of alveolar structure, and extensive pulmonary fibrosis (H and E; x 48).

but not with SOD or chemically inactivated catalase (Fig. 5). When either lactoperoxidase (LPO) or myeloperoxidase (MPO) is instilled with the glucose–glucose oxidase system, severe lung injury occurs, frequently progressing to diffuse pulmonary fibrosis by 4 days. These data suggest that a product (HOCl or $^1O_2$) of the MPO(LPO)–H_2O_2–halide system may play a significant role in the induction of pulmonary fibrosis (see Chapter 4). These observations demonstrate that oxygen-derived free radicals and their metabolites have the capacity to cause acute lung injury that may, under certain conditions, result in progressive lung injury with pulmonary fibrosis.

The direct toxic effects of H_2O_2 and products of the xanthine–xanthine oxidase system on lung parenchyma have been supported using an in-vitro system. When ^{51}Cr-labeled lung explants are incubated in the presence of either H_2O_2 or a xanthine–xanthine oxidase system, cell injury occurs as monitored by ^{51}Cr release and increased extracellular levels of lactate dehydrogenase (a cytoplasmic enzyme) (Marten et al. 1981). In both systems, catalase, but not SOD, is effective in blocking the cytotoxic effects, suggesting that H_2O_2 or a metabolite is the significant toxic agent. In addition, rat and human lung explants appear to be more susceptible to injury compared to rabbit lung explants, indicating a species difference in the susceptibility of lung parenchyma to injury by toxic oxygen metabolites. Additional studies are necessary to define the precise targets of the oxygen metabolites.

3.5. CHEMOTACTIC-FACTOR-MEDIATED LUNG INJURY

3.5.1. Intravascular effects of chemotactic factors

In recent years, there have been numerous studies attempting to determine the role of chemotactic factors in initiating lung injury. Intravascular activation of the complement system with the generation of chemotactic peptides and sequestration of neutrophils in the lung has been suggested as a mechanism of respiratory distress associated with extracorporal hemodialysis, severe burns and extensive trauma (Craddock et al. 1977a). In addition, circulating immune complexes, which have the ability to activate the complement system and generate chemotactic factors, have been associated with pulmonary injury (see below). When exposed to chemotactic factors (i.e. C5a, f-Met-Leu-Phe) in vitro, neutrophils respond with an increase in cell volume and the formation of multicellular aggregates (Jacob et al. 1980; O'Flaherty and Ward 1978). As described earlier, activated neutrophils produce O_2^- and other oxygen metabolites which have been shown to be cytotoxic for endothelial cells. When either chemotactic factors or cobra venom factor (an activator of the alternative complement pathway) are instilled intravenously into rabbits, a rapid, marked, and transient neutropenia develops reaching a nadir within 1–2 minutes and returning to normal levels within 15–30 minutes (O'Flaherty et al. 1977, 1978). The

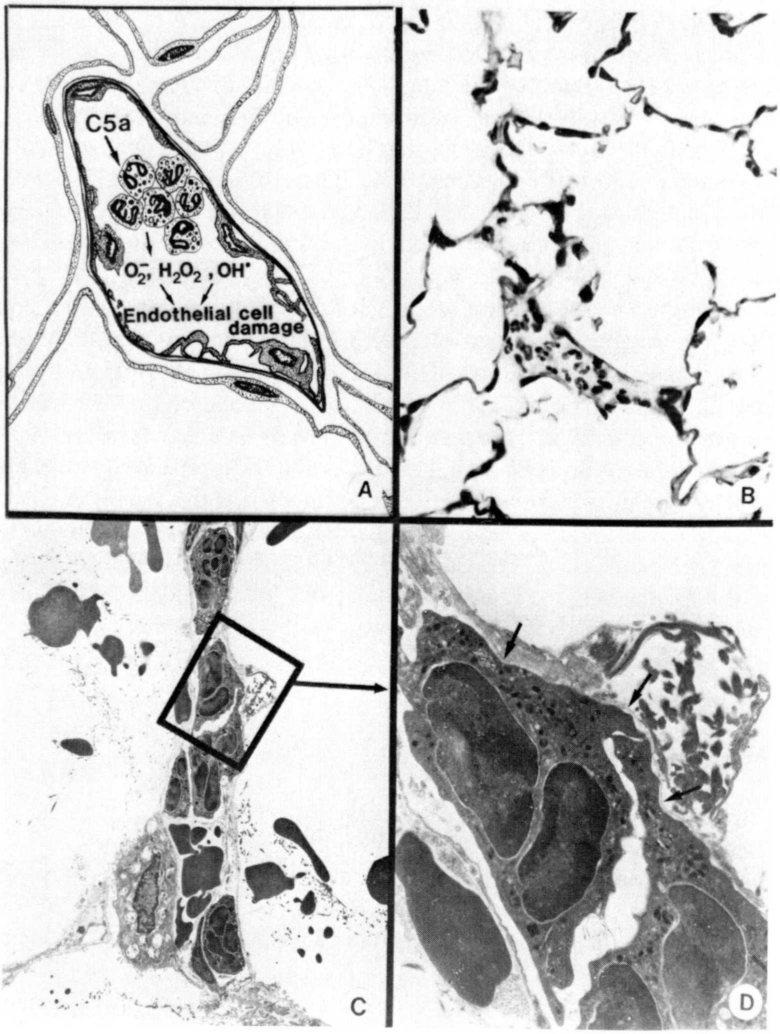

Fig. 6. Endothelial cell injury by polymorphonuclear leukocytes following intravascular complement activation. (A) Proposed mechanism(s) of intravascular complement activation and neutrophil-mediated endothelial cell injury by oxygen metabolites. (B) Section of rat lung 30 min after intravenous infusion of 80 μg cobra venom factor shows sequestration of neutrophils in alveolar capillaries (H and E; x 130). (C) Transmission electron micrograph of rat lung from animals treated as in Fig. 6B, showing interstitial capillaries containing neutrophils in contact with endothelium. Red blood cells and fibrin are present in alveolar spaces (x 3,000). (D) A higher magnification of the inset in Fig. 6C shows an area in which the capillary endothelial cell is absent and neutrophils (arrows) are in direct contact with vascular basement. Fibrin deposits are present on the extraluminal surface of the vascular wall (x 8,750).

neutrophils appear to sequester in the lung as a result of cell aggregation and embolization in capillaries, as well as increased adherence to vascular endothelial cells (margination). However, there does not appear to be significant intra-alveolar edema as assessed by increased serum proteins in bronchoalveolar lavage (Webster et al. 1982). When zymosan-activated serum is infused into sheep, there is marked pulmonary leukostasis and pulmonary edema (Binder et al. 1980). It has been proposed that the pulmonary edema may be the result of injury of the capillary endothelial cells by oxygen metabolites derived from activated neutrophils. A recent report has shown that intravascular infusion of cobra venom factor in rats results in neutrophil accumulation within the pulmonary vasculature and an increase in lung permeability with focal intra-alveolar hemorrhage (Till et al. 1982) (Fig. 6). These reactions are neutrophil-dependent, since depletion of blood neutrophils prior to infusion of cobra venom factor protects the lung from injury. Ultrastructural study shows evidence of endothelial cell damage that is prevented by prior treatment of animals with catalase. Therefore, it appears that endothelial cell injury after intravascular activation of complement can occur in certain species and is the result of the generation and cytotoxic effects of neutrophil-derived H_2O_2 or its metabolites.

Additional studies using models of endotoxin- or air-embolus-induced lung injury in sheep have demonstrated a dependence on neutrophils for the hemodynamic alterations as well as increased lung lymph flow (Heflin and Brigham 1981). A recent report substantiates the role of neutrophil-derived oxygen metabolites in vascular injury associated with air emboli in sheep. When SOD is administered to heparinized sheep prior to or during the time of air infusion, there is a marked decrease in the total lung lymph flow as compared with non-SOD-treated controls (Flick et al. 1981). It is not known whether catalase has similar effects in this model. Additional studies are necessary to define the precise relationship between these observations and lung injury in humans.

3.5.2. *Intra-alveolar chemotactic factors*

Since the local generation of chemotactic factors is believed to be responsible for the recruitment of neutrophils and other inflammatory cells into the lung, several groups have investigated the effects of intratracheal instillation of preformed chemotactic factors of the lung. When highly purified preparations of C5a or C5a-des-Arg are administered intratracheally, large accumulations of neutrophils occur within alveolar spaces. Intratracheal instillation of 200 μg of intact human C5 into hamster lung results in a marked, acute inflammatory reaction with large numbers of neutrophils (Desai et al. 1979). This reaction appears to be the result of intrapulmonary cleavage of C5 into chemotactically active fragments by lung-derived proteases and appears to be unique to the hamster. Intrapulmonary (airway) instillation into rabbits (Shaw et al. 1978) or hamsters (Kreutzer et al. 1979b) of small quantities (10–40 μg) of chemotactically active fragments derived from C5 produces a neutrophil-rich, diffuse inflammatory infiltrate which reaches a peak within 4 hours after instillation. This response is dose-related and provides direct evidence for the phlogistic properties of C5a and C5a-des-Arg in the lung.

Since C5a is rapidly converted to C5a-des-Arg in vivo by serum carboxypeptidase-N, additional studies have been undertaken to investigate the inflammatory potential of C5a-des-Arg in the lung (Stimler et al. 1980). After intratracheal instillation of C5a-des-Arg (10—20 g) into rabbit lungs, an intense acute inflammatory response develops, reaching a peak within 6 hours. In comparison to C5a, the rabbit lung is more susceptible to injury by C5a-des-Arg, suggesting that, in vivo, C5a-des-Arg may be the significant mediator of lung injury. Although C5a-des-Arg is less active than C5a in in-vitro systems, the possible formation of a C5a-des-Arg—"helper" factor complex (discussed above) could explain the in-vivo observations. These data demonstrate the strong phlogistic potential of C5-derived chemotactic peptides and support their potential role in inflammatory reactions in the lungs.

3.6. EXPERIMENTAL MODELS OF IMMUNE-COMPLEX LUNG INJURY

There is abundant evidence in both in-vivo and in-vitro models that immune complexes have the ability to elicit inflammatory responses by the generation of chemotactic factors derived from complement. The initial experimental studies which suggested a possible role of immune complexes in lung injury were described by Kniker and Cochrane (1965) using a model of acute ("one shot") serum sickness. After a single intravenous injection of antigen into rabbits, reversible inflammatory changes in medium-size pulmonary arteries were observed. The injury consisted of acute inflammatory reactions in the vessel wall with both medial and endothelial cell proliferation. Immunofluorescence studies of the vessel walls revealed the presence of both immunoglobulin (IgG), antigen, and complement components (C3). Complement depletion experiments using cobra venom factor markedly depressed vascular injury and neutrophil influx despite the deposition of immune complexes. Although the intrapulmonary changes in these studies were limited to the vascular compartment, the data implicate the role of complement in the initiation of neutrophil accumulation and lung injury.

Currently, the only evidence which suggests that circulating immune complexes can directly cause irreversible lung injury is in the model of chronic serum sickness in rabbits. Antigen injected daily over a period of weeks causes an intense inflammatory response with irreversible changes in the alveolar interstitium and basement membrane (Brentjens et al. 1974). Ultrastructural and immunofluorescence studies show an inflammatory reaction with fibrin deposition, interstitial fibrosis, thickening of capillary basement membrane, and deposits of immune complexes and complement in vascular basement membranes. The most intense reaction is associated with a marked and protracted antibody response in rabbits maintained in a state of relative antigen—antibody equivalence. These conditions produce immune complexes of optimal size and maximal complement-fixing activity. These studies suggest that circulating immune complexes can elicit inflammatory changes in the lung mediated by the local activation of complement and the generation of chemotactic factors. However, it is possible that other immune mechanisms are active in these models (e.g. cellular immune mechanisms), contributing to the inflammatory response and development of interstitial fibrosis.

Immune complexes formed within the alveolar compartment are also capable of producing inflammatory reactions in the lung. In a model similar to the reverse passive Arthus reaction in the skin, an acute inflammatory reaction in rat lung is produced after the intratracheal administration of heterologous rabbit antibody (IgG) and the simultaneous intravascular injection of antigen (Johnson and Ward

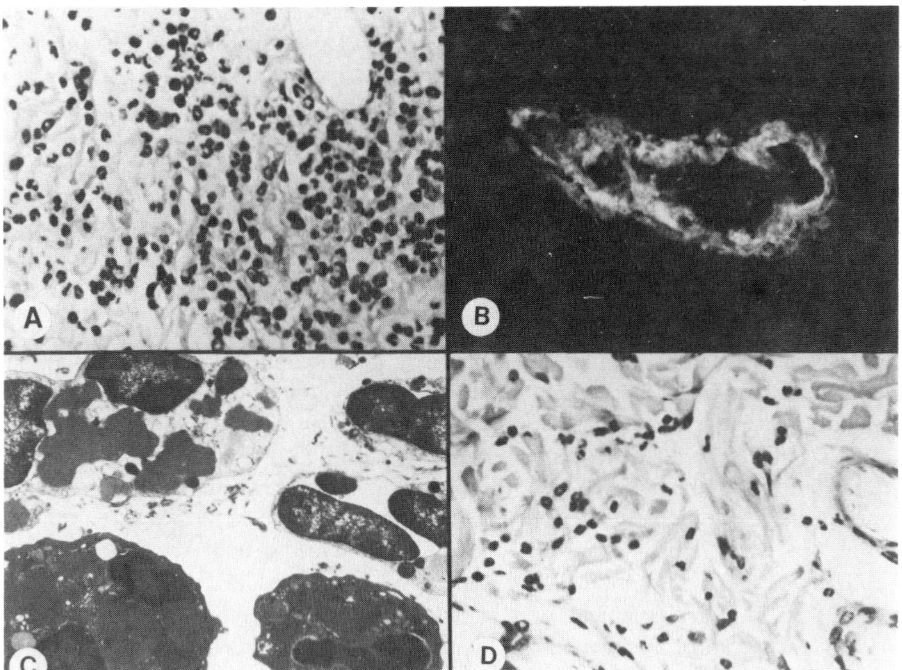

Fig. 7. Reverse passive Arthus reaction (immune complex inflammation) in the skin of untreated (A) and superoxide-dismutase-treated (D) rats (H and E; x 344). Bovine serum albumin (10 mg) was administered intravenously simultaneously with the intradermal injection of rabbit anti-BSA (IgG, 50 μg antibody N). Six hours later, the superoxide dismutase (1500 U i.d.) treated rats showed a depressed neutrophil infiltrate despite the presence of immune complex formation and complement fixation. (B) Demonstrates the presence of rabbit IgG at the reaction side. Immunofluorescence, fluorescein-conjugated goat anti-rabbit IgG. (C) Phagocytized electron-dense material (immune complexes) is present within neutrophils in the untreated animals (transmission electron micrograph, x 6,960).

1974). This reaction consists of both an intra-alveolar and interstitial reaction which is most intense 4–6 hours after antibody instillation (Fig. 7). The deposition of immune complexes and complement components occurs within alveolar walls. Complement depletion markedly inhibits the influx of neutrophils into the lung. The mechanism of neutrophil influx is thought to result from the diffusion of antibody and antigen from the alveoli and vascular compartments, respectively, forming immune complexes within alveolar walls. Chemotactic peptides (e.g. C5a) are generated from activation of the classical complement pathway, resulting in the recruitment of neutrophils from the circulation. The immune complexes are ingested by neutrophils, resulting in the release of proteolytic enzymes (from lysosomal granules) capable of causing both hydrolysis of lung structural proteins and generating additional chemotactic factors. In addition, oxygen-derived metabolites such as O_2^-, HOCl, $OH^{\cdot}$ and H_2O_2 are also generated. These products have the capacity to augment the inflammatory response as previously described. In these inflammatory reactions, alveolar macrophages are theoretically capable of phagocytizing immune complexes and generating products similar to those described for the neutrophil.

A similar inflammatory response has been seen in the lung following the intratracheal administration of preformed immune complexes into rats (Scherzer and Ward 1978a, b). An acute hemorrhagic inflammatory reaction with a marked neutrophil infiltrate is present within the alveolar compartment after airway instillation of preformed immune complexes. The reaction resembles the reverse passive Arthus reaction in the lung (as described above) and is both neutrophil- and complement-dependent. The critical property in the initiation of inflammatory reaction appears to be the ratio of antigen to antibody in the immune complexes. The most intense reaction occurs when the complexes are formed in antigen equivalence, corresponding to complexes with the greatest complement-fixing activity. Complexes formed at 6 times antigen excess are less phlogistic, smaller in size, and have minimal complement-fixing activity. This evidence supports the dependency of immune-complex-induced lung injury on complement activation and neutrophil influx. Additional experimental models of immune-complex-mediated lung injury have demonstrated both complement- and neutrophil-dependent mechanisms after aerosol challenge or intrapleural injection of antigen into actively immunized rabbits (Kaplan et al. 1980; Willoughby et al. 1979), and in guinea pigs (Richerson 1972; Roska 1979).

In recent studies, two groups have shown that systemic administration of superoxide dismutase (SOD) to rats will inhibit the reverse passive Arthus reaction in the skin (Petrone et al. 1980; McCormick et al. 1981). Immunofluorescence studies have shown that a suppressed inflammatory response occurs, despite the local formation of immune complexes and activation of complement (Fig. 7B). Further evidence implicating a role for O_2^- and H_2O_2 in acute immune-complex-induced injury has been demonstrated by catalase-induced inhibition of immune-complex-mediated acute inflammatory reactions in the lung (Johnson and Ward 1981). In this model, catalase is more effective than SOD, while antiproteases have little, if any, protective effects against lung injury. The inhibitory effects of SOD on inflammatory reactions are brief in duration (<2 hours) and are associated with a decreased influx of neutrophils. This is consistent with the experimental evidence demonstrating the production of lipid chemotactic factors by O_2^- which may serve as important amplifiers of the inflammatory response. The protective effects of catalase are not associated with blocking of the influx of neutrophils. This observation is consistent with the idea that catalase destroys H_2O_2 generated by immune-complex-activated cells, thus protecting the tissue from injury.

3.7. CLINICAL EXAMPLES OF NEUTROPHIL-DEPENDENT LUNG INJURY

An influx of neutrophils into the lung has long been recognized as an integral component of most acute bacterial pneumonias. Classical lobular and lobar pneumonia are associated with edema and intra-alveolar accumulations of neutrophils, resulting in phagocytosis and clearance of the pathogen. Several in-vivo studies have demonstrated a dependence on complement and neutrophils for the clearance of pneumococci and other bacteria in experimental models of bacterial pneumonia (Ansfield et al. 1977; Gross et al. 1978; Rehm 1980; Coonrod and Yoneda 1981). Pulmonary opsonins have also been shown to play a significant role in the modulation of *Klebsiella pneumoniae* and pneumococci in experimental animals (Guckian et al. 1980; Coonrod 1981; Hoff et al. 1980). In addition, pneumonias associated with aspiration and exposure to certain toxic gases are characterized by neutrophil infiltrates.

Adult respiratory distress syndrome is a clinically defined condition characterized by increasing hypoxemia, respiratory distress, tachypnea, tachycardia and cyanosis (Katzenstein 1976). These clinical findings may be the result of a variety of pathological insults with the basic lesion being that of diffuse alveolar damage with pulmonary edema and hyaline membrane formation, which may progress to interstitial fibrosis. Although the mechanism(s) of alveolar capillary damage is not known, several studies suggest that intravascular activation of the complement system and the generation of C5a may lead to intravascular neutrophil activation (Fearon et al. 1975; Hosea et al. 1980). Previously described experimental studies have shown that intravascular neutrophil activation by complement components leads to sequestration of polymorphonuclear leukocytes in the lung vasculature and to endothelial cell injury. Additional studies are necessary to determine if similar events occur in humans.

Several other less common diseases have been associated with an influx of neutrophils into the lung. In many cases, there is an association of the lung disease with the deposition and/or formation of immune complexes within the lung parenchyma and subsequent fixation of complement. In patients with idiopathic pulmonary fibrosis, immunofluorescent studies have revealed the presence of immunoglobulin and complement components in the lung interstitium (Dreisin et al. 1978). Immune complexes capable of activating complement have been identified both in serum (Dreisin et al. 1978; Haslam et al. 1979) and in bronchial lavage fluids (Hunninghake et al. 1978a) in patients with idiopathic pulmonary fibrosis. In addition, examination of bronchoalveolar lavage fluids has revealed an increased number of neutrophils in bronchial lavage fluids derived from patients with idiopathic pulmonary fibrosis as compared to normal controls and patients with sarcoidosis. The evidence suggests that the presence of neutrophils within the lavage fluid may serve as an indicator of disease activity.

The inflammatory pneumonitis associated with systemic lupus erythematosus and other collagen vascular diseases has been associated with immune complex and complement deposition in the lung (Brentjens et al. 1979; Inoue et al. 1979; Pertschuck et al. 1977). Immunohistopathological studies of lung tissues from patients with pneumonitis in systemic lupus erythematosus have revealed dense deposits of IgG, C3 and antigen in the alveolar interstitium. Also, pleural fluids from patients with systemic lupus erythematosus and rheumatoid arthritis contain immune complexes and decreased levels of complement activity (Halla et al. 1980; Hunder et al. 1972). In addition, the pleural fluid of one patient with rheumatoid arthritis has been shown to contain a substance capable of activating the classical complement pathway (Glovsky et al. 1976). Deposits of immune complexes with complement proteins have also been reported in lung tissue of patients with eosinophilic granuloma of the lung (King et al. 1979). In addition, there are selected reports of a decrease in serum complement levels after aerosol antigen challenge in asthmatic patients (Edwards 1976; Arroyave et al. 1981). These studies demonstrate the presence of immune complexes with evidence of activation of the complement cascade in several lung diseases, suggesting a role for the neutrophil in the evolution of these diseases.

Hypersensitivity pneumonitis (also known as extrinsic allergic alveolitis) is an inflammatory lung disease with components of both humoral and cell-mediated components. Several studies have implicated a role for cell-mediated immune responses (Type IV immunological injury) and a defect of suppressor cell mechanisms in the lungs of these patients (Roberts and Moore 1977). However, there is abundant evidence implicating immune complex mediation in the acute forms of hypersensitivity pneumonitis. In the acute phase of the illness, high titers of specific precipitating antibodies to the sensitizing antigen are present in patient's plasma and appears to correlate with the severity of the disease. Histological examination of lung tissue classically demonstrates the presence of lymphocytes, plasma cells, mononuclear cells, giant cells and non-caseating granulomas in the alveolar interstitium, consistent with a cell-mediated response. However, studies by Ghose et al. (1974b) and Barrowcliff and Arblaster (1968) suggest that the earliest lesion resembles a classic neutrophil-dependent necrotizing vasculitis characteristic of a Type III immune-complex-mediated tissue injury. In addition, skin tests with the appropriate antigen typically show a characteristic Arthus type of necrotizing vasculitis. Although immune complexes are rarely found in lung biopsy material from patients with hypersensitive pneumonitis, the time course of the development of the acute phase of the disease after antigen exposure is consistent with that of a classical Type III Arthus reaction.

Although most clinical conditions associated with a neutrophil influx (e.g. classic lobular pneumonia) are self-limited, with clearance of the pathogenic agent by the neutrophil, resolution of the inflammatory response and little residual tissue destruction, there is significant evidence suggesting a role for the neutrophil in both the development of adult respiratory distress syndrome and diffuse pulmonary fibrosis of the idiopathic variety or associated with collagen vascular disease. Further study is necessary to elucidate the precise role of the neutrophil in these diseases.

REFERENCES

Altman, L.C. (1978) Chemotactic lymphokines: a review. In: J.I. Gallin and P.G. Quie (Eds), *Leukocyte Chemotaxis, Methods, Physiology, and Clinical Implications,* Raven Press, New York.

Ansfield, M.J., Woods, D.E. and Johanson, W.G., Jr (1977) Lung bacterial clearance in murine pneumococcal pneumonia. *Infect. Immun. 17,* 195–204

Arroyave, C.M., Stevenson, D.D., Vaughan, J.H. and Tan, E.M. (1981) Plasma complement changes during provoked bronchospasm in asthmatic patients. *J. Clin. Allergy,* in press.

Babior, B.M. (1978) Oxygen-dependent microbial killing by phagocytes. I. *N. Engl. J. Med. 298,* 659–668.

Baehner, R.L., Boxer, L.A., Allen, J.M. and Davis, J. (1977) Autooxidation as a basis for altered function by polymorphonuclear leukocytes. *Blood 50,* 327–335

Barrowcliff, D.F. and Arblaster, P.G. (1968) Farmer's lung: a study of an early acute fatal case. *Thorax 23,* 490–500.

Becker, E.L., Sigman, M. and Oliver, J.M. (1979) Superoxide production induced in rabbit polymorphonuclear leukocytes by synthetic chemotactic peptides and A23187. *Am. J. Pathol. 95,* 81–97.

Beebe, D.P., Ward, P.A. and Spitznagel, S.K. (1980) Isolation and characterization of an acidic chemotactic factor from complement activated human serum. *Clin. Immunol. Immunopathol. 15,* 88–105.

Binder, A.S., Kageler, W., Perel, A., Flick, M.R. and Staub, N.C. (1980) Effect of platelet depletion on lung vascular permeability after micro-emboli in sheep. *J. Appl. Physiol. 48,* 414–420.

Brentjens, J.R., O'Connell, D.W., Pawlowski, I.B., Hsu, K.C. and Andres, G.A. (1974) Experimental immune complex disease of the lung: the pathogenesis of a laboratory model resembling certain human interstitial diseases. *J. Exp. Med. 140,* 105–125.

Brier, A.M., Snyderman, R., Mergenhagen, J.E. and Notkins, A.L. (1970) Inflammation and herpes simplex virus: release of a chemotaxis-generating factor from infected cells. *Science 170,* 1104–1106.

Burls, R.F., Lawrence, R.A. and Love, M.M. (1980) Liver necrosis and lipid peroxidation in the rat as a result of paraquot and diquot administration: effect of selenium deficiency. *J. Clin. Invest. 65,* 1024–1031.

Caldwell, J.R., Pearce, D.E., Spencer, C., Leder, R. and Waldman, R.H. (1973) Immunologic mechanisms in hypersensitivity pneumonitis: evidence for cell-mediated immunity and complement fixation in pigeon breeder's disease. *J. Allergy Clin. Immunol. 52,* 225–230.

Carp, H. and Janoff, A. (1978) Possible mechanisms of emphysema in smokers: in vitro suppression of serum elastase-inhibitory capacity by fresh cigarette smoke and its prevention by antioxidants. *Am. Rev. Respir. Dis. 118,* 617–621.

Carp, H. and Janoff, A. (1979) In vitro suppression of serum elastase inhibitory capacity by reactive oxygen species generated by phagocytosing polymorphonuclear leukocytes. *J. Clin. Invest. 63,* 793–797.

Chenoweth, D. E. and Hugli, T. F. (1980) Human C5a and C5a analogs as probes of the neutrophil C5a receptor. *Mol. Immunol. 17,* 151–157.

Clark, R.A. and Klebanoff, S.J. (1975) Neutrophil-mediated tumor cell cytotoxicity: role of the peroxidase system. *J. Exp. Med. 141,* 1442–1447.

Clark, R.A. and Klebanoff, S.J. (1979) Myeloperoxidase-mediated platelet release reaction. *J. Clin. Invest. 63,* 177–183.

Clark, R.A., Klebanoff, S.J., Einstein, A.B. and Fefer, A. (1975) Peroxidase–H_2O_2–halide system: cytotoxic effect on mammaliam tumor cells. *Blood 45,* 161–170.

Clark, R.A. and Szot, S. (1982) Chemotactic factor inactivation by stimulated human neutrophils mediated by myeloperoxidase-catalyzed methionine oxidation. *J. Immunol. 128,* 1507–1513.

Clark, R. A., Szot, S., Venkatasubramanian, K. and Schiffman, E. (1980) Chemotactic factor inactivation by myeloperoxidase mediated oxydation of methionine. *J. Immunol. 124,* 2020–2026.

Cline, M.J. and Territo, M.C. (1980) Phagocytosis. In: C.W. Parker (Ed.), *Textbook of Immunology, Vol. 1,* W.B. Saunders, Philadelphia, pp. 298–313.

Coonrod, J. D. (1981) Pulmonary opsonins in Klebsiella pneumoniae pneumonia in rats. *Infect. Immun. 33,* 533–539.

Coonrod, J. D. and Yoneda, K. (1981) Complement and opsonins in alveolar secretions and serum of rats with pneumonia due to Streptococcus pneumoniae. *Rev. Infect. Dis. 3,* 310–322.

Craddock, P.R., Fehr, J., Brigham, K.L., Kronenberg, R.S. and Jacob, H.S. (1977a) Complement and leukocyte-mediated pulmonary dysfunction in hemodialysis. *N. Engl. J. Med. 296,* 769–774.

Craddock, P.R., Fehr, J., Dalmasso, A.P., Brigham, K.L. and Jacob, H.S. (1977b) Pulmonary vascular leukostasis resulting from complement (Cl) activation by dialyzer cellophane membranes. *J. Clin. Invest. 59,* 879–888.

Curnette, J.T. and Babior, B.M. (1979) Biologic defense mechanisms: the effects of bacteria and serum on superoxide production of granulocytes. *J. Clin. Invest. 53,* 1662–1674.

Desai, U., Kreutzer, D. L., Showell, H. J., Arroyave, C. F. and Ward, P.A. (1979) Acute inflammatory pulmonary reactions induced by chemotactic factors. *Am. J. Pathol. 96,* 71–83.

Dewald, B., Rindler-Ludwig, R., Bretz, U. and Baggiolini, M. (1975) Subcellular localization and heterogeneity of neutral proteases neutrophilic polymorphonuclear leukocytes. *J. Exp. Med. 141,* 709–723.

Doroshow, J.H., Locker, G.Y. and Myers, C.E. (1980) Enzymatic defenses of the mouse heart against reactive oxygen metabolites: alterations produced by doxorubicin. *J. Clin. Invest. 65,* 128–135.

Dreisin, R.B., Schwarz, M.I., Theofilopoulos, A.N. and Stanford, R.E. (1978) Circulating immune complexes in the idiopathic interstitial pneumonias. *N. Engl. J. Med. 298,* 353–357.

Edwards, J.H. (1976) A quantitative study in the activation of the alternative pathway of complement by mouldy hay dust and thermophilic actinomycetes. *Clin. Allergy 6,* 19–25.

Fantone, J.C. and Ward, P.A. (1981) Experimental studies of immune complex injury in the lung. *Am. Rev. Respir. Dis. 124,* 743–748.

Fantone, J.C. and Ward, P.A. (1982) Role of oxygen derived free radicals and metabolites in leukocyte dependent inflammatory reactions. *Am. J. Pathol. 107,* 394–418.

Fearon, D.T., Ruddy, S., Schur, P.H. and McCabe, W.R. (1975) Activation of the properidin pathway of complement in patients with gram-negative bacteria. *N. Engl. J. Med. 292,* 937–940.

Fernandez, H.N., Henson, P.M., Otani, A. and Hugli, T.E. (1978) Chemotactic response of human C3a and C5a anaphylatoxins. I. Evaluation of C3a and C5a leukotaxis in vitro under simulated in vivo conditions. *J. Immunol. 120,* 109–115.

Fink, J.N., Moore, V.L. and Barboriak, J.J. (1975) Cell-mediated hypersensitivity in pigeon breeders. *Int. Arch. Allergy Appl. Immunol. 49,* 831–836.

Flick, M.R., Hoeffel, J. and Staub, N.L. (1981) Superoxide dismutase prevents increased lung vascular permeability after air emboli in unanesthetized sheep (Abstract). *Fed. Proc. 40,* 405.

Gell, P.G.H., Coombs, R.R.A. and Lachman, P.J. (1975) *Clinical Aspects of Immunology, 3rd edn.* Blackwell Scientific Pub., Oxford.

Ghose, T., Landrigan, P. and Asif, A. (1974a) Localization of immunoglobulin and complement in pulmonary sarcoid granulomas. *Chest 66,* 264–268.

Ghose, T., Landrigan, P., Killeen, R. and Dill, J. (1974b) Immunopathological studies in patients with farmer's lung. *Clin. Allergy 4,* 119–126.

Glovsky, M.M., Louise, J.G., Pitts, W.H. and Alenty, A. (1976) Reduction of pleural fluid complement activity in patients with systemic lupus erythematosus and rheumatoid arthritis. *Clin. Immunol. Immunopathol. 6,* 31–41.

Goetzl, E.J. (1980) Mediators of immediate hypersensitivity derived from arachidonic acid. *N. Engl. J. Med. 303,* 822–825.

Goetzl, E.J. and Austen, K.F. (1975) Purification and synthesis of eosinophilotactic tetrapeptides of human lung tissue: identification as eosinophil chemotactic factor of anaphylaxis. *Proc. Natl. Acad. Sci. USA 72,* 4123–4127.

Granelli-Piperno, A., Vassalli, J.D. and Reich, E. (1977) Secretion of plasminogen activator by human polymorphonuclear leukocytes: modulation by glucocorticoids and other effectors. *J. Exp. Med. 146,* 1693–1706.

Gross, G.N., Rehm, S.R. and Pierce, A.K. (1978) The effect of complement depletion on lung clearance of bacteria. *J. Clin. Invest. 62,* 373–378.

Guckian, J.D., Christensen, G.D. and Fine, D.P. (1980) The role of opsonins in recovery from experimental pneumococcal pneumonia. *J. Infect. Dis. 142,* 175–190.

Hafeman, D.D. and Lucas, Z.J. (1979) Polymorphonuclear leukocyte mediated antibody dependent cellular cytotoxicity against tumor cells: dependence on oxygen and the respiratory burst. *J. Immunol. 123,* 55–62.

Halla, J.T., Schrohenloher, R.E. and Volanakis, J.E. (1980) Immune complexes and other laboratory features of pleural effusions: a comparison of rheumatoid arthritis, systemic lupus erythematosus and other diseases. *Ann. Intern. Med. 92,* 748–752.

Hansen, P.J. and Penny, R. (1974) Pigeon breeder's disease: study of cell-mediated immune response to pigeon antigens by the lymphocyte culture technique. *Int. Arch. Allergy Appl. Immunol. 47,* 498–507.

Haslam, D.L., Thompson, B., Mohammed, I., Townsend, P.J., Hodson, M.E., Holbrow, E.J. and Turner-Warwick, M. (1979) Circulating immune complexes in patients with cryptogenic fibrosing alveolitis. *Clin. Exp. Immunol. 37,* 381–390.

Heflin, A.C. and Brigham, K.L. (1981) Prevention by granulocyte depletion of increased vascular permeability of sheep lung following endotoxemia. *J. Clin. Invest. 68,* 1253–1260.

Henson, P.M. (1980) Mechanisms of exocytosis in phagocytic inflammatory cells. *Am. J. Pathol. 101,* 494–511.

Henson, P.M., McCarthy, K., Larsen, G.L., Webster, R.O., Gickas, P.C., Dreisin, R.B., King, T.E. and Shaw, J.O. (1979) Complement fragments, alveolar macrophages, and alveolitis. *Am. J. Pathol. 97,* 93–110.

Hoff, D.G., Peterson, P.K., Repine, J.E. and Hoidal, J.R. (1980) Phagocytosis by human alveolar macrophages and neutrophils: qualitative differences in the opsonic requirements for uptake of Staphylococcus aureus and Streptococcus pneumoniae in vitro. *Am. Rev. Respir. Dis. 121,* 65–72.

Hosea, S., Brown, E., Hammer, C. and Frank, M. (1980) Role of complement activation in a model of adult respiratory distress syndrome. *J. Clin. Invest. 66,* 375–382.

Huber, W. and Saifer, M.G. (1977) Orgotein, the drug version of bovine Cu-Zn superoxide dismutase. I. A summary account of safety and pharmacology in laboratory animals. In: A.M. Michelson, J.M. McCord and I. Fridovich (Eds), *Superoxide and Superoxide Dismutases,* Academic Press, New York, pp. 517–534.

Hugli, T.E. (1978) Chemical aspects of the serum anaphylatoxins. *Contemp. Top. Mol. Immunol. 7,* 181–214.

Hugli, T.E. and Muller-Eberhard, H.J. (1978) Anaphylatoxins: C3a and C5a. *Adv. Immunol. 26,* 1.

Hunder, G.G., McDuffie, F.C. and Hepper, N.G.G. (1972) Pleural fluid complement in systemic lupus erythematosus and rheumatoid arthritis. *Ann. Intern. Med. 76,* 357–363.

Hunninghake, G.W. and Crystal, R.G. (1981) Mechanisms of hypergammaglobulinemia in pulmonary sarcoidosis: site of increased antibody production and role of T-lymphocytes. *J. Clin. Invest. 67,* 86–92.

Hunninghake, G.W., Gadek, J.E., Lawley, T.J., Kelman, J., Fulmer, J.D. and Crystal, R.G. (1978a) Role of immune complexes in amplifying the alveolitis of idiopathic pulmonary fibrosis (IPF) (Abstract). *Clin. Res. 26,* 446A.

Hunninghake, G.W., Gallin, J.I. and Fauci, A.S. (1978b) Immunologic reactivity of the lung: the in vivo and in vitro generation of a neutrophil chemotactic factor by alveolar macrophages. *Am. Rev. Resp. Dis. 117,* 15–23.

Hunninghake, G.W., Fulmer, J.D., Young, R.C., Gadek, J.E. and Crystal, R.G. (1979) Localization of the immune response in sarcoidosis. *Am. Rev. Resp. Dis. 120,* 49–57.

Hunninghake, G., Gadek, J. and Crystal, R. (1980a) Mechanisms by which cigarette smoke attracts polymorphonuclear leukocytes to lung. *Chest 77 (Suppl.)*, 273.

Hunninghake, G.W., Gadek, J.E., Fales, H.M. and Crystal, R.G. (1980b) Human alveolar macrophage-derived chemotactic factor for neutrophils: stimuli and partial characterization. *J. Clin. Invest. 66*, 473–483.

Hunninghake, G.W., Gadek, J.E., Young, R.C., Kawanami, O., Ferran, N.J. and Crystal, R. (1980c) Maintenance of granuloma formation in pulmonary sarcoidosis by T-lymphocytes within the lung. *N. Engl. J. Med. 302*,594–598.

Inoue, T., Kanayamo, Y., Akiko, O., Kato, N., Horiguchi, T., Ishii, M. and Zshiota, K. (1979) Immunopathologic studies of pneumonitis in systemic lupus erythematosus. *Ann. Intern. Med. 91*, 30–34.

Jacob, H.S., Craddock, P.R., Hammerschmidt, D.E. and Moldow, C.F. (1980) Complement-induced granulocyte aggregation: an unsuspected mechanism of disease *N. Engl. J. Med. 302*, 784–794.

Janoff, A., Sloan, B., Weinbaum, G., Damiano, V., Sandhaus, R.A., Elias, J. and Kimbel, P. (1977) Experimental emphysema produced by purified human neutrophil elastase: tissue localization of the instilled protease. *Am. Rev. Respir. Dis. 115*, 461–478.

Johnson, K.J. and Ward, P.A. (1974) Acute immunologic pulmonary alveolitis. *J. Clin. Invest. 54*, 349–357.

Johnson, K.J. and Ward, P.A. (1981) Role of oxygen metabolites in immune complex injury of lung. *J. Immunol. 126*, 2365–2369.

Johnson, K.J., Anderson, T.P. and Ward, P.A. (1977) Suppression of immune complex-induced inflammation by the chemotactic factor inactivator. *J. Clin. Invest. 59*, 951–958.

Johnson, K.J., Varani, J., Oliver, J. and Ward, P.A. (1979) Immunologic vasculitis in beige mice with deficiency of leukocytic neutral proteases. *J. Immunol. 122*, 1807–1812.

Johnson, K.J., Fantone, J.C., Kaplan, J. and Ward, P.A. (1981) In vivo damage of rat lungs by oxygen metabolites. *J. Clin. Invest. 67*, 983–993.

Kaplan, R.L., Schocket, A.L., King, T.E., Mawitz, R.M., Good, J.T., Stanford, R.E. and Sahn, S.A. (1980) A model of immune complex mediated pleuropulmonary injury: evidence of deposition of circulating immune complexes in the lung. *Am. J. Pathol. 100*, 115–128.

Katzenstein, A., Bloor, C.M. and Liebow, A. (1976) Diffuse alveolar damage: the role of oxygen, shock, and related factors. *Am. J. Pathol. 85*, 210–228.

Kay, A.B. and Austen, K.F. (1971) The IgE-mediated release of an eosinophil leukocyte chemotactic factor from human lung. *J. Immunol. 107*, 899–902.

Kazmierowski, J.A., Gallin, J.I. and Reynolds, N.Y. (1977) Mechanism for the inflammatory response in primate lungs: demonstration and partial characterization of an alveolar macrophage-derived chemotactic factor with preferential activity for polymorphonuclear leukocytes. *J. Clin. Invest. 59*, 273–281.

Kellogg, E.W. and Fridovich, I. (1977) Liposome oxidation and erythrocyte lysis by enzymatically generated superoxide and hydrogen peroxide. *J. Biol. Chem. 252*, 6721–6728.

King, T.E., Schwarz, M.I., Pratt, D.S., Dreisin, R.G. and Theofilopoulos, A.N. (1979) Circulating immune complexes with immunoglobulin and complement deposition in pulmonary tissue of patients with eosinophilic granuloma of the lung. *Ann. Intern. Med. 91*, 397–399.

Klebanoff, S. J. (1980) Oxygen metabolism and the toxic properties of phagocytes. *Ann. Intern. Med. 93,* 480–489.

Klebanoff, S.J. and Clark, R.A. (1975) Hemolysis and iodination of erythrocyte components by a myeloperoxidase-mediated system. *Blood 45,* 699–707.

Kniker, W.T. and Cochrane, G.G. (1965) Pathogenic factors in vascular lesions of experimental serum sickness. *J. Exp. Med. 122,* 83–98.

Kreutzer, D.L., Claypool, W.D., Jones, M.L. and Ward, P.A. (1979a) Isolation by hydrophobic chromatography of the chemotactic factor inactivators from human serum. *Clin. Immunol. Immunopathol. 12,* 162–176.

Kreutzer, D.L., Desai, U., Orr, W., Showell, H. and Ward, P.A. (1979b) Induction of acute inflammatory reactions in lung following intrapulmonary instillation of preformed chemotactic peptides and purified complement components. *Chest 755,* 2595–2625.

Kueppers, F. and Black, L.E. (1974) α_1-Antitrypsin and its deficiency. *Am. Rev. Respir. Dis. 110,* 176–194.

Kunkel, S.L., Thrall, R.S., Kunkel, R.G., McCormick, J.N., Ward, P.A. and Zurier, R.B. (1979) Suppression of immune complex vasculitis in rats by prostaglandin. *J. Clin. Invest. 64,* 1525–1531.

Leiberman, J. (1969) Heterozygous and homozygous α_1-antitrypsin deficiency in patients with pulmonary emphysema. *N. Engl. J. Med. 281,* 279–284.

Lynn, W.S. and Mukherjee S.P. (1979) Motility of rabbit alveolar cells: role of unsaturated fatty acids. *Am. J. Pathol. 96,* 663–672.

Marasco, W.A. and Becker, E.L. (1982) Anti-idiotype as antibody against the formyl peptide chemotaxis receptor of the neutrophil. *J. Immunol. 128,* 963–969.

Marasco, W.A., Showell, H.J., Freer, R.J. and Becker, E.L. (1982) Anti-f Met-Leu-Phe: similarities in fine specificity with the formyl peptide chemotaxis receptor of the neutrophils. *J. Immunol. 128,* 956–962.

Marten, W.J., Gadek, J.E., Hunninghake, G.W. and Crystal, R.G. (1981) Oxidant injury of lung parenchymal cells. *J. Clin. Invest. 68,* 1277–1288.

McCormick, J.R., Harkin, M.M., Johnson, K.J. and Ward, P.A. (1981) The effect of superoxide dismutase on pulmonary and dermal inflammation. *Am. J. Pathol. 102,* 55–61.

Merrill, W.W., Naegel, G.P., Matthey, R.A. and Reynolds, H. (1980) Alveolar macrophage-derived chemotactic factor: kinetics of in vitro production and partial characterization. *J. Clin. Invest. 65,* 268–276.

Nathan, C.F., Brukner, L., Silverstein, S.C. and Cohn, Z.A. (1979) Extracellular cytolysis by activated macrophages and granulocytes. *J. Exp. Med. 149,* 100–113.

O'Flaherty, J.T. and Ward, P.A. (1978) Leukocyte aggregation induced by chemotactic factors: a review. *Inflammation 3,* 177–194.

O'Flaherty, J.T., Showell, H.J. and Ward, P.A. (1977) Neutropenia induced by systemic infusion of chemotactic factors. *J. Immunol. 118,* 1586–1589.

O'Flaherty, J.T., Craddock, P.R. and Jacob, H.S. (1978) Effect of intravascular complement activation on granulocyte adhesiveness and distribution. *Blood 51,* 731–739.

Orr, F.W., Varani, J., Kreutzer, D.L., Senior, R.M. and Ward P.A. (1979) Digestion of the fifth component of complement by leukocytic enzymes: sequential generation of chemotactic activities for leukocytes and for tumor cells. *Am. J. Pathol. 94,* 75–84.

Oyanagui, Y. (1976) Participation of superoxide anions at the prostaglandins phase of carrageenin foot edema. *Biochem. Pharmacol. 25,* 1465–1472.

Perez, H.D. and Goldstein, J.M. (1980) Generation of a chemotactic lipid from arachidonic acid by exposure to a superoxide generating system (Abstract). *Fed. Proc. 39,* 1170.

Perez, H.D., Goldstein, I.M., Chernoff, D., Webster, R.O. and Henson, P.M. (1980) Chemotactic activity of C5a des-Arg: evidence of a requirement for an anionic peptide "helper factor" and inhibition by a cationic protein in serum from patients with systemic lupus erythematosus. *Mol. Immunol. 17,* 163–169.

Pertschuk, L.P., Morca, L.F. and Rosen, Y. (1977) Acute pulmonary complications in systemic lupus erythematosus: immunofluorescence and light microscopic study. *Am. J. Clin. Pathol. 68,* 553–557.

Petrone, W.F., English, D.K., Wong, K. and McCord, J.M. (1980) Free radicals and inflammation: the superoxide dependent activation of a neutrophil chemotactic factor in plasma. *Proc. Natl. Acad. Sci. USA 77,* 1159–1163.

Postlewaite, A.E. and Kang, A.H. (1976) Collagen and collagen peptide-induced chemotaxis of human blood monocytes. *J. Exp. Med. 143,* 1299–1307.

Postlewaite, A.E. and Snyderman, R. (1975) Characterization of chemotactic activity produced in vivo by a cell-mediated immune reaction in the guinea pig. *J. Immunol. 114,* 274–278.

Postlewaite, A.E., Seyer, J.M. and Kang, A.H. (1978) Chemotactic attraction of human fibroblasts to Type I, II and III collagens and collagen-derived peptides. *Proc. Natl. Acad. Sci. USA 75,* 871–875.

Rehm, S.R., Gross, G.N. and Pierce, A.K. (1980) Early bacterial clearance from murine lungs. *J. Clin. Invest. 66,* 194–199.

Richerson, H.B. (1972) Acute experimental hypersensitivity pneumonitis in the guinea pig. *J. Lab. Clin. Med. 79,* 745–757.

Rister, M. and Baehner, R.L. (1976) The alteration of superoxide dismutase, catalase, glutathione peroxidase, NAD(P)H, cytochrome c reductase in guinea pig polymorphonuclear leukocytes and alveolar macrophages during hyperoxia. *J. Clin. Invest. 58,* 1174–1184.

Roberts, R.C. and Moore, V.L. (1977) Immunopathogenesis of hypersensitivity pneumonitis. *Am. Rev. Respir. Dis. 116,* 1075–1090.

Robertson, J., Caldwell, J.R., Castle, J.R. and Waldman, R.I.I. (1976) Evidence for the presence of components of the alternative (properdin) pathway of complement activation in respiratory secretions. *J. Immunol. 117,* 900–903.

Rodriguez, R.J., White, R.R., Senior, R.M. and Levine, E.A. (1977) Elastase release from human alveolar macrophages: comparison between smokers and nonsmokers. *Science 198,* 313–314.

Roos, D. (1980) The metabolic response to phagocytosis. In: G. Weissman (Ed.), *Handbook of Inflammation, Vol. 2: Cell Biology of Inflammation,* Elsevier/North-Holland, Biomedical Press, Amsterdam, pp. 337–387.

Roos, D., Keller H.U., Hess, M.W. and Cottier, H. (1977) *Alveolar Macrophages: Phagocytosis-induced Release of Neutrophil Chemotactic Activity, Pulmonary Macrophages and Epithelial Cells,* C.L. Sanders et al (Eds), ERDA Technical Information Center Washington DC, pp. 326–339.

Roos, D., Weenig, R.S. and Voetman, A.A. (1980) Protection of human neutrophils against oxidation damage. *Agents Actions 10,* 528–535.

Root, R.K., Metcalf, J., Oshino, W. and Chance, B. (1975) H_2O_2 release from human granulocytes during phagocytosis. I. Documentation, quantitation and some regulating factors. *J. Clin. Invest. 55,* 945–955.

Roska, A.K.B., Moore, V.L. and Abramoff, P. (1979) Immune complex disease in guinea pig lungs: elicitation with pigeon serum. *Am. Rev. Respir. Dis. 120,* 129–136.

Sachs, T., Moldow, C.F., Craddock, P.R., Bowers, T.K. and Jacob, H.S. (1978) Oxygen radicals mediate endothelial cell damage by complement stimulated granulocytes: an in vitro model of immune vascular damage. *J. Clin. Invest. 61,* 1161–1167.

Saltzman, H.A. and Fridovich, I. (1975) Oxygen toxicity: introduction to a protective enzyme-superoxide dismutase. *Circulation 48,* 921–923.

Salvin, S.B., Youngner, J.S. and Lederer, W.H. (1973) Migration inhibitory factor and interferon in the circulation of mice with delayed hypersensitivity. *Infect. Immun. 7,* 68–75.

Scherzer, H. and Ward, P.A. (1978a) Lung injury produced by immune complexes of varying composition *J. Immunol. 121,* 947–952

Scherzer, H. and Ward, P.A. (1978b) Lung and dermal vascular injury produced by preformed immune complexes. *Am. Rev. Respir. Dis. 117,* 551–557

Schiffman, E.H., Showell, H.J., Corcoran, B.A., Weep, P.A., Smith, E. and Becker, E. L. (1975) The isolation and partial characterization of neutrophil chemotactic factors from Escherichia coli. *J. Immunol. 114,* 1831–1836

Schrieber, A.D., Kaplan, A.P. and Austen, K.F. (1973) Plasma inhibitors of the components of the fibrinolytic pathway in man. *J. Clin. Invest. 52,* 1394–1401

Senior, R.M., Griffin, G.L. and Mecham, R.P. (1980) Chemotactic activity of elastin-derived peptides. *J. Clin. Invest. 66,* 859–862

Senior, R.M., Tegner, H., Kuhn, C., Ohlsson, K., Stascher, B.C. and Pierce, J.A. (1977) The induction of pulmonary emphysema with human leukocyte elastase. *Am. Rev. Respir. Dis. 116,* 469–475

Shaw, J., Henson, J., Phillips, D. and Henson, P.M. (1978) Lung injury induced by intratracheal administration of a chemotactic fragment from the fifth component of complement. *Am. Rev. Respir. Dis. 117,* 80

Showell, H.J., Freer, R.J., Zigmond, S.H., Schiffman, E., Aswanikumar, J., Corcoran, P.A. and Becker, E.L. (1976) The structure–activity relations of synthetic peptides as chemotactic factors and inducers of lysosomal enzyme secretion for neutrophils. *J. Exp. Med. 14,* 1154–1159.

Simon, R.H., Scoggin, C.H. and Patterson, D. (1981) Hydrogen peroxide causes fatal injury to fibroblasts exposed to oxygen radicals. *J. Biol. Chem. 256,* 7181–7186

Stimler, N.P., Hugli, T.E. and Bloor, C.M. (1980) Pulmonary injury induced by C3a and C5a anaphylatoxins. *Am. J. Pathol. 100,* 327–348.

Sullivan, T.J. and Kulczycki, A. (1980) In: C.W. Parker (Ed.). Immediate Hypersensitivity Responses in Clinical Immunology, In: C.W. Parker (Ed.), *Clinical Immunology, Vol 1, Chapter 5,* W.B. Saunders Co., Philadelphia, pp 115–142.

Taylor, F.B., Jr. and Ward, P.A. (1967) Generation of chemotactic activity in rabbit serum by plasminogen streptokinase mixtures. *J. Exp. Med. 126,* 149–160

Till, G. and Ward, P.A. (1975) Two distinct chemotactic factor inactivators in human serum. *J. Immunol. 114,* 843–847.

Till, G., Johnson, K. and Ward, P.A. (1982) Intravascular activation of complement and acute lung injury: dependency of neutrophils and toxic oxygen metabolites. *J. Clin. Invest.,* in press.

Unkeless, J., Gordon, S. and Reich, E. (1974) Secretion of plasminogen activator by stimulated macrophages. *J. Exp. Med. 139,* 834–841.

Verge, P. and Olsson, I. (1975) Cationic proteins of human granulocytes. VI. Effects on the complement system and mediation of chemotactic activity. *J. Immunol. 115,* 1505–1508.

Vogt, W. (1974) Activation, activities, and pharmacologically active products of complement. *Pharmacol. Rev. 26,* 125.

Ward, P.A. (1980) Chemotaxis. In: C.W. Parker (Ed.), *Textbook of Immunology, Vol. 1,* W. B. Saunders Co., Philadelphia, pp. 272–297.

Ward, P.A. and Hill, J.H. (1970) C5 chemotactic fragments produced by an enzyme in lysosomal granules of neutrophils. *J. Immunol. 104,* 535–543.

Ward, P.A., Lepow, I.H. and Newman, L.J. (1960) Bacterial factors chemotactic for polymorphonuclear leukocytes. *Am. J. Pathol. 52,* 725–736.

Ward, P.A., Cohen, S. and Flanagan, T.D. (1972) Leukotactic factors elaborated by virus infected tissues. *J. Exp. Med. 135,* 1095–1103.

Ward, P.A., Chapitis, J., Conroy, M.C. and Lepow, T.H. (1973) Generation by bacterial proteinases of leukotactic factors from human C3 and C5. *J. Immunol. 110,* 1003–1009.

Ward, P.A., Hugli, J.E. and Chenoweth, D.P. (1979) Complement and chemotaxis. In: J.C. Houck (Ed.), *Handbook of Inflammation, Vol. 1,* Elsevier/North-Holland, Biomedical Press, Amsterdam, pp. 153–178.

Weiss, S.J., LoBuglio, A.F. and Kessler, H.B. (1980) Oxidative mechanisms of monocyte mediated cytotoxicity. *Proc. Natl. Acad. Sci. USA 77,* 584–587.

Weiss, J.J., Young, J., LoBuglio, A.F., Slivka, A. and Nimeh, N.F. (1981) Role of hydrogen peroxide in neutriophil mediated destruction of cultured endothelial cells. *J. Clin. Invest. 68,* 714–721.

Webster, R.O., Larsen, G.L., Mitchell, C., Goins, A.J. and Henson, P.M. (1982) Absence of inflammatory lung injury in rabbits challenged intravascularly with complement-derived chemotactic factors. *Am. Rev. Respir. Dis. 125,* 335–340.

Willoughby, W.F., Willoughby, J.B., Cantrell, B.B. and Wheelis, R. (1979) In vivo response to inhaled proteins. II. Induction of interstitial pneumonitis and enhancement of immune complex mediated alveolitis by inhaled concanavalin A. *Lab. Invest. 40,* 399–414.

CHAPTER 4

Fibrotic mechanisms in lung diseases

SEM H. PHAN
Department of Pathology, University of Michigan Medical School, Ann Arbor, Michigan 48109

4.1. INTRODUCTION

The lung is simultaneously exposed to both an internal, systemic, and an external, or extracorporeal, environment. Consequently, it is subject to injury by agents or processes occurring in both these environments. As the result of such interactions, events are initiated which may result in pulmonary fibrosis. In many cases, the initiating agent or event remains unidentified (so-called idiopathic pulmonary fibrosis; IPF). It is unclear why certain stimuli cause pulmonary fibrosis while others do not, despite similarities in the acute responses. Furthermore, a more intense inflammatory response cannot always be directly correlated with a greater or more severe fibrotic response. It also remains unclear why and how the fibrotic process can be arrested in a few of these diseases by certain therapeutic modalities not directly related to connective tissue metabolism. This chapter is an attempt at summarizing the latest advances made in the overall effort to provide some answers to these questions. The emphasis being on mechanistic considerations, no attempt has been made here to comprehensively list each and every known possible cause of pulmonary fibrosis. Instead, a few aspects on which sufficient data have been accumulated to provide certain insights into the underlying mechanism have been selected and discussed.

Fibrosis can be defined as the increased and/or the abnormal deposition of connective tissue. It can be desirable, as in wound healing, or it can be detrimental, when a vital organ is involved, with consequent loss of function. Since the ultimate event in each case is the increased production or disordered accumulation of connective tissue elements, the ability to unravel the mechanism of the fibrogenic response is limited by the extent of our knowledge of connective tissue cells and metabolism as well as of their regulation. This chapter has been organized to reflect this dependence and limitation. Following a brief review of normal connective tissue metabolism, known abnormalities of this process are described. Regulatory aspects of connective tissue elements are then reviewed.

4.2. CAUSES OF PULMONARY FIBROSIS

Pulmonary fibrosis is caused by and closely associated with numerous disease processes, representative categories of which are listed in Table 1. An additional category (IPF) has no known cause. The various histopathologic types of interstitial pneumonitis (IP) that can result in IPF have been described by Liebow (1967). The histologic differences are relatively distinct and they also differ in their responsiveness to steroid therapy. The desquamative form (DIP) appears to be more responsive to steroids than the usual variety (UIP) (Scadding and Hinson 1967; Carrington et al. 1978). Furthermore, IPF patients with large numbers of lymphocytes in their bronchoalveolar lavage fluid (BAL) also are more responsive to steroids (Haslam et al. 1980). The presence of circulating as well as lung-fixed immune complexes also improves their steroid responsiveness (Turner-Warwick et al. 1971; Dreisin et al. 1978; Haslam et al. 1979). This implies a multiplicity of mechanisms and suggests that IPF is far from being a single entity but is probably a heterogeneous collection of diseases. There are, however, some features of IPF that are more or less common to all of them. The majority of patients have peripheral lymphocytes that secrete macrophage migration inhibition factor (MIF) upon stimulation with Type I collagen (Kravis et al. 1976). They also have large numbers of neutrophils in their BAL (Haslam et al. 1980; Keogh et al. 1981), the relative number of which is related to their prognosis (Keogh et al. 1981). The presence of

TABLE 1.
Causes of pulmonary fibrosis

1. Physico-chemical injury
   a) Ionizing radiation
   b) Inhaled gases
      e.g. beryllium fumes, cadmium, mercury vapor, NO_2, oxygen toxicity
   c) Aspiration of acids, bases and organic solvents
2. Pneumoconioses and granulomatoses
   e.g. coal-dust, silica, asbestos, sarcoidosis
3. Inhalation of organic dusts (extrinsic allergic alveolitis)
   e.g. farmer's lung, pigeon breeder's disease
4. Viral pneumonias
5. Close association with certain systemic diseases
   e.g. systemic lupus erythematosus, rheumatoid arthritis, systemic sclerosis
6. Drug-induced
   e.g. bleomycin, cyclophosphamide, nitrofurantoin, busulfan, hydralazine
7. Miscellaneous
   e.g. left ventricular failure, uremia, shock lung, Dressler's syndrome
8. Idiopathic

detectable collagenase activity in their BAL (usually not detectable in patients without IPF) has also been reported (Gadek et al. 1979). Serological abnormalities have also been reported in these patients (Turner-Warwick et al. 1971; Nagaya and Sieker 1972; Haslam et al. 1975; Pearson et al. 1981). And most recently, it has been reported that IPF patients had a significantly greater incidence of the HLA type DrW2 (Libby et al. 1981), although previous attempts failed to show such an association due to inhomogeneity of the sampled population (Fulmer et al. 1973). A familial type of Hamman-Rich syndrome has also been described (Swaye et al. 1969; Solliday et al. 1973). These findings suggest both immunologic and non-immunologic factors regulating the fibrotic response, which will be further discussed in a subsequent section.

Diseases with major immune system involvement include the collagen vascular diseases (Divertie 1964; Petty and Wilkins 1966; Schwartz et al. 1976; Turner-Warwick 1981) and some of the pneumonitides due to inhaled dusts (e.g. pigeon breeder's disease and farmer's lung) and fumes (e.g. beryllium) (Pepys 1969; Marx and Burrell 1973). The offending antigen is either an auto- or a foreign antigen. In some of these diseases, both clinical and experimental findings have revealed immune complex deposition with activation of the complement pathways and subsequent tissue injury (Berrens et al. 1974; Ghose et al. 1974; Hensley et al. 1974; Edwards 1976). T-cell sensitization to some of these antigens has also been reported (Moore et al. 1974; Allen et al. 1977). The granulomatous component in sarcoidosis certainly suggests an immune phenomenon, although no antigen has been unequivocally identified (Hanngren et al. 1974; Mitchell 1976). Viral pneumonias occasionally result in pulmonary fibrosis (Finch and Bader 1974) and an Arthus type of phenomenon in the lung has been postulated as the mechanism (Turner-Warwick 1973). The survival of these patients, as in any immunopathologic process, would depend on the ability to suppress this immune responsiveness, either by effective immunosuppression or by removal of the offending antigen. The inability to achieve either of these would result in uncontrollable, diffuse and eventually fatal pulmonary fibrosis.

Physico-chemical causes of pulmonary fibrosis encompass a large number of agents which are directly injurious or toxic to tissue. Agents such as strong acids or bases can cause tissue necrosis with subsequent inflammation and healing, resulting usually in scar formation. The extent of injury determines the extent of fibrosis and, ultimately, survival. Radiation can also cause tissue necrosis and pulmonary fibrosis (Gross 1977). In experimental animal models this was, after a brief delay, accompanied by increased lung collagen (Pickrell et al. 1976). There also was some responsiveness to steroid therapy (Phillips et al. 1975; Gross 1980). Inhalation of certain inorganic dusts, usually encountered in the pneumoconioses, can also result in fibrosis. Silicosis and asbestosis are probably the more common and well-studied ones (Corrin and Price 1972; Heppleston 1973; Ziskind 1976). In the case of silicosis, ingestion of silica or quartz crystals by macrophages has been known to stimulate them to produce fibroblast-activating factor(s) (Heppleston and Styles

1967; Aalto et al. 1976). Exposure to oxidizing atmospheres such as ozone and high oxygen tensions can also result in pulmonary fibrosis (Clark and Lambertsen 1971; Freeman et al. 1973; Chvapil and Leng 1975). The disease process can be halted if the organism is removed from these atmospheres early enough, while in some cases the process becomes irreversible and fatal (as in "shock lung"). The toxicity is apparently due to generation of oxygen metabolites and free radicals (Crapo and Tierney 1974; Fridovich 1976). Ingestion of paraquat has been reported to cause fibrosis by similar mechanisms, i.e. reduction of O_2 by paraquat to generate superoxide anion and other subsequent O_2 metabolites (Fisher et al. 1973). It is not surprising, therefore, that the lung content of O_2 metabolite-detoxifying enzymes can affect the survival of an organism exposed to oxidizing atmospheres (Frank and Roberts 1979).

Drug-induced pulmonary fibrosis has been extensively reported (Rosenow 1972). Many of these cases, however, were based on limited numbers of patients, some of whom were concurrently being treated with other unrelated drugs or therapeutic modalities, thus making it difficult to isolate the offending agent. Among the many drugs, several have been well studied and their ability to induce pulmonary fibrosis has been well documented. Some of these, such as bleomycin, busulphan and methotrexate, have been reported to cause similar changes in animals, thus providing convenient models. This type of drug usually causes an interstitial pneumonitis resembling UIP (Luna et al. 1972). Other drugs, such as hydralazine, cause a lupus-like syndrome occasionally with associated pulmonary fibrosis (Alarcon-Segovia 1969; Estes and Christian 1971). The mechanism is presumably related to the lupus-associated pulmonary fibrosis. Others, such as nitrofurantoin on the other hand, have features of hypersensitivity with appearance of eosinophils in the lung (Cole 1976).

This brief survey of etiologies and associations emphasizes the fact that a multiplicity of causes, with varying mechanisms, can have the same outcome. The consequence of this resulting excessive and disordered connective tissue deposition in the lung is a decreased compliance, with shifting to the right of the pressure—volume curve, and an impairment of alveoar—capillary gas diffusivity. The extent of lung involvement ultimately determines the survival of the affected individual.

4.3. REVIEW OF CONNECTIVE TISSUE METABOLISM

Connective tissue consists of three major components: collagen, elastin and glycosaminoglycans (mostly in the form of proteoglycans), present in differing amounts in any one location. Their composition and the known physical properties of each have helped us understand the function of certain tissues. Excellent detailed reviews of connective tissue metabolism are available elsewhere (Lamberg and Stoolmiller 1974; Hance and Crystal 1975; Ramachandran and Reddi 1976; Fessler and Fessler 1978; Lennarz 1980; Vudi and Vuust 1980; Pickrell 1981) and therefore only the salient points of connective tissue metabolism will be discussed here. These steps of connective tissue metabolism which are subject to regulation and which may be rate-limiting, have been elucidated by data derived from studies with lung as well as with other organs. Steps unique to or absent in lung will be noted.

4.3.1. Collagen

It has been estimated that the total lung connective tissue mass is composed of 60–70% collagen (Hance and Crystal 1975). Collagen is also widely distributed in other organs, due to its importance in maintaining structural integrity and in providing a framework which is essential for organ growth and development. For instance, azetidine-2-carboxylic acid, a proline analogue, interferes with the normal development of mouse tooth germs and lung epithelial budding (Alescio 1973). This finding is further supported by the observation that the mesoderm is a major determinant or regulator of normal lung growth and development (Thurlbeck 1975). Because of this and its relative ease of isolation, collagen has been most extensively studied and is therefore the best understood among the components of connective tissue.

The basic mechanism of collagen synthesis is similar to that of other proteins, with incorporation of amino acids from the various pools into the peptidyl structure via t-RNA. The more unique features of collagen synthesis comprise (1) the greater content of certain amino acids such as proline, hydroxyproline, lysine, hydroxylysine and glycine; (2) the large number of post-translational modification steps due to its high content of hydroxyproline, hydroxylysine and carbohydrate residues; (3) the triple helical configuration of the assembled tropocollagen with non-helical extensions or terminal segments in both NH_2- and COOH-ends, which are cleaved by specific proteases in the conversion from procollagen to collagen; and (4) the extensive cross-linking which results in the final stable product.

Little is known at the level of transcription in the collagen biosynthetic pathway. It is clear, however, that several different genes, probably located in different chromosomes, direct the synthesis of the several types of collagen that have been identified up to now (Types I–V) (Sundar et al. 1977; Sykes and Solomon 1978; Bornstein and Sage 1980). Little is known about the importance of this step in the overall regulation of collagen synthesis, although viral transformations and the developmental stage of the organism have been known to affect the rate of transcription and the amount of m-RNA available for translation (Evans and Peterkovsky 1976; Miller 1976; Hata and Peterkovsky 1977). Even less is known concerning control at the translational level.

Prolyl and lysyl hydroxylation occurs on nascent chains, and is catalyzed by hydroxylases (Fessler and Fessler 1978). Prolyl hydroxylation is important for triple helical formation and thus for stabilization and fibril formation. Interference with this hydroxylation also inhibits overall collagen synthesis with intracellular breakdown of the procollagen chains (Grant and Prockop 1972; Bienkowski et al. 1978). This provides the rationale behind recent therapeutic strategies using proline analogues to inhibit fibrosis (Kelley et al. 1980; Riley et al. 1980, 1981b). However, prolyl hydroxylase activity cannot always be directly related to rate of collagen synthesis (Murad et al. 1981), suggesting that under certain conditions this step is not rate-limiting. The lungs contain abundant prolyl hydroxylase (Cutroneo et al. 1974). Lung collagen has similar degrees of prolyl hydroxylation to those of other tissue collagens (Bradley et al. 1974). Lysine, however, appears to be more hydroxylated in collagen from lung than from other tissues (Bradley et al. 1974; Seyer et al. 1976; McLees et al. 1977). Lysine and hydroxylysine residues are important in the cross-linking reactions (Piez 1968; Tanger 1973; Siegel 1976). The hydroxylysine residues are also important for the next post-translational modification step.

Glycosylation of hydroxylysine residues is catalyzed by several glycosyl transferases (Spiro and Spiro 1971; Hance and Crystal 1975), with further glycosylation occurring at the Golgi apparatus during the secretion process (Spiro and Spiro 1971). The functional significance of this glycosylation step is unclear, although its importance to fibril formation has been suggested (Spiro 1969).

The sequence of events following these modification steps is unclear, but the following steps occur prior to secretion: (a) inter-chain disulfide bond formation at the carboxy-terminal region; (b) assembly into triple helix with both amino and carboxy terminal non-helical extensions; and (c) translocation of this procollagen via the Golgi apparatus. The "procollagenous" state has been hypothesized as being conducive to initiation of triple helix formation and secretion to the extracellular space, as well as inhibition of intracellular fibril formation (Bornstein 1974). The secretory process is not dissimilar to that used by other secreted or exported proteins (Grant and Jackson 1976). It requires microtubules and is inhibited by agents, such as colchicine, which disrupt microtubule assembly (Ehrlich et al. 1974).

Conversion of procollagen to collagen occurs probably extracellularly, at least in tissue culture (Goldberg 1977). At least two specific proteases are involved in cleaving both amino- and carboxy-terminal non-helical extensions of Type I procollagen (Duksin et al. 1978; Tuderman et al. 1978). These enzymes, however, have not been well characterized. The amino-terminal digestion product of pro-α_1 (I) is known to have inhibitory effects on procollagen synthesis, thus providing possible feedback control of the entire pathway (Wiestner et al. 1979).

In the extracellular space, the formation of fibrils can occur with or without prior conversion of procollagen to collagen (Timpl et al. 1975). Lysyl oxidase then catalyzes the formation of inter- and intra-chain cross-links (Tanzer 1973).

Due to the complexity of the entire pathway, potentially numerous disorders of collagen metabolism can occur, affecting one or more of these steps, and some of these have been reported and reviewed in detail (Prockop et al. 1979). It is unclear at this time whether all the structurally distinct collagen Types I–V (controlled by different genes) utilize the same synthetic process as outlined here. The same tissue can synthesize several of these types of collagen, and furthermore certain cloned cells can synthesize the different collagen types simultaneously (Gay et al. 1976). For the most part, however, normal cells usually synthesize the type(s) of collagen which are appropriate for their physiologic function. For instance, fibroblasts synthesize mostly Types I and III collagen (Hance et al. 1976), while endothelial cells synthesize mostly basement membrane types of collagen (Jaffe et al. 1976); and chondrocytes predominantly produce Type II collagen (Dehm and Prockop 1973).

The adult lung contains all five types of collagen, but consists predominantly of Type I (Bradley et al. 1974). Type I collagen is composed of two α_1 (I) and one α_2 (I) chains forming the triple helical tropocollagen molecule (Bornstein and Sage 1980). It is found, together with Type III collagen, in the interstitial areas, in walls of blood vessels, but mostly in skin and tendons. Type II collagen is composed of three α_1 (II) chains and represents the major collagen in articular and other types of cartilage (Bornstein and Sage 1980). Type III collagen is composed of three α_1 (III) chains and is found mostly in blood vessel walls (Bornstein and Sage 1980). All Types I−III collagen α-chains have been studied in detail with complete amino acid sequences available for Types I and III, and a partial sequence available for Type II (Bornstein and Sage 1980). The distinct distribution of polar and hydrophobic residues along the helical region gives rise to the well-recognized cross-banding pattern seen in electron microscopy after staining with uranyl acetate (which is bound to the polar residues) (Fietzek and Kuhn 1976). Type IV collagen is less well characterized, primarily due to its insolubility in non-denaturing solvents. Solubilization usually requires pepsin digestion and the final preparation appears to be heterogeneous, possibly, and partially, due to proteolytic digestion (Crouch et al. 1980). Recently, Crouch et al. (1980) have shown that epithelioid amniotic fluid cells synthesized two genetically distinct Type IV procollagen chains, which they have termed pro-α_1 (IV) and pro-α_2 (IV) and which upon pepsin digestion resulted in various breakdown products resembling the purified Type IV collagen prepared by others using pepsin digestion of various basement membrane preparations. This association with basement membrane is also true of Type V collagen, initially thought to be composed of αA- and αB-chains (Burgeson et al. 1976), but which has also been reported to include αC-chains (Bornstein and Sage 1980).

The structural differences between these various collagen types are great enough to cause different susceptibilities to digestion by purified collagenases. For instance, Type I collagen is more susceptible to digestion by neutrophil collagenase than Type III (Horwitz et al. 1977). Furthermore, basement membrane-derived collagen is resistant to digestion by skin collagenase (Woolley et al. 1978; Liotta et al. 1979). Recent evidence indicates the existence of a novel collagenase, isolated from a murine fibrosarcoma, which is relatively specific for Type IV collagen and will not digest Type I, III, or V collagens (Liotta et al. 1979). The vertebrate collagenases (except for the Type IV collagen-specific enzyme) are well characterized and have been reviewed recently (Harper 1980). They are metalloenzymes having a preference for native collagen as substrate, which they cleave at neutral pH at a fairly specific site in the helical region containing the Gly-Ile (or Gly-Leu) bond of the α_1-CB7 peptide obtained by cyanogen bromide cleavage (Gross et al. 1974). This cleavage results in production of a large TC^A and a shorter TC^B fragment (Gross and Nagai 1965); these fragments are unstable at body temperature and would become susceptible to digestion by other non-specific proteases. These purified collagenases appear to be relatively specific for collagen (Woolley et al. 1975, 1978). The enzymes of this class appear to be synthesized *de novo* in zymogen form, but several inhibitors of the active enzyme have also been reported (Harper 1980), thus making it difficult to distinguish between a zymogen form and an enzyme–inhibitor complex. These enzymes are also probably the sole agent capable of digesting native triple helical collagen at neutral pH in vivo. Other proteases certainly can digest the non-helical telopeptide extensions (Weiss 1976). However, at sites of low pH (e.g. sites of tissue damage, phagolysosomes, etc.), several cathepsins have the capability of digesting native collagen (Burleigh et al. 1974; Coffey et al. 1976).

These data suggest that, in vivo, normal (undiseased) collagen breakdown or catabolism is initiated by a relatively specific collagenase secreted (by inflammatory and other cells) into the extracellular space where the substrate collagen is located. Following this initial cleavage, unraveling of the helical structure ensues, making it susceptible to further degradation by other proteases (Harper 1980). This process would be slow if the collagen is fibrillar and highly cross-linked (as it is in vivo), and would even be slower if highly substituted (e.g. by carbohydrate residues), since the cleavage site would be less accessible; this would probably account for its slow turnover (Harris and Farrell 1972) and the relative irreversibility of the fibrotic process, if this is not arrested prior to maturation of the collagen.

4.3.2. Elastin

The insolubility of elastin is a major obstacle in the attempt to characterize it. Proteolytic digestion is usually required in its solubilization. Furthermore, it remains unknown whether elastin is a homogeneous entity. Various tissues perform different functions, requiring different dimensions of elasticity or resiliency, which is the major recognizable attribute of elastin (Sandberg 1976). In the lung, the consequence of reduced elastin is a decreased resiliency of the alveolar walls resulting in some of the clinical manifestations of emphysema (Johanson and Pierce 1972; Janoff et al. 1977; Snider et al. 1977b). Alterations of lung elastin content also have been described in certain types of pulmonary fibrosis (Starcher et al. 1978), but the significance of these alterations remains unknown.

Elastin is generally described as being composed of an amorphous and a microfibrillar form (Gosline 1976). Upon maturation, the amorphous form is usually found in a cross-linked state, with tetrafunctional desmosines at the cross-linking sites (Francis et al. 1973). This cross-linking plays a major role in giving it the elasticity which is a major functional attribute of elastin (Sandberg 1976). Because of this unique content of desmosine, assays for total lung elastin content have relied on developing techniques for assaying desmosines (Starcher 1977). The primary structure of elastin has been partially characterized by the use of soluble non-cross-linked material (Foster et al. 1973). These studies reveal absence of methionine residues, and using tryptic peptides approximately 800 amino acid residues have been identified in an elastin "monomer" from copper-deficient swine. Frequent repetitions of several oligopeptides containing glycine, proline, valine and alanine account for the high content of glycine. But the collagenous Gly-X-Y sequences are not seen in elastin. Sequences of Lys-(Ala)n-Lys (n = 2 or 3) are frequently seen near cross-linking sites (Foster et al. 1974). Little is known about the microfibrillar form, aside from its being an elastic fiber and its close association with the amorphous form (Hance and Crystal 1975).

Synthesis of elastin has been demonstrated in the fibroblast and smooth muscle cell (Hance and Crystal 1975). The genes directing the two types of elastin have not been elucidated. Transcription and translation presumably utilize the usual machinery and their regulation is also poorly understood. Post-translational modification also includes hydroxylation of proline by prolyl hydroxylase. Varying degrees of prolyl hydroxylation have no apparent effect on elastin synthesis or secretion (Uitto et al. 1976), although there may be effects on final assembly and maturation of the secreted product (Urry et al. 1979). Promicrofibrillar elastin is a glycoprotein, and the glycosylation presumably occurs during transit through the Golgi apparatus (Hance and Crystal 1975). Secretion of the proelastin and promicrofibrillar elastin appears to occur via a process similar to that utilized by other secreted proteins (Uitto et al. 1976).

Cleavage of the proelastin, which has been reported to have a molecular weight of 90,000−135,000 (Foster et al. 1976; Rucker et al. 1979), occurs presumably in the extracellular space by proteases which remain to be identified and characterized (Foster et al. 1976). Several fragmentary products of this process have been reported, with the 72,000 molecular weight fragment being the tropoelastin molecule (Foster et al. 1976).

Interaction of the tropoelastin with microfibrillar elastin appears to precede cross-linking, catalyzed by lysyl oxidase, an enzyme which prefers an insoluble substrate (Siegel 1974). This interaction appears to be mediated by disulfide bonds since dithiothreitol enables the separation and isolation of microfibrils from this complex (Hance and Crystal 1975). Lysine appears to play the major role in this cross-linking process, which results in the formation of desmosines (Francis et al. 1973; Foster et al. 1974). This is also inhibitable by β-aminopropionitrile (Narayanan and Page 1976).

The highly cross-linked mature elastin is resistant to trypsin digestion, while soluble tropoelastin is digestible (Foster et al. 1976). This may explain the slow turnover rate of mature elastin in lung (Pierce et al. 1967). Despite active synthesis of elastin in the lung, the total amount of lung elastin remains relatively constant in the adult (Hance and Crystal 1975). This, and the loss of lung elastin in emphysema, may be due to the digestion of the more susceptible tropoelastin and other less mature forms of elastin (Christner et al. 1978). Mature elastin, however, is susceptible to degradation by elastases that have been purified from leukocytes and pancreas (Hartley and Shotton 1971; Ohlsson and Ohlsson 1974; Feinstein and Janoff 1975; Baugh and Travis 1976). These enzymes, however, lack the substrate specificity of a collagenase, because of the latter's ability to also degrade proteins other than elastin. The pancreatic enzyme is synthesized as an inactive proelastase, which is activated to elastase by cleavage of a single peptide bond near the amino terminus (Hartley and Shotton 1971). The pancreatic enzyme has a molecular weight of 25,000, is composed of 240 amino acid residues, and is inhibitable by NaCl, α_1-antitrypsin and other proteolytic inhibitors as well as unsaturated fatty acids (Hartley and Shotton 1971; Ohlsson and Ohlsson 1974; Ashe and Zimmerman (1977). Inactivation of inhibitors such as α_1-antitrypsin by oxidation of methionine residues may be important in the pathogenesis of emphysema (Johnson and Travis 1979; Carp and Janoff 1980).

4.3.3. Glycosaminoglycans and proteoglycans

The interaction between collagen and proteoglycans is unclear, but may be important in maintaining structural integrity. For instance, dermatan sulfate has a greater affinity for collagen than chondroitin sulfate (Laurent 1977). In connective tissue, the complex polysaccharides referred to as glycosaminoglycans are usually present as proteoglycans, with the exception of hyaluronic acid. These proteoglycans are generally composed of a protein core (molecular weight $\simeq$ 200,000), highly substituted by side chains composed of the various glycosaminoglycans (Hance and Crystal 1975). Link proteins with molecular weights of $\sim$ 60,000 stabilize the association of these proteoglycans to chains of hyaluronic acid in native aggregates (Hardingham and Muir 1977; Hascall 1977; Caterson and Baker 1979; Hardingham 1979).

Glycosaminoglycan side chain substitution to the protein core is either via an o-glycosidic linkage between xylose and the hydroxyl group of serine, as well as between N-acetylgalactosamine and the hydroxyl group of threonine (especially with keratan sulfate) and serine, or via an N-glycosylamine linkage between N-acetylglucosamine and the amide moiety of asparagine (Roden 1980). The common glycosaminoglycans (chondroitin 4 and 6 sulfates, hyaluronic acid, dermatan sulfate, keratan sulfate, heparin and heparan sulfate) are all found in the lung, except for keratan sulfate (Hance and Crystal 1975).

Synthesis of connective tissue glycosaminoglycans is tightly coupled to synthesis of the protein core to which they are attached, except possibly for hyaluronic acid (Roden 1980). Inhibition of protein synthesis by puromycin and chloramphenicol does not inhibit hyaluronic acid production (Stoolmiller and Dorfman 1969). The synthetic process is common to most glyco-conjugated proteins (Schachter 1978; Roden 1980). Following (or simultaneously with) synthesis of the protein core, the various nucleotide sugar transferases catalyze the stepwise addition of the glycosyl residues to acceptor sites on the growing molecule. More recent data also show that dolichol sugars are important in this process (Hart and Lennarz 1978).

Epimerization of glucuronic residues after incorporation into the growing polysaccharide chain results in iduronic residues found in heparin, heparan sulfate and dermatan sulfate (Lindahl et al. 1979). The various sugars are derived from interconversion of glucose (Schachter and Roseman 1980). Specificity of this initiation and polysaccharide chain elongation is determined by the substrate specificity of the particular nucleotide sugar transferase and the configuration of the acceptor site (Hagopian et al. 1968; Silbert 1973; Schachter and Roseman 1980). Sulfation and polymerization are also poorly understood processes, occurring in the endoplasmic reticulum and Golgi apparatus (Lindahl et al. 1977; Roden 1980). Knowledge concerning regulation of these various steps is lacking except for their dependence on the availability of the nucleotide sugar precursors (Silbert 1973).

Catabolism of proteoglycans is mediated by the various lysosomal hydrolases, with varying degrees of specificity for the configurations of the linkage sites between the monosaccharides (Dorfman and Matalon 1976). This has been reviewed in detail elsewhere (Dorfman and Matalon 1976; Neufeld et al. 1975; Hall et al. 1978). Several proteases are capable of degrading the protein core (Barrett 1972). The actual in-vivo degradative process, however, has not been elucidated, despite the characterization of the various exo- and endoenzymes capable of degrading the polysaccharides into monosaccharides.

4.4. ABNORMALITIES IN LUNG CONNECTIVE TISSUE COMPOSITION AND METABOLISM IN PULMONARY FIBROSIS

Due to the more extensive understanding of collagen structure, function and metabolism, and the larger concentration of collagen in connective tissue (up to as high as 70% of total lung connective tissue mass is made up of collagen (Hance and Crystal 1975)), more data are available describing the changes in lung collagen metabolism and composition during, or as a result of, the fibrotic process. Scanty data are available from human studies and most of the data to be discussed are derived from animal models of pulmonary fibrosis. There are several reasons for this lack of human data, aside from the ethical considerations regarding experimentation with humans. Some of these will be mentioned when possible causes of discrepancies between human- and non-human-derived data are discussed.

Analysis of both lung biopsy and autopsy material obtained from patients with IPF reveals no significant difference from normal non-fibrotic tissue, in terms of both lung collagen and protein syntheses per mg DNA, and in hydroxyproline content per mg dry weight of lung tissue (Fulmer et al. 1980). In contrast, morphologic evaluations show many areas with large accumulation of collagenous fibers as defined both by the Masson-trichrome stain and ultrastructurally with the electron microscope (Crystal et al. 1976; Fulmer et al. 1979). Physiologic parameters of lung-restrictive disease correlate well with the degree of fibrosis as evaluated histologically, using biopsy material (Fulmer et al. 1979). This correlation may be fortuitous, since small biopsy specimens are hardly representative of the whole lung, which in its totality determines the observed physiologic parameters such as lung volume, compliance and gas diffusing capacity. This discrepancy between morphologic (and physiologic) and biochemical parameters of pulmonary fibrosis has not been satisfactorily resolved. This is due to a sampling problem as well as to the inadequacy of both the biochemical and morphologic parameters. The sampling problem is obviated in smaller mammals in which the entire lung can be conveniently homogenized and used for analysis. Furthermore, especially with respect to such dynamic and time-dependent variables as collagen synthesis, single determinations from biopsy material are not helpful for our understanding of what is basically a dynamic process. This point becomes critical in view of data from studies with animals showing a *finite* period of increased lung collagen synthesis following various treatments known to cause pulmonary fibrosis (see below). Therefore, to merely categorize the patient samples into IPF and non-IPF groups (Fulmer et al. 1980) would be inadequate and probably is a contributory cause of the lack of statistical significance between the mean rate of lung collagen synthesis in the IPF biopsy specimens and those of the non-IPF group (Fulmer et al. 1980); i.e. inclusion of IPF patients in a quiescent (with respect to increased lung collagen synthesis) stage of the disease would lower the mean value for the entire IPF group. The high degree of scatter in the data for collagen synthesis in the IPF biopsy specimens (Fulmer et al. 1980) supports this possibility, although the alternative possibility of variation due to sampling sites with varying stages of disease activity cannot be ruled out. Another complication is in the manner of expressing biochemical variables of lung collagen content and synthesis. Normalizing rates of synthesis to "per unit total DNA mass in the sample" can result in artificially low or normal (diluted) values if more cells normally incapable of collagen synthesis (e.g. inflammatory cells) are present in the IPF sample, despite actual increases in synthesis by the connective tissue cells. Significant increases in cells, as determined morphologically, and in DNA have been noted in the biopsy samples from IPF patients when compared to non-IPF samples (Crystal et al. 1976), thus providing support for such a possibility. Similarly, normalizing collagen content to "per unit mass of sample dry weight" can result in the incorrect interpretation that IPF causes no absolute increase in lung collagen, since increased collagen (numerator) would also increase the overall dry weight (denominator). Due to these considerations, the available human-derived (IPF) biochemical data do not allow unequivocal conclusions to be drawn concerning the role of biochemically defined collagen in IPF.

Morphologic evaluation has consistently shown accumulation of interstitial as well as basement membrane-related collagens in fibrotic lungs. Techniques based on special stains (e.g. the Masson-trichrome), immunofluorescence (using purified antibodies to specific collagen types) and electron microscopy, have all confirmed the concept that IPF is a disease of abnormal and increased collagen (and other connective tissue) deposition (Fulmer et al. 1980; Madri and Furthmayr 1980; Bateman et al. 1981). Special stains and electron microscopy, however, visualize mainly Type I and possibly Type III collagen (Fulmer et al. 1980). The possibility that Type III collagen is present only as non-fibrillar "reticulin" is probably unlikely (Wiedermann et al. 1975; Ranterberg 1981). Furthermore, microscopic examination utilizes a minute amount of tissue as compared to the total lung mass, thus necessitating numerous samples for adequate analysis. Again, this sampling problem is obviated if the small lungs of rodents or other suitably small animals are used, since the entire lung can be processed for light microscopic evaluation. Despite these considerations the following explanation (Fulmer et al. 1980) has been proposed to resolve this apparent discrepancy between biochemical and morphologic data. On the assumption that the biochemical data are correct, the morphologic data can be interpreted as being due to a rearrangement of collagen types with respect to location, relative composition and physical properties, and not due to an absolute increase in collagen content and synthesis. The altered localization of the various collagen types as examined by immunofluorescence (Madri and Furthmayr 1980; Bateman et al. 1981) and the abnormal appearance of the collagen fibers of IPF lungs (Fulmer et al. 1980) would favor this conclusion. A relative decrease in lung Type III collagen (vs Type I collagen) in autopsy lungs from IPF patients also supports this possibility (Seyer et al. 1976; Madri and Furthmayr 1980; Bateman et al 1981). It is this alteration in collagen localization, composition and structure, rather than the generalized total increase in lung collagen, which eventually results in the observed altered physiologic parameters. The lack of correlation between the histologic appearance of biopsy material and physiologic parameters (Carrington et al. 1978) is partly due to the sampling problem described above.

The lack of correlation between total lung connective tissue content, as defined biochemically, and lung physiologic parameters is well documented (see below), despite the observation that chord compliance is a measure of lung function that is dependent on collagen's physical properties (Karlinsky et al. 1976). On the other hand, improvements in lung compliance and/or TLC_{25} (lung volume at 25 cm H_2O) are seen when specific inhibitors of collagen synthesis or cross-linking are given to animals insulted by various agents to induce pulmonary fibrosis (see below). Penicillamine, however, was not effective in improving lung compliance, despite significant reduction in the bleomycin-induced increase in lung collagen, elastin and glycosaminoglycan content (Fedullo et al. 1980). These conflicting results are not totally surprising since biochemical assays of total lung connective tissue bulk do not in any way reveal the tissue distribution, type composition, mutual interaction and three-dimensional configuration, i.e. higher structure, which together ultimately determine, along with other variables (e.g. degree of interstitial edema and alveolar surface tension) these observed physiologic parameters. It is more difficult, however, to reconcile the obvious increase in stainable (both by Masson-trichrome and immunofluorescence using purified type-specific antibodies) collagen with the lack of increase as assayed biochemically (Fulmer et al. 1980). It is indisputable that there is rearrangement and abnormal distribution of collagen as determined by light microscopy, but it would require significant reductions in "non-stainable" (at least by

Masson-trichrome) collagen before the morphologic data can be reconciled with the biochemically determined lack of increase. Such a major reduction has not been observed. Furthermore, Type III collagen can assume a fibrillar form in vitro, and the concept that Type III collagen in vivo is always amorphous and synonymous with reticulin, has not been supported by experimental data. Thus ultrastructural data showing increases in fibrillar collagen do not necessarily signify a *sole* increase in Type I collagen.

Aside from the possible increase in lung collagen content and synthesis in IPF, minor differences have also been noted in amino acid composition of some of the collagen α-chains. Amino acid analysis of α_1 (I) and α_1 (III) chains obtained from autopsy specimens of IPF patients by acidic pepsin digestion and salt fractionation reveal less hydroxylysine content, 7.1 per 1000 residues for α_1 (I) and 8.3 per 1000 residues for α_1 (III), when compared to non-fibrotic lungs, which contained 10.0 and 11.1 residues per 1000, respectively (Seyer et al. 1976). Otherwise, the collagens Types I and III from IPF patients are indistinguishable from those in control lungs (Seyer et al. 1976). However, the relative content of Type III collagen is reduced from 33% of total lung collagen, to 12–24% in various patients with IPF (Seyer et al. 1976). This relative reduction is also confirmed by immunochemical methods (Madri and Furthmayr 1980). Human lung fibroblasts in culture have an opposite effect at confluency, synthesizing 26–68% more Type III collagen than when they are analyzed at lower cell density (Trombley et al. 1981). This increase in relative Type III collagen content is also noted in early wound healing or other scarring processes (Bailey et al. 1972; Kent et al. 1976; Bailey 1977; Wick et al. 1978; Clore et al. 1979; Bateman et al. 1981).

Increases in lung dermatan sulfate have been observed in a case of IPF (Motomiya et al. 1975). The affinity of collagen for dermatan sulfate has been noted previously (Laurent 1977). Otherwise, very little is known about proteoglycan metabolism in IPF. The situation is similar with respect to elastin in IPF, although more is known about its changes in emphysema, a disease thought to be primarily due to uncontrolled elastolysis (Snider 1981).

In contrast to the lack of increase in biochemically detectable collagen in IPF lungs, patients with acute respiratory failure, who manage to survive for a period of two weeks, exhibit definite increase in biochemically assayed lung collagen when corrected for lung tissue hemoglobin content (Zapol et al. 1979). This underlines the importance of normalization of data to appropriate parameters.

Animal models of pulmonary fibrosis have been developed, with features resembling the human disease. Induction of pulmonary fibrosis by various known fibrogenic agents has been examined and extensive data have now been accumulated from studies using silica, radiation, bleomycin, paraquat and oxidizing atmospheres as the injurious agents.

Silicosis in humans is characterized by granulomatous inflammation and, eventually, pulmonary fibrosis. A similar disease has been induced in animals (Heppleston 1973). Inhalation of silica particles over a period of months causes an alveolar lipoproteinosis in rats, which eventually results in the formation of silicotic nodules and fibrosis (Heppleston 1973). This is confirmed biochemically by increased lung collagen content, prolyl hydroxylase (Stacy and King 1954; Halme et al. 1979), and also presumably synthesis. An increase in soluble hydroxyproline-containing peptides also suggests an increased rate of catabolism. In vitro, macrophages exposed to quartz crystals produce factor(s) capable of stimulating isolated fibroblasts (Heppleston and Styles 1967; Aalto et al. 1976). The fibrogenic response to silica is localized only to exposed lung tissue; thus, unexposed lobes are free of disease (Dale 1973), suggesting a localized (vs systemic) mechanism in accord with the in vitro data (Heppleston and Styles 1967; Aalto et al. 1976). The fibrogenic response is inhibited by steroids (Stacy and King 1954) and the cross-linking inhibitor is β-aminopropionitrile (Levene et al. 1968). Increased levels of lung carbohydrate and uronic acids suggest increased proteoglycan metabolism (Vasilyeva 1971). The in vitro counterpart is the observation that fibroblasts respond by increased glycosaminoglycan synthesis upon exposure to anthracite dust (Richards and Wusteman 1974). Elastin metabolism has not been studied in this disease, and so its role is unknown.

Pulmonary fibrosis upon exposure to radiation has been extensively studied (Eddy and Casarett 1972; Law et al. 1976; Pickrell et al. 1976; Gross 1977; Dubrawsky et al. 1978; Ward et al. 1979). Gamma- and X-irradiation have been used as inducing agents. There is a variable time course dependent upon the dose and type of radiation as well as the species of the target animal. In most cases however, lung collagen accumulation usually is delayed, e.g. by 2−3 months in the rat following ^{60}Co radiation exposure (Pickrell et al. 1975). In hamsters, following a 15-week delay, lung collagen synthesis is detectably increased, reaching a maximum at approximately 30 weeks, and then slowly declining towards normal rates at time points beyond 50 weeks (Pickrell et al. 1975, 1976). In this same species, lung collagen content is detectably increased from 20−25 weeks onwards, and begins to plateau at 30 weeks. Increases in non-collagenous protein synthesis parallel the increase in collagen synthesis. It is noteworthy that collagenolytic activity is also elevated, beginning at 20 weeks, peaking at 25 weeks, and slowly declining towards normal values by 50 weeks. The fibrotic response to ^{60}Co in rats is inhibitable by penicillamine as well as colchicine (Dubrawsky et al. 1978; Ward et al. 1979). Penicillamine is effective presumably due to its known inhibitory effects on cross-link formation (Deshmulch and Nimmi 1969). Colchicine is effective presumably due to its inhibition of procollagen secretion (Ehrlich et al. 1974; Harwood et al. 1976). The latter drug is also partially effective in reversing the radiation-induced decreased compliance (Dubrawsky et al. 1978). Decreased compliance in the rat is better correlated with increased lung weight than with the increased lung hydroxyproline content (Dubrawski et al. 1978). In mice exposed to X-irradiation, the increased compliance has been attributed to increased amounts of plasma proteins in the alveolar space (due to radiation-induced increased permeability) altering the alveolar surface characteristics (Gross 1980). Steroid treatment ameliorates this decreased compliance by increased production of surfactant which reduces the radiation-induced alterations in alveolar surface properties (Gross 1980). β-Aminopropionitrile is also effective in inhibiting radiation-induced fibrosis (Percarpio and Fischer 1976).

Increased lung glycosaminoglycans have been reported in animals exposed to radioactive plutonium (Tseleva 1974). The increase is mostly in dermatan (as in silicosis) and chondroitin sulfate. In-vitro alterations in cultured fibroblast glycosaminoglycan synthesis upon radiation exposure have also been reported (Yaron et al. 1972).

Bleomycin is a complex glycopeptide antibiotic with antitumor properties (Umezawa 1974). Pulmonary toxicity in the form of an interstitial pneumonitis (resembling UIP) with subsequent fibrosis occurs in humans when it is administered in high cumulative doses (Luna et al. 1972; Blum et al. 1973; Crooke and Bradner

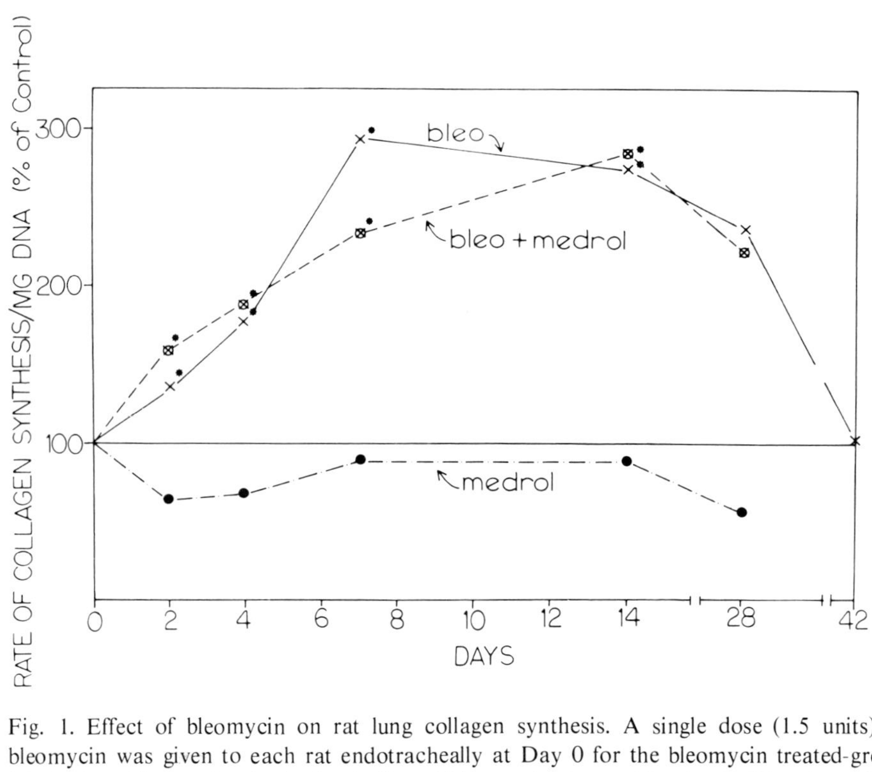

Fig. 1. Effect of bleomycin on rat lung collagen synthesis. A single dose (1.5 units) of bleomycin was given to each rat endotracheally at Day 0 for the bleomycin treated-group (bleo). Steroid-treated animals (medrol) and bleomycin + steroid animals (bleo + medrol) were treated with daily injections of methylprednisolone. For further experimental details, see Phan et al. (1981b). Asterisks indicate statistically significant ($p < 0.05$) differences from untreated control mean values. (From Phan et al. 1981b, with permission of the publisher.)

1973). Toxicity is more common in lung and skin, presumably due to lower levels of bleomycin hydrolase (Umezawa 1974). Biochemical evaluation of lung connective tissue in humans suffering from bleomycin toxicity has not been reported. The drug has been administered by several routes in various animals and results in similar lung toxicity (Fleischman et al. 1971; Adamson and Bowden 1974; Bedrossian et al. 1977; Snider et al. 1977a; McCullough et al. 1978; Sikic et al. 1978; Starcher et al. 1978; Thrall et al. 1979a; Phan et al. 1980). Increases in lung collagen content following bleomycin administration have been well documented (Snider et al. 1977a; McCullough et al. 1978; Sikic et al. 1978; Starcher et al. 1978; Thrall et al. 1979a). This is preceded in the rat by an increased rate of lung collagen synthesis (Fig. 1), first detectable at 4 days, reaching a maximum at approximately 7−10 days, and gradually returning to normal rates at 5−7 weeks after a single endotracheal dose of bleomycin (Phan et al. 1981b). Lung collagen content (Fig. 2) is first detectably increased at about 7−14 days and gradually increases to a maximum of 180−200% of normal, usually after one month, and remains at this level as long as two months after drug instillation (Phan et al. 1981b). Similar changes are seen in hamsters (Clark et al. 1980a). Lung collagenolytic activity is also decreased, especially at the later time points (Phan et al. 1981b).This is also seen in the skin of bleomycin-treated mice (Ichihashi et al. 1973). Various immunosuppressive, anti-inflammatory and antifibrotic (i.e. by collagen synthesis and/or maturation inhibitors) therapies have been partially successful in inhibiting the bleomycin-induced increase in lung collagen content and synthesis (Thrall et al. 1979b, 1980, 1981; Fedullo et al. 1980; Kelley et al. 1980; Zuckerman et al. 1980; Riley et al. 1981a, 1982; Phan and Thrall 1982).

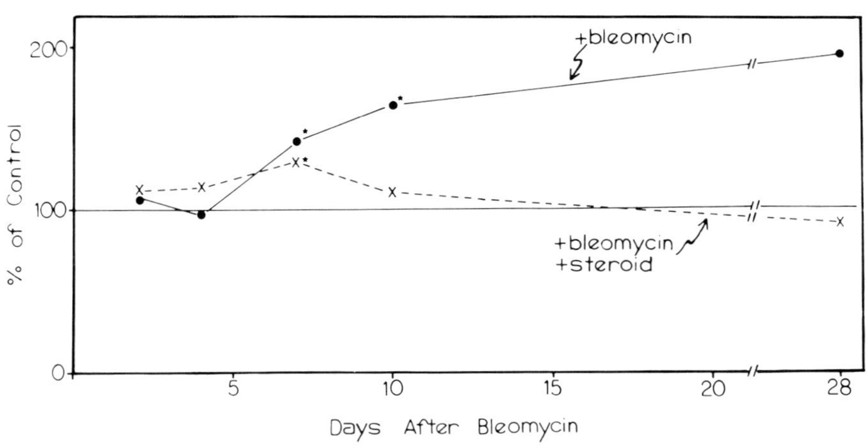

Fig. 2. Effect of bleomycin on rat total-lung hydroxyproline content. Bleomycin (1.5 units) is also given at Day 0. Steroid refers to daily injections of methylprednisolone. Asterisks refer to statistically significant ($p < 0.05$) differences from control mean values. For details see Phan et al. 1981b. (Reproduced from the same source, with permission of the publisher.)

These therapies, however, do not necessarily have an effect on the decreased lung compliance (Fedullo et al. 1980). Improvements in lung compliance are noted with the proline analogues, dehydroproline (Kelley et al. 1980), cis-4-hydroxy-L-proline (Riley et al. 1981a) and the cross-linking inhibitor, β-aminopropionitrile (Riley et al. 1982). Concomitant treatment with either of these drugs inhibits the bleomycin-induced lung collagen accumulation, with significant improvement in lung compliance. This, again, is consistent with the concept that lung compliance is the result of multiple factors which are less dependent on total bulk collagen, as they are on the physical state or properties of the collagenous product, its distribution or localization, and its composition. In vitro, bleomycin stimulates cultured fibroblasts to increase collagen as well as glycosaminoglycan syntheses (Otsuka et al. 1976, 1978; Clark et al. 1980b). The increased collagen synthesis is type specific, with a relative decrease in Type III/Type I ratio (Clark et al. 1980b).

Increases in lung elastin and glycosaminoglycan content also accompany the increased lung collagen (Starcher et al. 1978). Increased elastin is probably due to increased synthesis, but the significance of this increase to the physiologic manifestations is unclear. Increases in glycosaminoglycans are thought to be secondary to the increased rates of collagen, and possibly elastin biosynthesis (Fedullo et. al. 1980).

Chronic exposure to high oxygen tensions has been known to cause pulmonary fibrosis (Clark and Lambertsen 1971; Crapo and Tierney 1974; Chvapil and Leng 1975; Valimaki et al. 1975; Fridovich 1976; Riley et al. 1980). In rats, for instance, prolonged hyperoxia causes lung collagen content to be elevated by approximately 50% above unexposed animals within 14 days of initiation of exposure (Riley et al. 1980). Cis-4-hydroxy-L-proline, a proline analog, inhibits this increase and also prevents the development of abnormal lung physiologic parameters (Riley et al. 1980). Exposure to ozone causes both increased lung collagen synthesis and deposition in rats as well as monkeys, as early as seven days after intitiation of exposure (Last et al. 1979, 1981). Rates of synthesis depending on the ozone concentration, reach values as high as three times the control rate (Last et al. 1979). Lung organ cultures when exposed to hyperoxic atmospheres also react with increased rate of collagen synthesis with an increased Type III/Type I ratio, which is typical of early fibrotic processes (Bhatnagar et al. 1978). Other elements of connective tissue have not been studied in this model.

The herbicide paraquat (1,1′-dimethyl-4,4′-bipyridilium) has been known for some time to cause pulmonary toxicity in both humans and animals (Smith et al. 1974; Smith and Heath 1976; Autor 1977; Hollinger and Chvapil 1977; Smith and Rose 1977; Greenberg et al. 1978; Hollinger et al. 1978; Thompson and Patrick 1978; Griffin et al. 1979). Independent of route of administration (subcutaneously or intraperitoneally) pulmonary fibrosis develops if the animal survives for a long enough period. A single high dose or chronic exposure to low doses is effective in causing fibrosis (Autor 1977). Lung collagen synthesis is increased as early as three days after a single intraperitoneal injection (Greenberg et al. 1978). This is accompanied by increases in the tissue free proline pool size, as has been described in other fibrotic processes (Greenberg et al. 1978). Prolyl hydroxylase activity is also increased (Griffin et al. 1979), probably as part of the response resulting in increased collagen synthesis, rather than merely representing an increase in hydroxylation of prolyl residues.

More recently, endotracheal instillation of an enzyme system capable of producing H_2O_2 and hypohalous acids produces an intense acute reaction in the lung, resulting in consolidated and fibrotic areas as early as seven days after treatment (Johnson et al. 1981). This response is inhibitable only by concomitant endotracheal administration of catalase and not by superoxide dismutase, thus implicating H_2O_2 as the key toxic metabolite in this process.

In summary, pulmonary fibrosis is a disease of (1) heightened lung collagen metabolism with increased deposition and synthesis, (2) abnormal lung collagen type composition; (3) abnormal lung collagen distribution; and (4) increased elastin and proteoglycan metabolism. The different etiologies may not exhibit all these features equally, but they all have abnormal connective tissue metabolism. In view of the overwhelming animal data reviewed above and the data obtained from ARDS patients (Zapol et al. 1979), the biochemical data – and especially the method of normalizing them – obtained from IPF patients (Fulmer et al. 1980) should be interpreted with caution and re-evaluated with comparable normalizing factors before it can be concluded that IPF is unique in its fibrotic manifestation; i.e. fibrosis with normal lung collagen content and synthesis.

4.5. ABNORMALITIES OF REGULATION OF CONNECTIVE TISSUE METABOLISM IN PULMONARY FIBROSIS

Abnormalities in connective tissue metabolism are the result of abnormal connective tissue cell function and/or an altered internal milieu which affects the physicochemical state of the connective tissue cells and their products. In fibrotic lesions, most of the collagen is of the interstitial type (Types I and III), the greater part of which is formed by products of fibroblasts and smooth muscle cells (Hance and Crystal 1975; Hance et al. 1976). This, plus the ease of isolating and maintaining them in culture, has made fibroblasts the appropriate connective tissue cell prototype in studies of connective tissue metabolism. Their growth and metabolism are subject to regulation by numerous factors, which have been listed and reviewed (Ristow et al. 1978), and only those that are relevant to the topic of pulmonary fibrosis will be discussed here. The factors governing the composition of the internal milieu are also numerous and complex, and thus, discussion will be restricted only to those elements which have a bearing on the fate of (mature) connective tissue. The division into non-immune and immune mechanisms of regulation is artificial and merely serves to emphasize another consequence of immunologically mediated tissue injury.

Initiation of the fibrotic process can result in a reversible or an irreversible heightened and abnormal state of connective tissue metabolism. A spontaneously reversible process is wound healing, wherein cessation of fibroblast proliferation occurs after a finite period (Ross 1968; Raff and Houck 1969). Another reversible initiating mechanism is dependent on removal of the noxious stimulus (e.g. hyperoxia, ozone, etc.). However, chronic exposure to the stimuli can eventually result in the irreversible course to end-stage fibrosis. Thus, the questions that need to be asked in order to understand the mechanisms operative in pulmonary fibrosis are the following: (1) How does a noxious stimulus initiate the reversible phase, and what is the mechanism that converts it into an irreversible phase? (2) How do other noxious stimuli cause the irreversible phase upon a single exposure — even after the stimuli have been removed? (3) Is the irreversibility a result of an irreversible change in the ultimate target connective tissue cell, or is it a result of a permanent or chronic alteration in the various factors (cellular and/or acellular elements) regulating connective tissue cell function? The answers to these questions are not completely available, but data suggestive of possible clues are being actively accumulated.

4.5.1. Non-immune mechanisms

In-vitro evidence, using either cultured fibroblast (or other mesenchymal cells) or lung organ cultures, has shown that a multiplicity of factors can directly stimulate fibroblasts and connective tissue synthesis. Lung organ cultures exposed to hyperoxic atmospheres and paraquat synthesize collagen at a higher rate than unexposed controls (Bhatnagar et al. 1978; Hussain and Bhatnagar 1979). The newly synthesized product contains a higher ratio of Type III/Type I collagen, which is consistent with the composition of early fibrotic lesions (Bailey 1977; Clore et al. 1979). As the fibrotic tissue matures, there is usually a shift to predominantly Type I vs Type III collagen (Seyer et al. 1976; Madri and Furthmayr 1980; Bateman et al. 1981). The mechanism causing this shift in composition is not completely understood (Trombley et al. 1981). The increase in collagen synthesis can be prevented by superoxide dismutase (Hussain and Bhatnagar 1979), suggesting the superoxide anion as a key intermediate. Since the in-vitro system is presumably free of inflammatory or immune system effects (or at least lacks the ability to recruit systemic defences) other than what is locally present in the organ slices, the mechanism is probably due to a direct effect of superoxide on the connective tissue cell. This suggestion is further supported by the observation that the same paraquat dose does not cause any morphologic evidence of cellular or tissue injury. Higher doses of paraquat (1 mmol l^{-1}) are more effective in causing lung tissue injury in vitro (Martin et al. 1981). The injury in rat lung slices is preventable or ameliorated by concomitant exposure to superoxide dismutase, catalase, ascorbate or α-tocopherol, and only by catalase and α-tocopherol in rabbit lung slices. Superoxide has been implicated as the active form of O_2 in the prolyl and lysyl hydroxylase reactions (and thus, increased superoxide levels presumably would lead to an increase in collagen synthesis) (Myllyla et al. 1979). Nevertheless, the effects on fibroblast proliferation and collagen metabolism of lipid peroxidation, and other oxidative processes not directly related to collagen synthesis, cannot be ruled out. The latter events may be more important in the in-vivo situation, where harmful products of the oxidative process can incite a further destructive inflammatory response with a greater stimulation of the connective tissue cells. This possibility is suggested by evidence that paraquat can deplete cellular levels of NADPH, thus depriving cells of this cofactor, which plays a major role in the overall defence against lipid hydroperoxide formation (Autor 1977). These processes, which are dependent on the superoxide anion, are presumably common to all initiating agents which can bring about the production of this anion. Other in-vitro data, based on studies with isolated homogeneous populations of cells in culture, show that H_2O_2, but not O_2^-, is effective in causing cellular injury (Simon et al. 1981; Weiss et al. 1981). Furthermore, both in vivo and in vitro, H_2O_2 (and hypohalous acids) is significantly more effective than O_2^- in causing injury to rat lungs (Hollinger and Chvapil 1977; Johnson et al. 1981). These data suggest the following: (1) O_2^- can directly stimulate lung collagen synthesis without causing cellular injury, possibly and partly by stimulating the prolyl and lysyl hydroxylase reactions. (2) O_2^- can also contribute to oxidative cellular injury; e.g. the cyclical oxidation and reduction of paraquat consumes NADPH with production of O_2^-, which may be an important intermediate (especially upon dismutation into H_2O_2) in injury of cell membranes (Autor 1977). (3) H_2O_2 (a product of the dismutation of O_2^-), and hypohalous acids are toxic to cells, but their ability to directly stimulate connective tissue metabolism has not been investigated. Since intensity of lung injury is not always directly correlatable to activation and intensity of the fibrotic response it is impossible to predict fibrogenic potential of an agent on basis of its effectiveness in causing lung injury. Studies using in-vitro lung organ cultures are limited by their short-term survival, thus precluding experiments designed to analyze the long-term consequences of the injurious stimulus.

Other in-vitro data based on studies using isolated fibroblasts show that bleomycin can directly stimulate them to synthesize more collagen and glycosaminoglycans (Otsuka et al. 1976, 1978; Clark et al. 1980b). The collagenous product, in contrast to the situation in which lung organ cultures are exposed to hyperoxia or paraquat (Bhatnagar et al. 1978; Hussain and Bhatnagar 1979), shows a lower Type III/Type I collagen ratio (Clark et al. 1980b). The mechanism of this stimulation is unknown, but may be due to bleomycin's ability in the presence of Fe (II) to produce O_2 metabolites (Obserley and Bueltner 1979), which subsequently activate the fibroblasts via a mechanism similar to that utilized by hyperoxia-induced fibrosis (Bhatnagar et al. 1978; Hussain and Bhatnagar 1979). Alternatively, bleomycin-induced cellular injury could cause a non-specific response to toxic stimuli by increasing collagen synthesis. This bleomycin-induced stimulation may be irreversible, as suggested by data showing that lung fibroblasts isolated from bleomycin-treated animals synthesize collagen at an approximately 50% higher rate than do fibroblasts isolated from untreated normal animals (Phan et al. 1981c). Bleomycin-mediated selection of a fibroblast population with heightened collagen metabolism cannot be ruled out. Both possibilities could explain the observed data.

In-vivo studies of hyperoxia and paraquat-induced lung injury in animals as well as in human subjects, all reveal interstitial edema and endothelial cell injury as early events (Smith et al. 1974; Smith and Rose 1977). This is usually accompanied by Type I pneumocyte injury and subsequent proliferation of Type II pneumocytes. This appears to be a common response of the lung to any injurious stimulus (Freeman et al. 1973; Adamson and Bowden 1974, 1976; Hirai et al. 1977; Thrall et al. 1979a). Additionally, in silicosis, inhalation of indigestible material such as silica is a phagocytic cell problem, with consequent production of fibrogenic factors by the cell (Heppleston and Styles 1967; Aalto et al. 1976). Radiation pneumonitis in addition exhibits an alveolar lipoproteinosis, whose significance is probably greater on the observed decreased lung compliance than on the fibrogenic response (Gross 1980). Aside from these few additional unique features, most modes of lung injury result in this stereotypic response.

It has been suggested that irreversibility (i.e. the development of progressive fibrosis) is dependent upon the ability of Type II pneumocytes to proliferate and replace the epithelial barrier which normally consists of mostly Type I pneumocytes (Adamson and Bowden 1976; Witschi et al. 1981). This suggestion is based on the observation that pulmonary fibrosis develops after BHT (butylated hydroxytoluene)-induced lung injury if proliferation of Type II pneumocytes is inhibited by subsequent exposure to hyperoxic atmospheres (Witschi and Cote 1977; Witschi et al. 1981). According to this hypothesis, injury per se does not necessarily result in fibrosis, but injury severe enough to impair the ability of Type II pneumocytes to proliferate and eventually differentiate to Type I pneumocytes is the ultimate event triggering the fibrotic response. This injury to Type II pneumocytes would result in denudation of the epithelium, with consequent exposure of the interstitium and basement membranes to the alveolar space. This would in turn expose the interstitial connective tissue cells to influences which are normally excluded by both intact epithelial and endothelial cell linings. The presence of stimulatory (mitogenic) factors in serum is well known (Ristow et al. 1978) and is partially attributable to platelet-derived factors (Kohler and Lipton 1974; Ross et al. 1974; Rutherford and Ross 1976). The importance of serum proteins and their conversion products is underlined by the observation that urokinase is effective in inhibiting bleomycin-induced pulmonary fibrosis in dogs (Shigematsu et al. 1980). Factors from alveolar compartment cells, especially alveolar macrophages, will also exert their stimulatory influence on the interstitial mesenchymal (connective tissue) cells, if re-epithelialization is inhibited. In summary, according to this scenario, abrogation of the epithelial and/or endothelial barrier can expose the interstitial connective tissue cells to (activated) serum and/or alveolar stimulatory factors, thus triggering the fibrogenic response. Re-establishment of these barriers will result in a successful repair process, with the connective tissue cells returning to their quiescent state. Thus, in prolonged hyperoxia, paraquat and bleomycin toxicity, radiation pneumonitis, etc., injury to the epithelial and endothelial lining is severe enough to inhibit their proliferation in a normal healing process, which results in the prolonged exposure of interstitial cells to normally "forbidden" stimuli, with resultant progressive fibrosis. The cellular source of some of these stimuli constitutes the immune and inflammatory systems, and these factors will be discussed in the following Section 4.5.2.

4.5.2. Immune mechanisms

Involvement of the immune and inflammatory systems in the fibrogenic response is now well documented; however, its exact role remains to be defined. Evaluation of patients with pulmonary fibrosis has revealed a high incidence of circulating and lung-fixed immune complexes (which may also occur in bronchoalveolar lavage fluid), and other serological abnormalities (Turner-Warwick et al. 1971; Nagaya and Sieker 1972; Haslam et al. 1975, 1979; Dreisin et al. 1978; Pearson et al. 1981). In the most recent study, 60% of patients with UIP without any known risk of developing hypersensitivity pneumonitis, were found to have circulating immune complexes, some of which were positive for *Thermoactinomyces vulgaris* antigen (Cocchiara et al. 1981); 60% of these patients also have antibodies to *T. vulgaris* but the presence of precipitating antibodies in serum is poorly correlated with presence of disease. The ability of immune complexes — especially those that are fixed in the tissues — to cause inflammatory reactions and tissue injury, has been extensively documented and reviewed elsewhere (Daniele et al. 1981).

Data from human studies reveal good correlation between levels of circulating immune complexes and disease activity in a group of patients with steroid-responsive IPF (Dreisin et al. 1978). Such correlation however, is not observed in another study, which uses a different method of assaying for immune complexes (Haslam et al. 1979). Furthermore, circulating immune complexes have also been reported in other diseases without any evidence of pneumonitis or pulmonary fibrosis. To analyze further the role of immune complex injury in the fibrotic response, several animal models have been developed. Rabbits have been immunized against BSA (bovine serum albumin) and repeatedly challenged with high intravenous doses of the antigen to achieve a proliferative pneumonitis with morphologic evidence of fibrosis (Brentjens et al. 1974). In the rat, a single episode of passive Arthus reaction in the lung as well as endotracheal administration of preformed immune complexes are effective in causing reversible acute lung injury, but without chronic sequelae (Johnson and Ward 1974; Scherzer and Ward 1978). Similarly stimulated rabbit lungs, however, produce no such reaction (Willoughby and Willoughby 1977). The lack of fibrosis is also observed in similar models, using a variety of animals (Daniele et al. 1981). On the other hand, concomitant endotracheal administration of concanavalin A with antigen in previously hyperimmunized animal results in an intense pneumonitis with morphologic evidence of fibrosis (Willoughby et al. 1979), which is inhibitable by cholera toxin and cobra venom factor (Shenker et al. 1980).

These data have been interpreted as indicating a specific role of polyclonal pulmonary lymphocyte activation in enhancing the immune complex-mediated injury (Shenker et al. 1980). The evidence therefore suggests that immune complexes per se do not play a decisive role in the fibrotic process despite their efficacy in causing tissue injury. It appears, however, that immune complexes as a measure of immune reactivity are more correlatable to a fibrotic outcome. Thus, enhancing reactivity by repeated high-dose challenge and by polyclonal activation (with concanavalin A) is effective in causing pulmonary fibrosis. Similarly, chronic exposure to pigeon droppings, fungi and other organic dusts can result in fibrosis, whereas timely removal of some of these hypersensitive patients from the offending antigen can reverse some of the early changes without fibrosis ever developing (Pepys 1969). Thus, immune complexes are important in the fibrogenic response, only to the extent that they are a manifestation or a by-product of immune reactivity.

The importance of immune reactivity is supported by evidence showing that immunosuppressive therapy is effective in certain forms of pulmonary fibrosis. The effectiveness of steroids in inhibiting pulmonary fibrosis in (1) certain IPF, sarcoid and collagen vascular disease patients (Crystal et al. 1976; Carrington et al. 1978; Dreisin et al. 1978; De Reniee and Rohrbach 1980; Haslam et al. 1980); (2) ozone-exposed animals (Hesterberg and Last 1981); and (3) bleomycin-treated rats (Figs 1 and 2) (Phan et al. 1981b), has been reported. Anti-lymphocyte globulin and thymectomy also are partially effective in ameliorating bleomycin-induced pulmonary fibrosis in rats (Thrall et al. 1979b, 1980). On the other hand, the athymic nude mouse develops bleomycin-induced pulmonary fibrosis with an intensity equal to that seen in the normal background strain as judged morphologically (Szapiel et al. 1979). Differences in method of bleomycin administration (endotracheal vs intraperitoneal), in species (rat vs mouse), and in method of evaluating fibrosis (total lung hydroxyproline vs morphometry) may account for the apparent discrepancy concerning the role of cell-mediated immune reactivity in the fibrogenic response. Association of IPF with presence of the *HLA-DrW2* in humans (Libby et al. 1981), and the ability of *H-2* haplotype in mice to modulate the intensity of response to bleomycin and ovalbumin challenge in immunized animals (Rossi et al. 1981) further suggest a role for the immune system.

The antigen(s) involved in this immune reactivity has not always been identified, especially when no obvious heterologous agent is involved. For instance, in hypersensitivity pneumonitis, the heterologous antigens are the organic dusts, such as pigeon droppings (pigeon serum proteins being the actual antigens) in pigeon breeder's disease (Moore et al. 1974; Allen et al. 1977). In IPF, antibodies to *T. vulgaris* (Cocchiara et al. 1981) and macrophage migration inhibition factor (MIF) production upon exposure of peripheral lymphocytes to Type I collagen (Kravis et al. 1976), have been reported. Reactivity to collagen has also been reported in scleroderma (Stuart et al. 1976), other collagen vascular diseases (Andriopoulos et al. 1976; Foidait et al. 1978; Trentham et al. 1978), chronic liver disease (Menzel et al. 1980; Suou and Hirayama 1980), emphysema (Michaeli and Fudenberg 1974) and leprosy (McAdam et al. 1978). Cell-mediated immunity to beryllium has also been reported in berylliosis (Elias et al. 1981; Moritz et al. 1981). The ability to achieve resolution upon removal of the offending extrinsic or heterologous antigen is presumably dependent on the stage of disease progression. The extent of injury is not directly correlated with the intensity of the fibrogenic response, although it may play a greater role in simple self-limited wound healing or repair. Thus, these data suggest that the injury as a consequence of an activated immune system is probably not the trigger (or sufficient condition) for the diffuse and irreversible fibrogenic response.

A more direct role for the immune system in the connective tissue response or fibrosis is suggested by in-vitro data. Lymphocytes under certain conditions can (1) produce factors chemotactic for fibroblasts (Postlethwaite et al. 1976); (2) produce fibroblast-activating factors (Johnson and Ziff 1976; Wahl et al. 1978; Neilson et al. 1980; Schmidt and Green 1980); (3) produce fibroblast-inhibitory factors (Jimenez et al. 1979); (4) produce factors capable of stimulating collagenase production in macrophages (Wahl et al. 1975); and (5) produce macrophage-activating factor(s) (Hadden et al. 1981). Resting, as well as phytohemagglutinin-stimulated blood mononuclear cells produce and secrete a factor or factors capable of inhibiting fibroblast collagen synthesis (Jimenez et al. 1979). Other investigators, on the other hand, have reported increased fibroblast proliferation, collagen and non-collagenous protein synthesis by conditioned medium of sensitized lymphocytes exposed to antigen (Wahl et al 1978; Neilson et al. 1980). To examine the role of immunoregulation of fibroblasts in vivo, a model of interstitial nephritis, which can result in scar formation, has been utilized (Neilson et al. 1980). Upon injection of a preparation of tubular basement membrane, cell-mediated immunity to the antigen preparation can be demonstrated. The time course of disease evolution can be correlated with the time course of production of fibroblast stimulatory factors by mononuclear cells upon exposure to tubular antigen. A return to production of fibroblast-inhibitory factor(s) is observed when the disease becomes quiescent. The physico-chemical characteristics of these factors are not available, but may be similar to the 22,000 molecular weight lymphocyte-derived chemotactic factor for fibroblasts (LDCF-F) (Postlethwaite et al. 1976). Soluble factors with inhibitory activity toward collagen synthesis in lung explant cultures have also been obtained from normal rat lungs (Phan and Thrall 1981a). There is a marked loss of this activity in lung homogenates from animals with bleomycin-induced pulmonary fibrosis, suggesting decreased activity of normal inhibitory regulatory factors (and/or presence of a compensating stimulatory factor(s)) as the cause for increased collagen synthesis (Leibovich and Ross 1975). The cellular source of this factor(s) is uncertain. Production of collagenase is increased in macrophages when exposed to factors derived from lymphocytes (or mononuclear cells) (Wahl et al. 1975). Collagenase can potentially be beneficial by digesting the collagen due to excessive production, but can also be damaging by digestion of normal tissue collagen (i.e. normal tissue architecture) and thus exposing collagenous proteins and derivatives thereof to the immune system, with potential auto-immune consequences. Integration of these data provides possible mechanisms by which a heightened immune state can result in a fibrogenic response: (1) by direct lymphocyte-induced connective tissue cell chemotaxis and activation with consequent fibrosis; (2) by mononuclear cell-induced inflammatory cell activition, especially macrophages, which in turn are capable of producing fibroblast-activating factors (see below); and (3) exacerbation of injury and inflammation by immune complex formation and deposition as well as by increased collagenase production, which could expose the collagen and collagen derivatives for an autoimmune response, thus further amplifying these mechanisms in a manner reminiscent of a positive feedback loop. This latter mechanism could account for the observed irreversibility of the process after a certain degree of lung injury is attained. On the basis of these data, it is clear that cells of the immune system potentially can serve both as initiators and as facilitators of the fibrogenic response (i.e. in being capable of maintaining the fibrotic process via continuous connective tissue cell stimulation). The role of humoral immunity is probably indirect, via such mechanisms as immune complex formation and enhancing tissue injury, as noted above. Thus, in those diseases in which there is evidence of involvement by cell-mediated immunity, one would expect to see amelioration by immunosuppressive therapies or by removal of the offending antigen — only during early phases of the disease. It is interesting to note in this regard that IPF patients with high lymphocyte counts in their bronchoalveolar lavage fluid are more responsive to steroid therapy, as reported by Haslam et al. (1980). On the other hand, another group reports the lack of significant change in the bronchoalveolar lavage fluid lymphocyte population in IPF, but notes, instead, the remarkably large increases in the neutrophil population (Keogh et al. 1981), thus suggesting the importance of inflammatory mechanisms (Gadek et al.1979).

Inflammation usually precedes the fibrotic process. Because of its close association with the fibrotic process, an obvious assumption is that it should have an influence on connective tissue cell function and growth. Early studies on wound healing reveal the importance of the macrophage in fibroplasia (Leibovich and Ross 1975). Antineutrophil serum has no effect on fibroplasia, but antimacrophage serum inhibits the process. Antineutrophil serum also has no effect on bleomycin-induced pulmonary fibrosis in rats, while cobra venom factor is highly effective (Thrall et al. 1981; Phan and Thrall 1982). This suggests the importance of complement function other than that related to neutrophils in the fibrogenic response. Macrophages produce fibroblast-activating factors upon exposure to silica or quartz crystals (Heppleston and Styles 1967; Aalto et al. 1976). These macrophage-conditioned media cause increased DNA and protein (including collagen) synthesis in the target fibroblasts. Most recently, activated macrophage-derived fibronectin has been reported to be chemotactic for fibroblasts (Tsukamoto et al. 1981). Fibroblasts can also be recruited by collagenous peptides and fragment(s) derived from the fifth component of complement (C5) (Postlethwaite et al. 1978, 1979). In vivo, these fragments are presumably the products of proteolysis by various proteases and collagenase released by activated neutrophils and macrophages. Thus, macrophages and neutrophils can initiate fibroblast recruitment (and possibly activation) accompanied by activation of the macrophages (directly, e.g. quartz crystals, or indirectly, e.g. via lymphokine(s)), with consequent fibroblast proliferation and activation, by both collagen synthesis — with fibrotic consequences — and increased collagenase production — with destructive consequences. The ability of macrophages to also regulate lymphocyte function is also well documented and reviewed elsewhere (Mizel 1981), and presumably will also have an impact on lymphocyte regulation of fibroblast function. Thus, a complex mutual interaction between both immune and inflammatory cells influences the balance between stimulation and inhibition of fibroblast or connective tissue cell function. The net effect of these, plus the non-immune factors, ultimately determines whether or not progressive fibrosis will ensue.

4.6. CONCLUSION

A review of the in-vitro data reveals that a variety of factors can directly activate fibroblasts and other connective tissue cells. Immune mechanisms can serve both as initiators of lung injury and as propagators of fibrosis. Experimental evidence, however, suggests that they play a more significant role as modulators of the intensity of the fibrogenic response than as initiators. As such, they can modulate the severity of the response, and thus immunosuppressive therapy (including removal of offending antigen, if possible) would be effective in those cases. On the other hand, non-immune mechanisms can also be effective in propagating the fibrogenic response (e.g. silicosis, with persistence of silica particles). This divergence is reflected by the large number of stimuli capable of stimulating fibroblasts (and other connective tissue cells) and, to a lesser degree, inhibiting them. It is the net effect of these stimuli that will decide the final outcome. Due to this complex interaction, it is difficult to predict which stimulus is predominant, or if any one stimulus is predominant at all. For instance, initial injury by hyperoxia can directly activate fibroblasts to proliferate and synthesize more collagen, but at the same time causes a pneumonitis with cellular and tissue injury, with a potential for an autoimmune process t develop, thus also activating the immune/inflammatory mechanism of connective tissue cell activation. In summary, the fibrogenic response is the result of a disruption in the complex regulatory interaction between immune and non-immune factors on the one hand, and the connective tissue cell on the other. It remains uncertain whether irreversibility of the fibrogenic response is a reflection of the permanence in the change of the regulatory forces or in the activation state of the target connective tissue cell. The disruption in this regulatory interaction is partially attributable to disruption of the normal architecture and abrogation of the endothelial/epithelial barrier, with consequent exposure of the interstitially located connective tissue cells to normally restricted stimuli. Examination of the effects on the fibrogenic response of selective systematic abrogation of discrete components of the immune and inflammatory systems, either by pharmacologic manipulation and/or genetic (strain) variation (and mutations), should provide further insight into the actual role of these systems.

ACKNOWLEDGEMENT

The author wishes to thank Jeny Breakstone for her excellent secretarial assistance during the preparation of this chapter, and for typing the manuscript.

REFERENCES

Aalto, M., Potila, M. and Kulonen, E. (1976) The effect of Silica-treated macrophages on the synthesis of collagen and other proteins in vitro. *Exp. Cell Res. 97,* 193.

Adamson, I.Y.R. and Bowden, D.H. (1974) The pathogenesis of bleomycin-induced pulmonary fibrosis in mice. *Am. J. Pathol. 77,* 185.

Adamson, I.Y.R. and Bowden, D.H. (1976) Pulmonary injury and repair. Organ culture studies of murine lung after oxygen. *Arch. Pathol. Lab. Med. 100,* 640.

Alarcon-Segovia, D. (1969) Drug-induced lupus syndromes. *Mayo Clin. Proc. 44,* 664.

Alescio, T. (1973) Effect of a proline analogue, azetidine-2-carboxylic acid, on the morphogenesis in vitro of mouse embryonic lung. *J. Embryol. Exp. Morphol. 29,* 439.

Allen, D.H., Basten, A. and Wookock, A.J. (1977) Studies of cell mediated and humoral immunity in bird breeder's hypersensitivity pneumonitis. *Am. Rev. Resp. Dis. 115,* 45.

Andriopoulos, N.A., Mestecky, J., Wright, P. and Miller, E.J. (1976) Characterization of antibodies to the native human collagens and to their component α-chains in the sera and the joint fluids of patients with rheumatoid arthritis. *Immunochemistry 13,* 709.

Ashe, B.M. and Zimmerman, M. (1977) Specific inhibition of human granulocyte elastase by unsaturated fatty acids. *Fed. Proc. 36,* 678.

Autor, A.P. (1977) *Biochemical Mechanisms of Paraquat Toxicity.* Academic Press, New York.

Bailey, A.J. (1977) Some aspects of collagen maturation and fibrosis. *Ann. Rheum. Dis. 36 (Suppl),* 5.

Bailey, A.J., Sims, T.J., LeLous, M. and Bazin, S. (1972) Collagen polymorphism in experimental granulation tissue. *Biochem. Biophys. Res. Commun. 66,* 1160.

Barrett, A. (1972) In: J.T. Dingle (Ed.), *Lysosomes: A Laboratory Handbook,* North-Holland Publishing Co., Amsterdam, p. 46.

Bateman, E., Turner-Warwick, M. and Adelman-Grill, B.C. (1981) Immuno-histochemical study of collagen types in human foetal lung and fibrotic lung disease. *Thorax 36,* 645.

Baugh, R.J. and Travis, J. (1976) Human leukocyte granule elastase: Rapid isolation and characterization. *Biochemistry 15,* 836.

Bedrossian, C.W.M., Greenberg, S.D., Yawn, D.H. and O'Neal, R.M. (1977) Experimentally induced bleomycin sulfate pulmonary toxicity. *Arch. Pathol. Lab. Med. 101,* 248.

Berrens, L., Guikers, C.L.H. and Van Dijk, A. (1974) The antigens in pigeon breeder's disease and their interactions with human complement. *Ann. NY Acad. Sci. 221,* 153.

Bhatnagar, R.S., Hussain, M.Z., Streifel, J.A., Tolentino, M. and Enriquez, B. (1978) Alteration of collagen synthesis in lung organ cultures by hyperoxic environments. *Biochem. Biophys. Res. Commun. 83,* 392.

Bienkowski, R.S., Baum, B.J. and Crystal, R.G. (1978) Fibroblasts degrade newly synthesized collagen within the cell before secretion. *Nature (London) 276,* 413.

Blum, R.H., Carter, S.K. and Agre, K. (1973) A clinical review of bleomycin – a new antineoplastic agent. *Cancer 31,* 903.

Bornstein, P. (1974) The biosynthesis of collagen. *Ann. Rev. Biochem. 43,* 567.

Bornstein, P. and Sage, H. (1980) Structurally distinct collagen types. *Ann. Rev. Biochem. 49,* 957.

Bradley, K.H., McConnell, S.D. and Crystal, R.G. (1974) Lung collagen composition and synthesis: characterization and changes with age. *J. Biol. Chem. 249,* 2674.

Brentjens, J.R., O'Connell, D.W., Pawlowski, I.B., Hsu, K.C. and Andres, G.A. (1974) Experimental immune complex disease of the lung. The pathogenesis of a laboratory model resembling certain human interstitial lung diseases. *J. Exp. Med. 140,* 105.

Burgeson, R.E., Eradli, F.A., Kaitila, I.I. and Hollister, D.W. (1976) Fetal membrane collagens: Identification of two new collagen α-chains. *Proc. Natl Acad. Sci. USA 73,* 2579.

Burleigh, M.C., Barrett, A.J. and Lazarus, G.S. (1974) Cathepsin Bl: A lysosomal enzyme that degrades native collagen. *Biochem. J. 137,* 387.

Carp, H. and Janoff, A. (1980) Potential mediator of inflammation: Phagocyte-derived oxidants suppress the elastase-inhibitory capacity of alpha-1-proteinase inhibitor in vitro. *J. Clin. Invest. 66,* 987.

Carrington, C.B., Gaensler, E.A., Coutu, R.E., Fitzgerald, M.X. and Gupta, R.G. (1978) Natural history and treated course of usual and desquamative interstitial pneumonia. *N. Engl. J. Med. 298,* 801.

Caterson, B. and Baker, J.R. (1979) The link proteins as specific components of cartilage proteoglycan aggregates in vivo. *J. Biol. Chem. 254,* 2394.

Christner, P., Weinbaum, G., Sloan, B. and Rosenbloom, J. (1978) Degradation of tropoelastin by proteases. *Analyt. Biochem. 88,* 682.

Chvapil, M. and Leng, Y.M. (1975) Oxygen and lung fibrosis. *Arch. Environ. Health 30,* 528.

Clark, J.M. and Lambertsen, C.J. (1971) Pulmonary oxygen toxicity: a review. *Pharmacol. Rev. 23,* 57.

Clark, J.G., Overton, J.E., Marino, B.A., Uitto, J. and Starcher, B.C. (1980a) Collagen biosynthesis in bleomycin-induced pulmonary fibrosis in hamsters. *J. Lab. Clin. Med. 96,* 943.

Clark, J.G., Starcher, B.C. and Uitto, J. (1980b) Bleomycin-induced synthesis of type I procollagen by human lung and skin fibroblasts in culture. *Biochim. Biophys. Acta 631,* 359.

Clore, J.N., Cohen, I.K. and Diegelmann, R.F. (1979) Quantitation of collagen types I and III during wound healing in rat skin. *Proc. Soc. Exp. Biol. Med. 161,* 337.

Cocchiara, R., Giallongo, A., Amoroso, S., Spina, G., Stancampiano, R. and Geraci, D. (1981) Circulating immune complexes in patients with usual interstitial pulmonary fibrosis partial characterization and relationship with Thermoactinomyces vulgaris. *Immunology 44,* 817.

Coffey, J.W., Fiedler-Nagy, C., Georgiadis, A.G. and Salavador, R.S. (1976) Digestion of native collagen, denatured collagen and collagen fragments by extracts of rat liver lysosomes. *J Biol. Chem. 251,* 5280.

Cole, P.J. (1976) Possible mechanisms in pathogenesis of nitrofurantoin-induced lung disease. *Chemotherapy 4,* 279.

Corrin, B. and Price, A.B. (1972) Electron microscopic studies in desquamative interstitial pneumonia associated with asbestos. *Thorax 27,* 324.

Crapo, J.D. and Tierney, D.F. (1974) Superoxide dismutase and pulmonary oxygen toxicity. *Am. J. Physiol. 226,* 1401.

Crooke, S.T. and Bradner, W.T. (1973) Bleomycin, a review. *J. Med. 7,* 903.

Crouch, E., Sage, H. and Bornstein, P. (1980) Structural basis for apparent heterogeneity of collagens in human basement membranes: Type IV procollagen contains two distinct chains. *Proc. Natl Acad. Sci. USA 77,* 745.

Crystal, R.G., Fulmer, J.D., Roberts, W.C., Moss, M.L., Line, B.R. and Reynolds, H.Y. (1976) Idiopathic pulmonary fibrosis: Clinical, histologic, radiologic, physiologic, scintigraphic, cytologic and biochemical aspects. *Ann. Intern. Med. 85,* 769.

Cutroneo, K.R., Guzman, N.A. and Sharaway, M.M. (1974) Evidence for a subcellular vesicular site of collagen prolyl hydroxylation. *J. Biol. Chem. 249,* 5989.

Dale, K. (1973) A method for inducing unilateral silicosis in rabbits by an injection technique with some observations on lung clearance and quantitative ȅvaluation of experimental silicosis. *Scand. J. Respir. Dis. 54,* 157.

Daniele, R.P., Henson, P.M., Fantone, J.C., Ward, P.A. and Dreisin, R.B. (1981) Immune complex injury of the lung. *Am. Rev. Respir. Dis. 124,* 738.

Dehm, P. and Prockop, D.J. (1973) Biosynthesis of cartilage procollagen *Eur. J. Biochem. 35,* 159.

DeRemee, R.A. and Rohrbach, M.S. (1980) Serum angiotensin-converting enzyme activity in evaluating the clinical course of sarcoidosis. *Ann. Intern. Med. 92,* 361.

Deshmulch, K. and Nimmi, M. (1969) A defect in intramolecular and intermolecular cross-linking of collagen caused by penicillamine. Functional groups involved in the interaction process. *J. Biol. Chem. 244,* 1787.

Divertie, M.B. (1964) Lung involvement in the connective tissue disorders. *Med. Clin. N. Amer. 48,* 1015.

Dorfman, A. and Matalon, R. (1976) The mucopolysaccharidoses. *Proc. Natl Acad. Sci. USA 73,* 630.

Dreisin, R.B., Schwarz, M.I., Theofilopoulos, A.N. and Stanford, R.E. (1978) Circulating immune complexes in the idiopathic interstitial pneumonias. *N. Engl. J. Med. 298,* 5353.

Dubrawsky, C., Dubrawsky, N.B. and Withers, H.R. (1978) The effect of colchicine on the accumulation of hydroxyproline and on lung compliance. *Radiat. Res. 73,* 111.

Duksin, D., Davidson. J.M. and Bornstein, P. (1978) The role of glycosylation in the enzymatic conversion of procollagen to collagen: Studies using tanicamycin and concanavalin A. *Arch. Biochem. Biophys. 185,* 326.

Eddy, H.A. and Casarett, G.W. (1972) Pathology of radiation syndromes in the hamster. *Prog. Exp. Tumor Res. 16,* 98.

Edwards, J.H. (1976) A quantitative study on the activation of the alternative pathway of complement by mouldy hay dust and thermophilic actinomycetes. *Clin. Allergy 6,* 19.

Ehrlich, H.P., Ross, R. and Bornstein, P. (1974) Effects of antimicrotubular agents on the secretion of collagen. *J. Cell Biol. 62,* 390.

Elias, J.A., Rossman, M.D., Atkinson, B.J., Phillips, S.M. and Daniele, R.P. (1981) Experimental berylliosis and beryllium-induced interstitial fibrosis. *Am. Rev. Respir. Dis. 123,* 141.

Estes, D. and Christian, C.L. (1971) The natural history of systemic lupus erythematosus by prospective analysis. *Medicine 50,* 85.

Evans, C.A. and Peterkovsky, B. (1976) Ascorbate-dependent proline hydroxylation resulting from viral transformation of BALB 3T3 cells and unaffected by dibutyryl cAMP treatment. *J.Cell. Physiol. 89,* 355.

Fedullo. A.J., Karlinsky, J.B., Snider, G.L. and Goldstein, R.H. (1980) Lung statics and connective tissues after penicillamine in bleomycin-treated hamsters. *J. Appl. Physiol. 49,* 1083.

Feinstein, G. and Janoff, A. (1975) A rapid method for purification of human granulocyte cationic neutral proteases: Purification and further characterization of human granulocyte elastase. *Biochim. Biophys. Acta 403,* 493.

Fessler, J.H. and Fessler, L.I. (1978) Biosynthesis of procollagen. *Ann. Rev. Biochem. 47,* 129.

Fietzek, P.P. and Kuhn, K. (1976) The primary structure of collagen. *Int. Rev. Connect. Tissue Res. 7,* 1.

Finch, E.S. and Bader, L. (1974) Pulmonary damage from Hong Kong influenza. *Aust. NZ J. Med. 4,* 16.

Fisher, H.K. Clements, J.A. and Wright, R.R. (1973) Enhancement of oxygen toxicity by the herbicide paraquat. *Am. Rev. Respir. Dis. 107,* 246.

Fleischman, R.W., Baber, J.R., Thompson, G.R., Schaeppi, M.H., Ilievski, V.R., Cooney, D.A. and Davis, R.D. (1971) Bleomycin-induced interstitial pneumonia in dogs. *Thorax 26,* 675.

Foidart, J.M., Shigeto, A., Martin, G.R., Zizic, T.M., Barnett, E.V., Lawley, T.J. and Katz, S.I.L. (1978) Antibodies to type II collagen in relapsing polychondritis. *N. Engl. J. Med. 299,* 1203.

Foster, J.A., Bruenger. E., Gray, W.R. and Sandberg, L.B. (1973) Isolation and amino acid sequences of tropoelastin peptides from elastin. *J. Biol. Chem. 249,* 6191.

Foster, J.A., Rubin, L., Kagan, H.M. and Franzblau, C. (1974) Isolation and characterization of cross-linked peptides from elastin. *J. Biol. Chem. 249,* 6191.

Foster, J.A., Mecham, R.P. and Franzblau, C. (1976) A high molecular weight species of soluble elastin. *Biochem. Biophys. Res. Commun. 72,* 1399.

Francis, G., John, R. and Thomas, J. (1973) Biosynthetic pathway of desmosines in elastin. *Biochem. J. 136,* 45.

Frank, L. and Roberts, R.J. (1979) Endotoxin protection against oxygen-induced acute and chronic lung injury. *J. Appl. Physiol. 47,* 577.

Freeman, G., Stephens, R.J., Coffin, D.L. and Stara, J.F. (1973) Changes in dogs lungs after long term exposure to ozone. *Arch. Environ. Health 26,* 209.

Fridovich, I. (1976) Oxygen radicals, hydrogen peroxide, and oxygen toxicity. In: W.A. Pryor (Ed.), *Free Radicals in Biology, Vol. 1,* Academic Press, New York, *p. 239.*

Fulmer, J.D., Spasovska, M.S., Von Gal, E.R. and Crystal, R.G. (1973) Distribution of HLA antigens in idiopathic pulmonary fibrosis. *Am. Rev. Respir. Dis. 118,* 141.

Fulmer, J.D., Von Gal, E.R., Roberts, W.C. and Crystal, R.G. (1979) Morphologic correlates of the severity of fibrosis in idiopathic pulmonary fibrosis. *J. Clin. Invest. 63,* 665.

Fulmer, J.D., Bienkowski, R.S., Cowan. M.J., Breul, S.D., Bradley, K.M., Ferrans, V.J., Roberts, W.C. and Crystal, R.G. (1980) Collagen concentration and rates of synthesis in idiopathic pulmonary fibrosis. *Am. Rev. Respir. Dis. 122,* 289.

Gadek, J.E., Kelman, J.A., Fells, G., Weinberger, S.T., Horwitz, A.L., Reynolds, H.Y., Fulmer, J.D. and Crystal, R.G. (1979) Collagenase in the lower respiratory tract of patients with idiopathic pulmonary fibrosis. *N. Engl. J. Med. 301,* 734.

Gay, S., Martin, G.R., Muller, P.K., Timpl, R. and Kuhn, K. (1976) Simultaneous synthesis of type I and III collagen by fibroblasts in culture. *Proc. Natl Acad. Sci. USA 73,* 4037.

Ghose, T., Landrigan, P., Killeen, R. and Dill, J. (1974) Immunopathological studies in patients with farmer's lung. *Clin. Allergy 4,* 119.

Goldberg, B. (1977) Kinetics of processing of type I and type III procollagens in fibroblast cultures. *Proc. Natl Acad. Sci. USA 74,* 3322.

Gosline, J.M. (1976) The physical properties of elastic tissue. *Int. Rev. Connect. Tissue Res. 7,* 211.

Grant, M.E. and Jackson, D.S. (1976) The biosynthesis of procollagen. *Essays Biochem. 12,* 77.

Grant, M.E. and Prockop, D.J. (1972) The biosynthesis of collagen. *N. Engl. J. Med. 286,* 194, 242 and 291.

Greenberg, D.B., Lyons, S.A. and Last, J.A. (1978) Paraquat-induced changes in the rate of collagen biosynthesis by rat lung explants. *J. Lab. Clin. Med. 92,* 1033.

Griffin, M., Smith, L.L. and Wynne, J. (1979) Changes in transglutaminase activity in an experimental model of pulmonary fibrosis induced by paraquat. *Br. J. Exp. Pathol. 60,* 653.

Gross, N.J. (1977) Pulmonary effects of radiation therapy. *Ann. Intern. Med. 86,* 81.

Gross, N.J. (1980) Radiation pneumonitis in mice: some effects of corticosteroids on mortality and pulmonary physiology. *J. Clin. Invest. 66,* 504.

Gross, J. and Nagai, Y. (1965) Specific degradation of the collagen molecule by tadpole collagenolytic enzyme. *Proc. Natl Acad. Sci. USA 54,* 1197.

Gross, J., Harper, E., Harris, E.D. Jr, McCroskery, P.A., Highberger, J.H., Corbett, C. and Kanh, A.H. (1974) Animal collagenases: specificity of action and structures of the substrate cleavage site. *Biochem. Biophys. Res. Commun. 61,* 605.

Hadden, J.W., Sadlik, J.R. and Warfel, A.H. (1981) Characterization of lymphokines acting on the macrophage. In: J.W. Hadden and W.E. Stewart II (Eds.), *The Lymphokines,* Humana Press, Clifton, NJ, p. 73.

Hagopian, A., Bosmann, H.B. and Eylar, E.H. (1968) Glycoprotein biosynthesis: The localization of polypeptidyl:N-acetyl-galactosaminyl, collagen:glucosyl, and glycoprotein:galactosyl transferases in HeLa cell membrane fractions. *Arch. Biochem. Biophys. 128,* 387.

Hall, C.W., Liebaers, I., DiNatale, P. and Neufeld E.F. (1978) Enzymic diagnosis of the genetic mucopolysaccharide storage disorders. *Methods Enzymol. 50,* 349.

Halme, J., Uitto, J., Kahanpaa, K., Karhumen, P. and Lindy, S. (1979) Protocollagen proline hydroxylase activity in experimental pulmonary fibrosis of rats. *J. Lab. Clin. Med. 75,* 535.

Hance, A.J. and Crystal, R.G. (1975) The connective tissue of lung. *Am. Rev. Respir. Dis. 112,* 657.

Hance, A.J. and Crystal, R.G. (1976) Collagen. In: R.G. Crystal (Ed.), *The Biochemical Basis of Pulmonary Function.* Marcel Dekker, New York, p. 197.

Hance, A.J., Bradley, K. and Crystal, R.G. (1976) Lung collagen heterogeneity – Synthesis of type I and type III collagen by rabbit and human lung cells in culture. *J. Clin. Invest. 57,* 102.

Hanngren, A., Biberfeldt, G., Carlens, E., Hedfors, E., Nilsson, B.S., Ripe, E. and Wakren, B. (1974) Ossarcoidosis due to an infectious interaction between virus and mycobacterium? In: K. Iwai and Y. Hosoda (Eds.), *Proceedings of the Sixth International Conference on Sarcoidosis,* 1974, University of Tokyo Press, Tokyo, p.8.

Hardingham, T.E. (1979) The role of link-protein in the structure of cartilage proteoglycan aggregates. *Biochem. J. 177,* 237.

Hardingham, T.E. and Muir, H. (1974) Hyaluronic acid in cartilage and proteoglycan aggregation. *Biochem. J. 139,* 565.

Harper, E. (1980) Collagenases. *Ann. Rev. Biochem. 49,* 1063.

Harris, Jr. E.D. and Farrell, M.E. (1972) Resistance to collagenase: a characteristic of collagen fibrils cross-linked by formaldehyde. *Biochim. Biophys. Acta 278,* 133.

Hart, G.W. and Lennarz, W.J. (1978) Effects of tunicarrycin on the biosynthesis of glycosaminoglycans by embryonic chick cornea. *J. Biol. Chem. 253,* 5795.

Hartley, B.S. and Shotton, D.M. (1971) Pancreatic elastase. In: P.D. Boyer (Ed.), *The Enzymes, Vol. 3,* Academic Press, New York, p. 323.

Harwood, R., Grant, L.L.E. and Jackson, D.S. (1976) The route of secretion of procollagen. *Biochem. J. 156,* 81.

Hascall, V.A. (1977) Interaction of cartilage proteoglycans with hyaluronic acid. *J. Supramol. Struct. 7,* 101.

Haslam, P., Turner-Warwick, M. and Lukoszek, A. (1975) Antinuclear antibody and lymphocyte responses to nuclear antigens in patients with lung disease. *Clin. Exp. Immunol. 20,* 379.

Haslam, P., Thompson, B., Mohammed, I. and Turner-Warwick, M. (1979) Circulating immune complexes in patients with cryptogenic fibrosing alveolitis. *J. Immunol. 37,* 381.

Haslam, P.L., Turton, C.W.G., Lukoszek, A., Salisbury, A.J., Dewar, A., Collins, J.V. and Turner-Warwick, M. (1980) Bronchoalveolar lavage fluid cell counts in cryptogenic fibrosing alveolitis and their relation to therapy. *Thorax 35,* 328.

Hata, R.-I. and Peterkovsky, B. (1977) Specific changes in the collagen phenotype of BALB 3T3 cells as a result of transformation by sarcoma viruses or a chemical carcinogen. *Proc. Natl Acad. Sci. USA 74,* 2933.

Hensley, G.T., Fink, J.N. and Barboriak, J.J. (1974) Hypersensitivity pneumonitis in the monkey. *Arch. Pathol. 97,* 33.

Heppleston, A.G. (1973) The biological response to silica. In: E. Kulonen and J. Pikkarainen (Eds.), *Biology of the Fibroblast.* Academic Press, New York, p. 529.

Heppleston, A.G. and Styles, J.A. (1967) Activity of a macrophage factor in collagen formation by silica. *Nature (London) 214,* 521.

Hesterberg, T.W. and Last, J.A. (1981) Ozone-induced acute pulmonary fibrosis in rats: Prevention of increased rates of collagen synthesis by methyl-prednisolone. *Am. Rev. Respir. Dis. 123,* 47.

Hirai, K.I., Witschi, H.P. and Cote, M.G. (1977) Electron microscopy of butylated hydroxytoluene-induced lung damage in mice. *Exp. Mol. Pathol. 27,* 295.

Hollinger, M.A. and Chvapil, M. (1977) Effect of paraquat on lung prolyl hydroxylase activity. *Res. Commun. Chem. Pathol. Pharmacol. 16,* 159.

Hollinger, M.A., Zuckerman, J.E. and Giri, S.N. (1978) Effect of acute and chronic paraquat on rat lung collagen content. *Res. Commun. Chem. Pathol. Pharmacol. 21,* 295.

Horwitz, A.L., Hance, A.J. and Crystal, R.G. (1977) Granulocyte collagenase: Selective digestion of type I relative to type III collagen. *Proc. Natl Acad. Sci. USA 74,* 879.

Hussain, M.Z. and Bhatnagar, R.S. (1979) Involvement of superoxide in the paraquat-induced enhancement of lung collagen synthesis in organ culture. *Biochem. Biophys. Res. Commun. 89,* 71.

Ichihashi, M., Shinkai, H., Takei, M. and Sano, S. (1973) Analysis of the mechanism of bleomycin-induced cutaneous fibrosis in mice. *J. Antibiot. 26,* 238.

Jaffe, E.A., Minick, C.R., Adelman, B., Becker, C.G. and Nachman, R. (1976) Synthesis of basement membrane collagen by cultured human endothelial cells. *J. Exp. Med. 144,* 209.

Janoff, A., Sloan, B., Weinbaum, G., Damiano, V., Sandhaus, R.A., Elias, J. and Kimbal, P. (1977) Experimental emphysema induced with purified human neutrophil elastase: tissue localization of the instilled protease. *Am. Rev. Respir. Dis. 115, 461.*

Jimenez, S.A., McArthur, W. and Rosenbloom, J. (1979) Inhibition of collagen synthesis by mononuclear cell supernatants. *J. Exp. Med. 150,* 1421.

Johanson, W.G. and Pierce, A.K. (1972) Effects of elastase, collagenase and papain on structure and function of rat lungs in vitro. *J. Clin. Invest. 51,* 288.

Johnson, D. and Travis, J. (1979) The oxidative inactivation of human alpha-1-proteinase inhibitor: Further evidence for methionine at the reactive center. *J. Biol. Chem. 254,* 4022.

Johnson, K.J. and Ward, P.A. (1974) Acute immunologic pulmonary alveolitis. *J. Clin. Invest. 54,* 349.

Johnson, R.L. and Ziff, M. (1976) Lymphokine stimulation of collagen accumulation. *J. Clin. Invest. 58,* 240.

Johnson, K.J., Fantone, J.C. III, Kaplan, J. and Ward, P.A. (1981) In vivo damage of rat lungs by oxygen metabolites. *J. Clin. Invest. 67,* 983.

Karlinsky, J.B., Snider, G.L., Franzblau, C., Stone, P.J. and Hoppin, F.G. Jr. (1976) In vitro effects of elastase lungs. *Am. Rev. Respir. Dis. 113,* 769.

Kelley, J., Newman, R.A. and Evans, J.N. (1980) Bleomycin-induced pulmonary fibrosis in the rat: prevention with an inhibitor of collagen synthesis. *J. Lab. Clin. Med. 96,* 954.

Kent, G., Gay, S., Inouye, T., Bahu, R., Minick, O.T. and Popper, H. (1976) Vitamin A-containing lipocytes and formation of type III collagen in liver injury. *Proc. Natl Acad. Sci. USA 73,* 3719.

Keogh, B., Line, A., Rust, M., Hunninghake, G., Meier-Sydow, J. and Crystal, R.G. (1981) Clinical staging of patients with idiopathic pulmonary fibrosis. *Am. Rev. Respir. Dis. 123,* 89.

Kohler, N. and Lipton, A. (1974) Platelets as a source of fibroblast growth-promoting activity. *Exp. Cell Res. 87,* 297.

Kravis, T.C., Ahmed, A., Brown, T.E., Fulmer, J.D., Crystal, R.G., (1976) Pathogenic mechanisms in pulmonary fibrosis: Collagen-induced migration inhibition factor production and cytotoxicity mediated by lymphocytes. *J. Clin. Invest. 58,* 1223.

Lamberg, S.I. and Stoolmiller, A.C. (1974) Glycosaminoglycans: a biochemical and clinical review. *J. Invest. Dermatol. 63,* 433.

Last, J.A., Greenberg, D.B. and Castleman, W.L. (1979) Ozone-induced alterations in collagen metabolism of rat lungs. *Toxicol. Appl. Pharmacol. 51,* 247.

Last, J.A., Hesterberg, T.W., Reiser, K.M., Cross, C.E., Amis, T.C., Gunn, C., Steffey, E.P., Grandy, J. and Henrickson, R. (1981) Ozone-induced alterations in collagen metabolism of monkey lungs. Use of biopsy-obtained lung tissue. *Toxicol. Appl. Pharmacol. 60,* 579.

Laurent, T.C. (1977) Interaction between proteins and glycosaminoglycans. *Fed. Proc. 36,* 24.

Law, M.P., Hornsey, S. and Field, S.B. (1976) Collagen content of mice after X-ray irradiation. *Radiat. Res. 65,* 60.

Leibovich, S.J. and Ross, R. (1975) The role of the macrophage in wound repair. A study with hydrocortisone and antimacrophage serum. *Am. J. Pathol. 78,* 71.

Lennarz, W.J. (Ed.) (1980) *The Biochemistry of Glycoproteins and Proteoglycans,* Plenum Press, New York.

Levene, C.I., Bye, I. and Saffriotti, U. (1968): The effect of β-aminopropionitrile on silicotic pulmonary fibrosis in the rat. *Br. J. Exp. Pathol. 49,* 152.

Libby, D.M., Gibofsky, A., Fotino, M. and Smith, J.P. (1981) Immunogenetic and clinicopathologic correlations in idiopathic pulmonary fibrosis. *Am. Rev. Respir. Dis. 123,* 45.

Liebow, A.A. (1967) Definition and classification of interstitial pneumonias in human pathology. *Prog. Respir. Res. 8,* 1.

Lindahl, U., Hook, M., Backstrom, G., Jacobsson, I., Riesenfeld, J., Malmstrom, A., Roden, L. and Feingold, D.S. (1977) Structure and biosynthesis of heparin-like polysaccharides. *Fed. Proc. 36,* 19.

Liotta, L.A., Abe, S., Robey, P.G. and Martin, G.R. (1979) Preferential digestion of basement membrane collagen by an enzyme derived from a metastatic murine tumor. *Proc. Natl Acad. Sci. USA 76,* 2268.

Luna, M.A., Bedrossian, C.W.M., Lichtiger, B. and Salem, P.A. (1972) Interstitial pneumonitis associated with bleomycin therapy. *Am. J. Clin. Pathol. 58,* 501.

Madri, J.A. and Furthmayr, H. (1980) Collagen polymorphism in the lung: an immunochemical study of pulmonary fibrosis. *Human Pathol. 11,* 353.

Martin, W.J., Gadek, J.E., Hunninghake, G.W. and Crystal, R.G. (1981) Oxidant injury of lung parenchymal cells. *J. Clin. Invest. 68,* 1277.

Marx, J.J. and Burrell, R. (1973) Delayed hypersensitivity to beryllium compounds. *J. Immunol. 111,* 590.

McAdam, K.P.W.J., Fudenberg, H.H. and Michaeli, O. (1978) Antibodies to collagen in patients with leprosy. *Clin. Immunol. Immunopathol. 9,* 16.

McCullough, B., Collins, J.F., Johanson, W.G. Jr and Grover, F.L. (1978) Bleomycin-induced diffuse interstitial pulmonary fibrosis in baboons. *J. Clin. Invest. 61,* 79.

McLees, B.D., Schleiter, G. and Pinnell, S.R. (1977) Isolation of type III collagen from human adult parenchymal lung. *Biochemistry. 16,* 185.

Menzel, E.J., Smolen, J.S., Renner, F., Steffen, C. and Horak, W. (1980) Autoantibodies to collagen in patients with chronic liver diseases. *Int. Arch. Allergy Appl. Immunol. 63,* 424.

Michaeli, D. and Fudenberg, H.H. (1974) Antibodies to collagen in patients with emphysema. *Clin. Immunol. Immunopathol 3,* 187.

Miller, E.J. (1976) Biochemical characteristic and biological significance of the genetically-distinct collagens. *Mol. Cell. Biochem. 13,* 165.

Mitchell, D.N. (1976) The nature and the physical characteristics of a transmissible agent from human sarcoid tissue. *Ann. NY Acad. Sci. 278,* 333.

Mizel, S.B. (1981) Biochemical characteristics of macrophage derived lymphostimulatory factors. In: J.W. Hadden and W.E. Stewart II (Eds.), *The Lymphokines,* Humana Press, Clifton, NJ, p. 347.

Moore, V.L., Fink, J.N., Barboriak, J.J., Ruff, L.L. and Schleuter, D.P. (1974) Immunologic events in pigeon breeder's disease. *J. Allergy Clin. Immunol. 33,* 319.

Moritz, E.D., Hunninghake, G.W. and Crystal, R.G. (1981) Activation of lung immune effector cells: A possible precursor to beryllium lung disease. *Am. Rev. Respir. Dis. 123,* 140.

Motomiya, M., Arai, H., Sato, H., Yokosawa, A., Nagai, H. and Konno, K. (1975) Increase of dermatan sulfate in a case of pulmonary fibrosis. *Tohoku J. Exp. Med. 115,* 361.

Murad, S., Sivarajah, A. and Pinnell, S.R. (1981) Regulation of prolyl and lysyl hydroxylase activities in cultured human skin fibroblasts by ascorbic acid. *Biochem. Biophys. Res. Commun. 101,* 868.

Myllyla, R., Schubotz, L.M., Weser, U. and Kivirikko, K.I. (1979) Involvement of superoxide in the prolyl and lysyl hydroxylase reactions. *Biochem. Biophys. Res. Commun. 89,* 98.

Nagaya, H. and Sieker, H.O. (1972) Pathogenetic mechanisms of interstitial pulmonary fibrosis in patients with serum antinuclear factor: A histologic and clinical correlation. *Am. J. Med. 52,* 51.

Narayanan, A.S. and Page, R.C. (1976) Demonstration of a precursor-product relationship between soluble and cross-linked elastin, and the biosynthesis of the desmosines in vitro. *J. Biol. Chem. 251,* 1125.

Neilson, E.G., Jimenez, S.A. and Phillips, S.M. (1980) Cell-mediated immunity in interstitial nephritis III. T lymphocyte-mediated fibroblast proliferation and collagen synthesis: An immune mechanism for renal fibrogenesis. *J. Immunol. 125,* 1708.

Neufeld, E.F., Lim, T.W. and Shapiro, L.J. (1975) Inherited disorders of lysosomal metabolism. *Ann. Rev. Biochem. 44,* 357.

Obserley, L.W. and Bueltner, G.R. (1979) The production of hydroxyl radical by bleomycin and iron (II). *FEBS Lett. 97,* 47.

Ohlsson, K. and Ohlsson, I. (1974) The neutral proteases of human granulocytes. Isolation and partial characterization of granulocyte elastases. *Eur. J. Biochem. 42,* 519.

Otsuka, K., Murota, S. and Mori, Y. (1976) Stimulatory effect of bleomycin on the synthesis of acidic glycosaminoglycans in cultured fibroblasts derived from rat carrageenin granuloma. *Biochim. Biophys. Acta 444,* 359.

Otsuka, K., Murota, S. and Mori, Y. (1978) Stimulatory effect of bleomycin on the hyaluronic acid synthetase in cultured fibroblasts. *Biochem. Pharmacol. 27,* 1551.

Pearson, D.J., Mentnech, M.S., Elliott, J.A., Price, C.D., Taylor, G. and Major, P.C. (1981) Serologic changes in pneumoconiosis and progressive massive fibrosis of coal workers. *Am. Rev. Respir. Dis. 124,* 696.

Pepys, J. (1969) Hypersensitivity diseases of the lung to fungi and other organic dusts. *Monogr. Allergy, 4.*

Percarpio, B. and Fischer, J.J. (1976) Beta-aminopropionitrile as a radiation reaction preventive agent. *Radiology 121,* 737.

Petty, T.L. and Wilkins, M. (1966) The five manifestations of rheumatoid lung. *Dis. Chest 49,* 75.

Phan, S.H. and Thrall, R.S. (1981a) The role of soluble factors in bleomycin-induced pulmonary fibrosis. *Am. J. Pathol., 106,* 156.

Phan, S.H. and Thrall, R.S. (1982) Inhibition of bleomycin-induced pulmonary fibrosis by cobra venom factor. *Am. J. Pathol., 107,* 25.

Phan, S.H., Thrall, R.S. and Ward, P.A. (1980) Bleomycin-induced pulmonary fibrosis in rats: Biochemical demonstration of increased rate of collagen synthesis. *Am. Rev. Respir. Dis. 121,* 501.

Phan, S.H., Thrall, R.S. and Williams, C. (1981b) Bleomycin-induced pulmonary fibrosis: Effects of steroid on lung collagen metabolism. *Am. Rev. Respir. Dis. 124,* 428.

Phan, S.H., Varani, J., Lovett, E.J. III and Schrier, D. (1981c) Isolation and characterization of fibroblasts from bleomycin-induced fibrotic lungs. *Fed. Proc. 40,* 793.

Phillips, T.L., Wharam, M.D. and Margolis, L.W. (1975) Modification of radiation injury to normal tissues by chemotherapeutic agents. *Cancer 35,* 1678.

Pickrell, J.A. (1981) *Lung Connective Tissue: Location, Metabolism and Response to Injury,* CRC Press, Boca Raton.

Pickrell, J.A., Harris, D.V., Hahn, F.F., Belasich, J.J. and Jones, R.K. (1975) Biological alterations resulting from chronic lung irradition. III Effect of partial (^{60}Co) thoracic irradiation upon pulmonary collagen metabolism and fractionation in syrian hamsters. *Radiat. Res. 62,* 133.

Pickrell, J.A., Harris, D.V., Mauderly, J.L. and Hahn F.F. (1976) Altered collagen metabolism in radiation-induced interstitial pulmonary fibrosis. *Chest 69,* 311.

Pierce, J.A., Resnick, H. and Henry, P.M. (1967) Collagen and elastin metabolism in the lungs, skin and bones of adult rats. *J. Lab. Clin. Med. 69,* 485.

Piez, K.A. (1968) Cross-linking of collagen and elastin. *Ann. Rev. Biochem. 37,* 547.

Postlethwaite, A.E., Snyderman, R. and Kang, A.H. (1976) The chemotactic attraction of human fibroblasts to a lymphocyte derived factor. *J. Exp. Med. 144,* 1188.

Postlethwaite, A.E., Seyes, J.M. and Kang, A.H. (1978) Induction of fibroblast chemotaxis by type I, II, III collagens, and collagen degradation peptides. *Proc. Natl Acad. Sci. USA 75,* 871.

Postlethwaite, A.E., Snyderman, R. and Kang, A.H. (1979) Generation of a fibroblast chemotactic factor in serum by activation of complement. *J. Clin. Invest. 64,* 1379.

Prockop, D.J., Kivirikko, K.I., Tuderman, L. and Guzman, N.A. (1979) The biosynthesis of collagen and its disorders. *N. Engl. J. Med. 301,* 13 and 77.

Raff, E.C. and Houck, J.C. (1969) Migration and proliferation of diploid human fibroblasts following "wounding" of confluent monolayers. *J. Cell. Physiol. 74,* 235.

Ramachandran, G.N. and Reddi, A.H. (1976) *Biochemistry of Collagen,* Academic Press, New York.

Ranterberg, J. (1981) Tissue specific differences of collagen. In: Z. Deyl and M. Adam (Eds), *Connective Tissue Research: Chemistry, Biology and Physiology,* Alan R. Liss, Inc., New York, p. 125.

Richards, R.J. and Wusteman, F.S. (1974) The effects of silica dust and alveolar macrophages on lung fibroblast growth in vitro. *Life Sci. 14,* 355.

Riley, D.J., Berg, R.A., Edelman, N.H. and Prockop, D.J. (1980) Prevention of collagen deposition following pulmonary oxygen toxicity in the rat by cis-4-hydroxy-L-proline. *J. Clin. Invest. 65,* 643.

Riley, D.J., Kerr, J.S., Berg, R.A., Ianni, B.D., Pietra, G.G., Edelman, N.H. and Prockop, D.J. (1981a) Prevention of bleomycin-induced pulmonary fibrosis in the hamster by cis-4-hydroxy-L-proline. *Am. Rev. Respir. Dis. 123,* 221.

Riley, D.J., Kerr, J.S., Berg, R.A., Ianni, B.D., Pietra, G.G., Edelman, N.H. and Prockop, D.J. (1981b) Prevention of bleomycin-induced pulmonary fibrosis in the hamster by cis-4-hydroxy-L-proline. *Am. Rev. Respir. Dis. 123,* 388.

Riley, D.J., Kerr, J.S., Berg, R.A., Iami, B.D., Pietra, G.G., Edelman, N.H. and Prockop, D.J. (1982) Beta-aminopropionitrile prevents bleomycin-induced pulmonary fibrosis in the hamster. *Am. Rev. Respir. Dis. 125,* 67.

Ristow, H., Holley, R.W. and Messmer, T.O. (1978) Regulation of growth of fibroblasts. *J. Invest. Dermatol. 71,* 18.

Roden, L. (1980) Structure and metabolism of connective tissue proteoglycans. In: W.J. Lennarz (Ed.), *The Biochemistry of Glycoproteins and Proteoglycans,* Plenum Press, New York, p. 267.

Rosenow, E.C. III (1972) The spectrum of drug-induced pulmonary disease. *Ann. Intern. Med. 77,* 977.

Ross, R. (1968) The fibroblast and wound repair. *Biol. Rev. Biol. Proc. Cambridge Philos. Soc. 43,* 5196.

Ross, R., Glomset, J., Kariya, B. and Harker, L. (1974) A platelet-dependent serum factor that stimulates the proliferation of arterial smooth muscle cells in vitro. *Proc. Natl Acad. Sci. USA 71,* 1207.

Rossi, G.A., Hunninghake, G.W., Szapiel, S.V. and Crystal, R.G. (1981) Pulmonary response to environmental agents and drugs are influenced by immune response and non-immune response genes. *Am. Rev. Respir. Dis. 123,* 144.

Rucker, R.B., Heng-Khoo, C.S., Dubrick, M., Lefevre, M. and Cross, C.E. (1979) Partial characterization of a tropoelastin precursor isolated from chick aorta. *Biochemistry 18,* 3854.

Rutherford, R.B. and Ross, R. (1976) Platelet factors stimulated fibroblasts and smooth muscle cells quiescent in plama-serum to proliferate. *J. Cell Biol. 69,* 196.

Sanberg, L.B. (1976) Elastin structure in health and disease. *Int. Rev. Connect. Tissue Res. 7,* 159.

Scadding, J.B. and Hinson, K.F.W. (1976) Diffuse fibrosing alveolitis correlation of histology at biopsy with prognosis. *Thorax 22,* 291.

Schachter, H. (1978) Glycoprotein biosynthesis. In: M.I. Horowitz and W. Pigman (Eds.), *The Glycoconjugates, Vol. 2,* Academic Press, New York, p. 87.

Schachter, H. and Roseman, S. (1980) Mammalian glycosyltransferases: Their role in the synthesis and function of complex carbohydrates and glycolipids. In: W.J. Lennarz (Ed.) *The Biochemistry of Glycoproteins and Proteoglycans,* Plenum Press, New York, p. 85.

Scherzer, H. and Ward, P.A. (1978) Lung and dermal vascular injury produced by preformed immune complexes. *Am. Rev. Respir. Dis. 117,* 551.

Schmidt, J.A. and Green, L. (1980) Secondary MLR supernatants stimulate fibroblast proliferation. *Fed. Proc. 39,* 1158.

Schwartz, M.I., Matthay, R.A. and Sahn, S.A. (1976) Interstitial lung disease in polymyositis and dermatomyositis: Analysis of six cases and review of the literature. *Medicine 55,* 89.

Seyer, J.M., Hutcheson, E.T. and Kang, A.H. (1976) Collagen polymorphism in idiopathic chronic pulmonary fibrosis. *J. Clin. Invest. 57,* 1498.

Shenker, B.J. Willoughby, W.F. Hollingdale, M.R. and Mann, T.N. (1980) In vivo responses to inhaled proteins. III. Inhibition of experimental immune complex pneumonitis after suppression of peripheral blood lymphocytes. *J. Immunol. 124,* 1763.

Shigematsu, N., Matsuba, K., Shirakusa, T., Sham, L.D. and Tanaka, K. (1980) The preventive effect of urokinase on experimental bleomycin-induced interstitial pneumonia. *Am. Rev. Respir. Dis. 121,* 188.

Siegel, R.C. (1974) Biosynthesis of collagen cross-links: increased activity of purified lysyloxidase with reconstituted collagen fibrils. *Proc. Natl Acad. Sci. USA 71,* 4826.

Siegel, R.C. (1976) Collagen cross-linking, synthesis of collagen cross-links in vitro with highly purified lysyloxidase. *J. Biol. Chem. 251,* 5786.

Sikic, B.I, Yound, D.M., Mimnaugh, E.G. and Gram, T.E. (1978) Quantification of bleomycin pulmonary toxicity in mice by changes in lung hydroxyproline content and morphometric histopathology. *Cancer Res. 38,* 787.

Silbert, J.E. (1973) Biosynthesis of mucopolysaccharides and protein-polysaccharides. In: R. Perez-Tamayo and M. Rojkind (Eds), *Molecular Pathology of Connective Tissues,* Marcel Dekker, New York, p. 323.

Simon, R.H., Scoggin, C.H. and Patterson, D. (1981) Hydrogen peroxide causes the fatal injury to human fibroblasts exposed to oxygen radicals. *J. Biol. Chem. 256,* 7181.

Smith, P. and Heath, D. (1976) Paraquat. *CRC Crit. Rev. Toxicol. 4,* 411.

Smith, L.L. and Rose, M.S. (1977) A comparison of the effect of paraquat and diquat on the water content of rat lung and the incorporation of thymidine into lung DNA. *Toxicology 8,* 223.

Smith, P., Heath, D. and Kay, J.M. (1974) The pathogenesis and structure of paraquat-induced pulmonary fibrosis in rats. *J. Pathol. 114,* 57.

Snider, G.L. (1981) The pathogenesis of emphysema — Twenty years of progress. *Am. Rev. Respir. Dis. 124,* 211.

Snider, G.L. Celli, B.R., Goldstein, R.H. and Hayes, J.A. (1977a) Endotracheal bleomycin in hamsters: a model of chronic interstitial pulmonary fibrosis. *Am. Rev. Respir. Dis. 115,* 245.

Snider, G.L., Sherter, C.B., Kook, W., Karlinsky, J.B., Hayes, J.A. and Franzblau, C. (1977b) Respiratory mechanics in hamsters following treatment with endotracheal elastase or collagenase. *J. Appl. Physiol. 42,* 206.

Solliday, N.H., Williams, J.A., Gaemsler, E.A., Coutu, R.E. and Carrington, C.B. (1973) Familial chronic interstitial pneumonia. *Am. Rev. Respir. Dis. 108,* 193.

Spiro, R.G. (1969) Characterization and quantitative determination of the hydroxylysine-linked carbohydrate units of several collagens. *J. Biol. Chem. 244,* 602.

Spiro, R.G. and Spiro, M.J. (1971) Studies on the biosynthesis of the hydroxylysine-linked disaccharide unit of basement membranes and collagens. III. Tissue and subcellular distribution of glycosyltransferases and the effect of various conditions on the enzyme levels. *J. Biol. Chem. 246,* 4919.

Stacy, B.D. and King, E.J. (1954) Silica and collagen in the lungs of silicotic rats treated with cortisone. *Br. J. Ind. Med. 11,* 192.

Starcher, B.C. (1977) Determination of the elastin content of tissues by measuring desmosine and isodesmosine. *Analyt. Biochem. 79,* 11.

Starcher, B.C., Kuhn, C. and Overton, J.E. (1978) Increased elastin and collagen content in the lungs of hamsters receiving an intratracheal injection of bleomycin. *Am. Rev. Respir. Dis. 117,* 299.

Stoolmiller, A.C. and Dorfman, A. (1969) The biosynthesis of hyaluronic acid by streptococcus. *J. Biol. Chem. 244,* 236.

Stuart, J.M., Postlethwaite, A.E. and Kang, A.H. (1976) Evidence for cell-mediated immunity to collagen in progressive systemic sclerosis. *J. Lab. Clin. Med. 88,* 601.

Sundar, R., Church, C.V., Klobutcher, L.A. and Ruddle, F.H. (1977) Genetics of the connective tissue proteins: assignment of the gene for human type I procollagen to chromosome 17 by analysis of cell hybrids and microcell hybrids. *Proc. Natl Acad. Sci. USA 74,* 444.

Suou, T. and Hirayama, C. (1980) Antibodies to denatured bovine collagens in sera of patients with liver disease. *Clin. Exp. Immunol. 39,* 119.

Swaye, P., Von Ordstrand, H.S., McCormack, J.J. and Wolpow, S.E. (1969) Familial Hamman-Rich syndrome. *Dis. Chest 55,* 7.

Sykes, B. and Solomon, E. (1978) Assignment of a type I collagen structural gene to human chromosome T. *Nature (London) 272,* 548.

Szapiel, S.V., Elson, N.A., Fulmer, J.D., Hunninghake, G.W. and Crystal, R.G. (1979) Bleomycin-induced interstitial pulmonary disease in the nude athymic mouse. *Am. Rev. Respir. Dis. 120,* 893.

Tanzer, M.L. (1973) Cross-linking of collagen. *Science 180,* 561.

Thompson, W.D. and Patrick, R.S. (1978) Collagen prolyl hydroxylase levels in experimental paraquat poisoning. *Br. J. Exp. Pathol. 59,* 288.

Thrall, R.S., McCormick, J.R., Jack, R.M., McReynolds, R.A. and Ward, P.A. (1979a) Bleomycin-induced pulmonary fibrosis in the rat. *Am. J. Pathol. 95,* 117.

Thrall, R.S., McCormick, J.R., Phan, S.H., Jack, R.H. and Ward, P.A. (1979b) The effect of antilymphocyte globulin on the development of bleomycin-induced pulmonary fibrosis in the rat. *Am. Rev. Respir. Dis. 119,* 83.

Thrall, R.S., Lovett, E.J. III, Barton, R.W., McCormick, J.R., Phan, S.H. and Ward, P.A. (1980) The effect of T-cell depletion on the development of bleomycin-induced pulmonary fibrosis in the rat. *Am. Rev. Respir. Dis. 121,* 99.

Thrall, R.S., Phan, S.H., McCormick, J.R. and Ward, P.A. (1981) The development of bleomycin-induced pulmonary fibrosis in neutrophil-depleted and complement-depleted rats. *Am. J. Pathol. 105,* 76.

Thurlbeck, W.M. (1975) Postnatal growth and development of the lung. *Am. Rev. Respir. Dis. 111,* 803.

Timpl, R., Glanville, R.W., Nowack, H., Wiedemann, H., Fietzek, P.P. and Kuhn, K. (1975) Isolation chemical and electron microscopical characterization of neutral salt-soluble type III collagen and procollagen from fetal skin. *Hoppe-Seyler's Z. Physiol. Chem. 356,* 1783.

Trentham, D.E., Dynesins, R.A., Rocklin, R.E. and David, J.R. (1978) Cellular sensitivity to collagen in rheumatoid arthritis. *N. Engl. J. Med. 299,* 327.

Trombley, L., Absher, M. and Kelley, J. (1981) Lung cell population density determines the ratio of type III to type I collagens. *Am. Rev. Respir. Dis. 123,* 694.
Tseleva, I.A. (1974) Collagen biosynthesis in the lungs of rats with radiation injury. *Vopr. Med. Khim. 20,* 640.
Tsukamoto, Y., Helsel, W.E. and Wahl, S.M. (1981) Macrophage production of fibronectin, a chemoattractant for fibroblasts. *J. Immunol. 127,* 673.
Tuderman, L., Kivirikko, K.I. and Prockop, D.J. (1978) Partial purification and characterization of a neutral protease which cleaves the N-terminal propeptides 120 m procollagen. *Biochemistry 17,* 2948.
Turner-Warwick, M. (1973) Immunology of the lower respiratory tract. *Clin. Allergy 3,* 653.
Turner-Warwick, M. (1981) Interstitial pulmonary fibrosis with and without associated "collagen vascular disease". *Am. Rev. Respir. Dis. 123,* 73.
Turner-Warwick, M., Haslam, P. and Weeks, J. (1971) Antibodies in some chronic fibrosing lung diseases. *Clin. Allergy 1,* 209.
Uitto, J., Hoffman, H.P. and Prockop, D.J. (1976) Synthesis of elastin and procollagen by cells from embryonic aorta: differences in the role of hydroxyproline and the effects of proline analogs on the secretion of the two proteins. *Arch. Biochem. Biophys. 173,* 187.
Umezawa, H. (1974) Chemistry and mechanism of action of bleomycin. *Fed. Proc. 33,* 2296.
Urry, D.W., Bhatnagar, R.S, Suzano, H. and Prasad, K.U. (1979) A molecular basis for defective elastic tissue in environmentally induced lung disease. In: R.E. Bhatnagar (Ed.), *The Molecular Basis of Environmental Toxicity,* Ann Arbor Scientific, Ann Arbor, MI.
Valimaki, M., Juva, K., Rantanen, J. and Ekfors, T. (1975) Collagen metabolism in rat lungs during chronic intermittent exposure to oxygen. *Aviat. Space Environ. Med. 46,* 684.
Vasilyeva, G.N. (1971) Soluble collagen and protein carbohydrate component content in the lungs of rats with experimental silicosis. *Vopr. Med. Khim. 17,* 277.
Vudi, A. and Vuust, J. (1980) *Biology of Collagen,* Academic Press, New York.
Wahl, L.M., Wahl, S.M., Mergenhagen, S. and Martin, C.E. (1975) Collagenase production by lymphokine-activated macrophages. *Science 187,* 261.
Wahl, S.M., Wahl, L.M. and McCarthy, J.B. (1978) Lymphocyte mediated activation of fibroblast proliferation and collagen production. *J. Immunol. 121,* 442.
Ward, W.F., Shih-Hoellwarth, A., Port, C.D. and Kim, Y.T. (1979) Modification of radiation-induced pulmonary fibrosis in rats. *Radiology 131,* 751.
Weiss, J.B. (1976) Enzymic degradation of collagen. *Int. Rev. Connect. Tissue Res. 7,* 101.
Weiss, S.J. Yound, J., LoBuglio, A.F., Slivka, A. and Nimeh, N.F. (1981) Role of hydrogen peroxide in neutrophil mediated destruction of cultured endothelial cells. *J. Clin. Invest. 68,* 714.
Wick, G., Brunner, H., Penner, E. and Timpl, R. (1978) The diagnostic application of specific antiprocollagen sera: II Analysis of liver biopsies. *Int. Arch. Allergy Appl. Immunol. 56,* 316.
Wiedermann, H., Chung, E., Fufii, T., Miller, E.J. and Kuhn, K. (1975) Comparative electron microscopic studies on type III and type I collagens. *Eur. J. Biochem. 51,* 363.
Wiestner, M., Krieg, T., Horlein, D., Glanville, R.W., Fietzek, P. and Muller, P.K. (1979) Inhibiting effect of procollagen peptides on collagen biosynthesis in fibroblast cultures. *J. Biol. Chem. 254,* 7016.

Willoughby, J.B. and Willoughby, W.F. (1977) In vivo responses to inhaled proteins. I. Quantitative analysis of antigen uptake, fate and immunogenicity in a rabbit model system. *J. Immunol. 119,* 2137.

Willoughby, W.F., Willoughby, J.B. Cantrell, B.B. and Wheelis, R. (1979) In vivo responses to inhaled proteins. II. Induction of interstitial pneumonitis and enhancement of immune complex-mediated alveolitis by inhaled concanavalin A. *Lab. Invest. 40,* 399.

Witschi, H.R. and Cote, M.G. (1977) Inhibition of butylated hydroxytoluene induced mouse lung cell division by oxygen: time-effect and dose-effect relationships. *Chem. Biol Interact. 19,* 279.

Witschi, H.R. Hascek, W.M., Klein-Szanto, A.J.P. and Hakkinen, P.J. (1981) Potentiation of diffuse lung damage by oxygen: Determining variables. *Am. Rev. Respir. Dis. 123,* 98.

Woolley, D.E., Glanville, R.W., Crossley, M.J. and Evanson, J.M. (1975) Purification of rheumatoid synovial collagenase and its action on soluble and insoluble collagen. *Eur. J. Biochem. 54,* 611.

Woolley D.E., Glanville, R.W., Roberts, D.R. and Evanson J.M. (1978) Purification, characterization and inhibition of human skin collagenase. *Biochem. J. 169,* 265.

Yaron, M., Yaron, I. and Allalouf, D. (1972) Effect of ionizing radiation on hyaluronic acid production by cultured human synovial fibroblasts. *Isr. J. Med. Sci. 8,* 1751.

Zapol, W.M., Trelstad, R.L., Coffey, J.W., Tsai, I. and Salvador, R.A. (1979) Pulmonary fibrosis in severe acute respiratory failure. *Am. Rev. Respir. Dis. 119,* 547.

Ziskind, M., Jones, R.N. and Weill, H. (1976) Silicosis. *Am. Rev. Respir. Dis. 113,* 643.

Zuckerman, J.E., Hollinger, M.A. and Giri, S.N. (1980) Evaluation of antifibrotic drugs in bleomycin-induced pulmonary fibrosis in hamsters. *J. Pharmacol. Exp. Ther. 213,* 425.

CHAPTER 5

Mediation and modulation of immediate hypersensitivity and inflammation by products of the oxygenation of arachidonic acid

DANIEL W. GOLDMAN

and

EDWARD J. GOETZL

Howard Hughes Medical Institute Laboratories at the University of California Medical Center, Department of Medicine, San Francisco, California 94143

5.1. INTRODUCTION

The universal involvement of lipids as mediators of inflammation and hypersensitivity reactions has become increasingly evident over the past decade. In many different types of cells, arachidonic acid is released from membrane phospholipids in response to specific stimuli and is converted by the cyclo-oxygenase pathway to diverse prostaglandins and thromboxanes. The predominant effects of the cyclo-oxygenase products of arachidonic acid in inflammation and hypersensitivity are smooth muscle contraction, altered vascular permeability and tone, and modulation of cellular responsiveness to other stimuli. Arachidonic acid metabolites of the more recently characterized lipoxygenase pathways are also critical mediators of hypersensitivity and inflammation and, in many instances, are 100- to 1000-fold more potent than the cyclo-oxygenase products with respect to a specific activity. Cross-linking by antigen of IgE on the surface of basophils initiates the synthesis and release of several unique peptide-lipid products of the 5-lipoxygenase pathway, termed leukotrienes, which constitute the smooth muscle contractile factor known as the slow-reacting substance of anaphylaxis (SRS-A). In response to inflammatory stimuli, the polymorphonuclear (PMN) and mononuclear leukocytes secrete a series of monohydroxy-eicosa-6,8,11,14-tetraenoic acid (mono-HETE) isomers and several dihydroxy-eicosa-6,8,11,14-tetraenoic acids (di-HETEs), which exhibit chemotactic activity for leukocytes and exert other humoral and cellular activities. The mechanisms of synthesis and release of lipoxygenase products of arachidonic acid, the individual biological activities expressed by the products, and the overall roles of these products in normal host responsiveness and in disease states are all areas currently under investigation. The present review is directed to the biochemical pathways and cellular mechanisms of release and oxygenation of arachidonic acid in relation to hypersensitivity reactions and inflammation. The relevant functions of the products of oxygenation of arachidonic acid will be considered in terms of their roles both as extracellular mediators and as cellular constituents critical to the activation of leukocytes.

5.2. PRODUCTS OF ARACHIDONIC ACID METABOLISM

Unstimulated PMN and mononuclear leukocytes, mast cells, and basophils from several species produce amounts of arachidonic acid metabolites that are only barely detectable by chemical techniques. Addition of exogenous arachidonic acid, calcium ionophores, or stimuli specific for each type of leukocyte greatly enhances the production of oxygenated metabolites of arachidonic acid to the level of nanograms per 10^7 cells (Kuehl and Egan 1980; Smith 1980; Lewis et al. 1981c; Goetzl et al. 1981b, see Fig. 1). The first step in the cyclo-oxygenase pathway is catalyzed by prostaglandin synthetase which forms the two unstable endoperoxides PGG_2 and PGH_2. In rat and human (Lewis et al. 1981c) mast cells these intermediates are converted predominantly to PGD_2, with relatively smaller amounts of other cyclo-oxygenase metabolites. In PMN and mononuclear leukocytes from several species, the predominant cyclo-oxygenase metabolite is PGE_2, with lesser quantities of PGE_1, $PGF_{2\alpha}$, 6-keto $PGF_{1\alpha}$, and thromboxane B_2 (Smith 1980; Morley et al. 1979; Bokoch and Reed 1980; Rouzer et al. 1980; Humes et al. 1977; Goldstein et al. 1978).

The 5-lipoxygenase pathway of arachidonic acid metabolism predominates both on a quantitative and functional basis in neutrophils and eosinophils and, under some conditions, in other types of leukocytes (Samuelsson 1980, 1981). The major initial metabolite of the 5-lipoxygenase pathway in leukocytes is the unstable intermediate 5-hydroperoxy-ETE (5-OOHETE). In most types of leukocytes, 5-OOHETE is converted predominantly to 5-HETE and to lesser quantities of leukotrienes, which are a family of complex 5-HETEs that contain additional polar substituents and three conjugated double bonds. 5-OOHETE first is converted to the highly reactive 5,6-epoxy-eicosa-7,9,11,14-tetraenoic acid (leukotriene A or LTA_4, where the subscript 4 indicates the total number of double bonds in the molecule). LTA_4 is hydrated enzymatically to yield 5(S),12(R)-dihydroxy-6,14-cis-8,10-trans-ETE (LTB_4), which is a potent chemotactic factor for PMN leukocytes (Goetzl and Pickett 1980). Non-enzymatic hydration of LTA_4 yields other stereoisomers of 5,12-di-HETE, which are far less potent chemotactic factors than LTB_4 (Samuelson

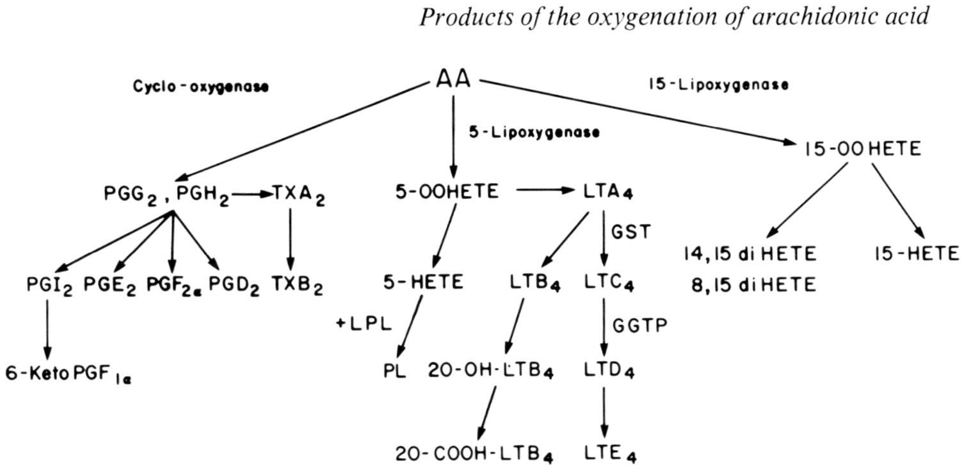

Fig. 1. Cyclo-oxygenase and lipoxygenase products of arachidonic acid produced by leukocytes. AA = arachidonic acid; PGG_2 and PGH_2 = prostaglandin endoperoxides; PG = prostaglandin; TXA_2 and TXB_2 = thromboxanes; -OOHETE = hydroperoxyeicosatetraenoic acid; HETE = hydroxyeicosatetraenoic acid; LPL = lysophospholipid; PL = phospholipid; LTA_4, LTB_4, LTC_4, LTD_4, and LTE_4 = leukotrienes (see text for structural names of each compound); GST = glutathione-S-transferase; and GGTP = γ-glutamyl-transpeptidase.

1981). LTB_4 is further metabolized in stimulated leukocytes to 20-hydroxy-LTB_4 and subsequently to 20-carboxy-LTB_4 (Hansson et al. 1981). In basophils, macrophages, and some other types of leukocytes, glutathione-S-transferase catalyzes the reaction of LTA_4 and glutathione, which generates 5-hydroxy-6-sulfido-glutathionyl-ETE (LTC_4). LTC_4 is metabolized by γ-glutamyl-transpeptidase to 5-hydroxy-6-sulfido-cysteinyl-glycinyl-ETE (LTD_4) and subsequently is degraded to 5-hydroxy-6-sulfido-cysteine-ETE (LTE_4). LTC_4, LTD_4 and LTE_4 are the major constituents of the smooth muscle contractile factor of immediate-type hypersensitivity reactions, designated the slow-reacting substance of anaphylaxis (SRS-A) (Samuelsson 1981).

Several other products of the lipoxygenation of arachidonic acid have been identified in leukocytes. Human PMN leukocytes and T-lymphocytes generate 15-OOHETE, which is reduced to 15-HETE. Four isomers of 8,15-di-HETE and two isomers of 14,15-di-HETE have been identified in PMN leukocytes, in addition to the 15-HETE product (Goetzl 1981; Maas et al. 1981; Jubiz et al. 1981; Lundberg et al. 1981). There has been no evidence for a glutathionyl adduct of 15-OOHETE. The 15-di-HETE isomers have not as yet been tested for biological activity. 15-HETE appears to play an important role as an endogenous inhibitor of lipoxygenation in PMN leukocytes (Vanderhoek et al. 1980a), T-lymphocytes (Goetzl 1981), and platelets (Vanderhoek et al. 1980b). Several other mono-HETE isomers are produced by human PMN leukocytes (Goetz and Sun 1980), while 12-HETE is the primary lipoxygenase product of platelets (Kuehl and Egan 1980).

5.3. CONTROL OF ARACHIDONIC ACID RELEASE AND METABOLISM

A variety of inflammatory stimuli initiate the release and rapid oxygenation of arachidonic acid. Considerable evidence suggests that the rate of metabolism of arachidonic acid by oxidative pathways is controlled primarily by the rate of release of arachidonic acid from phospholipids. The events which initiate the release of arachidonic acid may be unique for each type of cell, but three general pathways of phospholipid metabolism in leukocytes have been implicated in the release of arachidonic acid (Fig. 2).

The primary mechanism for the release of arachidonic acid in PMN leukocytes and mast cells is the degradation of phospholipids by phospholipase A_2 (PLA_2) (Hirata and Axelrod 1980; Hirata et al. 1979). PLA_2 hydrolyzes phospholipids almost exclusively at the 2-position and generates equimolar quantities of free unsaturated fatty acids and lysophospholipids. The results of studies with leukocytes that were preincubated with radiolabeled arachidonic acid prior to stimulation indicate that phosphatidylcholine (PC) is the principal source of the arachidonic acid released by PLA_2. Two other major phospholipid classes, phosphatidylethanolamine

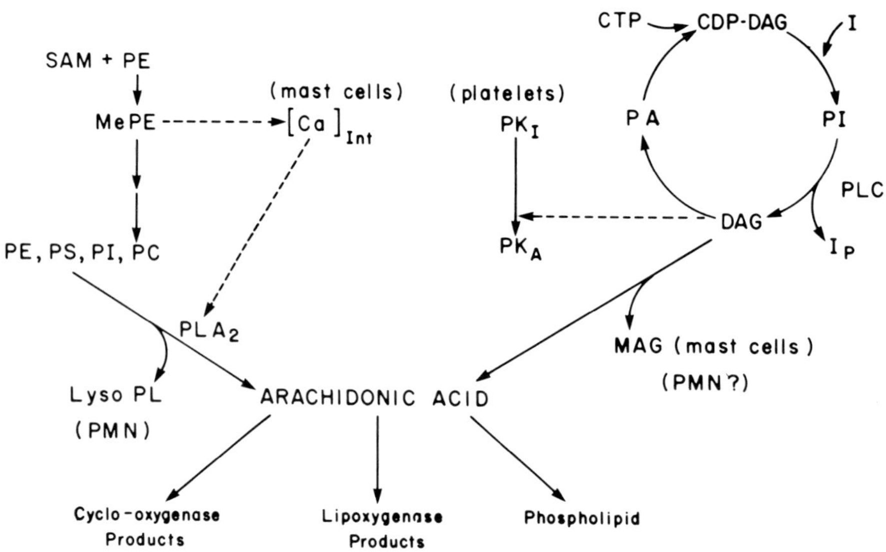

Fig. 2. Phospholipid metabolic pathways involved in the mobilization of arachidonic acid. PE = phosphatidylethanolamine; PS = phosphatidylserine; PI = phosphatidylinositol; PC = phosphatidylcholine; SAM = S-adenosylmethionine; MePE = monomethyl PE; PLA_2 = phospholipase A_2; LysoPL = lysophospholipid; PLC = phospholipase C; DAG = diacylglycerol; MAG = monoacylglycerol; PA = phosphatidic acid; CTP = cytidine triphosphate; CDP-DAG = cytidine diphosphate diacylglycerol; I = inositol; I_p = phosphorylinositol and PK_I and PK_A = protein kinase; --➤ = stimulation or enhancement.

(PE) and phosphatidylserine (PS) contribute lesser amounts of arachidonic acid, depending on the type of leukocyte and the experimental conditions. Phosphatidylinositol (PI), the fourth major phospholipid class, donates free arachidonic acid at a significantly enhanced rate during the stimulation of leukocytes, which may reflect greater activity of either PLA_2 or a PI-specific pathway (Goetzl et al. 1981c; Bonser et al. 1981; Walsh et al. 1981a; Rubin et al. 1981a). Several lines of evidence implicate PLA_2 as the predominant pathway for arachidonic acid release. Firstly, inhibitors of PLA_2 activity in leukocytes inhibit concomitantly the release of arachidonic acid (Hirata et al. 1979). Further, the levels of lysoPC, a product of PLA_2 activity, were found to be elevated at the time of increased arachidonic acid release in rabbit PMN leukocytes (Hirata et al. 1979). In addition, the rate of release of arachidonic acid varies inversely with the activity of an endogenous PLA_2 inhibitory protein of 30,000 to 40,000 m.w., termed lipomodulin (Hirata et al. 1980; Hirata 1981). When the expression of lipomodulin is increased in PMN leukocytes by treatment with corticosteroids, a parallel decrease in arachidonic acid release is observed (Hirata et al. 1980). Similarly, the release of arachidonic acid by PMN leukocytes stimulated with chemotactic factors is associated temporally with the phosphorylation of lipomodulin and its conversion to a form which does not inhibit PLA_2. (Hirata 1981).

Marked increases in the rates of release and re-incorporation of arachidonic acid into PI were noted in several studies of leukocyte phospholipid metabolism (Goetzl et al. 1981c; Walsh et al. 1981a; Rubin et al. 1981a). PI metabolism in other systems is characterized by a specific cycle of degradation and synthesis that is initiated by the action of a PI-specific phospholipase C (Michell 1975). The diacylglycerol (DAG) generated by this enzyme then is hydrolyzed by a diacylglycerol A_2 lipase, which releases arachidonic acid. PI is considered to be a significant source of arachidonic acid, as mammalian PI is highly enriched in arachidonic acid at the 2-position. The rapid phosphorylation of excess DAG to phosphatidic acid (PA) is followed by the conversion of PA to cytidine diphosphate diacylglycerol, which then is restored to PI (Michell 1975).

It is difficult to assess to what extent PI serves as a source of arachidonic acid in leukocytes responding to natural challenges. Stimulation of PMN leukocytes from several species with formyl-methionyl peptides or with calcium ionophore A23187 leads to significant increases in the rate of turnover of arachidonic acid and of the phosphate head group (Goetzl et al. 1981c; Walsh et al. 1981a; Rubin et al. 1981a, b; Tou 1978; Cockcroft et al. 1980). A transient increase in the content of radiolabeled arachidonic acid in PA also has been observed in horse PMN leukocytes stimulated by A23187 (Lapetina et al. 1980). However, such approaches were unable to differentiate between a net release of arachidonic acid and an increased rate of turnover of PI. In rat mast cells, the increased rate of turnover of the phosphate head group of PI and PA evoked by the cross-linking of IgE receptors or by A23187 correlated closely in time with the release of histamine (Kennerly et al. 1979). Significantly, the increases in the total amount of DAG and of DAG-containing arachidonic acid also were detected during histamine release. The presence of significant DAG lipase activity in mast cell homogenates was shown by the release of free fatty acids from DAG, which consequently suggested a role for PI as a source of free arachidonic acid (Sullivan 1981).

The increased metabolism of PI in stimulated leukocytes may activate biochemical pathways other than the metabolism of arachidonic acid. Products of PI metabolism appear to be involved in the modulation of the intracellular concentration of calcium in non-leukocytic cell types by altering membrane permeability to calcium. PA may act as a calcium ionophore, whereas DAG can regulate the expression of protein kinase activity in platelets and thus provides a potential mechanism for altering the activity of a wide range of enzymes, including those which control membrane permeability to calcium (Putney 1981). In PMN leukocytes, the increase in PI metabolism stimulated by chemotactic factors does not appear to be a prerequisite for enhancing membrane permeability to calcium. Inhibition of calcium influx also inhibits chemotactic factor stimulation of PI metabolism, which suggests that increased calcium influx is a prerequisite for the stimulation of PI metabolism (Cockcroft et al. 1980).

The sequential methylation of PE by S-adenosyl methionine (SAM)-dependent methyltransferases to form PC also has been implicated in the release of arachidonic acid in rabbit PMN leukocytes (Hirata et al. 1979). Formyl-methionyl peptides enhanced the rate of degradation of PC formed by methylation of PE, but had no effect on PC synthesized from exogenously added choline. The time course of formyl-methionyl peptide-induced degradation of the PC formed by methylation of PE closely paralleled the time course of enhancement of release of arachidonic acid, which suggested that methylated PE is the preferred PL source of arachidonic acid (Hirata et al. 1979). Inhibition of the pathway for methylation of PE in mononuclear leukocytes and rat mast cells results in the suppression of chemotaxis and histamine release, respectively (Hirata and Axelrod 1980; Pike et al. 1979), which suggests that the rate of methylation of PE is crucial to the activation of some leukocyte functions. In rat mast cells, increases in the rate of methylation of PE appear to be part of a sequence of biochemical events which couples perturbation of the IgE receptor to increased calcium influx. It is the resulting increase in the concentration of intracellular calcium which presumably initiates the release of arachidonic acid (Hirata and Axelrod 1980). Methylated PE may not be the principal source of free arachidonic acid in mast cells, as it is in PMN leukocytes. Although the link between PE methylation and the release of arachidonic acid has not yet been defined in mononuclear leukocytes, some data imply that PE methylation may be a prerequisite for alteration in the biophysical properties of the plasma membrane adjacent to occupied chemotactic factor receptors (Pike and Snyderman 1981).

While many mechanisms that may contribute to the release of arachidonic acid from phospholipids have been elucidated, little is known about the modulation of the re-acylation pathway or of the oxygenase pathways. The major fate of exogenous arachidonic acid added to PMN leukocytes from several species is acylation into phospholipids. Inhibition of the acylation pathway could play a major role in the enhancement of the net release of arachidonic acid and subsequent oxygenation. Studies of macrophages (Kroner et al. 1981) and PMN leukocytes (Lapetina et al. 1980) show that stimulation of cells with A23187 inhibits the acylation of exogenously added arachidonic acid into most classes of phospholipids. Analyses of the lipoxygenation of arachidonic acid indicate that increases in calcium influx stimulate the rate of lipoxygenation even when excess exogenous arachidonic acid is provided to maintain a high level of free arachidonic acid (Goetzl et al. 1981b; Lapetina et al. 1980; Borgeat and Samuelsson 1979). These studies imply that calcium acts not only to increase the rate of release of arachidonic, but also to direct arachidonic acid away from the reacylation pathway and into the lipoxygenation pathway. That SRS-A synthesis in homogenates of rat leukemic basophils was stimulated significantly by 2 mM calcium (Jakschik and Lee 1980), supports the possibility that the lipoxygenase pathway is regulated by intracellular levels of calcium.

5.4. PHARMACOLOGIC MODULATION OF ARACHIDONIC ACID METABOLISM

Diverse endogenous principles and pharmacologic agents modulate the release and oxygenation of arachidonic acid (Fig. 3). Agents which inhibit arachidonic acid release, and consequently the synthesis of both the cyclo-oxygenase and lipoxygenase products of arachidonic acid, appear to act primarily by blocking PLA_2 activity. Indomethacin, more commonly known for its effects on cyclo-oxygenase activity, acts directly on PLA_2 to inhibit arachidonic acid release in rabbit PMN leukocytes (Kaplan et al. 1978). The glucocorticoids induce the synthesis of the protein lipomodulin, which inhibits PLA_2 activity (Hirata et al. 1980). Some patients with rheumatoid arthritis have an autoantibody against lipomodulin but the pathogenic significance of this finding is uncertain (Hirata et al. 1981).

Neither the natural nor the pharmacologic modulators of arachidonic acid oxygenation are perfectly specific for the lipoxygenase or the cyclo-oxygenase pathways. Some show a certain degree of specificity, depending on the concentrations tested and on the target cell or tissue. Vitamin E enhances the production of 5-HETE and LTB_4 by human neutrophils at physiological concentrations in vitro (Goetzl 1980a), but its effects on the cyclo-oxygenase pathway are controversial. At higher concentrations vitamin E inhibits the activity of both the cyclo-oxygenase and lipoxygenase pathways (Goetzl et al. 1981b). At concentrations higher than those found normally in blood and most tissues, vitamin C stimulates cyclo-oxygenase activity in fibroblasts and platelets and, in the latter cells, favors the synthesis of $PGF_{2\alpha}$ as compared to other prostaglandins (Nugteren 1975). Recently, a factor of m.w. 18,000 has been isolated from explant cultures of rheumatoid synovial cell tissue and shown to stimulate PGE_2 and PGI_2 synthesis in

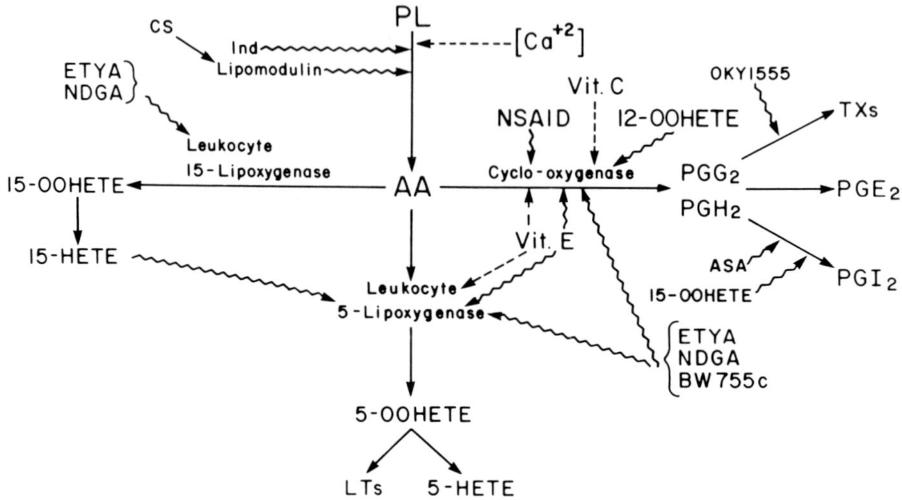

Fig. 3. Pharmacologic modulation of arachidonic acid metabolism. Ind = indomethacin; vit. = vitamin; NSAID = non-steroidal anti-inflammatory drugs; ASA = aspirin, ETYA = 5,8,11,14-eicosatetraynoic acid; NDGA = nordihydroguaiaretic acid; CS = corticosteroid, ⟶ = release or generation; ---▶ = enhancement; ⁓▶ = inhibition; other abbreviations as in the text and previous figures.

synovial cells (Robinson et al. 1981). This protein acts selectively to increase cyclo-oxygenase activity, without an increase in phospholipase activity. Of the pharmacological agents, the non-steroidal anti-inflammatory drugs block cyclo-oxygenase activity in numerous cell types and may also inhibit the conversion of 12-OOHETE to 12-HETE in platelets (Siegel et al. 1980a) and of 5-OOHETE to 5-HETE in PMN leukocytes (Siegel et al. 1980b). ETYA, NDGA and BW755C suppress the activity of the lipoxygenase and cyclo-oxygenase pathways, with different potencies for each pathway in different types of cells. Benoxaprofen inhibited the lipoxygenase pathway of macrophages that were exposed to the calcium ionophore A23187, without affecting the cyclo-oxygenase pathway. However, no inhibition of the lipoxygenase pathway was observed in macrophages that had been stimulated by C5a or f-Met-Leu-Phe (Walker and Dawson 1979). The vast differences in the susceptibility of the cyclo-oxygenases and lipoxygenases from different cell types to inhibition by pharmacologic agents imply that selective control of the oxygenation of arachidonic acid at localized sites may be possible.

Some of the products of arachidonic acid can act as feedback modulators of enzymatic oxygenation. The hydroperoxy-metabolites are the most active in this regard. 12-OOHETE in platelets enhances lipoxygenation of arachidonic acid to 12-OOHETE, while concurrently inhibiting the cyclo-oxygenase pathway (Siegel et al.

1979). 15-OOHETE modulates the distribution of the products of the cyclo-oxygenase pathway by the inactivation of platelet prostacyclin synthetase, but not thromboxane A_2 synthetase (Ham et al. 1979). 15-HETE from several sources blocks the lipoxygenase activity of platelets (Vanderhoek et al. 1980b), PMN leukocytes (Vanderhoek et al. 1980a), and lymphocytes (Goetzl 1981).

5.5. LIPID MEDIATORS IN HYPERSENSITIVITY

Presentation of antigen systemically to sensitized individuals initiates a chain of events in the blood and tissues, which culminates in an immediate hypersensitivity or anaphylactic reaction. This reaction consists of rapidly induced bronchoconstriction, vasodilatation, and increased vasopermeability, followed by the infiltration of leukocytes, with a predominance of eosinophils, and on some occasions tissue destruction. The leukotrienes LTC_4, LTD_4 and LTE_4, which comprise SRS-A, are primary lipid mediators of the anaphylactic response. SRS-A mediates many of the same humoral activities as histamine, but with far greater potency and a characteristically slower rate of contraction and relaxation of bronchial and other smooth muscles. Products of the cyclo-oxygenase pathway of arachidonic acid metabolism also mediate some of the humoral effects observed in hypersensitivity reactions, but their principal contributions may be in the modulation of responses to the leukotrienes (Table 1).

SRS-A is synthesized and released from purified preparations of basophils, mononuclear leukocytes, and lung tissue in response to challenge by immunological stimuli, as well as calcium ionophores (Austen et al. 1974; Lewis and Austen 1981; Lewis et al. 1979, 1981a). Unlike histamine, ECF-A and other preformed granule-associated mediators, SRS-A can only be extracted from lung tissue after immunologic challenge (Brocklehurst 1960). SRS-A synthesis in human lung fragments or enzymatically dispersed parenchymal cells is initiated simultaneously with histamine release, but SRS-A release from the cell does not begin until histamine release is almost complete (Austen et al. 1974). Three lines of evidence suggest that the generation of SRS-A and prostaglandins occurs in more than one type of cell in lung tissue. Firstly, lung tissue releases LTC_4, LTD_4, $PGF_{2\alpha}$, PGE_2, and PGD_2, during pulmonary anaphylaxis (Lewis and Austen 1981; Lewis et al. 1979), whereas purified mast cells challenged by similar IgE-dependent mechanisms generate predominantly PGD_2 and far lesser amounts of other prostaglandins and lipoxygenase products (Lewis et al. 1981a, c). Significantly, the amount of LTC_4 and LTD_4 produced by enzymatically dispersed human lung cells decreases as the preparation becomes more highly enriched in mast cells (Lewis et al. 1981a). Secondly, both SRS-A and histamine evoke prostaglandin release in some lung models, suggesting that at least a part of the prostaglandins produced during anaphylaxis is a secondary response to the SRS-A and histamine released initially (Yen et al. 1976; Mathe et al. 1977). Thirdly, SRS-A synthesis in human lung tissue

TABLE 1.
Humoral effects of the products of oxygenation of arachidonic acid

Constriction of pulmonary airways		Microvascular permeability		Microvascular tone	
		Increase	Decrease	Increase	Decrease
TXA_2		PGD_2	PGF_2 (slight)	TXA_2	PGD_2
PGD_2	small large	PGI_2		$PGF_{2\alpha}$	PGI_2
$PGF_{2\alpha}$		PGE_2		LTC_4	PGE_2
		LTC_4 (slight)			LTB_4
LTB_4	small only low potency	LTD_4			LTD_4
LTC_4		LTE_4			LTE_4
LTD_4	small > large				
LTE_4					

PGD_2, PGF_2 , PGE_2, PGI_2, = prostaglandins; TXA_2 = thromboxane A_2; LTB_4, LTC_4, LTD_4, LTE_4 = leukotrienes (for structural names, see Section 5.2).

and isolated lung cells is biphasic, including an initial phase that begins with histamine release and a second phase, which starts 10 minutes later, after histamine release is completed (Austen et al. 1974). Pulmonary interstitial mononuclear cells that have been stimulated by mediators of the first phase may be an important source of the SRS-A observed in the second phase (Lewis and Austen 1981).

The structural studies establishing that SRS-A is a mixture of LTC_4, LTD_4, and LDE_2 were only recently completed, largely because of the difficulties associated with purifying sufficient quantities. Early work demonstrated that SRS-A is an acidic, highly polar lipid derived from arachidonic acid (Lewis and Austen 1981). SRS-A appeared to be synthesized by the lipoxygenase pathway because inhibitors of the cyclo-oxygenase and lipoxygenase pathways, but not the cyclo-oxygenase pathway alone, blocked the incorporation of radiolabeled arachidonic acid into SRS-A (Bach et al. 1979). Similarities between the UV absorption spectra of 5,12-di-HETE and the UV absorption spectra previously determined for SRS-A implied that 5,12-di-HETE and SRS-A both contain three conjugated double bonds. Chemical analyses established initially that LTC_4 and LTD_4 are the functionally critical components of SRS-A generated by rat leukemic basophils stimulated with calcium ionophore. That LTC_4 and LTD_4 account for the activity of SRS-A was proven, and the stereochemistry of the molecules confirmed, by total synthesis of the component mediators. Subsequent studies demonstrated that 5-OOHETE and LTA_4 are biosynthetic precursors of LTC_4, and that the SRS-A from rat mononuclear leukocytes and human lung is a mixture of three leukotrienes: LTC_4, LTD_4, and LTE_4 (Samuelsson 1981; Lewis and Austen 1981).

Purified and synthetic LTC_4, LTD_4, and other peptide-containing leukotrienes are potent mediators of smooth muscle contraction. Leukotrienes contract guinea pig ileum and other smooth muscles with the characteristically slow onset and relaxation times which serve to differentiate "slow-reacting" substances from histamine, bradykinin, $PGF_{2\alpha}$ and some other contractile factors. Dose–response studies have shown that LTD_4 is 5–20 times more potent than LTC_4 and LTE_4 and approximately 50–500 times more potent than histamine in contracting the smooth muscle of guinea pig ileum (Lewis et al. 1979; Drazen et al. 1980). Studies of the contractile potency of a series of synthetic analogs of LTC_4 with respect to guinea pig ileal smooth muscle established that the location of the glutathionyl peptide at the 6-position of the hydrocarbon chain is critical for activity and that the length and hydrophobicity of the C7 to C20 portion of LTC_4 is far more important than the actual conformational state of the double bonds in determining potency (Drazen et al. 1981).

The important role that SRS-A plays in the homeostatic regulation and disease-associated abnormalities of airway tone was suggested by in vivo and in vitro studies of the responses of guinea pig lung. The intravenous administration of partially purified SRS-A (Drazen and Austen 1974) and synthetic leukotrienes (Drazen et al. 1980) resulted in a marked decrease in the dynamic compliance of peripheral airways in unanesthetized guinea pigs while smaller decreases occurred in the conductance of the large central airways. In contrast, the ratio of the decrease in pulmonary compliance to the decrease in airway conductance was significantly smaller and of shorter duration for histamine than for SRS-A, indicating a greater activity of histamine on large airways (Drazen and Austen 1974). These in vivo results have been borne out by in vitro studies on the effects of SRS-A, the leukotrienes and histamine in the contraction of parenchymal strips of guinea pig lung, a model for small airways, and the constriction of guinea pig trachea, a model for large airways (Lewis et al. 1979, 1980, 1981b; Drazen et al. 1979, 1980). LTC_4 and LTD_4 are approximately 200-fold and 20,000-fold more potent than histamine, respectively, in contracting parenchymal strips of guinea pig lung (Drazen et al. 1980). LTB_4 exhibited a potency 1/10,000 to 1/1000 that of LTD_4 in the same assay system (Lewis et al. 1981b). Synthetic analogs of LTC_4 demonstrated the same structural requirements for activity in the guinea pig lung parenchymal strips as in the guinea pig ileal assay (Drazen and Austen 1974; Drazen et al. 1981). LTC_4 and LTD_4 were 30- to 100-fold more potent than histamine in constricting segments of guinea pig trachea, which confirmed the generally greater effect of leukotrienes on small airways than on large airways (Drazen et al. 1980). LTB_4 had no effect on tracheal segments at concentrations as high as 2×10^{-8} mol l^{-1} (Lewis et al. 1981b).

SRS-A and the purified leukotrienes also alter vascular tone and vasopermeability. LTD_4 was slightly more potent than LTC_4 and SRS-A in evoking a transient decrease in arterial blood pressure, when intravenously administered to unanesthetized guinea pigs (Drazen et al. 1980). Native SRS-A, synthetic LTD_4, LTE_4 and, to a lesser extent, LTC_4 similarly alter the permeability of the cutaneous microvasculature in guinea pigs and some other animals, which results in the leakage of intravascular fluid and proteins into the tissue (Drazen et al. 1980; Lewis et al. 1981b). LTE_4 and LTD_4 are each 100 times more potent than histamine in inducing an increase in vasopermeability in guinea pig skin (Drazen and Austen 1974; Drazen et al. 1980). While the decrease in arterial blood pressure induced in unanesthetized guinea pigs by LTD_4 and LTC_4 implies that these mediators may dilate arterioles as well as other blood vessels, current data from studies in guinea pigs, monkeys, and humans are consistent with constriction of small cutaneous vessels by LTC_4 and dilatation by LTD_4 (Drazen et al. 1980; Lewis et al. 1981b). LTB_4 is a weaker vasodilator than LTD_4 (Lewis et al. 1981b).

The major role of cyclo-oxygenase products in hypersensitivity reactions is a modulatory one, although certain prostaglandins directly mediate humoral effects. In the pulmonary airways, different prostaglandins exert opposing influences, but the bronchoconstrictor activities of $PGF_{2\alpha}$, PGD_2, and thromboxane A_2 appear to prevail over the bronchodilatory actions of PGE_2 (Moncada and Vane 1979). However, these prostaglandins are considerably less potent than the leukotrienes. In the unanesthetized guinea pig, $PGF_{2\alpha}$ was 1/100–1/1000 as active as histamine, LTC_4, LTE_4 or LTD_4 in decreasing dynamic compliance (Lewis et al. 1980). PGE_2, PGD_2, and PGI_2 alone did not elicit significant edema in several experimental models, but were capable of significantly augmenting the plasma exudation and increase in blood flow elicited by bradykinin and histamine (Davidson et al. 1978; Williams 1979). Similarly, the administration of $PGE_{2\alpha}$ along with LTD_4 synergistically enhanced the increase in cutaneous microvascular permeability achieved by LTD_4 alone in guinea pigs, rats, and rabbits (Bray et al. 1981). At the cellular level, certain prostaglandins can increase cyclic nucleotide levels in mast cells, which in turn inhibits the release of histamine and the generation and release of SRS-A. PGE_1 and PGI_2 increase cyclic AMP levels in mast cells, which results in the inhibition of histamine release in vitro, while $PGF_{2\alpha}$, which increases cyclic GMP levels, can enhance histamine release. Pretreatment of human lung with PGE_1 and $PGF_{2\alpha}$ suppressed and enhanced, respectively, the subsequent generation of SRS-A. In the rat peritoneal cavity and guinea pig lung tissue, pretreatment with PGI_2 suppressed SRS-A generation (Lewis and Austen 1981).

5.6. LIPID MEDIATORS OF THE CELLULAR ELEMENTS OF HYPERSENSITIVITY AND INFLAMMATION

The discovery that aspirin and other non-steroidal anti-inflammatory drugs, such as indomethacin, are effective inhibitors of the cyclo-oxygenation of arachidonic acid increased interest in the role of prostaglandins in inflammatory reactions. The more recent appreciation that leukocytes metabolize arachidonic acid by lipoxygenase pathways and that PMN leukocytes respond chemotactically to LTB_4 and mono-HETEs has led to studies of the contributions of these products to inflammation. Preliminary evidence supports the concept that LTB_4 and 5-HETE are primary mediators that can attract leukocytes to sites of inflammation in vivo, and that prostaglandins enhance leukocyte infiltration primarily through vasodilatation and enhancement of vasopermeability which augment the local availability of the leukocytes.

The chemotactically most potent lipid mediators of inflammation are derived from the 5-lipoxygenation of arachidonic acid. Peptide chemotactic factors such as formyl-methionyl peptides and C5a stimulate a 2- to 3-fold increase in the intracellular content of 5-HETE and LTB_4 in human PMN leukocytes, rabbit leukocytes, and human eosinophils by 5 minutes, with maximal release attained by 15 to 30 minutes (Goetzl et al. 1980; Goetzl 1980b). Phagocytic stimuli also enhance the release from PMN leukocytes of 5-HETE and LTB_4 (Walsh et al. 1981c; Ford-Hutchinson 1981). Human PMN leukocytes also release minor amounts of PGE_2, TXB_2, LTC_4, and LTD_4 (Smith 1980; Henderson et al. 1981). Monocytes and macrophages release PGE_2 and thromboxanes (Morley et al. 1979; Rouzer et al. 1980; Humes et al. 1977), in addition to lipoxygenase products (Bach et al. 1979; Doig and Ford-Hutchinson 1980; Valone et al. 1980), during the phagocytosis of particles opsonized with IgG and components of complement. Mononuclear cells produce greater amounts of arachidonic acid metabolites than PMN leukocytes, but peak levels are not achieved for up to 2–4 hours (Valone et al. 1980).

The results of investigations of the leukocyte-directed activities of the lipoxygenase products of arachidonic acid in vitro demonstrated that mono-HETEs stimulate the chemotaxis of human eosinophils and neutrophils, but not mononuclear leukocytes, in modified Boyden micropore filter chambers (Goetzl and Sun 1979; Goetzl et al. 1977). The maximal responses elicited by the mono-HETEs are similar in magnitude to those evoked by peptide chemotactic factors, such as C5a and synthetic formyl-methionyl peptides. A rank order of potency is manifested in the series of mono-HETEs, such that 5-HETE $>>$ 8-HETE $=$ 9-HETE $>$ 11-HETE $=$ 12-HETE, while 15-HETE had no chemotactic activity (Samuelsson 1980; Goetzl et al. 1980a). Of the other stable lipoxygenase products which have been purified, LTB_4 is by far the most potent lipid chemotactic factor for human PMN leukocytes, while tri-hydroxy-eicosatetraenoic acids from platelets, LTC_4 and LTD_4 are inactive (Goetzl and Pickett 1980; Goetzl et al. 1981c). The chemotactic activity of LTB is detectable in some in vitro systems at a concentration of 10^{-9} mol l^{-1} and is maximal at 2 x 10^{-8} mol l^{-1} to 10^{-7} mol l^{-1}, which defines a potency that is similar to that of C5a and some of the synthetic formyl-methionyl peptide chemotactic factors (Goetzl and Pickett 1980; Ford-Hutchinson et al. 1980; Palmer et al. 1980). The free hydroxyl groups and the conjugated double bonds of LTB_4 appear to be critical determinants of the chemotactic potency of LTB_4. The PMN leukocyte chemotactic potency of LTB_4 is decreased 4- to 10-fold by acetylation of the free hydroxyl

TABLE 2.
Comparison of the PMN leukocyte-directed activity of LTB_4 and N-formyl-Met-Leu-Phe (fMLP)

Function	LTB_4*	fMLP*
Chemokinesis**	++	+
Chemotaxis	++	++
Enzyme release	+	++
Chemotactic deactivation***	+	++
Adherence	++	++
Aggregation	++	++
Early biochemical events (hexose uptake, Ca^{2+} permeability, cyclic nucleotides)	++	++
Oxidative metabolism	±	++

* ++ = maximal activation; + = submaximal activation; ± = borderline effect.
** LTB_4 stimulates a greater chemokinetic response than does fMLP. Also, the concentration of LTB_4 for maximal chemokinesis is half of that required for maximal chemotaxis whereas the concentration of fMLP for maximal chemokinesis is the same as that required for maximal chemotaxis.
*** Higher concentrations of LTB_4 are required to achieve deactivation compared to fMLP.

groups and 30- to 300-fold by changes in the double-bond geometry, as found in several natural di-HETE isomers, such as 5(S),12(R)-dihydroxy-eicosa-6,8,10-(all-trans)-14(cis)-tetraenoic acid, which lacks a 6-cis-double bond (Goetzl and Pickett 1981).

The mono-HETEs and LTB_4 differ significantly from the peptide chemotactic factors in that they selectively modify only a few activities of neutrophils and eosinophils in contrast to the broad range of functions modified by C5a and the formyl-methionyl peptides (Table 2). The HETEs stimulate neutrophil and eosinophil chemokinesis in the absence of a concentration gradient and at concentrations that are lower than those required to evoke an optimal chemotactic response (Goetzl and Pickett 1980; Goetzl et al. 1980a). The HETEs at the same low concentrations also increase the intracellular level of cyclic GMP to a maximal value within one minute and for up to 20 minutes (Goetzl et al. 1980b). Both 5-HETE and LTB_4 activate metabolic pathways which also are activated by the peptide chemotactic factors and which may be a part of the biochemical sequence of activation of leukocyte functions. In human neutrophils (Bass et al. 1982) and eosinophils (Bass et al. 1981), 5-HETE and LTB_4 stimulate hexose uptake stereospecifically. In rabbit and human PMN leukocytes, LTB_4 stimulates both the intracellular mobilization of calcium and the increase in plasma membrane permeability that leads to enhanced calcium influx (Naccache et al. 1981). The expression of C3b receptors on human neutrophils and eosinophils in vitro is also enhanced by LTB_4 and 5-HETE with lesser increases in the expression of IgG-Fc receptors, as assessed by rosetting techniques (Goetzl et al. 1980a). PGE_2, which stimulates the expression of erythrocyte receptors on human T-lymphocytes (Venza-Teti et al. 1980), had no effect on the PMN leukocyte receptors. None of the mono-HETEs or leukotrienes modify PMN leukocyte oxidative metabolism to the same extent as peptide chemotactic factors (Goetzl and Pickett 1980; Goetzl et al. 1980a). LTB_4 and mono-HETEs do enhance to a certain extent the release of lysosomal enzymes in the presence or absence of cytochalasin B, but degranulation evoked by peptide chemotactic factors is significantly greater than that evoked by chemotactically equivalent concentrations of LTB_4 and mono-HETEs (Goetzl and Pickett 1980; Goetzl et al. 1980a). The selective stimulation of PMN leukocyte functions by lipoxygenase products of arachidonic acid compared to the more global stimulation elicited by peptide chemotactic factors may reflect differences in the structure, number, or cellular distribution of the receptors committed selectively to each of the classes of factors.

Unlike the peptide chemotactic factors C5a and formyl-methionyl peptides, the lipoxygenase products of arachidonic acid are synthesized by stimulated PMN leukocytes and a role for these products as functional intracellular constituents has been proposed. Inhibitors selective for the lipoxygenase pathways suppress PMN leukocyte migration, hexose transport, aggregation and lysosomal enzyme release. In certain instances, the addition of exogenous 5-HETE can restore function (Goetzl 1980b; Goetzl et al. 1980c; Walsh et al. 1981b). While the mechanism of the lipoxygenase dependence of some PMN leukocyte functions has not been identified, two distinct possibilities have been proposed. Human PMN leukocytes reincorporate into cellular phospholipids a variable fraction of the 5-HETE generated, which would alter the properties of the plasma membrane, possibly at specific sites of prior deacylation (Stenson and Parker 1979). Alternatively, the reactive intermediates, such as 5-OOHETE and LTA_4, can covalently derivatize intracellular peptides, proteins, and other constituents critical to cell function, some of which have been recovered by chromatographic procedures from specifically stimulated cells (Goldman and Goetzl 1981).

Certain features of the interactions of LTB_4 and 5-HETE with human PMN leukocytes suggest that these lipids bind to specific receptor sites on the cell. Small changes in the chemical structure of LTB_4 produce significant decrements in chemotactic potency (Goetzl and Pickett 1981), implying that LTB_4 interacts in a stereospecific manner with PMN leukocytes. Similarly, the ability of the methyl esters of mono-HETEs, which lack chemotactic activity, to suppress selectively the chemotactic response of PMN leukocytes to mono-HETEs in vitro argues for a receptor-mediated interaction between the mono-HETEs and PMN leukocytes (Goetzl et al. 1979a). Considerable similarities between stimulus-specific deactivation by LTB_4 and 5-HETE and by the peptide chemotactic factors also suggest that PMN leukocytes may express specific receptors for LTB_4 and 5-HETE. Preincubation of leukocytes with fully chemotactic concentrations of LTB_4 or 5-

HETE significantly reduces the chemotactic response of these cells to the same factor present during the preincubation period, but not to the other lipid factor or to peptide chemotactic factors (Goetzl et al. 1981a). A study of the mechanisms of "stimulus-specific deactivation" toward formyl-methionyl peptides demonstrated that the decrease in chemotactic responsiveness correlated temporally with the decrease in the number of receptor binding sites expressed on the cell surface (Vitkauskas et al. 1980). This suggests that stimulus-specific deactivation towards LTB_4 and 5-HETE also may be due to the loss of cell surface receptors specific for each of these lipids. Preincubation of PMN leukocytes with 5-OOHETE reduced the subsequent chemotactic response towards both lipid and peptide chemotactic factors, implying that the presence of a reactive hydroperoxy-substituent inhibits chemotaxis by a non-receptor mediated mechanism (Goetzl et al 1981a). Specific LTB_4 receptors have been demonstrated recently by the binding of ^3H-LTB_4 to human PMN leukocytes. Human PMN leukocytes bound ^3H-LTB_4 in a time-dependent, reversible and saturable manner at 4°C. The Scatchard plot of binding data was a straight line with a dissociation constant between $1.0-2.0 \times 10^{-8}$ mol l^{-1} and 20,000−40,000 binding sites per PMN leukocyte. These binding sites probably mediate the functional effects of LTB_4 on PMN leukocytes because the dissociation constant for LTB_4 binding closely correlates with the concentration of LTB_4 which elicits either a half-maximal chemotactic response ($3-9 \times 10^{-9}$ mol l^{-1}) or a half-maximal increase in adherence ($3-9 \times 10^{-9}$ mol l^{-1}) (Goldman and Goetzl 1982).

Lipoxygenase products of arachidonic acid also serve as chemotactic factors in vivo. Microgram quantities of 12-HETE (Goetzl et al. 1979a), a fraction of 1 μg of 5-HETE, and 10−30 ng of LTB_4 (Ford-Hutchinson 1981) elicit a rapid accumulation of eosinophils and a later influx of neutrophils in the guinea pig peritoneal cavity. Similarly, a fraction of 1 μg of LTB_4 led to the rapid accumulation of PMN leukocytes in the eyes and skin of rabbits (Ford-Hutchinson 1981). In rhesus monkey and human skin, 500 ng of natural or synthetic LTB_4 led to maximal infiltration of PMN leukocytes within 4 hours (Lewis et al. 1981b). Application of LTB_4 in skin chambers to skin abrasions on the human forearm resulted in similar accumulations of PMN leukocytes (Ford-Hutchinson 1981). The infiltration of PMN leukocytes in monkey and human skin stimulated by LTB_4 is accelerated and augmented by the presence of the vasodilating agent PGD_2 (Lewis et al. 1981b). The vasodilator PGE_2 has a similar effect on LTB_4-induced PMN leukocyte infiltration in rabbit, rat and guinea pig skin (Bray et al. 1981). The enhancement of vasopermeability by LTB_4 may result from an interaction between accumulating PMN leukocytes and the vascular endothelial cells, since similar effects are observed with the peptide chemotactic factors C5a and f-Met-Leu-Phe (Wedmore and Williams 1981), the increase in vasopermeability exactly parallels the increase in PMN leukocyte accumulation (Ford-Hutchinson 1981; Issekutz 1981), and the effect is not observed in neutropenic subjects (Issekutz 1981).

The ability of LTB_4 and mono-HETEs to stimulate PMN leukocyte chemotaxis in vitro strongly implies a role for these lipoxygenase products of arachidonic acid as mediators of inflammation in vivo. Elevated levels of mono-HETEs have been detected in psoriatic skin lesions (Hammarstrom et al. 1975). Patients with rheumatoid arthritis or spondyloarthritis showed increased levels of LTB_4 in synovial fluid, while 5-HETE also was elevated in rheumatoid synovial tissue (Klickstein et al. 1980). Although the presence of elevated levels of lipoxygenase products of arachidonic acid in inflammation lesions suggests that these products may contribute to the inflammatory response, proof that these products contribute significantly is lacking due to the paucity of non-toxic inhibitors specific for the lipoxygenase pathway. Indomethacin, which blocks the cyclo-oxygenase pathway specifically, effectively reduces the erythema, edema, and hyperalgesia associated with inflammation, but has little effect on the leukocyte influx. This is in contrast to inhibitors of both pathways of oxidative metabolism of arachidonic acid, where the leukocyte influx as well as the humoral effects are inhibited significantly (Higgs et al. 1980).

The important role that the cyclo-oxygenase products of arachidonic acid play in homeostasis and inflammation have been reviewed recently (Kuehl and Egan 1980; Moncada and Vane 1979; Trang 1980). That prostaglandins may be involved in inflammatory reactions was first appreciated when the anti-inflammatory drugs aspirin and indomethacin were shown to inhibit prostaglandin synthesis (Kuehl and Egan 1980). This observation has led to the demonstration that inflammatory states are associated with increased levels of cyclo-oxygenase products of arachidonic acid, both in animal models and in some human diseases (Kuehl and Egan 1980; Trang 1980; Robinson et al. 1979). For example, the concentrations of PGE_2, $PGF_{2\alpha}$ and arachidonic acid, as well as HETEs, were highly significantly increased in human psoriatic lesions as compared to uninvolved skin of the same patients (Hammarstrom et al. 1975). Concurrent studies indicated that the synovial fluid of patients with rheumatoid arthritis contains higher concentrations of PGE_2, and, to a lesser extent, $PGF_{2\alpha}$ and thromboxane B_2 than synovial fluid of subjects with non-inflammatory arthropathies (Robinson et al. 1979). The role of PGE_2 in rheumatoid arthritis is further supported by the observation that explants of synovial tissues and cultures of adherent synovial cells from patients with rheumatoid arthritis produce greater quantities of PGE_2 and some other cyclo-oxygenase products in vitro than comparable tissues and cells from subjects with non-rheumatoid arthropathies (Robinson et al. 1979).

Intracutaneous injection of various cyclo-oxygenase products of arachidonic acid evoke the inflammatory symptoms of erythema, edema, and pain (Table 1). Different prostaglandins will cause either vasodilatation or vasoconstriction, depending on the system (Trang 1980). The vasodilatory action of PGE_2 was established when intracutaneous administration in animals and humans was shown to result in erythema, termed the flare response, and pruritus. PGFs were inactive in these systems (Horton 1963; Kaley and Weiner 1971). PGE_2, PGD_2 and PGI_2 significantly enhance the edema evoked by histamine and bradykinin, although they have little effect alone (Davidson et al. 1978; Williams 1979). None of the prostaglandins alone appear to account for the intense pain characteristic of inflammatory reactions. PGI_2 and PGE_2 evoke moderate pain and enhance the capacity of other mediators to induce hyperalgesia and tenderness to pressure (Trang 1980). PGE_2 is less potent than PGI_2, but PGI_2 sustains the painful response for a longer interval (Ferreira and Nakamura 1979). Both thromboxane A_2 and $PGF_{2\alpha}$ increase microvascular tone in some systems, but none of these effects are comparable in magnitude to the decrease in microvascular tone evoked by PGE_2, PGI_2 and PGD_2 (Moncada and Vane 1979). PGE_2 also stimulates bone resorption by synoviocytes and the secretion of collagenase by macrophages, and inhibits the production of proteoglycans by synoviocytes and articular chondrocytes (Fahey et al. 1977; Lippiello et al. 1978). Such activities of prostaglandins together contribute to the extensive tissue damage seen in chronically inflamed joints of patients with rheumatoid arthritis.

The cyclo-oxygenase-derived metabolites of arachidonic acid do not directly activate PMN leukocyte functions, but they can significantly modulate PMN leukocyte responses to other inflammatory stimuli. Non-directed migration of human neutrophils and eosinophils, a phenomenon termed chemokinesis, is enhanced by PGD_2, PGI_2, and, with a lower potency, PGE_2 (Goetzl et al. 1979b). The same prostaglandins fail to stimulate PMN leukocyte degranulation, but do inhibit the release of lysosomal enzymes in response to chemotactic factors and other defined stimuli (Weissmann et al. 1980). The effects of prostaglandins on PMN leukocyte migration and degranulation appear to parallel the effects of PGE_2, PGD_2, and PGI_2 on the intracellular concentrations of cyclic AMP. PGI_2 also inhibits the adherence of human PMN leukocytes to nylon fibers, endothelial cells and other surfaces in vitro (Boxer et al. 1980), while thromboxane A_2 (Spagnulo et al. 1980) enhances adherence.

5.7. CONCLUSIONS

Cyclo-oxygenase and lipoxygenase products of arachidonic acid have been identified which are potent mediators of the humoral and cellular components of allergic and inflammatory reactions. Leukotrienes C, D and E, which are cysteine or cysteine-peptide adducts of 5-hydroperoxyeicosatetraenoic acid, respresent the principal constituents of SRS-A. These factors are 100- to 10,000 times more potent than histamine in constricting peripheral pulmonary airways and altering vascular tone and permeability. LTB_4 and 5-HETE are potent chemotactic factors for neutrophils and eosinophils. The cyclo-oxygenase products of arachidonic acid exert their effects primarily on the humoral component of hypersensitivity and inflammation, in addition to modulating the leukocytic, chemotactic, vascular, and non-vascular smooth muscle responses to the leukotrienes. While many endogenous principles and pharmacological agents regulate the mobilization and oxygenation of arachidonic acid, the present range of drugs are not specific enough in their inhibitory effects to permit an understanding of the precise role of individual products in pathological reactions. However, the presence of elevated levels of arachidonic acid metabolites in tissues and fluids of patients with hypersensitivity reactions or arthritis supports the contention that such products may act as primary mediators of some components of hypersensitivity and inflammation.

ACKNOWLEDGMENT

Dr. Goldman is the recipient of a postdoctoral fellowship from the Arthritis Foundation.

REFERENCES

Austen, K.F., Lewis, R.A., Stechschulte, D.J., Wasserman, S.I., Leid Jr R.W. and Goetzl, E.J. (1974) Generation and release of chemical mediators of immediate hypersensitivity. In: L. Brent and J. Holborow (Eds), *Progress in Immunology II, Vol. 2,* North-Holland Publishing Co., New York, pp. 61–71.

Bach, M.K. Brashler, J.R., Brooks, C.D. and Neerken, J.A. (1979) Slow-reacting substance: comparison of some properties of human lung SRS-A and two distinct fractions from ionophore-induced rat mononuclear cell SRS. *J. Immunol. 122*, 160–165.

Bass, D.A., Szedja, P., Goetzl, E.J., Love, S., O'Flaherty, J.T. and McCall, C.E. (1981) Stimulation of hexose uptake by human eosinophils with chemotactic factors. *J. Infect. Dis. 143*, 719–725.

Bass, D.A., O'Flaherty, J.T., Goetzl, E.J., DeChatelet, L.R. and McCall, C.E. (1981). Arachidonic acid and hexose transport in human polymorphonuclear leukocytes. *Prog. Lipid Res. 20,* 735–737.

Bokoch, G.M. and Reed, P.W. (1980) Stimulation of arachidonic acid metabolism in the polymorphonuclear leukocyte by an N-formylated peptide: comparison with ionophore A23187. *J. Biol. Chem. 255,* 10223–10226.

Bonser, R.W., Siegel, M.I., Chung, S.M., McConnell, R.T. and Cuatrecasas, P. (1981) Esterification of an endogenously synthesized lipoxygenase product into granulocyte cellular lipids. *Biochemistry 20*, 5297–5301.

Borgeat, P. and Samuelsson (1979) Arachidonic acid metabolism in polymorphonuclear leukocytes: Effects of ionophore A23187. *Proc. Natl Acad. Sci. USA 76,* 2148–2152.

Boxer, L.A., Allen, J.M., Schmidt, M., Yoder, M. and Baehner, R.L. (1980) Inhibition of polymorphonuclear leukocyte adherence by prostacyclin. *J. Lab. Clin. Med. 95,* 672–678.

Bray, M.A., Cunningham, F.M., Ford-Hutchinson, A.W. and Smith, M.J.H. (1981) Leukotriene B_4: a mediator of vascular permeability. *Br. J. Pharmacol. 72,* 483–486.

Brocklehurst, W.E. (1960) The release of histamine and the formation of a slow-reacting substance (SRS-A) during anaphylactic shock. *J. Physiol. (London) 151,* 416–435.

Cockcroft, S., Bennett, J.P. and Gomperts, B.D. (1980) f-MetLeuPhe-induced phosphatidylinositol turnover in rabbit neutrophils is dependent on extracellular calcium. *FEBS Lett. 110,* 115–118.

Davidson, E.M., Ford-Hutchinson, A.W., Smith, M.J.H. and Walker, J.R. (1978) Prostacyclin (PGI_2): a potential mediator of inflammation. *Br. J. Pharmacol. 64,* 437P.

Doig, M.V. and Ford-Hutchinson, A.W. (1980) The production and characterization of products of the lipoxygenase enzyme system released by rat peritoneal macrophages. *Prostaglandins 20,* 1007–1019.

Drazen, J.M. and Austen, K.F. (1974) Effects of intravenous administration of slow-reacting substance of anaphylaxis, histamine, bradykinin, and prostaglandin $F_{2\alpha}$ on pulmonary mechanics in the guinea pig. *J. Clin. Invest. 53,* 1679–1685.

Drazen, J.M., Lewis, R.A., Wasserman, S.I., Orange, R.P. and Austen, K.F. (1979) Differential effects of a partially purified preparation of slow-reacting substance of anaphylaxis on guinea pig tracheal spirals and parenchymal strips. *J. Clin. Invest. 63,* 1–5.

Drazen, J.M., Austen, K.F., Lewis, R.A., Clark, D.A., Goto, G., Marfat, A.M. and Corey, E.J. (1980) Comparative airway and vascular activities of leukotrienes C-1 and D in vivo and in vitro. *Proc. Natl Acad. Sci. USA 77,* 4354–4358.

Drazen, J.M., Lewis, R.A., Austen, K.F., Toda, M., Brion, F., Marfat, A. and Corey, E.J. (1981) Contractile activities of structural analogs of leukotrienes C and D: necessity of a hydrophobic region. *Proc. Natl Acad. Sci. USA 78,* 3195–3198.

Fahey, J.V., Ciosek, C.P. and Newcombe, D.S. (1977) Human synovial fibroblasts: the relationship between cyclic AMP, bradykinin and prostaglandins. *Agents Actions 7,* 255–264.

Ferreira, S.H. and Nakamura, M. (1979) I-Prostaglandin hyperalgesia, a cAMP/Ca^{2+} dependent process. *Prostaglandins 18,* 179–190.

Ford-Hutchinson, A.W. (1981) Leukotriene B_4 and neutrophil function: A review. *J. R. Soc. Med. 74,* 831–833.

Ford-Hutchinson, A.W., Bray, M.A., Doig, M.V., Shipley, M.E. and Smith, M.J.H. (1980) Leukotriene B_4, a potent chemotactic and aggregating substance released from polymorphonuclear leukocytes. *Nature (London) 286,* 264–265.

Goetzl, E.J. (1980a) Vitamin E modulates the lipoxygenation of arachidonic acid in leukocytes. *Nature (London) 288,* 183–185.

Goetzl, E.J. (1980b) A role for endogenous mono-hydroxy-eicosatetraenoic acids (HETEs) in the regulation of human neutrophil migration. *Immunology 40,* 709–726.

Goetzl, E.J. (1981) Selective feed-back inhibition of the 5-lipoxygenation of arachidonic acid in human T-lymphocytes. *Biochem. Biophys. Res. Commun. 101,* 344–350.

Goetzl, E.J. and Pickett, W.C. (1980) The human PMN leukocyte chemotactic activity of complex hydroxy-eicosatetraenoic acids (HETEs). *J. Immunol. 125,* 1789–1791.

Goetzl, E.J. and Pickett, W.C. (1981) Novel structural determinants of the human neutrophil chemotactic activity of leukotriene B. *J. Exp. Med. 153,* 482–487.

Goetzl, E.J. and Sun, F.F. (1979) Generation of unique mono-hydroxy-eicosatetraenoic acids from arachidonic acid by human neutrophils. *J. Exp. Med. 150,* 406–411.

Goetzl, E.J., Woods, J.M. and Gorman, R.R. (1977) Stimulation of human eosinophil and neutrophil polymorphonuclear leukocyte chemotaxis and random migration by 12-L-hydroxy-5,8,10,14-eicosatetraenoic acid (HETE). *J. Clin. Invest. 59,* 179–183.

Goetzl, E.J., Valone, F.H., Reinhold, V.N. and Gorman, R.R. (1979a) Specific inhibition of the PMN leukocyte chemotactic response to hydroxy-fatty acid metabolites of arachidonic acid by methyl ester derivatives. *J. Clin. Invest. 63,* 1181–1186.

Goetzl, E.J., Weller, P.F. and Valone, F.H. (1979b) Biochemical and functional basis of the regulatory and protective roles of the human eosinophil. In: G. Weissmann, B. Samuelsson and R. Paoletti (Eds), *Advances in Inflammation Research, Vol. 14,* Raven Press, New York, pp. 157–167.

Goetzl, E.J., Brash, A.R., Tauber, A.I., Oates, J.A. and Hubbard, W.C. (1980a) Modulation of human neutrophil function by monohydroxyeicosatetraenoic acids. *Immunology 39,* 491–501.

Goetzl, E.J., Hill, H.R. and Gorman, R.R. (1980b) Unique aspects of the modulation of human neutrophil function by 12-L-hydroperoxy-5,8,10,14-eicosatetraenoic acid. *Prostaglandins 19,* 71–85.

Goetzl, E.J., Weller, P.F. and Sun, F.F. (1980c) The regulation of human eosinophil function by endogenous mono-hydroxy-eicosatetraenoic acids (HETEs). *J. Immunol. 124,* 926–933.

Goetzl, E.J., Boeynaems, J.M., Oates, J.A. and Hubbard, W.C. (1981a) Stimulus-specificity of the chemotactic deactivation of human neutrophils by lipoxygenase products of arachidonic acid. *Prostaglandins 22,* 279–288.

Goetzl, E.J., Derian, C.K., Owens, C.J. and Valone, F.H. (1981b) Modulation of the PMN leukocyte component of hypersensitivity reaction by lipoxygenase products of arachidonic acid. In: J. Hadden, L. Chedid, P. Mullen and F. Spreafico (Eds), *Advances in Immunopharmacology,* Pergamon Press, New York, pp. 343–353.

Goetzl, E.J., Goldman, D.W. and Valone, F.H. (1981c) Lipid mediators of leukocyte function in immediate-type hypersensitivity reactions. In: E.L. Becker, A.S. Simon and K.F. Austen (Eds), *Biochemistry of the Acute Allergic Reaction, Fourth International Symposium,* Alan R. Liss, Inc., New York, pp. 169–182.

Goldman, D.W. and Goetzl, E.J. (1981) Novel metabolites of arachidonic acid (AA) in human neutrophils (N). *Fed. Proc. 40,* 1004a.

Goldman, D.W. and Goetzl, E.J. (1982) Characterization of a receptor on human neutrophils for the chemotactic mediator 5,12-di-hydroxy-6,14 cis-8,10-trans-eicosatetraenoic acid (leukotriene B_4). *J. Immunol. 129,* 1600–1604.

Goldstein, I.M., Malmsten, C.L., Kindahl, H., Kaplan, H.B., Radmark, O., Samuelsson, B. and Weissmann, G. (1978) Thromboxane generation by human peripheral blood polymorphonuclear leukocytes. *J. Exp. Med. 148,* 787–792.

Ham, E.A., Egan, R.W., Soderman, D.D., Gale, P.H. and Kuehl Jr, F.A. (1979) Peroxidase-dependent deactivation of prostacyclin synthetase. *J. Biol. Chem. 254,* 2191–2194.

Hammarstrom, S., Hamberg, M., Samuelsson, B., Duell, E.A., Stawiski, M. and Voorhees, J.J. (1975) Increased concentrations of nonesterified arachidonic acid, 12-L-hydroxy-5,8,10,14-eicosatetraenoic acid, prostaglandin E, and prostaglandin $F_{2\alpha}$ in epidermis of psoriasis. *Proc. Natl Acad. Sci. USA 72,* 5130–5134.

Hansson, G., Lindgren, J.A., Dahlen, S., Hedqvist, P. and Samuelsson, B. (1981) Identification and biological activity of novel ω-oxidized metabolites of leukotriene B_4 from human leukocytes. *FEBS Lett. 130,* 107–112.

Henderson, W.R., Joerg, A. and Klebanoff, S.J. (1981) Slow-reacting substance generation by eosinophils and its inactivation by peroxidase. *Clin. Res. 29,* 491A.

Higgs, G.A., Eakins, K.E., Mugridge, K.G., Moncada, S. and Vane, J.R. (1980) The effects of non-steroid anti-inflammatory drugs on leukocyte migration in carrageenin-induced inflammation. *Eur. J. Pharmacol. 66,* 81–86.

Hirata, F. (1981) The regulation of lipomodulin, a phospholipase inhibitory protein, in rabbit neutrophils by phosphorylation. *J. Biol. Chem. 256,* 7730–7733.

Hirata, F. and Axelrod, J. (1980) Phospholipid methylation and biological signal transmission. *Science 209,* 1082–1090.

Hirata, F., Corcoran, B.A., Venkatasubramanian, K., Schiffmann, E. and Axelrod, J. (1979) Chemoattractants stimulate degradation of methylated phospholipids and release of arachidonic acid in rabbit leukocytes. *Proc. Natl Acad. Sci. USA 76,* 2640–2643.

Hirata, F., Schiffmann, E., Venkatasubramanian, K., Salomon, D. and Axelrod, J. (1980) A phospholipase A_2 inhibitory protein in rabbit neutrophils induced by glucocorticoids. *Proc. Natl Acad. Sci. USA 77,* 2533–2536.

Hirata, F., Del Carmine, R., Nelson, C.A., Axelrod, J., Schiffmann, E., Warabi, A., DeBlas, A.L., Nirenberg, M., Manganiello, V., Vaughan, M., Kumegi, S., Green, I., Decker, J.L. and Steinberg, A.D. (1981) Presence of autoantibody for phospholipase inhibitory protein, lipomodulin, in patients with rheumatic diseases. *Proc. Natl Acad. Sci. USA 78,* 3190–3194.

Horton, E.W. (1963) Action of prostaglandin E_1 on tissues which respond to bradykinin. *Nature (London) 200,* 892–893.

Humes, J.L., Bonney, R.J., Pelus, L., Dahlgren, M.E., Sadowski, S.L., Kuehl Jr. F.A. and Davies, P. (1977) Macrophages synthesize and release prostaglandins in response to inflammatory stimuli. *Nature (London) 269,* 149–151.

Issekutz, A.C. (1981) Vascular responses during acute neutrophilic inflammation: their relationship to in vivo neutrophilic emigration. *Lab. Invest. 45,* 435–441.

Jakschik, B.A. and Lee, L.H. (1980) Enzymatic assembly of slow reacting substance. *Nature (London) 287,* 51–52.

Jubiz, W., Radmark, O., Lindgren, J.A., Malmsten, C. and Samuelsson, B. (1981) Novel leukotrienes: products formed by initial oxygenation of arachidonic acid at C-15. *Biochem. Biophys. Res. Commun. 99,* 976–986.

Kaley, G. and Weiner, R. (1971) Prostaglandin E_1: a potential mediator of the inflammatory response. *Ann. NY Acad. Sci. 180,* 338–350.

Kaplan, L., Weiss, J. and Elsbach, P. (1978) Low concentrations of indomethacin inhibit phospholipase A_2 of rabbit polymorphonuclear leukocytes. *Proc. Natl Acad. Sci. USA 75,* 2955–2958.

Kennerly, D.A., Sullivan, T.J. and Parker, C.W. (1979) Activation of phospholipid metabolism during mediator release from stimulated rat mast cells. *J. Immunol. 122,* 152–159.

Klickstein, L.B., Shapleigh, C. and Goetzl, E.J. (1980) Lipoxygenation of arachidonic acid as a source of polymorphonuclear leukocyte chemotactic factors in synovial fluid and tissue in rheumatoid arthritis and spondyloarthritis. *J. Clin. Invest. 66,* 1166–1170.

Kroner, E.E., Peskar, B.A., Fischer, H. and Ferber, E. (1981) Control of arachidonic acid accumulation in bone marrow-derived macrophages by acyltransferases. *J. Biol. Chem. 256,* 3690–3697.

Kuehl Jr, F.A. and Egan, R.W. (1980) Prostaglandins, arachidonic acid and inflammation. *Science 210,* 978–984.

Lapetina, E.G., Billah, M.M. and Cuatrecasas, P. (1980) Rapid acylation and deacylation of arachidonic acid into phosphatidic acid of horse neutrophils. *J. Biol. Chem. 225,* 10966–10970.

Lewis, R.A. and Austen, K.F. (1981) Mediation of local homeostasis and inflammation by leukotrienes and other mast cell-dependent compounds. *Nature (London) 293,* 103–108.

Lewis, R.A., Austen, K.F., Drazen, J.M., Clark, D.A., Marfat, A.M. and Corey, E.J. (1979) Slow reacting substances of anaphylaxis: identification of leukotrienes C-1 and D from human and rat sources. *Proc. Natl Acad. Sci. USA 77,* 3710–3714.

Lewis, R.A., Drazen, J.M., Austen, K.F., Clark, D.A. and Corey, E.J. (1980) Identification of the C(6)-S-conjugate of leukotriene A with cysteine as a naturally occurring slow reacting substance of anaphylaxis (SRS-A). Importance of the 11-cis-geometry for biological activity. *Biochem. Biophys. Res. Commun. 96,* 271–277.

Lewis, R.A., Drazen, J.M., Corey, E.J. and Austen, K.F. (1981a) Structural and functional characteristics of the leukotriene components of slow reacting substance of anaphylaxis (SRS-A). In: P.J. Piper (Ed.), *SRS-A and the Leukotrienes,* Wiley, London, pp. 101–117.

Lewis, R.A., Goetzl, E.J., Soter, N.A., Corey, E.J. and Austen, K.F. (1981b) Leukotriene (LT) B_4: stereochemical dependence of chemotactic and spasmogenic activities. *Fed. Proc. 40,* 791a.

Lewis, R.A., Holgate, S.T., Roberts II, L.J., Oates, J.A. and Austen, K.F. (1981c) Preferential generation of prostaglandin D_2 in rat and human mast cells. In: E.L. Becker, A.S. Simon and K.F. Austen (Eds), *Biochemistry of the Acute Allergic Reaction, Fourth International Symposium,* Alan R. Liss, Inc., New York, pp. 239–354.

Lippiello, L., Yamamoto, K., Robinson, D. and Mankin, H.J. (1978) Involvement of prostaglandins from rheumatoid synovium in inhibition of articular cartilage metabolism. *Arthritis Rheum. 21,* 909–917.

Lundberg, U., Radmark, O., Malmsten, C. and Samuelsson, B. (1981) Transformation of 15-hydroperoxy-5,9,11,13-eicosatetraenoic acid into novel leukotrienes. *FEBS Lett. 126,* 127–132.

Maas, R.L., Brash, A.R. and Oates, J.A. (1981) A second pathway of leukotriene biosynthesis in porcine leukocytes. *Proc. Natl Acad. Sci. USA 78,* 5523–5527.

Mathe, A.A., Strandberg, K. and Yen, S.-S. (1977) Prostaglandin release by slow-reacting substance from guinea pig and human lung tissue. *Prostaglandins 14,* 1105–1115.

Michell, R.H. (1975) Inositol phospholipids and cell surface receptor function. *Biochim. Biophys. Acta 415,* 81–147.

Moncada, S. and Vane, J.R. (1979) Pharmacology and endogenous roles of prostaglandin endoperoxides, thromboxane A_2 and prostacyclin. *Pharmacol. Rev. 30,* 293–331.

Morley, J., Bray, M.A., Jones, R.W., Nugteren, D.H. and Van Dorp, D.A. (1979) Prostaglandin and thromboxane production by human and guinea-pig macrophages and leukocytes. *Prostaglandins 17,* 729–736.

Naccache, P.H., Sha'afi, R.I., Borgeat, P. and Goetzl, E.J. (1981) Mono- and di-hydroxyeicosatetraenoic acids alter calcium homeostasis in rabbit neutrophils. *J. Clin. Invest. 67,* 1584–1587.

Nugteren, H. (1975) Arachidonic lipoxygenase in blood platelets. *Biochim. Biophys. Acta 380,* 299–307.

Palmer, R.M.J., Stepney, R.J., Higgs, G.A. and Eakins, K.E. (1980) Chemokinetic activity of arachidonic acid lipoxygenase products on leukocytes of different species. *Prostaglandins 20,* 411−418.

Pike, M.C. and Snyderman, R. (1981) Alterations of new methylated phospholipid synthesis in the plasma membranes of macrophages exposed to chemoattractants. *J. Cell Biol. 91,* 221−226.

Pike, M.C., Kredich, N.M. and Snyderman, R. (1979) Phospholipid methylation in macrophages is inhibited by chemotactic factors. *Proc. Natl Acad. Sci. USA 76,* 2922−2926.

Putney Jr, J.W. (1981) Recent hypotheses regarding the phosphatidylinositol effect. *Life Sci. 29,* 1183−1194.

Robinson, D.R., Dayer, J.-M. and Krane, S.M. (1979) Prostaglandins and their regulation in rheumatoid inflammation. *Ann. NY Acad. Sci. 332,* 279−294.

Robinson, D.R., Bastian, D., Hamer, R.J., Pichiarallo, D. and Stephenson, M.L. (1981) Mechanism of stimulation of prostaglandin synthesis by a factor from rheumatoid synovial tissue. *Proc. Natl Acad. Sci. USA 78,* 5160−5164.

Rouzer, C.A., Scott, W.A., Kempe, J. and Cohn, Z.A. (1980) Prostaglandin synthesis by macrophages requires a specific receptor-ligand interaction. *Proc. Natl Acad. Sci. USA 77,* 4279−4282.

Rubin, R.P., Sink, L.E. and Freer, R.J. (1981a) Activation of (arachidonyl) phosphatidylinositol turnover in rabbit neutrophils by the calcium ionophore A23187. *Biochem. J. 194,* 497−505.

Rubin, R.P., Sink, L.E. and Freer, R.J. (1981b) On the relationship between formylmethionyl-leucyl-phenylalanine stimulation of arachidonyl phosphatidylinositol turnover and lysosomal enzyme secretion by rabbit neutrophils. *Mol. Pharmacol. 19,* 31−37.

Samuelsson, B. (1980) The leukotrienes: a new group of biologically active compounds including SRS-A. *Trends Pharmacol. Sci. 1,* 227−230.

Samuelsson, B. (1980) Oxidative products of arachidonate: leukotrienes, a new group of compounds including SRS-A. In: E.L. Becker, A.S. Simon and K.F. Austen (Eds), *Biochemistry of the Acute Allergic Reaction, Fourth International Symposium,* Alan R. Liss, Inc., New York, pp. 1−12.

Siegel, M.I., McConnell, R.T., Abrahams, S.L., Porter, N.A. and Cuatrecasas, P. (1979) Regulation of arachidonate metabolism via lipoxygenase and cyclo-oxygenase by 12-HPETE, the product of human platelet lipoxygenase. *Biochem. Biophys. Res. Commun. 89,* 1273−1280.

Siegel, M.I., McConnell, R.T., Porter, N.A. and Cuatrecasas, P. (1980a) Arachidonate metabolism via lipoxygenase and 12-L-hydroperoxy-5,8,10,14-eicosatetraenoic acid peroxidase sensitive to anti-inflammatory drugs. *Proc. Natl Acad. Sci. USA 77,* 308−312.

Siegel, M.I., McConnell, R.T., Porter, N.A., Selph, J.L., Turax, J.F., Vinegar, R. and Cuatrecasas, P. (1980b) Aspirin-like drugs inhibit arachidonic acid metabolism via lipoxygenase and cyclo-oxygenase in rat neutrophils from carrageenan pleural exudates. *Biochem. Biophys. Res. Commun. 92,* 688−695.

Smith, M.J.H. (1980) Prostaglandins and the polymorphonuclear leukocyte. In: A.W. Ford-Hutchinson and K.D. Rainsford (Eds), *Prostaglandins and Inflammation,* Birkhauser Verlag, Basel, pp. 91−103.

Spagnulo, P.J., Ellner, J.J., Hassid, A. and Dunn, M.J. (1980) Thromboxane A_2 mediates augmented polymorphonuclear leukocyte adhesiveness. *J. Clin. Invest. 66,* 406–414.

Stenson, W.F. and Parker, C.W. (1979) Metabolism of arachidonic acid in ionophore stimulated neutrophils. *J. Clin. Invest. 64,* 1457–1465.

Sullivan, T.J. (1981) Diacylglycerol metabolism and the release of mediators from mast cells. In: E.L. Becker, A.S. Simon and K.F. Austen, (Eds), *Biochemistry of the Acute Allergic Reaction, Fourth International Symposium,* Alan R. Liss, Inc., New York, pp. 229–238.

Tou, J. (1978) Modulation of ^{32}Pi incorporation into phospholipids of polymorphonuclear leukocytes by ionophore A23187. *Biochim. Biophys. Acta 531,* 167–178.

Trang, L.E. (1980) Prostaglandins and inflammation. *Semin. Arthritis Rheum. 9,* 153–190.

Valone, F.H., Franklin, M., Sun, F.F. and Goetzl, E.J. (1980) Alveolar macrophage lipoxygenase products of arachidonic acid. Isolation and recognition as the predominant constituents of the neutrophil chemotactic activity elaborated by alveolar macrophages. *Cell. Immunol. 54,* 390–401.

Vanderhoek, J.Y., Bryant, R.W. and Bailey, J.M. (1980a) Inhibition of leukotriene biosynthesis by the leukocyte product 15-hydroxy-5,8,11,13-eicosatetraenoic acid. *J. Biol. Chem. 255,* 10064–10065.

Vanderhoek, J.K., Bryant, R.W. and Bailey, J.M. (1980b) 15-hydroxy-5,8,11,13-eicosatetraenoic acid: a potent and selective inhibitor of platelet lipoxygenase. *J. Biol. Chem. 255,* 5996–5998.

Venza-Teti, D., Misefari, A., Sofo, V., Fimiani, V. and LaVia, M.F. (1980) Interaction between prostaglandin and human T lymphocytes: effect of PGE_2 on E-receptor expression. *Immunopharmacology 2,* 165–171.

Vitkauskas, G., Showell, H.J. and Becker, E.L. (1980) Specific binding of synthetic chemotactic peptides to rabbit peritoneal neutrophils: effects on dissociability of bound peptide, receptor activity and subsequent biologic responsiveness (deactivation). *Mol. Immunol. 17,* 171–180.

Walker, J.R. and Dawson, W. (1979) Inhibition of rabbit PMN lipoxygenase activity by benoxaprofen. *J. Pharm. Pharmacol. 31,* 778–780.

Walsh, C.E., DeChatelet, L.R., Thomas, M.J., O'Flaherty, J.T. and Waite, M. (1981a) Effect of phagocytosis and ionophores on release and metabolism of arachidonic acid from human neutrophils. *Lipids 16,* 120–127.

Walsh, C.E., Waite, B.M., Thomas, M.J. and DeChatelet, L.R. (1981b) Release and metabolism of arachidonic acid in human neutrophils. *J. Biol. Chem. 256,* 7228–7234.

Wedmore, C.V. and Williams, T.J. (1981) Control of vascular permeability by polymorphonuclear leukocytes in inflammation. *Nature (London) 289,* 646–650.

Weissmann, G., Smolen, J.E. and Korchak, H. (1980) Prostaglandins and inflammation: receptor/cyclase coupling as an explanation of why PGEs and PGI_2 inhibit functions of inflammatory cells. In: B. Samuelsson, P.W. Ramwell and R. Paoletti (Eds), *Advances in Prostaglandin and Thromboxane Research, Vol. 8,* Raven Press, New York, pp. 1637–1646.

Williams, J.T. (1979) Prostaglandin E_2, prostaglandin I_2 and the vascular changes of inflammation. *Br. J. Pharmacol. 65,* 517–524.

Yen, S.-S., Mathe, A.A. and Dugan, J.J. (1976) Release of prostaglandins from healthy and sensitized guinea pig lung and trachea by histamine. *Prostaglandins 11,* 227–239.

CHAPTER 6

Cyclic nucleotides and arachidonate metabolites in psoriasis

CYNTHIA L. MARCELO

and

JOHN J. VOORHEES

Department of Dermatology, University of Michigan Medical School, Ann Arbor, Michigan 48109

6.1. INTRODUCTION

Psoriasis is a multifactorial hereditary skin disease (Watson et al. 1971; Farber et al. 1974; Woodrow et al. 1975; Beckman et al. 1977). Persons with psoriasis develop cutaneous lesions, either spontaneously or in an area of skin damage, which show seemingly uncontrolled, non-malignant growth of the epidermis. The involved epidermal areas are characterized by markedly increased proliferative rates (Weinstein and McCullough 1973; Marks 1978), reduced morphological differentiation in the outer one-third of the epidermis (Voorhees et al. 1968; Stankler 1977), and frequently by an intense inflammatory cell infiltrate. Neutrophils and mononuclear leukocytes are often present in the upper dermis and dermal papillae of the lesion, and neutrophils may percolate up through the epidermis to form microabscesses (Stankler 1977). Often, the histology of clinically uninvolved skin immediately adjacent to the lesion also shows foci of accumulated lymphocytic cells in the upper dermis and adjacent to the basal zone of the epidermis (Stankler 1977; Fitzpatrick et al. 1979).

The epidermal abnormality is not restricted to the lesional area since the normal-appearing skin of the psoriatic patient shows a 48% increase in DNA synthesis when compared to the normal skin of non-psoriatic individuals (Marks 1978). This suggests that a psoriatic individual may have an imbalance of a variety of intracellular biochemical systems that results in expression of epidermal lesional psoriasis when skin damage or other unknown changes in the cutaneous microenvironment occur.

Various inflammatory disorders of the skin such as allergic contact dermatitis and atopic dermatitis also have increased epithelial proliferation as a major feature of the lesion. At present, it can be reasoned that many of the described abnormal mechanisms in the psoriatic epithelium will be present, in general, in the hyperplastic epidermis. This chapter will discuss known mediators of skin function, using psoriasis as a model, and inflammatory systems, with the expectation that this information may describe general inflammatory mechanisms in the skin.

6.2. THE CYCLIC NUCLEOTIDE SYSTEM

6.2.1. *Cyclic AMP*

In the skin, as in other tissues, the cytoplasmic level of cyclic AMP (adenosine 3′,5′-monophospate) is controlled by the rate of synthesis and of degradation. Cyclic AMP is formed from ATP by the cell membrane-bound enzyme adenylate cyclase (Duell et al. 1971; Marks and Rebien 1972) and is degraded by the enzyme cyclic nucleotide phosphodiesterase(s) to 5′-AMP (Marks and Raab 1974; Adachi et al. 1976). At present, all the effects of cyclic AMP are thought to be mediated by the activation of specific protein kinases which then catalyze the phosphorylation by ATP of protein substrates (Kumar et al. 1971, 1972, 1973).

Cyclic AMP-dependent protein kinase is a dimer of associated regulatory (R) plus catalytic (C) subunits, i.e. $(RC)^2$. In this form, the enzymatic activity of the catalytic unit is inhibited. When cyclic AMP specifically binds to the R-component, the R- and C-units dissociate; the catalytic unit then phosphorylates various protein substrates, thus causing the cyclic AMP effect (George and Ignarro 1977). At the present time, the specific substrates for cyclic AMP-dependent protein kinase phosphorylation in the skin are unknown.

Epidermal cell cyclic AMP can be increased through specific β-adrenergic receptor activation of adenylate cyclase by epinephrine, norepinephrine and isoproterenol (Marks and Rebien 1972; Powell et al. 1971; Yoshikawa et al. 1975a; Iizuka et al. 1978a). Prostaglandin (PG)E_1 and E_2, also by specific receptor binding (Adachi et al. 1975; Lord et al. 1978), stimulate cyclic AMP synthesis in pig and human epidermis as does histamine, through H_2-receptor activation (Iizuka et al. 1977). Specific refractoriness to epinephrine, PGE, histamine and to 5′-AMP (another receptor-mediated adenylate cyclase activator) (Weinstein and McCullough 1973; Farber et al. 1974) occurs in the epidermis (Adachi et al. 1977). Recovery from the epinephrine-induced refractoriness, in vivo, begins only after 48 hours and is not completely relieved until one week after injection of the hormone into the skin (Iizuka et al. 1978a). These studies demonstrate that specific receptor-mediated activation of epidermal cyclic AMP can occur, but because of prolonged cell refractory states, long-term changes in epidermal cyclic AMP levels are probably not induced by β-adrenergic agonists, nor by histamine nor PGE_1 and PGE_2. Cholera toxin, an irreversible stimulator of adenylate cyclase (Moss and Vaughan 1977), does cause a long-term elevation of epidermal cyclic AMP levels (Marcelo 1979). As will be discussed in a later section, the irreversibility of the cholera toxin stimulation has been used to study the effect of cyclic AMP on epidermal function.

6.2.2. *Cyclic GMP*

The other cyclic nucleotide that has a known biological function is cyclic GMP (guanosine 3′,5′-monophosphate). In the skin, cyclic GMP is synthesized from GTP by the enzyme guanylate cyclase (Marks 1973). This enzyme is not stimulated by α-adrenergic agonists, acetylcholine, serotonin, thyroxine or somatotropin (Marks 1973). Our own studies showed that norepinephrine, $PGF_{2\alpha}$, triamcinolone acetonide, the phosphodiesterase inhibitors 1-methyl-3-isobutylxanthine and papaverine, indomethacin and injury also do not change epidermal cyclic GMP (Marcelo and Voorhees 1980). The only consistent increases in epidermal cyclic GMP that have been reported are induced by application of high doses of the tumor promoter and epidermal irritant 12-O-tetradecanoyl phorbol-13-acetate (TPA), or by keratotome removal of epidermis that is immediately snap-frozen (instead of floated in buffer for 1−30 minutes) (Marcelo and Voorhees 1980). This lack of receptor-mediated response of epidermal cyclic GMP levels suggests that the cyclic GMP system of this tissue can be stimulated by cell membrane perturbations, possibly related to injury (Marcelo and Voorhees 1980). The cyclic GMP phosphodiesterase activity in supernatants from mouse epidermis homogenates has been characterized by Marks and Raab (1974) and Rusin et al. (1978). This enzyme is present in addition to the cyclic AMP phosphodiesterase.

6.2.3. *Cyclic AMP and cyclic GMP in psoriasis*

The first reports suggesting that changes in epidermal cyclic AMP could be involved in the pathophysiology of the psoriatic lesion were based on protein kinase binding assay data that showed a 30−40% decrease in lesional cyclic AMP levels (Voorhees et al. 1972a). Since that time, over 100 psoriatic-lesional, psoriatic-uninvolved, and normal-subject epidermal samples have been processed and assayed for cyclic AMP levels (Halprin et al. 1975; Wadskov and Sondergaard 1978; Marcelo et al. 1979; Wadskov et al. 1979; Adachi et al. 1980; Aoyagi et al. 1980; Saihan et al. 1980); 70 to 80 of these assays were done by this laboratory, over a 6-year time span (Voorhees et al. 1972a, c; Marcello et al. 1979). There is no consensus among these studies as to the level of cyclic AMP in the psoriatic-lesional tissue. In the last analysis, the data indicate that some abnormality probably occurs in the cyclic AMP system of the psoriatic epidermis. The results of these assays suggest that in the onset, steady state and regression of a lesion there are times when normal basal, decreased and increased epidermal cyclic AMP levels can be observed. The association of specific, absolute amounts of cyclic AMP with the disease state of a lesion has at present not been shown, although cyclic AMP is both a positive and negative modulator of epidermal growth, as will be discussed later.

Additionally, investigations have suggested that changes in cyclic AMP-synthesizing and -degrading enzymes, and in cell surface receptors occur in the lesional epidermis. Lesional tissue has been reported to demonstrate decreased responsiveness to β-adrenergic stimuli (Yoshikawa et al. 1975b; Iizuka et al. 1978b) and to PGE_1 (Aso et al. 1975), and increased responsiveness to histamine (Iizuka et al. 1978b) when assayed under appropriate conditions in vitro. In addition, Iizuka et al. (1978c) have reported that epidermis from lesional tissue contains greater amounts of both high- and low-km cyclic AMP and cyclic GMP phosphodiesterase activity. These data led to the idea that an altered lesional cyclic AMP level was secondary to changes in cyclic AMP synthesizing and degrading enzyme activities. However, in view of the pronounced and prolonged refractory states characteristic of the β-adrenergic, PGE and histamine receptors of the epidermis (Adachi et al. 1977; Iizuka et al 1978a; Duell 1980), it is not probable that slight shifts in receptor responsiveness and, concomitantly, of the cyclic AMP levels of lesional psoriasis, could account for the abnormal function of psoriatic-lesional epidermis. We also cannot easily dismiss the possibility that a change in response of whole lesional tissue to hormonal activation and the presence of altered cyclic nucleotide phosphodiesterase activity actually reflect the presence of a large portion of germinative cells in the population, and not an actual change in per-cell enzyme activity.

Other studies, however, do implicate changes in cyclic AMP at the onset and during exacerbation of psoriasis. Topical application of papaverine, a phosphodiesterase inhibitor that can elevate epidermal cyclic AMP, induces regression of psoriatic lesions (Adachi et al. 1981). Topical use of propranolol, a β-receptor antagonist (Gaylarde et al. 1978), causes psoriasiform changes in guinea pig skin. Injection of propranolol induced a proliferative response in psoriatic-uninvolved skin but had no effect on normal volunteer skin (Wiley and Weinstein 1979). It is possible that the psoriasis-like skin changes seen with the β-adrenergic antagonists reflect some receptor abnormality in psoriatic skin, although these agents may be affecting cyclic AMP changes in other tissue compartments involved in the expression of cutaneous psoriatic lesions, i.e., the inflammatory component of the disease.

The levels of cyclic GMP have been assayed in 65−70 lesional and normal appearing psoriatic epidermal samples (Voorhees et al. 1973; Marcelo et al. 1979; Saihan et al. 1980; Adachi et al. 1981). All the studies show that the level of cyclic GMP is increased in psoriatic-lesional tissue. Additionally, Saihan et al. (1980) have shown that dithranol, which is an effective drug in psoriasis, decreases the stimulated cyclic GMP levels. However, the still unanswered question is whether the increased cyclic GMP levels induce the lesional state as has been suggested (Voorhees et al. 1973; Adachi et al. 1981), or whether the increase in cyclic GMP reflects the abnormal state of the epidermis. Conceivably, the elevated cyclic GMP level in the lesional tissue could also be a negative feedback signal and reflects a part of the regression phase of a lesion.

6.2.4. *The function of cyclic nucleotides in in-vitro and in-situ systems*

The first studies done to determine the effect of cyclic AMP on epidermal cell proliferation showed that very large doses of cyclic AMP analogs, i.e., dibutyryl cyclic AMP, inhibited the G_2 and G_1 phases of the epidermal cell cycle (Voorhees et al. 1972b; Flaxman and Harper 1975). These studies used a 5-hour mouse ear assay (Voorhees et al. 1972b) and explant human epidermal cultures (Flaxman and Harper 1975). More recently, cyclic AMP has been shown to be a stimulator of neonatal mouse (Marcelo 1979), neonatal human (Green 1978) and adult human (Marcelo and Duell 1979) epidermal cell proliferation. The cyclic AMP mitogenic effect is dose-dependent: cyclic AMP both stimulates and inhibits adult human keratinocyte culture proliferation, the effect depending on the concentration of the added cyclic AMP (high inhibits, low stimulates) (Marcelo and Duell 1979). However, all doses of cyclic AMP stimulate the neonatal epidermal cell (Marcelo 1979). This same dose-dependent stimulation-inhibition of proliferation by cyclic AMP has been reported by Peters and White (1978) in studying sequential changes in rat skin induced to hyperplasia by hexadecane.

Moreover, Kuroki (1981a, b) has recently reported that subcutaneous injection of cholera toxin, an irreversible stimulator of epidermal adenylate cyclase (Moss and Vaughan 1977; Marcelo 1979), stimulates mouse epidermal proliferation and induces hyperplasia. In a similarly designed study, Jumblatt et al. (1980) showed that cholera toxin stimulated corneal wound closure. Therefore, the in-situ effect of consistently elevated cyclic AMP levels is to stimulate epidermal proliferation and growth. Our own most recent studies indicated that cyclic AMP, in addition to being an epidermal cell mitogen (Marcelo 1979), stimulated epidermal cell synthesis of keratohyalin granule, keratin and cell envelope proteins, these being indicative of epidermal cell differentiation (Tong and Marcelo 1981).

Cyclic GMP had been proposed as a proliferative stimulator of epidermal proliferation (Voorhees et al. 1973), since it was demonstrated to be elevated in the psoriatic-lesional tissue (Voorhees et al. 1973; Adachi et al. 1981). However, addition of cyclic GMP analogs to in-vitro epidermal cell cultures has no stimulatory effect on proliferation (Marcelo 1979). Instead, cyclic GMP appears to stimulate epidermal cell differentiation (Marcelo 1979; Tong and Marcelo, unpublished data).

6.3. INFLAMMATION

Inflammation can be induced by physical, chemical or immunologic stimuli. The skin response to such stimuli is progressive, from vascular permeability, edema, and cell migration to cell death (Winkelmann 1971; Cochrane 1978; Fitzpatrick et al. 1979). All these components of cutaneous inflammation can occur immediately, if the stimulus is severe, or progressively with chronic stimuli, or even in isolated steps, i.e., leukocyte migration may occur without changes in vasopermeability (Winkelmann

1971). Complement fragments, i.e., C5a (Ward et al. 1968; Winkelmann 1971; Fitzpatrick et al. 1979), plasma protein factors, and proteases are protein inflammatory mediators, while kinin, histamine (Greaves et al. 1976; Stenson et al. 1980), serotonin, and arachidonic acid metabolites are molecular mediators of inflammation (Flaxman and Harper 1975; Fitzpatrick et al. 1979).

In our discussion, we shall limit ourselves to those mediators and systems that have been reported to be involved in the exacerbation of psoriasis. These are the arachidonic acid metabolites, chemotactic and chemokinetic factors, and proteases.

6.3.1. Arachidonic acid metabolism

The precursor to the polyunsaturated fatty acid metabolites that are active in the inflammatory process is arachidonic acid. The precursor acid for the synthesis of oxygenated metabolites arises from several intracellular lipid pools; one such pool is the cell membrane phospholipids (Galli et al. 1978). The enzyme responsible for release of the fatty acid precursor is phospholipase A_2 (Galli et al. 1978). Phospholipase A_2 releases arachidonic acid from phosphatidyl choline, and also from phosphatidyl ethanolamine and phosphatidyl inositol (Lapetina et al. 1981); arachidonic acid is introduced into membrane phospholipids by esterification. When arachidonic acid is in the free non-membrane-bound form, it is acted upon by several enzyme systems to form the biologically active oxygenated metabolites (see Fig. 1). Cyclo-oxygenase forms the endoperoxides (PGG_2 and PGH_2) and the products thromboxane A_2 and B_2, and PGD_2, PGE_2, $PGF_{2\alpha}$ and PGI_2 (Samuelsson and Paolette 1976). The other enzyme system, the lipoxygenases, forms hydroperoxy- and hydroeicosatetraenoic acids (HPETEs and HETEs). These products are mediators of more importance than the cyclo-oxygenase products in a number of allergic and inflammatory states (Goetzl 1980). For example, the slow-reacting substance of anaphylaxis (SRS-A), which contracts smooth muscle and alters microvascular permeability, is composed of two or more cysteine-peptide adducts of 5-HETE derived from lipoxygenation of arachidonic acid (Samuelsson 1979, 1980; Bach et al. 1980; Hammarstrom et al. 1980; Orning et al. 1980; Radmark et al. 1980a, b, c; Lewis et al. 1981).

There are a number of HETEs generated in mammalian cells. Platelets synthesize 12-L-HETE; 11-HETE and 12-L-HETE are produced by mast cells; rabbit polymorphonuclear leukocytes generate 5-D-HETE while human PMN leukocytes are capable of producing 5-, 8-, 9-, 11- and 12-HETE (Goetzl et al. 1980b). The HETEs are chemotactic, that is, they induce directed movement for PMN and mononuclear leukocytes (Goetzl et al. 1980a). Although all the HETEs are chemotactic for PMN leukocytes, their potencies exhibit a rank order: 5-HETE $>>$ 8-HETE: 9-HETE $>$ 11-HETE$=$12-L-HETE (Goetzl et al. 1977; Lewis et al. 1981). Besides being chemoattractants, both 5-HETE and 12-L-HETE have been shown to also induce lysozyme release from specific leukocyte granules (Stenson and Parker 1980), which is part of the overall phenomenon of PMN leukocyte activation.

Another product of the lipoxygenase pathway, 5,12-di-HETE (LTB_4; see Fig. 1) is the most potent PMN leukocyte chemotactic factor generated via this system (Borgeat and Samuelsson 1979a; Goetzl and Pickett 1980; Ford-Hutchinson et al. 1980; Palmer et al. 1980; Bokoch and Reed 1981). New lipoxygenation products are currently being described: new dihydroxy acids (Hammarstrom et al. 1980; Jubiz et al. 1981), new unstable intermediate forms of dihydroxy acids (Borgeat and Samuelsson 1979b) and isomers of known di-HETEs (Goetzl and Pickett 1981; Ford-Hutchinson et al. 1981) are currently being synthesized and characterized.

Steroids inhibit PMN leukocyte phospholipase A_2 activity, probably through the induced synthesis by the hormone of a protein that has been named lipomodulin (Hirata et al. 1979, 1980, 1981) or macrocortin (Carnuccio et al. 1981). This inhibitory protein has not yet been described in other cells.

The non-steroidal anti-inflammatory drugs aspirin and indomethacin decrease prostaglandin synthesis by inhibiting cyclo-oxygenase activity. Additionally, these drugs also inhibit the conversion of 12-hydroperoxy-ETE (HPETE) to 12-L-HETE (Siegel et al. 1979, 1980). Thus, the overall effect of the non-steroidal anti-inflammatory drugs would be to increase the 12-L-HPETE production of a tissue. Most recently, the cytochrome P-450 system has been shown to be involved in lipoxygenase types of oxidation of arachidonic acid (Capdevila et al. 1981a, b). This additional pathway for the oxidative transformation of arachidonic acid must therefore be considered when discussing the control of arachidonic acid metabolism in the skin, since the epidermis has a very active and inducible aryl hydrocarbon hydroxylase enzyme system (Bickers and Kappas 1978).

6.3.2. Cyclic nucleotides in leukocytes

Polymorphonuclear leukocytes (PMN) form part of the inflammatory cell infiltrate that is often observed in psoriatic-lesional skin (Stankler 1977) and most probably contribute to these inflammatory events. PMN functions, at least in part, result from surface stimulation of these cells by a variety of factors that induce directed migration of PMNs (chemotaxis) and increase the speed of movement of the leukocytes (chemokinesis). Chemotactic factors such as the peptide N-formyl methionyl leucyl phenylalanine (FMLP), the complement-derived fragment C5a, and immune complexes induce a very rapid (10–45 sec) increase in PMN cyclic AMP that declines and vanishes by 5 minutes (Smolen et al. 1979; Simchowitz et al. 1980; Snyderman and Goetzl 1981). The peak elevation of cyclic AMP briefly proceeds the generation of superoxide radicals (O_2^-) and granule enzyme (lysosomal) release, which are two mechanisms by which PMN function is mediated. Sustained high levels of PMN cyclic AMP, however, inhibit chemotactic stimuli-induced O_2^- generation and granule enzyme release (Simchowitz et al. 1980), suggesting that the timing and extent of PMN cyclic AMP stimulation determines the final function, i.e., a stimulation or inhibition of PMN O_2^- generation and lysosomal enzyme release (Smolen et al. 1979; Simchowitz et al. 1980). Moreover, there may be differences between cyclic AMP induction of PMN O_2^- formation and lysosomal degranulation since chemoattractants can stimulate PMN movement at concentrations 1/10 to 1/100th less than are necessary to produce the 2- to 3-fold spike of cyclic AMP in these cells (Snyderman and Goetzl 1981).

Similar chemotactic and chemokinetic responses are associated with more prolonged increases in cyclic GMP (30 minutes). The chemoattractants used in this study were 12-HPETE and 12-HETE, two arachidonc acid lipoxygenase products (see Fig. 1). Both 12-HPETE and 12-HETE induced PMN chemotactic and chemokinetic responses, enhanced expression of PMN C3b receptors (another element of PMN function) along with increased cyclic GMP levels (Goetzl et al. 1981), although no increases in O_2^- radical and lysosomal degranulations were seen (Goetzl et al. 1981). 12-HPETE is a more potent stimulator of PMN chemotaxis, chemokinesis and C3b receptor expression than its more stable product, 12-HETE; 12-HPETE, but not 12-HETE augments the release of PMN lysosomal enzymes by C5a (Goetzl et al. 1981). So apparently chemotactic, chemokinetic and other associated PMN leukocyte functions can be controlled by short-term cyclic AMP and longer cyclic GMP concentrations (Smolen et al. 1979; Simchowitz et al. 1980; Snyderman and Goetzl 1981; Goetzl et al. 1981).

How cyclic AMP might control PMN leukocyte function has recently been described (Hirata et al. 1979, 1980, 1981; Siegel et al. 1979; Hirata 1981; Carnuccio et al. 1981). Hirata et al. (1979) suggested that part of the leukocyte response to chemoattractants might be modulated by release of arachidonic acid from membrane phospholipids (phosphatidyl choline). They suggested that the changes in ionic flux and in PMN membrane potential that precede the other changes associated with PMN activation resulted from increased phospholipid metabolism. Increased phospholipase A_2 activity caused the increase in arachidonic acid content of activated leukocytes (Hirata et al. 1979). As we previously discussed, phospholipase A_2 activity is modulated by the protein inhibitor lipomodulin (Hirata et al. 1980; Carnuccio et al. 1981 (or macrocortin)). In PMN leukocytes, lipomodulin normally controls, by inhibition, phospholipase A_2 enzyme release of arachidonic acid from phosphatidyl choline. Glucocorticoid treatment induces the synthesis of lipomodulin. The net increase in cellular lipomodulin decreases the amount of arachidonic acid released from the cell membranes. This inhibition of phospholipase A_2 release of arachidonic acid correlates with an inhibition of FMLP peptide induction of chemotaxis by glucocorticoid (Hirata et al. 1980). This showed that free arachidonic acid and its metabolites are involved in PMN leukocyte activation by the FMLP peptide.

Cyclic AMP, which, in short-lived bursts, is associated with chemoattractant induction of PMN leukocytes, stimulates the phosphorylation of lipomodulin using a cyclic AMP-dependent protein kinase. The phosphorylated lipomodulin does not inhibit phospholipase A_2 activity, so that the net result of this "inhibition of an inhibitor" is the release of arachidonic acid. This suggests that the phosphorylation–dephosphorylation of lipomodulin via a cyclic AMP-dependent

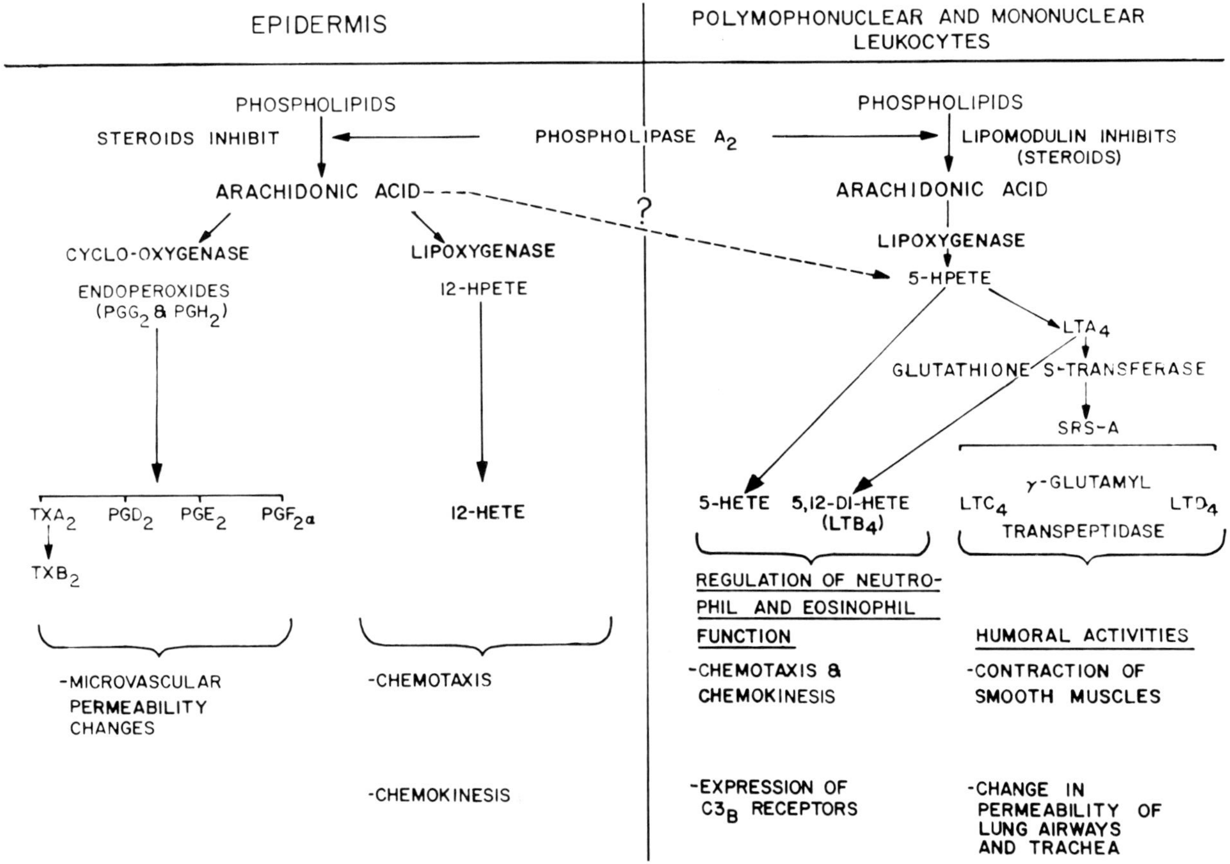

Fig. 1. Arachidonic acid metabolism in the epidermis and in leukocytes. SRS-A = slow reacting substance of anaphylaxis.

protein kinase is an important mechanism for chemotactic regulation of PMN leukocyte functions. A defect in the cyclic nucleotide system of the cells of a psoriatic individual might manifest itself in this component of the inflammatory response.

6.3.3. *Arachidonic acid metabolism in the skin*

In rat skin, both linoleic and arachidonic acids are found in the phospholipid component, with arachidonic acid being the most important precursor of the polyunsaturated fatty acid metabolites (Prottey 1977). Both human and mouse epidermis converts arachidonic acid to 12-L-HETE, PGE_2, $PGF_{2\alpha}$ and PGD_2 (Kingston and Greaves 1976; Hammarstrom et al. 1979); PGE_2 is apparently the major prostaglandin synthesized by skin (Jonsson and Anggard 1972; Ziboh 1973). No thromboxane A_2 and B_2 (TXA_2, TXB_2), nor PGI_2 or 6-keto-$PGF_{1\alpha}$ were detected (Hammarstrom et al. 1979). Additionally, Wilkinson and Walsh (1977) have reported the conversion of linoleic acid to PGE_1, PGD_2 and $PGF_{1\alpha}$ by mouse skin homogenates.

Phospholipase A_2 has been identified in human and rat skin (Ziboh and Lord 1979). The isolated enzyme is inhibited when cortisol and triamcinoline acetonide are directly added in vitro. However, it is unknown at present if protein inhibitors to phospholipase A_2, i.e., lipomodulin, are present in the skin, although inhibitors of PG synthesis (Penneys et al. 1977) and arachidonic acid oxidation have been reported (Penneys et al. 1980). The enzymes that degrade PG have also been identified in skin (Camp and Greaves 1980).

The essential fatty acid-deficient rat (Ziboh and Blank 1973) and hairless mouse (Lowe and Stoughton 1977a) systems are used to study the effect of arachidonic and linoleic acid and their metabolites on epidermal function. Animals deficient in these two fatty acids show thickening of the skin, scaling, acanthosis and hyperkeratosis and an increased basal cell mitotic index. These cutaneous manifestations are relieved by topical application of PGE_2 and linoleic acid (Ziboh and Blank 1973; Lowe and Stoughton 1977a, b). This effect of PGE_2 suggests that this prostaglandin can control epidermal proliferation and growth. How this may occur is unknown, although the epidermis has specific prostaglandin receptors (Lord et al. 1978).

Early studies on the functional effects of the prostaglandins on skin implicated PGE_2 in cutaneous inflammatory responses to injury. PGE_2 is formed in the skin following burn injury (Anggard and Jonsson 1972) to such a large extent that the urinary excretion of the PGE_1 and PGE_2 break-down metabolite was increased 5–9 fold (Hamberg and Jonsson 1973). In a more recent burn injury study, PGE_2, $PGF_{2\alpha}$, TXB_2 and efflux of cyclic AMP have been found (Jonsson et al. 1979). These studies all suggest a role for arachidonic acid metabolites in inflammatory injury.

Jorgensen and Sondergaard (1973) reported that intradermal injection of prostaglandin E_1 mediated vascular permeability and helped sustain an acute inflammation of the skin. More recently, prostaglandins have been shown to have their effect, not by increasing vascular permeability, but by increasing vasodilation (Williams and Peck 1979) and, possibly, by attracting polymorphonuclear leukocytes to the damaged area where the cells themselves interact with vascular endothelial cells to regulate permeability (Wedmore and Williams 1981).

The lipoxygenase arachidonic acid products have also been shown to be involved in inflammatory mechanisms of the skin. Indomethacin has been reported to be a poor inhibitor of chronic inflammatory skin lesions induced by carrageenan, although a significant decrease in PGE_2, $PGF_{2\alpha}$, PGB_2 and HETE was recorded (Bragt and Bonta 1980). These investigators most probably were increasing the amounts of HPETE (see Fig. 1) in the tissue via indomethacin inhibition of HPETE conversion to HETE (Siegel et al. 1979, 1980). Both HETE and HPETE have been reported to potentiate inflammatory responses (Higgs et al. 1981), with HPETE being more potent than HETE. In this same study, leukotriene B_4 was found to be a more effective potentiator of the inflammatory response. Intradermal injection of LTB_4 alone into skin produces little or no change in plasma vascular permeability and dilation as measured by plasma exudation (Bray et al. 1981a). Intradermal injection of PGE_2 also has little or no effect on plasma exudation at the skin injection site. However, if the LTB_4 and PGE_2 are injected together, there is a significant increase in plasma exudation in the skin. Therefore, when the vasodilating effect of PGE_2 is combined with a mediator of vasopermeability, as is LTB_4, a pronounced inflammatory skin response is seen. LTB_4 may be the mechanism used by polymorphonuclear leukocytes to induce vasopermeability in inflammation (Wedmore and Williams 1981; Bray et al. 1981b), but at the same time may potentiate the inflammatory response since this leukotriene is a chemotactic and chemokinetic factor.

The skin and epidermis synthesize LTB_4 (Ziboh et al. 1981; Ziboh et al. 1983a, b). The production of LTB_4 by the psoriatic epidermis could induce an inflammatory reaction that could self-potentiate the epidermal abnormality. It is possible that a HETE or HPETE product, if synthesized in vast amounts, might also cause such an inflammatory event. At present, this is one promising hypothesis.

6.3.4. Arachidonic acid metabolites in psoriasis

When psoriatic-lesional and uninvolved epidermis were assayed for arachidonic acid metabolites, it was found that there is a 40 and 80% increase in the lesional levels of PGE_2 and $PGF_{2\alpha}$, respectively (Hammarstrom et al. 1975). The changes in these two prostaglandins were not as pronounced as the 26-fold increase in free arachidonic acid and the 82-fold increase in 12-L-HETE in the lesional tissue. One possible explanation for this vast change in the arachidonic acid and 12-L-HETE levels in the lesion is the presence of an endogenous inhibitor of prostaglandin synthesis, as has been described in the skin (Penneys et al. 1977), which might shift an accelerated arachidonic acid metabolism to the lipoxygenase pathway.

Recently, it has been reported that both arachidonic acid and 12-L-HETE stimulate the soluble guanylate cyclase of human epidermis (Cantieri et al. 1980). This fact, plus the observation that psoriatic lesional epidermis has a 10-fold increased specific activity of guanylate cyclase, apparently explains the elevated cyclic GMP levels seen in psoriatic epidermis (Voorhees et al. 1973; Marcelo et al. 1979; Saihan et al. 1980; Adachi et al. 1981). Whether or not the increased cyclic GMP alters epidermal cell function is unknown. It is possible that the increase in psoriatic lesional cyclic GMP is an accidental and inconsequential by-product of a more biologically relevant change in arachidonic acid metabolism.

This shift to a predominantly 12-L-HETE metabolism in the tissue may be a critical factor in the chronic inflammation of the psoriatic lesion. Even though 12-L-HETE is not a very potent chemoattractant or inducer of vasopermeability, 82-fold increased amounts of this HETE, possibly in synergism with the increased PGE_2 levels, could induce or initiate a chronic inflammatory effect. The fact that glucocorticoids, which reduce the levels of both arachidonic acid and 12-L-HETE in the tissue, is therapeutic in psoriasis (Hammarstrom et al. 1977) is consistent with this theory. Moreover, indomethacin, which inhibits prostaglandin and 12-L-HETE synthesis and would shift an exaggerated lesional 12-L-HETE production to the more potent 12-L-HPETE, has been shown to exacerbate psoriasis (Katayama and Kawda 1981). Additionally, lithium, which exacerbates psoriasis to such an extent that the disease becomes highly resistant to treatment (Lazarus and Gilgor 1979), augments leukocyte functions (Spitzer et al. 1979; Gelfand et al. 1979; Lyman et al. 1980).

A number of studies have shown leukocyte function to be abnormal in this disease. Psoriatic persons appear to have altered polymorphonuclear leukocyte (Wahba et al. 1978; Michaelson 1980; Herlin and Kragballe 1981), monocyte (Krueger et al. 1978a, b; Bar-Eli et al. 1979; Herlin and Kragballe 1981) and T lymphocyte functions (Krueger et al. 1978a; Glinski et al. 1978; Sander et al. 1980). The lesional epidermis itself has also been shown to contain leukotactic factors (Tagami and Ofuji 1977), and sera from psoriatic patients have been reported to increase polymorphonuclear leukocyte activation (Kawohl et al. 1980; Sedgwick et al. 1981).

In addition to the inflammatory mechanism that we have discussed, human epidermis contains a number of proteinases that can contribute significantly to the chronic inflammation, and possibly to the hyperproliferation of the lesion (Lazarus 1974; Levine et al. 1976; Thomas et al. 1977; Hopsu-Have and Fraki 1981). These proteinases have been suggested to contribute to the pathology of the psoriatic lesion (Lazarus et al. 1977; Fraki et al. 1978; Glinski et al. 1980).

6.4. SUMMARY

It is appropriate to hypothesize that defective cyclic AMP, possibly cyclic GMP, and arachidonic acid metabolite systems combine to produce the hyperproliferative, inflammatory state of lesional psoriasis. Psoriatic individuals probably have an inherited susceptibility to a reversible loss of the coordination of these mediators, possibly both in the epidermal and leukocyte compartments of the disease. A better understanding of these basic underlying mechanisms and their interactions will allow the design of specific therapeutic agents.

REFERENCES

Adachi, K., Yoshikawa, K., Halprin, K. and Levine, V. (1975) Prostaglandins and cyclic AMP in epidermis. *Br. J. Dermatol. 92,* 381–388.

Adachi, K., Levine, V., Halprin, K., Iizuka, H. and Yoshikawa, K. (1976) Multiple forms of cyclic nucleotide phosphodiesterase in pig epidermis. *Biochim. Biophys. Acta 429,* 498–507.

Adachi, K., Iizuka, H., Halprin, K. and Levine, V. (1977) Specific refractoriness of adenylate cyclase in skin to epinephrine, prostaglandin E, histamine and AMP. *Biochim. Biophys. Acta 497,* 428–436.

Adachi, K., Iizuka, J., Halprin, K. and Levine, V. (1980) Epidermal cyclic AMP is not decreased in psoriasis lesions. *J. Invest. Dermatol. 74,* 74–76.

Adachi, K., Aoyagi, T., Nemoto, O., Halprin, K. and Levine, V. (1981) Epidermal cyclic GMP is increased in psoriasis lesions. *J. Invest. Dermatol. 76.* 19–20.

Anggard, E. and Jonsson, C. (1972) Formation of prostaglandins in the skin following a burn injury. In: P. Ramwell and B. Plauriss (Eds), *Prostaglandins in Cellular Biology,* Plenum Press, New York, p. 269.

Aoyagi, T., Kamigaki, K. and Miura, Y. (1980) Cyclic AMP level in different layers of psoriatic epidermis. *J. Dermatol. 7,* 131–136.

Aso, K., Orenburg, E. and Farber, E. (1975) Reduced epidermal cyclic AMP accumulation following prostaglandin stimulation: its possible role in the pathophysiology of psoriasis. *J. Invest. Dermatol. 65,* 375–378.

Bach, M., Brashler, J., Hammarstrom, S. and Samuelsson, B. (1980) Identification of a component of rat mononuclear cells SRS as leukotriene D. *Biochem. Biophys. Res. Commun. 93,* 1121–1126.

Bar-Eli, M., Gallily, R., Cohen, H. and Wahba, A. (1979) Monocyte function in psoriasis. *J. Invest. Dermatol. 73,* 147–149.

Beckman, L., Bergdahl, K., Cedergren, B. and Liden, S. (1977) Genetic markers in psoriasis. *Acta Derm. Venereol. 57,* 247–251.

Bickers, D. and Kappas, A. (1978) Human skin aryl hydrocarbon hydroxylase induction by coal tar. *J. Clin. Invest. 62,* 1061–1068.

Bokoch, G. and Reed, P. (1981) Effect of various lipoxygenase metabolites arachidonic acid on degranulation of polymorphonuclear leukocytes. *J. Biol. Chem. 256,* 5317–5320.

Borgeat, P. and Samuelsson, B. (1979a) Transformation of arachidonic acid by rabbit polymorphonuclear leukocytes. *J. Biol. Chem. 254,* 2643–2646.

Borgeat, P. and Samuelsson, B. (1979b) Arachidonic acid metabolism in polymorphonuclear leukocytes: unstable intermediate in formation of dihydroxy acids. *Proc. Natl Acad. Sci. USA 76,* 3213–3217.

Bragt, P. and Bonta, I. (1980) Indomethacin inhibits the in vitro formation of the lipoxygenase product HETE (12-hydroxy-5,8,10,14-eicosatetraenoic acid) during granulomatous inflammation in the rat. *J. Pharm. Pharmacol. 32,* 143–144.

Bray, M., Cunningham, F., Ford-Hutchinson, A. and Smith, J. (1981a) Leukotriene B_4: a mediator of vascular permeability. *Br. J. Pharmacol. 72,* 483–486.

Bray, M., Ford-Hutchinson, A. and Smith, M. (1981b) Leukotriene B_4: an inflammatory mediator in vivo. *Prostaglandins 22,* 213–222.

Camp, R. and Greaves, M. (1980) The metabolism of prostaglandins by rat skin. *Biochem. J. 186,* 153–160.

Cantieri, J., Graff, G. and Goldberg, N. (1980) Cyclic GMP metabolism in psoriasis: activation of soluble epidermal guanylate cyclase by arachidonic acid and 12-hydroxy-5,8,10,14-eicosatetraenoic acid. *J. Invest. Dermatol. 74,* 234–237.

Capdevila, J., Parkhill, L., Chacos, N., Okita, R., Masters, B. and Estabrook, R. (1981a) The oxidative metabolism of arachidonic acid by purified cytochromes P-450. *Biochem. Biophys. Res. Commun. 101,* 1357–1363.

Capdevila, J., Chacos, N., Werringloer, J., Prough, R. and Estabrook R. (1981b) Liver microsomal cytochrome P-450 and the oxidative metabolism of arachidonic acid. *Proc. Natl Acad. Sci. USA 78,* 5362–5366.

Carnuccio, R., Di Rosa, M., Flower, R. and Pinto, A. (1981) The inhibition by hydrocortisone of prostaglandin biosynthesis in rat peritoneal leucocytes is correlated with intracellular macrocortins levels. *Br. J. Pharmacol. 74,* 322–324.

Cochrane, C. (1978) Mediating systems in inflammatory disease. *J. Invest. Dermatol. 71,* 40–48.

Duell, E. (1980) Adenosine-induced alterations in the adenosine 3,5-monophosphate levels in mammalian epidermis. *Mol. Pharmacol. 18,* 49–52.

Duell, E., Voorhees, J., Kelsey, W.H. and Hayes, E. (1971) Isoproterenol-sensitive adenyl cyclase in a particulate fraction of epidermis. *Arch. Dermatol. 104,* 601–610.

Farber, E., Nall, L. and Watson, W. (1974) Natural history of psoriasis in 61 twin pairs. *Arch. Dermatol. 109,* 207–211.

Fitzpatrick, T., Eisen, A., Wolff, K., Freedberg, I. and Austen, K. (Eds) (1979) *Dermatology in General Medicine, 2nd ed.,* McGraw-Hill, New York, p.234.

Flaxman, B. and Harper, R. (1975) In vitro analysis of the control of keratinocyte proliferation in human epidermis by physiology and pharmacologic agents. *J. Invest. Dermatol. 65,* 52–59.

Ford-Hutchinson, A., Bray, M., Doig, M., Shipley, M. and Smith, M. (1980) Leukotriene B, a potent chemokinetic and aggregating substance released from polymorphonuclear leukocytes. *Nature (London) 286,* 264–265.

Ford-Hutchinson, A., Bray, M., Cunningham, F., Davidson, E. and Smith, M. (1980) Isomers of leukotriene B_4 possess different biological potencies. *Prostaglandins, 21,* 143–152.

Fraki, J., Djupsund, B. and Hopsu-Havu, V. (1978) Plasminogen activators of psoriatic scale extracts. *Arch. Dermatol. Res. 261,* 259–266.

Galli, C., Galli, G. and Porcellati, G. (Eds) (1978) Phospholipases and prostaglandins. In: *Advances in Prostaglandin Research, Vol. 3,* Raven Press, New York.

Gaylarde, P., Brock, A. and Sarkany, I. (1978) Psoriasiform changes in guinea-pig skin from propranolol. *Clin. Exp. Dermatol. 3,* 157–159.

Gelfand, E., Dosch, H., Hastings, D. and Shore, A. (1979) Lithium: a modulator of cyclic AMP-dependent events in lymphocytes. *Science 203,* 265–367.

George, W. and Ignarro G. (Eds) (1977) *Advances in Cyclic Nucleotide Research, Vol. 9,* Raven Press, New York.

Glinski, W., Obalek, S., Langner, A., Jablonska, S. and Haftek, M. (1978) Defective function of T lymphocytes in psoriasis. *J. Invest. Dermatol. 70,* 105–110.

Glinski, W., Zarebska, Z., Jablonska, S., Imiela, J. and Nosarzewski, J. (1980) The activity of polymorphonuclear leukocyte neutral proteinases and their inhibitors in patients with psoriasis treated with a continuous peritoneal dialysis. *J. Invest. Dermatol. 75,* 481–487.

Goetzl, E. (1980) Mediators of immediate hypersensitivity derived from arachidonic acid. *N. Engl. J. Med. 303,* 822–825.

Goetzl, E. and Pickett, W. (1980) The human PMN leukocyte chemotactic activity of complex hydroxy-eicosatetraenoic acids (HETEs). *J. Immunol. 124,* 1789–1791.

Goetzl, E. and Pickett, W. (1981) Novel structural determinants of the human neutrophil chemotactic activity of leukotriene B. *J. Exp. Med. 153,* 482–487.

Goetzl, E., Woods, J. and Gorman, R. (1977) Stimulation of human eosinophil and neutrophil polymorphonuclear leukocyte chemotaxis and random migration by 12-L-hydroxy-5,8,10,14-eicosatetraenoic acid. *J. Clin. Invest. 59,* 179–183.

Goetzl, E., Brash, A., Tauber, J., Oates, A. and Hubbard, W. (1980a) Modulation of human neutrophil function by monohydroxy-eicosatetraenoic acids. *Immunology 39,* 491–501.

Goetzl, E., Weller, P. and Sun, F. (1980b) The regulation of human eosinophil function by endogenous mono-hydroxy-eicosatetraenoic acids (HETEs). *J. Immunol. 124,* 926–933.

Goetzl, E., Hill, H. and Gorman, R. (1981) Unique aspects of the modulation of neutrophil function by 12-L-hydroperoxy-5,8,10,14-eicosatetraenoic acid. *Prostaglandins 19,* 71–85.

Greaves, M., Yamamoto, S. and Mahzoon, B. (1976) The mast cell: interrelationships between histamine and prostaglandins. *Clin. Exp. Dermatol. 1,* 327–329.

Green, H. (1978) Cyclic AMP in relation to proliferation of the epidermal cell: a new view. *Cell 15,* 801–811.

Halperin, K., Adachi, K., Yoshikawa, K., Levine, V., Mui, M. and Hsia, S. (1975) Cyclic AMP and psoriasis. *J. Invest. Dermatol. 65,* 170–178.

Hamberg, M. and Jonsson, C. (1973) Increased synthesis of prostaglandins in the guinea pig following scalding injury. *Acta Physiol. Scand. 87,* 240–245.

Hammarstrom, S. (1980) Leukotriene C_5: a slow reaction substance derived from eicosapentaenoic acid. *J. Biol. Chem. 255,* 7093–7094.

Hammarstrom, S., Hamberg, M., Samuelsson, B., Duell, E., Stawiski, M. and Voorhees, J. (1975) Increased concentrations of nonesterified arachidonic acid, 12-L-hydroxy-5,8,10,14-eicosatetraenoic acid, prostaglandin E_2, and prostaglandin $F_{2\alpha}$ in epidermis of psoriasis. *Proc. Natl Acad. Sci. USA 72,* 5130–5134.

Hammarstrom, S., Hamberg, M., Duell, E., Stawiski, M., Anderson, T. and Voorhees, J. (1977) Glucocorticoid in inflammatory proliferative skin disease reduces arachidonic and hydroxyeicosatetraenoic acids. *Science 197,* 994–996.

Hammarstrom, S., Lindgren, J., Marcelo, C., Duell, E., Anderson, T. and Voorhees,

J. (1979) Arachidonic acid transformations in normal and psoriatic skin. *J. Invest. Dermatol. 73,* 180–183.

Hammarstrom, S., Samuelsson, B., Clark, D., Goto, G., Marfat, A., Mioskowski, C. and Corey, E. (1980) Stereochemistry of leukotriene C-1. *Biochem. Biophys. Res. Comm. 92,* 946–953.

Herlin, T. and Kragballe, K. (1981) Enhanced monocyte and neutrophil cytotoxicity and normal cyclic nucleotide levels in severe psoriasis. *Br. J. Dermatol. 105,* 405–414.

Higgs, G., Salmon, J. and Spayne, J. (1981) The inflammatory effects of hydroperoxy and hydroxy acid products of arachidonate lipoxygenase in rabbit skin. *Br. J. Pharmacol. 74,* 429–433.

Hirata, F. (1981) The regulation of lipomodulin, a phospholipase inhibitory protein, in rabbit neutrophils by phosphorylation. *J. Biol. Chem. 256,* 7730–7733.

Hirata, F., Corcoran, B., Venkatasubramanian, K., Schiffmann, E. and Axelrod, J. (1979) Chemoattractants stimulate degradation of methylated phospholipids and release of arachidonic acid in rabbit leukocytes. *Proc. Natl Acad. Sci. USA 76,* 2640–2643.

Hirata, F., Schiffmann, E., Venkatasubramanian, Salomon, D. and Axelrod, J. (1980) A phospholipase A_2 inhibitory protein in rabbit neutrophils induced by glucocorticoids. *Proc. Natl Acad. Sci. USA. 77,* 2533–2536.

Hirata, F., Carmine, R., Nelson, C., Axelrod, J., Schiffman, E., Warabi, A., De Blas, A., Nirenberg, M., Manganiello, V., Vaughan, M., Kumagai, S., Green, I., Decker, J. and Steinberg, A. (1981) Presence of autoantibody for phospholipase inhibitory protein, lipomodulin, in patients with rheumatic diseases. *Proc. Natl Acad. Sci. USA. 78,* 3190–3194.

Hopsu-Have, V. and Fraki, J. (1981) Proteinases and their inhibitors in skin diseases. *J. Dermatol. 20,* 159–163.

Iizuka, H., Adachi, K., Halprin, K. and Levine, V. (1977) Epidermal adenylate cyclase: stimulation of the histamine (H_2) receptor by tolazoline. *J. Invest. Dermatol. 69,* 442–445.

Iizuka, H., Adachi, K., Halprin, K. and Levine, V. (1978a) Epinephrine activation of pig skin adenylate cyclase in vivo and subsequent refractoriness to activation. *J. Invest. Dermatol. 70,* 119–122.

Iizuka, H., Adachi, K., Halprin, K. and Levine, V. (1978b) Cyclic AMP accumulation in psoriatic skin: differential responses to histamine, AMP and epinephrine by the uninvolved and involved epidermis. *J. Invest. Dermatol. 70,* 250–253.

Iizuka, H., Adachi, K., Halprin, K. and Levine, V. (1978c) Cyclic nucleotide-phosphodiesterase in the uninvolved and involved skin of psoriasis. *J. Invest. Dermatol. 70,* 246–249.

Jonsson, C. and Anggard, E. (1972) Biosynthesis and metabolism of prostaglandin E_2 in human skin. *Scand. J. Clin. Lab. Invest. 29,* 289–296.

Jonsson, C., Shimizu, Y., Fredholm, B., Granstrom, E. and Oliw, E. (1979) Efflux of cyclic AMP, prostaglandin E_2 and $F_{2\alpha}$ and thromboxane B_2 in leg lymph of rabbits after scalding injury. *Acta Physiol. Scand. 107,* 377–384.

Jorgensen, H. and Sondergaard, J. (1973) Vascular response to prostaglandin E_1. *Acta Derm. Venereol. 53,* 203–206.

Jubiz, W., Radmark, O., Lindgren, J., Malmsten, C. and Samuelsson, B. (1981) Novel leukotrienes: products formed by initial oxygenation of arachidonic acid at C-15. *Biochem. Biophys. Res. Commun. 99,* 976–986.

Jumblatt, M., Fogle, J. and Neufeld, A. (1980) Cholera toxin stimulates adenosine 3′,5′-monophosphate synthesis and epithelial wound closure in the rabbit cornea. *Assoc. Res. Vision Ophthalmol. 19,* 1321–1327.

Katayama, H. and Kawada, A. (1981) Exacerbation of psoriasis induced by indomethacin. *J. Dermatol. 8,* 323–327.

Kawohl, F., Szperalski, B., Schroder, J. and Christophers, E. (1980) Polymorphonuclear leukocyte chemotaxis in psoriasis: enhancement by self-activated serum. *Br. J. Dermatol. 103,* 527–533.

Kingston, W. and Greaves, M. (1976) Factors affecting prostaglandin synthesis by rat skin microsomes. *Prostaglandins 12,* 51–69.

Krueger, G., Hill, H. and Jederberg, W. (1978a) Inflammatory and immune cell function in psoriasis-a subtle disorder. I. In vivo and in vitro survey. *J. Invest. Dermatol. 71,* 189–194.

Krueger, G., Jederberg, W., Ogden, B. and Reese, D. (1978b) Inflammatory and immune cell function in psoriasis. II. Monocyte function, lymphokine production. *J. Invest. Dermatol. 71,* 195–201.

Kumar, R., Tao, M. and Solomon, L. (1971) Cyclic 3′,5′-adenosine monophosphate-stimulated protein kinase from human skin. *J. Invest. Dermatol 57,* 312–315.

Kumar, R., Tao, M. and Solomon, L. (1972) Adenosine 3′,5′-cyclic monophosphate-stimulated protein kinase from human skin. *J. Invest. Dermatol. 59,* 196–200.

Kumar, R., Tao, M., Piotrowski, R. and Solomon, L. (1973) Multiple forms of adenosine-3′,5′-cyclic monophosphate-dependent protein kinase from monkey skin. *Biochim. Biophys. Acta 315,* 66–72.

Kuroki, T. (1981a) Induction by cholera toxin of synchronous divisions in vivo in the epidermis resulting in hyperplasia. *Proc. Natl Acad. Sci. USA. 78,* 6958–6962.

Kuroki, T. (1981b) Induction of hyperplasia of mouse epidermis by cholera toxin. *Proc. Jpn Acad. 57,* 100–104.

Lapetina, E., Billah, M. and Cuatrecasas, P. (1981) The phosphatidylinositol cycli and the regulation of arachidonic acid production. *Nature (London) 292,* 367–369.

Lazarus, G. (1974) The role of neutral proteinase and cathepsin D in turpentine-induced inflammation. *J. Invest. Dermatol. 62,* 367–371.

Lazarus, G. and Gilgor, R. (1979) Psoriasis, polymorphonuclear leukocytes, and lithium carbonate. *Arch. Dermatol. 115,* 1183–1184.

Lazarus, G., Yost, F. and Thomas, C. (1979) Polymorphonuclear leukocytes: possible mechanism of accumulation in psoriasis. *Science 198,* 1162–1163.

Levine, N., Hatcher, V. and Lazarus, G. (1976) Proteinases of human epidermis; a possible mechanism for polymorphonuclear leukocyte chemotaxis. *Biochim. Biophys. Acta 452,* 458–467.

Lewis, R., Drazen, J., Austen, K., Toda, M., Brion, F., Marfat, A. and Corey, E. (1981) Contractile activities of structural analogs of leukotrienes C and D: Role of the polar substituents. *Proc. Natl Acad. Sci. 78,* 4579–4583.

Lord, J., Ziboh, A. and Warren, S. (1978) Specific binding of prostaglandins E_2 and $F_{2\alpha}$ by membrane preparations from rat skin. *Endocrinology 102,* 1300–1308.

Lowe, N. and Stoughton, R. (1977a) Essential fatty acid deficient hairless mouse: a

model of chronic epidermal hyperproliferation. *Br. J. Dermatol. 96,* 155–162.
Lowe, N. and Stoughton, R. (1977b) Effects of topical prostaglandin E_2 analogue on normal hairless mouse epidermal DNA synthesis. *J. Invest. Dermatol. 68,* 134–137.
Lyman, G., Williams, C. and Preston, D. (1980) The use of lithium carbonate to reduce infection and leukopenia during systemic chemotheraphy. *N. Engl. J. Med. 302,* 257–260.
Marcelo, C. (1979) Differential effects of cAMP and cGMP on in vitro epidermal cell growth. *Exp. Cell Res. 120,* 201–210.
Marcelo, C. and Duell, E. (1979) Cyclic AMP stimulates and inhibits adult human epidermal cell growth. *J. Invest. Dermatol. 72,* 279.
Marcelo, C. and Voorhees, J. (1980) Cyclic nucleotides, prostaglandins and polyamines in psoriasis. *Pharmacol. Ther. 9,* 297–310.
Marcelo, C., Duell, E., Stawiski, M., Anderson, T. and Voorhees, J. (1979) Cyclic nucleotide levels in psoriatic and normal keratomed epidermis. *J. Invest. Dermatol. 72,* 20–24.
Marks, F. (1973) The second messenger system of mouse epidermis III. Guanyl cyclase. *Biochim. Biophys. Acta 309,* 349–356.
Marks, R. (1978) Epidermal activity in the involved and uninvolved skin of patients with psoriasis. *Br. J. Dermatol. 98,* 399–403.
Marks, F. and Raab, I. (1974) The second messenger system of mouse epidermis, IV. Cyclic AMP and cyclic GMP phosphodiesterase. *Biochim. Biophys. Acta 334,* 368–377.
Marks, F. and Rebien, W. (1972) The second messenger system of mouse epidermis, I. Properties and β-adrenergic activation of adenylase cyclase in vitro. *Biochim. Biophys. Acta 284,* 556–567.
Michaelsson, G. (1980) Increased chemotactic activity of neutrophil leukocytes in psoriasis. *Br. J. Dermatol. 103,* 351–356.
Moss, J. and Vaughan, M. (1977) Choleragen activation of solubilized adenylate cyclase: requirement for GTP and protein activator for demonstration of enzymatic activity. *Proc. Natl Acad. Sci. USA 74,* 4396–4400.
Orning, L., Hammarstrom, S. and Samuelsson, B. (1980) Leukotriene D: a slow reacting substance from rat basophilic leukemia cells. *Proc. Natl Acad. Sci. 77,* 2014–2017.
Palmer, R., Stepney, G., Higgs, G. and Eakins, K. (1980) Chemokinetic activity of arachidonic acid lipoxygenase products on leucocytes of different species. *Prostaglandins 20,* 411–417.
Penneys, N., Lord, J., Ziboh, V. and Simon, P. (1977) Inhibitor(s) of prostaglandin biosynthesis and epidermal injury. *Prostaglandins 14,* 355–362.
Penneys, N., Eaglstein, W. and Ziboh, V. (1980) Petrolatum: interference with the oxidation of arachidonic acid. *Br. J. Dermatol. 103.* 257–362.
Peters, R. and White, A. (1978) The relationship between cyclic adenosine 3′,5′-monophosphate and biochemical events in rat skin after the induction of epidermal hyperplasia using hexadecane. *Br. J. Dermatol. 98,* 301–313.
Powell, J., Duell, E. and Voorhees, J. (1971) Beta adrenergic stimulation of endogenous epidermal cyclic AMP formation. *Arch. Dermatol. 104,* 359–365.
Prottey, C. (1977) Investigation of functions of essential fatty acids in the skin. *Br. J. Dermatol. 97,* 29–38.

Radmark, O., Malmsten, C. and Samuelsson, B. (1980a) Leukotriene A: isolation from human polymorphonuclear leukocytes. *J. Biochem. 255,* 11828–11831.

Radmark, O., Malmsten, C. and Samuelsson, B. (1980b) Leukotriene A: stereochemistry and enzymatic conversion to leukotriene B. *Biochem. Biophys. Res. Commun. 92,* 954–961.

Radmark, O., Malmsten, C. and Samuelsson, B. (1980c) Leukotriene A_4: enzymatic conversion to leukotriene C_4. *Biochem. Biophys. Res. Commun. 96,* 1679–1687.

Rusin, L.J., Duell, E.A. and Voorhees, J.J. (1978) Papaverine and Ro. 20-1724 inhibit cyclic nucleotide phosphodiesterase activity and increase cyclic AMP levels in psoriatic epidermis in vitro. *J. Invest. Dermatol. 71,* 154–156.

Saihan, E., Albano, J. and Burton, J. (1980) The effect of steroid and dithranol therapy on cyclic nucleotides in psoriatic epidermis. *Br. J. Dermatol. 102,* 565–569.

Samuelsson, B. and Paolette, R. (Eds) (1976) *Advances in Prostaglandin and Thromboxane Research, Vol. 1,* Raven Press, New York.

Samuelsson, B., Borgeat, P., Hammarstrom, S. and Murphy, R. (1979) Introduction of a nomenclature: leukotrienes. *Prostaglandins 17,* 785–787.

Samuelsson, B., Borgeat, P., Hammarstrom, S. and Murphy, R. (1980) Leukotrienes: a new group of biologically active compounds. In: B. Samuelsson, P. Ramwell, and R. Paoletti (Eds), *Advances in Prostaglandin and Thromboxane Research,* Raven Press, New York, pp. 1–18.

Sauder, D., Bailin, P., Sundeen, J., Randall, M. and Krakauer, S. (1980) Suppressor cell function in psoriasis. *Arch. Dermatol. 116,* 51–55.

Sedgwick, J., Bergstresser, P. and Hurd, E. (1981) Increased superoxide generation by normal granulocytes incubated in sera from patients with psoriasis. *J. Invest. Dermatol. 76,* 158–163.

Siegel, M., McConnell, R. and Cuatrecasas, P. (1979) Aspirin-like drugs interfere with arachidonate metabolism by inhibition of the 12-hydroperoxy-5,8,10,14-eicosatetraenoic acid peroxidase activity of the lipoxygenase pathway. *Proc. Natl Acad. Sci. USA 76,* 3774–3778.

Siegel, M., McConnell, R., Porter, N. and Cuatrecasas, P. (1980) Arachidonic metabolism via lipoxygenase and 12-L-hydroperoxy-5,8,10,14-eicosatetraenoic acid peroxidase sensitive to anti-inflammatory drugs. *Proc. Natl Acad. Sci. USA 77,* 308–312.

Simchowitz, L., Fischbein, L., Spilberg, I. and Atkinson, J. (1980) Induction of a transient elevation in intracellular levels of adenosine-3′,5′-cyclic monophosphate by chemotactic factors: an early event in human neutrophil activation. *J. Immunol. 124,* 1482–1491.

Smolen, J., Korchak, H. and Weissmann, G. (1979) Increased levels of cyclic adenosine-3′,5′-monophosphate in human polymorphonuclear leukocytes after surface stimulation. *J. Clin. Invest. 65,* 1077–1085.

Snyderman, R. and Goetzl, E. (1981) Molecular and cellular mechanisms of leukocyte chemotaxis. *Science 213,* 830–837.

Spitzer, G., Verma, D., Barlogie, B., Beran, M. and Dicke, A. (1979) Possible mechanisms of action of lithium on augmentation of in vitro spontaneous myeloid colony formation. *Cancer Res. 39,* 3215–3219.

Stankler, L. (1977) Histological findings in clinically normal palmar skin of patients with psoriasis. *Br. J. Dermatol. 97,* 131–134.

Stawiski, M., Powell, J., Lang, P., Schork, A., Duell, E. and Voorhees, J. (1975) Papaverine: its effects on cyclic AMP in vitro and psoriasis in vivo. *J. Invest. Dermatol. 64,* 124–127.

Stenson, W. and Parker, C. (1980) Monohydroxyeicosatetraenoic acids (HETEs) induce degranulation of human neutrophils. *J. Immunol. 124,* 2100–2104.

Stenson, W., Parker, C. and Sulivan, T. (1980) Augmentation of IgE-mediated release of histamine by 5-hydroxyeicosatetraenoic acid and 12-hydroxyeicosatetraenoic acid. *Biochem. Biophys. Res. Commun. 96,* 1045–1052.

Tagami, H. and Ofuji, S. (1977) Characterization of a leukotactic factor derived from psoriatic scale. *Br. J. Dermatol. 97,* 509–518.

Thomas, C., Yost, F., Snyderman, R., Hatcher, V. and Lazarus, G. (1977) Cellular serine proteinase induces chemotaxis by complement activation. *Nature (London) 269,* 521–522.

Tong, P. and Marcelo, C. (1981) Protein synthesis and keratin disulfide cross-linking in epidermal cell cultures and induction of differentiation by 8-bromoadenosine 3′,5′-cyclic monophosphoic acid (8-BrcAMP). *Clin. Res. 29,* 790A.

Voorhees, J., Chakrabarti, S. and Bernstein, I. (1968) The metabolism of "histidine-rich" protein in normal and psoriatic keratinization. *J. Invest. Dermatol. 51,* 344–354.

Voorhees, J., Duell, E., Bass, L., Powell, J. and Harrell, R. (1972a) The cyclic AMP system in normal and psoriatic epidermis. *J. Invest. Dermatol. 59,* 114–120.

Voorhees, J., Duell, E. and Kelsey, W. (1972b) Dibutyryl cyclic AMP inhibition of epidermal cell division. *Arch. Dermatol. 105,* 384–386.

Voorhees, J., Duell, E., Bass, L., Powell, J. and Harrell, E. (1972c) Decreased cyclic AMP in the epidermis of lesions of psoriasis. *Arch. Dermatol. 105,* 695–701.

Voorhees, J., Kelsey, W., Stawiski, M., Smith, E., Duell, E., Haddox, M. and Goldberg, N. (1973) Increased cyclic GMP and decreased cyclic AMP levels in the rapidly proliferating epithelium of psoriasis. In: Schultz J. and Gratzner H.G. (Eds), *The Role of Cyclic Nucleotides in Carcinogenesis,* Academic Press, New York, pp. 325–371.

Wadskov, S. and Sondergaard, J. (1978) Determination of cyclic AMP in heat-separated human epidermal tissue. *Acta Derm. Venereol. 58,* 191–195.

Wadskov, S., Kassis, V. and Sondergaard, J. (1979) Cyclic AMP and psoriasis once more. *Acta Derm. Venereol. 59,* 525–559.

Wahba, A., Cohen, H., Bar-Eli, M. and Gallily, R. (1978) Enhanced chemotactic and phagocytic activities of leukocytes in psoriasis vulgaris. *J. Invest. Dermatol. 71,* 186–188.

Ward, P. and Becker, E. (1968) The deactivation of rabbit neutrophils by chemotactic factor and the nature of the activatable esterase. *J. Exp. Med. 127,* 693–709.

Watson, W., Cann, H.M., Farber, E. and Hall, M.L. (1971) The genetics of psoriasis. *Arch. Dermatol. 105,* 197–207.

Wedmore, C. and Williams, T. (1981) Control of vascular permeability by polymorphonuclear leukocytes in inflammation. *Nature (London) 289,* 646–650.

Weinstein, G.D. and McCullough, J.L. (1973) Cytokinetics in diseases of epidermal hyperplasia. *Ann. Rev. Med. 24,* 345–352.

Wiley, H. and Weinstein, G. (1979) Abnormal proliferation of uninvolved psoriatic epidermis: differential induction by saline, propranolol, and tape stripping in vivo. *J. Invest. Dermatol. 73,* 545–547.

Wilkinson, D. and Walsh, J. (1977) Prostaglandin biosynthesis in the epidermis and dermis of young mouse skin, and the effects of calcium and cyclic nucleotides. *J. Invest. Dermatol. 68,* 210–214.

Williams, T. and Peck, M. (1977) Role of prostaglandin-mediated vasodilation in inflammation. *Nature (London) 270,* 530–532.

Winkelmann, R. (1971) Molecular inflammation of the skin. *J. Invest. Dermatol. 57,* 197–208.

Woodrow, J.D., Dave, V.K., Usher, N. and Anderson, J. (1975) The HL-A system and psoriasis. *Br. J. Dermatol. 92,* 427–435.

Yoshikawa, K., Adachi, K., Halprin, K. and Levine, V. (1975a) The effects of catecholamine and related compounds on the adenyl cyclase system in the epidermis. *Br. J. Dermatol 93,* 29–36.

Yoshikawa, K., Adachi, I., Halprin, K. and Levine, V. (1975b) On the lack of response to catecholamine stimulation by the adenyl cyclase system in psoriatic lesions. *Br. J. Dermatol. 92,* 619–624.

Ziboh, V. (1973) Biosynthesis of prostaglandin E_2 in human skin: subcellular localization and inhibition by unsaturated fatty acids and anti-inflammatory drugs. *J. Lipid Res. 14,* 377–384.

Ziboh, V. and Blank, H. (1973) Die Rolle der Prostaglandine in der Haut. *Hautarzt 24,* 519–522.

Ziboh, V. and Lord, J. (1979) Phospholipase A activity in the skin: modulators of arachidonic acid release from phosphatidylcholine. *Biochem. J. 184,* 283–290.

Ziboh, V., Marcelo, C. and Voorhees, J. (1981) Induced lipoxygenation of arachidonic acid in mouse epidermal keratinocytes by calcium ionophore. *Clin. Res. 29,* 619A.

Ziboh, V., Casebol, T.T., Marcelo, C. and Voorhees, J. (1983a) Lipoxygenation of arachidonic acid by subcellular preparations from murine keratinocytes. *Clin. Res. 31,* 152A.

Ziboh, V., Casebol, T.T., Marcelo, C. and Voorhees, J. (1983b) Enhancement of 5-lipoxygenase activity in soluble preparations of human psoriatic plague. *J. Invest. Dermatol. 80,* 359.

CHAPTER 7

Chemotaxis in non-leukocytic cells

JAMES VARANI
Department of Pathology, University of Michigan Medical School
Ann Arbor, Michigan

and

F. WILLIAM ORR
Department of Pathology, University of Manitoba School of Medicine
Winnipeg, Manitoba, Canada

7.1. INTRODUCTION

Active cell motility occurs in a variety of biological processes. Well-known examples include fertilization (spermatozoa); embryonic development (whole germ layers, neural crest cells, lymphoid cells); wound healing and tissue repair (fibroblasts, epithelial cells, endothelial cells); inflammation (leukocytes, lymphocytes) and tumor cell invasion and metastasis (tumor cells of various types). Cell motility does not occur in an unregulated manner in any of these processes. Rather, the movement of cells is under the influence of several broad categories of regulatory factors. Factors have been identified which stimulate motility in quiescent cells. Other factors inhibit the movement of moving cells. In addition to factors which turn cell movement on or off, there are factors which influence the direction in which cell movement will occur. Contact inhibition of movement, contact guidance, haptotaxis and chemotaxis are all terms that describe the regulation of the directional movement of cells.

This review will discuss the regulation of directional motility in various non-leukocytic cells and suggest how this might influence the biological behavior of the cells in vivo. While most of the information to be discussed will focus on the process of chemotaxis, the review will not be strictly limited to it. The regulation of locomotion in leukocytes will not be covered here simply because so much has already been written about it and a recent good review is available (Snyderman and Goetzl 1981). Nonetheless, other cell types are invariably compared to leukocytes. In this context, pertinent findings relative to control of leukocyte motility will be considered. It should be pointed out that most of our understanding of the regulation of cell motility is derived from in-vitro studies. The significance of these findings to the regulation of cell motility in vivo can, for the most part, only be inferred. Nevertheless, recent studies suggest that these same regulatory mechanisms may play very important roles in vivo.

7.2. CELL MOTILITY IN VITRO

Cell motility has been observed in culture since the time that isolated cells were first established on glass. In spite of the fact that we still do not have a complete understanding of the mechanics involved, continued investigation has shed light on many essential features of the process. Translocation by most mammalian cell types (and indeed most eukaryotic cells) occurs as a result of the cell "pulling" itself over the surface of a substrate, rather than by swimming freely, as do bacteria and certain types of protozoa.

The fact that the cells move in contact with a solid surface insures, therefore, that the processes of cell-substrate adhesiveness and cell motility will be intimately linked. Indeed, nearly all of the factors that can be shown to alter the motility of cells in culture also affect the adhesiveness of the cells. The role of adhesiveness in the regulation of cell movement will be discussed in some detail later in this review. The ability of the cells to migrate over the substrate implies a continued making and breaking of cell-substrate contacts. In addition to this, there is the necessity for a locomotory apparatus capable of converting the chemical energy produced by the cell into mechanical energy. It is not the aim of this review to cover the voluminous literature on how cell movement occurs. Suffice it to say, however, that the finding of nearly all of the contractile proteins of muscle cells in various, non-muscle cell types (Lazarides and Weber 1974; Weber and Gröschel-Stewart 1974; Lazarides 1975; Lazarides and Burridge 1975; Isenberg et al. 1976) has led to the widespread belief that cell movements in non-muscle cells occur in the same way as in muscle cell (i.e. with energy generated by actin–myosin interaction). Information on how cells move can be found in recent reviews and chapters (Dunn 1980; Stossel 1978).

A variety of methodologies have been used to study cell motility in vitro. Included among these are the fragment culture technique (Abercrombie and Heaysman 1953), the wound culture technique (Burk 1973), the agarose assay (Carpenter 1963; Varani et al. 1978), and the Boyden Chamber micropore filter assay (Kreutzer et al. 1978). The first three of these assays are similar in that each measures cell migration in two dimensions across the surface of a culture dish. In the fragment culture technique pieces of tissue are allowed to attach to the surface of the dish and cells migrate out from the tissue fragment over the surface. The agarose assay is similar but instead of using a tissue fragment, a single-cell suspension of cells is centrifuged into a pellet in agarose. Drops of agarose containing the cells are placed on the dish and cells migrate out from the agarose. In the wound culture technique a monolayer of cells is traumatized so as to remove the cells from a small area. As a result of this denuding process, cells at the periphery of the wound migrate over the open space and repopulate the area. These techniques have all proved useful in studying various aspects of the motility response. A schematic view of the agarose assay is depicted in Figure 1. The type of data obtained with this assay is shown in Figures 2 and 3.

In contrast to the above techniques, which measure cell migration in two dimensions across the surface of a culture dish, the Boyden Chamber technique measures the migration of cells into the pores of micropore filters. This technique has been widely used in studies of leukocyte chemotaxis and has also been used in the study of random and chemotactic motility of non-leukocytic cells. In this technique a suspension of cells is placed on the upper surface of a micropore filter. Commercially available filters made from nitrocellulose, cellulose acetate or polycarbonate have all been used. The cells migrate into the pores of the filters and after an appropriate length of time, the filters are stained; the number of migrating cells is counted and the

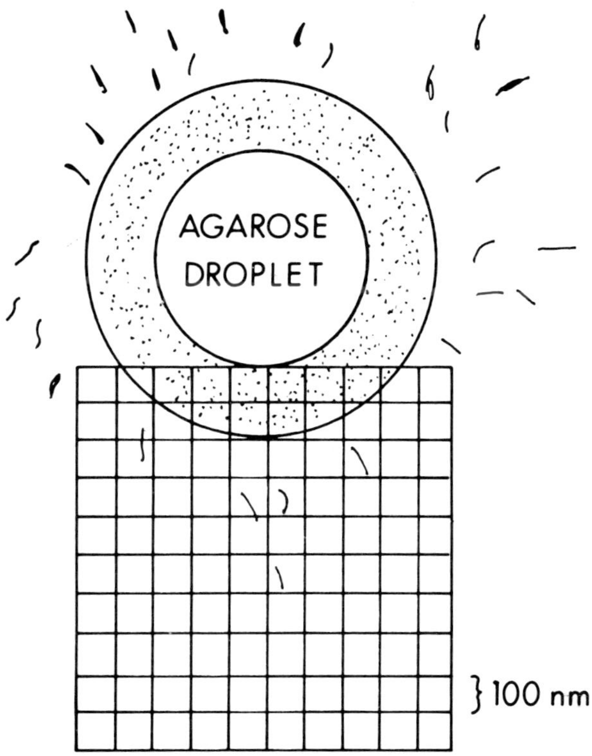

Fig. 1. Schematic diagram of the agarose assay. When examined with an inverted microscope the central agarose droplet is seen surrounded by a corona of cells which have migrated outward from the central focus. Individual cells which have migrated beyond the corona can also be seen.

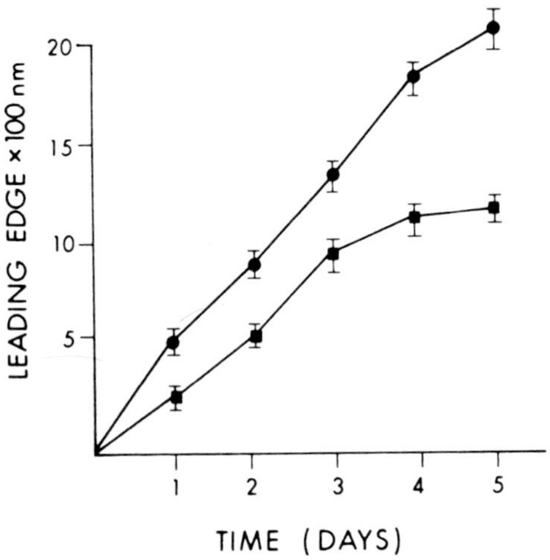

Fig. 2. Cell migration can be quantitated by placing a calibrated grid in the eyepiece of the microscope and measuring the distance from the edge of the agarose droplet to the leading edge of cell migration. The dots represent the distance migrated by a population of normal fibroblasts; they have migrated a greater distance per unit of time than a corresponding population of murine fibrosarcoma cells (squares).

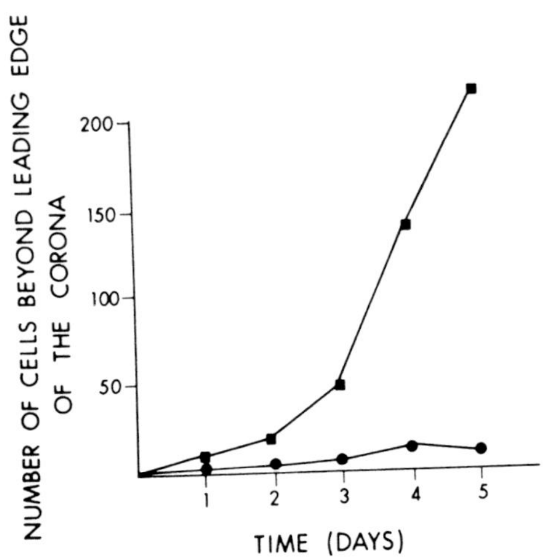

Fig. 3. The number of cells migrating beyond the corona can also be counted. In contrast to what is seen in Fig. 2, a much larger number of fibrosarcoma cells than fibroblasts migrate beyond the corona. See for details Varani et al. (1978).

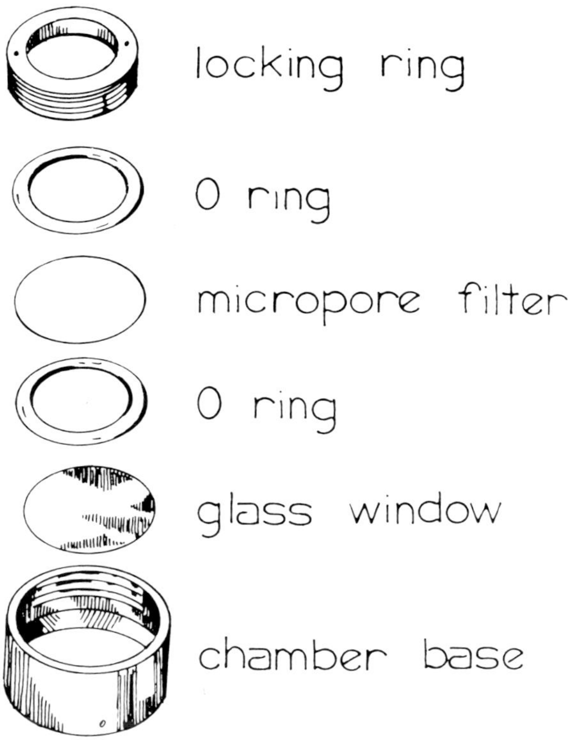

Fig. 4. Diagrammatic representation of a modified Boyden Chamber routinely used to measure chemotaxis. When fully assembled, a micropore filter separates the chamber into an upper and lower compartment. The lower compartment is filled with isotonic buffer containing the chemotactic factor. The upper compartment contains the identical buffer but without the chemotactic factor and a concentration gradient is formed as the chemotactic factor diffuses across the filter. Cells are added to the upper compartment and allowed to settle onto the upper surface of the micropore filter. The cells migrate into the pores of the filter. After a period of time, the filters are stained and the number of cells migrating (as well as the distance migrated) is determined.

distance migrated is measured. In the micropore filter assay, the cells must squeeze through very small pores in the filters. Therefore, cell deformability, along with the other properties governing cell migration, is important in this technique.

Because the filters are arranged in such a way as to separate two fluid-filled compartments, it is possible to establish a concentration gradient by the addition of appropriate diffusable substances to one side of the membrane. This produces a situation in which chemotactic migration (as opposed to random migration) can be assessed. Indeed, the difference in migration of a group of cells in two parallel

Boyden Chambers (one of which has a chemotactic factor added to it and the other which has none) is the basis on which the chemotactic response is evaluated. A schematic diagram of a modified Boyden Chamber is shown in Figure 4. Cell migration in the Boyden Chamber assay is shown in Figures 5 and 6.

A characteristic of many chemotactic factors is that they stimulate random migratory activity in addition to chemotaxis (Zigmond and Hirsch 1973). It is necessary, therefore, to separate these two effects. This can be done by systematically varying the concentrations of the putative chemotactic factor on both sides of the micropore filter and analyzing the effects on cell migration. If the factor stimulates random migration, there will be an increased movement of cells into the filters as the concentration of the factor is increased. This will occur regardless of whether the factor is added to the top half of the chamber (along with the cells) or to the bottom half of the chamber (distal to the cells). If the factor is chemotactic, maximum stimulation will occur when the factor is added to the bottom half of the chamber, since this establishes a concentration gradient across the membrane. Since

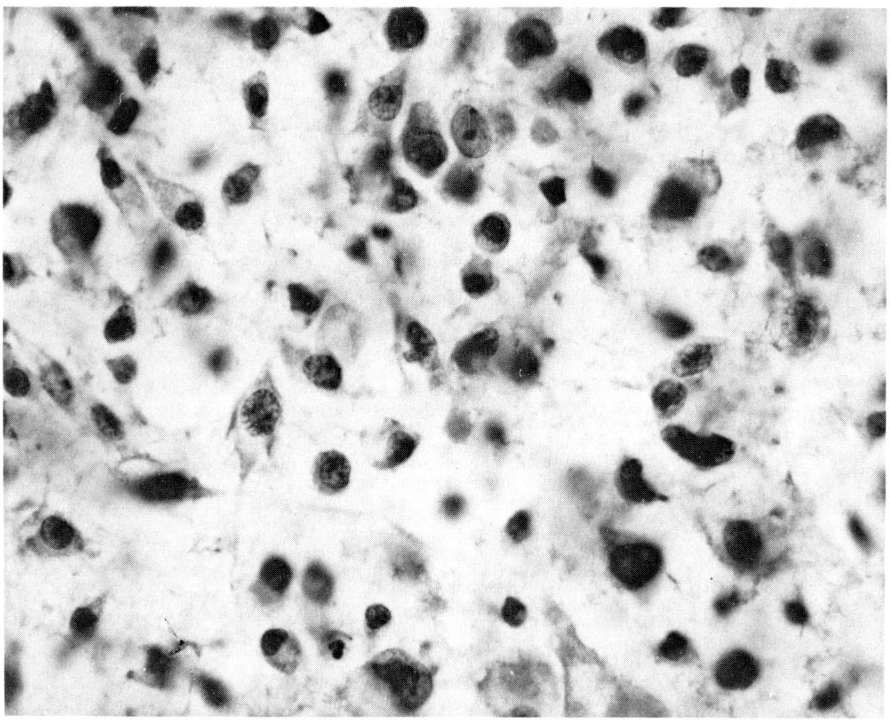

Fig. 5. Walker 256 carcinosarcoma cells attached to the upper surface of the micropore filter.

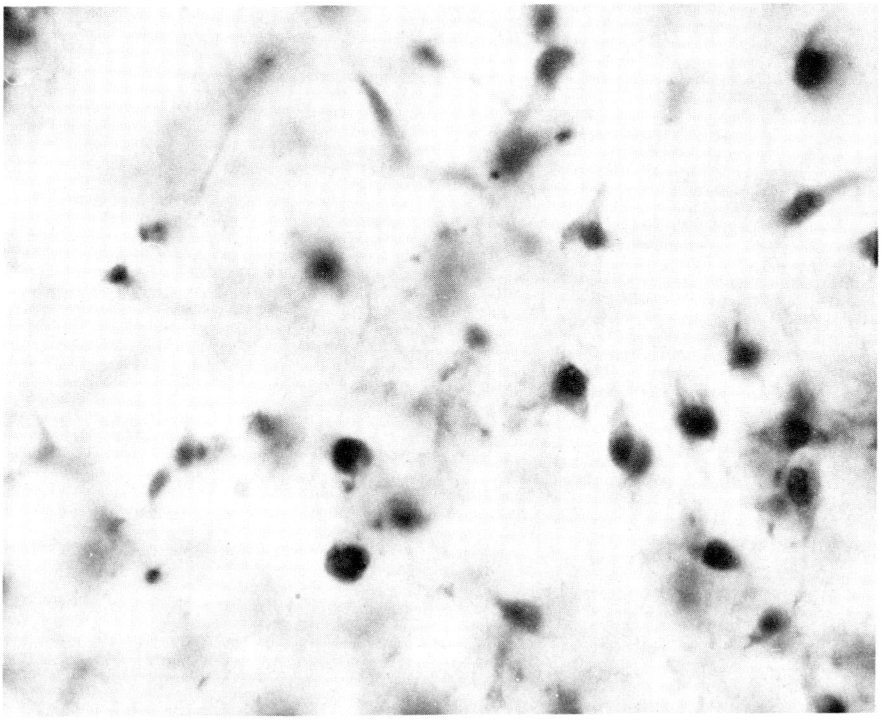

Fig. 6. Walker 256 carcinosarcoma cells which have migrated 25 μm into the pores of the filter. Approximately 18 cells are located at this level in the photograph. See Orr et al. (1978) for details.

many chemotactic factors also enhance random migration, what is normally observed is that maximum stimulation occurs when the factor is added to the bottom half of the chamber but, in addition, some stimulation of movement is also observed when the factor is added to the top half of the chamber or when it is added to both compartments.

Conventional application of the Boyden Chamber or agarose assays analyzes the mass movements of large populations of cells. However, by coupling these methods with transmission electron microscopy or scanning electron microscopy it is possible to study the effect of a chemoattractant on the structure of single cells (Malech et al. 1977; Nelson et al. 1976). This approach has provided information concerning the effects of chemotactic gradients on cell shape, cytoskeletal organization and exocytosis. Another means for examining the action of chemotactic gradients on single living cells is to generate the gradient across the surface of a microscope slide which can be examined by time-lapse photography (Zigmond 1977). This method has been used to examine the orientation of cells in chemotactic gradients and to study the separate cationic requirements for leukocyte orientation and locomotion (Marasco et al. 1980).

7.3. CHEMOTACTIC RESPONSES IN BIOLOGICAL SYSTEMS

7.3.1. Fertilization

Spermatozoan motility, one of the most dramatic forms of movement in mammalian cells, is essential for the passage of sperm cells through the cervical mucus, their entry into the oviduct and finally, their penetration of the corona radiata to fertilize the ovum (Tampion and Gibbons 1963; Blandau and Rumery 1964; Yanagimachi 1966). Unlike the other cell types described in this review, whose motility depend largely on actin and myosin based cytoskeletel microfilaments, the movement of sperm is a function of the tubulin and dynein-based microtubular axoneme which makes up the sperm tail. Despite this basic difference in the machinery of movement, it seems likely that the control of movement may be similar, at least in certain respects.

Subjective assessments of sperm movement are difficult, largely because of very rapid beating of the sperm tail (~10 times/second) and the corresponding velocities of cell movement (60 μm/second) (Katz and Overstreet 1979). Nevertheless, the direct microscopic examination of sperm remains the standard means in clinical practice for evaluating the percentage of motile cells and their direction of movement. More precise measurements of movement are now possible through the use of computer-assisted microscopy (for example, see Atherton et al. 1978).

The acquisition of the capability for sustained movement in a forward direction appears to be the consequence of maturation in the epididymis. Testicular sperm and those in the head of the epididymis are immobile or exhibit a thrashing movement in a circular fashion, while those in the tail of the epididymis or vas deferens exhibit persistent, directional movement associated with a characteristic reduction in tail flexibility (Fray et al. 1972; Bedford et al. 1973; Bedford 1975). What factors in the epididymal microenvironment are responsible for maturation has not been determined. The enzyme, neutral α-glucosidase may be one such epididymal factor, as its absence from seminal plasma is correlated with defective motility (Tremblay et al. 1979). Carnitine and acetylcarnitine are vitamin-like putative epididymal control factors (Tanphaichitr 1977; Casillas and Erickson 1975).

In vitro, a number of agents are capable of modulating spermatozoan motility. Stimulation of forward motility has been obtained by the addition of methyl xanthine or by the direct addition of cAMP. This suggests a role for cyclic nucleotides, possibly via activation of cAMP-dependent protein kinase and/or the phosphorylation of regulatory proteins (Schoenfeld et al. 1975; Haskins and Casillas 1975; Lindemann 1980). L-arginine and kallikrein also cause enhancement of sperm movement in vitro, the latter possibly by liberation of the pharmacologically active peptide kallidin from seminal kininogen (Schill 1975; Schill et al. 1979).

To what extent is the movement of sperm random and to what extent is it directed? Do spermatozoa actively seek out the ovum in response to a factor(s) released by the female gamete? The answer to these questions is unknown but recent studies suggest the fascinating possibility that, like many other free moving cells, sperm are able to sense and respond to gradients of specific chemotactic signals in their environment. Using an assay in which sperm moved from a buffered suspension into a capillary tube placed into the suspension, Vijayasarathy et al. (1980) and Lqbal et al. (1980) have shown that synthetic peptide chemoattractants caused an increased movement in bull sperm and also induced the release of acrosomal enzymes. As with leukocytes, various formyl peptides were active as chemoattractants while the corresponding t-butyloxycarbamyl peptides were inactive. The specific amino acid sequence did not appear important but studies with a panel of different peptides indicated that the presence of three consecutive hydrophobic residues was critical to the ability of the sperm to sense the attractant. These observations raise the possibility of specific membrane—ligand interactions, i.e. a chemotactic receptor on sperm, although this has not been proven formally.

Many questions remain to be answered. The nature of the naturally occurring chemoattractants (if these exist) has not been determined. If spermatozoa do respond to chemoattractants released by ova, the molecular mechanisms controlling these responses will require elucidation. For example, an intriguing problem will be to determine the means by which the sperm cells sense the chemotactic concentration gradient and orient themselves within it. The molecular mechanisms linking the chemoreceptors to the microtubular axoneme will require definition also. If sperm are proved to be chemotactically responsive cells, they will provide another example of a biological system in which invasive properties, conferred by directional movement and release of degradative enzymes, are under the influence of specific chemical messages present in the cellular environment.

7.3.2. Embryologic development of dorsal root ganglia

The direction of the various cell migrations which occur during embryogenesis are remarkably reproducible from one individual to the next. The mechanisms which control these movements can be related to intrinsic cellular properties, as for example, specializations of the cell surface, and to features in the extracellular environment such as the connective tissue matrix or factors present in the extracellular fluid.

The innervation of peripheral tissues, which depends upon the embryonic outgrowth of axons from dorsal root ganglia is one example of such coordinated growth. The importance to axonal development of relationships between the external substrate and the neurone is illustrated by variation observed in the numbers of axons exhibiting growth and the rate of elongation when neurons are cultured on plastic or agar surfaces (Letourneau 1975). Furthermore, it has been shown that the direction of neurite growth can be guided by contact with an aligned collagen matrix (Ebendal 1976). The outgrowth of axons from dorsal root and sympathetic ganglia is also promoted by trophic or growth-promoting factors, among them Nerve Growth Factor. This is a 13,250 dalton subunit of a larger (130,000 dalton) protein complex which maintains neuronal viability, enhances axonal outgrowth, and stimulates differentiation in vitro (reviewed by Mobley et al. 1977). In vitro, extension of nerve fibers from explanted ganglia is directed towards pieces of tissue innervated by these ganglia (Chamley and Dowel 1975; Ebendal and Jacobson 1977) or towards capillary tubes containing Nerve Growth Factor (Ebendal and Jacobson 1977), and it has therefore been postulated that chemotactic mechanisms may be involved in the control of neuronal outgrowth but early experiments have not examined the directional nature of these responses or the effects of concentration gradients. More recent studies provide direct evidence that nerve growth factor is able to guide both the direction of growth in addition to causing an enhanced growth rate. The most dramatic evidence is seen in the work of Gundersen and Barrett (1979, 1980), who found that 100% of chick embryo dorsal root growth cones turned and grew towards a localized source of nerve growth factor within 9 to 21 minutes of initiating a gradient. Lateral displacement of 5−30 μm (3.3 ± 0.2 degrees/minute) was accompanied by an increase in the number of microspikes and lamellipodia on the sides of the growth cones proximal, but not distal, to the nerve growth factor gradient. The turning response, effected by moving the point source of the nerve growth factor gradient, was not associated with an increased rate of growth as control axons did not demonstrate turning or significant lateral displacement and both grew at the same rate. Nor did the patterns of neurite initiation at the nerve cell body or survival appear to be altered by the presence of the gradient. Other proteins (fetal calf serum or bovine albumin) did not initiate the turning response and neurites which do not require nerve growth factor in vivo or in vitro for growth and survival (spinal cord neurones) did not exhibit a turning response under the experimental conditions. In these experiments the trophic and growth-promoting effects of nerve growth factor were exemplified by the necessity for uniform low concentrations in order to demonstrate the gradient-induced response.

In other experiments, Letourneau (1978) has demonstrated the orientation of circa 60% of growing nerve fiber tips towards increasing concentrations of nerve growth factor in agar gels. This was in contrast to circa 50% orientation observed in the absence of a gradient. More fibers extended towards the increasing concentration of nerve growth factor than away from it and the average distance fibers extended up the gradient was greater than distances down. The orientation of the point of axonal initiation on the nerve cell body did not appear to be under the influence of the nerve growth factor gradient.

The mechanisms responsible for the chemotactic response in nerve fiber extension have not been studied extensively. Both high and low affinity receptors for nerve growth factor have been reported on cells from sympathetic and sensory ganglia

(Sutter et al. 1977) and may exist on nerve tips (Campenot 1977). It is not known whether the trophic and chemotactic actions of nerve growth factor can be related to functions of these separate receptors. Cyclic nucleotides may be involved in the chemotactic response of neurite tips since dorsal root neurites will turn towards point sources of the lipid-soluble cAMP analogues, mono- and dibutyryl-cAMP or towards 1 mmol cGMP, or phosphodiesterase inhibitors including caffein and theophylline. A role for calcium also seems possible since, in the presence of the calcium ionophore A23187, growth cones turned towards a 20 mM point source of calcium, suggesting that the turning response could be related to local increase in internal calcium, such as that caused by a calcium influx. The response could also depend upon release of intracellular calcium stores since it can be observed in medium depleted of calcium but is blocked by the addition of dantrolene, an agent which reduces the release of calcium from intracellular stores in skeletal muscle (Gundersen and Barrett 1980).

As observed in other chemotactically responsive cell types, e.g. leukocytes (O'Flaherty et al. 1978b) and tumor cells (Varani et al. 1981b; Varani and Fantone 1982), agents which initiate or modify the chemotactic response (in this case nerve growth factor, cyclic nucleotides, and calcium) appear able to modulate adherence of the responsive cell (growth cone) to the adjacent substrate. It has been observed (Letourneau 1975) that large relative increases in the adhesion of growth cones to the substratum can guide the direction of neurite growth. However, in the case of the neurite, simple correlations between adhesion of the entire growth cone and turning do not appear to exist (Gundersen and Barrett 1980), suggesting that the mechanisms involved in the turning response are not related entirely to alterations in adherence of the growth cone to the substrate. Differential increases in growth cone adhesion, related to formation of microspikes on the side of the cone proximal to the stimulus, could be one mechanism for guiding neurite growth. One way in which this could occur is via tension generated in the filopodia on the proximal side of the growth cone. As in other cells, this would likely depend upon coordinated function of the cytoskeletal components of these processes.

In cultures of spinal ganglia, Krystosek and Seeds (1981) have noted plasminogen activator release around neuronal growth cones. These workers postulate that the release of this enzyme could facilitate localized tissue remodeling and invasion of these tissues by the growing axon. It is interesting to speculate that the release of this enzyme could be under the influence of chemotactic signals, leading to membrane shedding, potentiated by the formation and movement of microspikes during chemotaxis.

7.3.3. Tissue repair

In any significant tissue injury or inflammatory process, damage occurs to a variety of structures. The repair process which follows therefore, involves the coordinated efforts of several cell types. Parenchymal cells (in various internal organs), epithelial cells, fibroblasts, smooth muscle cells and endothelial cells all undergo activation during the repair process. Activation involves at least three distinct components: cell proliferation, migration and differentiation. Cell migration is prominent during wound healing. Epithelial cells migrate in sheets to close surface wounds. Beneath the surface, fibroblasts migrate into the connective tissue. The neovascularization process involves active migration of endothelial and smooth muscle cells. Because cell proliferation is going on simultaneously with cell migration, it is sometimes difficult to determine whether the repopulation of cells at the injured site is due mainly to active migration or due to the pressure exerted by the increasing number of cells as a result of proliferation. However, the effects of cell migration can be clearly distinguished when proliferation is prevented by irradiation or other means (Sholley et al. 1977; Thorgeirsson and Robertson 1978a, b). Wound healing occurs under these conditions although its progress may be delayed somewhat (Thorgeirsson et al. 1979).

7.3.3.1. Fibroblasts

Although each cell type must do its job during tissue repair, the fibroblasts play a particularly important role. While they are few in number and for the most part quiescent in normal, uninjured connective tissue, the response to inflammation and tissue injury results in the active migration of fibroblasts to the site of injury, the proliferation of these cells at the site and the laying down of new collagen and other connective tissue components which will constitute the scar tissue (Van Winkle 1967). The mechanism(s) by which these processes are regulated is the subject of much current research — not only because of its relevance to normal, physiological repair processes but also because of its possible involvement in conditions in which fibroblast activation occurs in an unchecked form. A hyperactivation of fibroblasts may account for some of the damage seen in conditions such as pulmonary fibrosis (Kravis et al. 1976), *Mycobacterium tuberculosis* and *Schistosoma mansoni* granulomas (Poole 1970; Cheever 1965) and Arthus type inflammatory lesions (Cochrane and Janoff 1974). In some persons, hyperactive repair processes can result in the formation of keloid scars and possibly low-grade fibromatoses such as desmoid tumors.

The accumulation of fibroblasts at tissue injury sites may occur as a result of the chemotactic attraction of cells to the site. Recent studies by Postlethwaite and his colleagues have shown that fibroblasts are capable of responding by chemotaxis to a variety of unrelated factors that may be present at the site of tissue injury. Among these are a factor obtained from lymphocytes during the process of transformation (Postlethwaite et al. 1976; Postlethwaite and Kang, 1980), collagen and collagen-derived peptides (Postlethwaite et al. 1978), a complement factor (Postlethwaite et al. 1979) and fibronectin (Postlethwaite et al. 1980). The lymphocyte-derived factor was the first to be described. It could be isolated from the culture supernatant fluid of phytohemagglutinin (PHA)-stimulated and streptokinase/streptodornase-stimulated mononuclear cells. The production of chemotactic activity was correlated (in terms of the amount produced as well as the time sequence of production) directly with the degree of the lymphocyte response to stimulation (as indicated by thymidine uptake). In addition, lymphocytes from tuberculin-positive individuals (but not lymphocytes from tuberculin-negative individuals) produced the fibroblast chemotactic factor upon stimulation with purified protein derivative. Population enrichment studies indicated that T-lymphocytes were the cells that elaborated the factor but that production was dependent on the presence of macrophages. Gel filtration studies indicated that the chemotactic factor had a molecular weight of 22,000 daltons and was proteinaceous in nature. In a later study (Postlethwaite and Kang 1980), a chemotactic factor for guinea pig fibroblasts was identified in the culture supernatant fluids of stimulated guinea pig lymphocytes. In many respects the chemotactic factor obtained from guinea pig lymphocytes was similar to the one obtained from the human lymphocytes.

Native Types I, II and III collagen were later identified as being chemotactic for the same human fibroblast cells (Postlethwaite et al. 1978). In addition to the intact molecules, the constituent α-chains as well as collagenolytic breakdown products and synthetic peptides with amino acids sequences common to collagen were also chemotactic. The fact that small collagen fragments as well as the intact molecule could induce the chemotactic response suggests that the cells may recognize a very small, highly specific portion of the collagen molecule. Unlike many chemotactic factors, the collagen peptides apparently do not enhance random migration because when they were added to both sides of the micropore filter in the chemotaxis assay, no enhancement of motility over baseline values was observed. It was interesting that either Type I, II or III collagen added to the upper chamber completely inhibited the cells from responding to any of the collagen types. This suggests that all of the collagen types act on the cells at a common point. In contrast, the lymphocyte-derived chemotactic factor, when added to the upper chamber, did not alter the cellular response to any of the collagen types.

The complement proteins were later identified as a third source of chemotactic factors for fibroblasts (Postlethwaite et al. 1979). This is of interest because of the fact that these proteins are a source of chemotactic factor for various leukocytic and non-leukocytic cell types (Ward and Cochrane 1965; Romualdez and Ward 1975). The fifth complement component (C5) was the most likely source of the activity. The chemotactic activity could be inhibited by antibodies to human C5 and the activity could not be generated in C5-deficient human serum. The C5-derived fibroblast chemotactic factor has a molecular weight of about 80,000 daltons as estimated by gel filtration and is clearly distinguishable from the much smaller leukocyte and tumor cell chemotactic factors derived from C5 (Romualdez et al. 1976; Orr et al. 1978). However, it is possible that all of the C5-derived chemotactic factors contain the same small sequence of amino acids at their active site. It was interesting that the complement-derived fibroblast chemotactic factors induced random as well as chemotactic migration; this was in contrast to both the lymphocyte-derived chemotactic factor and the collagen peptides.

Fibroblasts accumulate at sites of inflammatory reactions having diverse etiologies. It is tempting to speculate that they are drawn to these lesions as a result of chemotactic factor production at the site. In antigen–antibody induced inflammation, fibroblast accumulation could occur as a result of complement activation. In granulomatous lesions, the lymphocyte-derived factor may play the same role. In conditions such as pulmonary fibrosis, where collagen turnover is occurring more rapidly than normal, it is possible that the collagen molecules themselves or collagen breakdown products serve as the stimulus to attract additional fibroblasts to the site. Furthermore, the classic fibrotic disease states themselves may be the result of immunologic mechanisms (Kravis et al. 1976). Thus, it is likely that the lymphocyte-derived and complement-derived chemotactic factor could be generated in these lesions as well.

An interesting question that remains unanswered is the relationship between the stimulation of fibroblast migration and stimulation of other fibroblast functions. Do the chemotactic factors stimulate proliferation? Do they stimulate the synthesis of collagen and other connective tissue components? It is not unreasonable to suspect that they might, since studies with leukocytes (Kreutzer et al. 1978) and with a variety of tumor cell types (Varani 1982) have shown that chemotactic factors induce a number of functions in addition to stimulating motility. Whether or not activation of fibroblasts by chemotactic factors leads to a number of responses in addition to stimulating motility, it is known that lymphokine-rich supernatants of stimulated lymphocyte do produce factors that alter proliferation (Wahl et al. 1978) and induce the accumulation of collagen (Wahl et al. 1978; Johnson and Ziff 1976). It remains to be seen what relationship the factors that stimulate these activities have to those that stimulate chemotaxis.

7.3.3.2. Platelets

Vascular and endothelial injury are potential consequences of diverse etiologic agents and exposure of vessel wall collagen is a likely result (Adamson et al. 1970; Adamson 1976; Haudenschild and Schwartz 1979). Repair is usually initiated by the formation of a platelet plug at the site of the endothelial defect, a process associated with aggregation of circulating thrombocytes and their adhesion to the damaged surface (Marcus and Zucker 1965). It may be that platelet motility contributes to sealing off the endothelial defect since platelets are also capable of active migration, a process dependent upon calcium concentration, temperature and pH (Valone et al. 1974; Lowenhaupt et al. 1977). In addition to being random in direction, these migratory movements can also be specifically directed towards collagen, i.e. they may be chemotactic in character (Lowenhaupt et al. 1973). Thus it has been postulated that the formation of the platelet plug on an injured endothelial surface could be controlled by platelets recognizing chemical signals released from an exposed collagen surface.

This hypothesis has been formulated following the observation that platelets placed into a capillary tube migrated from the tube and towards adjacent capillary tubes containing various collagens. In the absence of the latter, active but non-directional migration was seen (Lowenhaupt et al. 1973). Similarly, in a two-dimensional chemotaxis assay there was streaming of platelets from one compartment of a "microscopic maze" to the entrance of another compartment which contained collagen. Platelets migrated toward several native Type I and Type III collagen preparations but directed movement was not observed when collagen was absent from the second compartment or was replaced by heat-denatured or chemically modified collagen or by cotton fibers (Lowenhaupt 1978). These studies did not include an analysis of the gradients formed in the microscopic maze assay, as has been done in the Boyden Chamber and the two-dimensional leukocyte chemotaxis chamber (Lauffenburger and Zigmond 1981), or the chamber devised to study movement of neural crest cells (Gundersen and Barrett 1980). Nor were concentrations of the chemotactic factors in various chambers varied to produce positive and negative gradients, as has been used in studies of leukocytes (Zigmond and Hirsch 1973), sperm (Lqbal et al. 1980) and tumor cell chemotaxis (Orr et al. 1978; Mundy et al. 1981). Thus "formal" evidence of the chemotactic nature of these platelet responses has not been provided although the photographic data presented is strongly in favor of the idea that these movements are indeed directed towards collagen-derived factors.

Plasma constituents may regulate the chemotaxis of platelets to collagen. Although they exhibited normal random movements, platelets from a patient deficient in clotting Factor XI did not exhibit chemotaxis towards collagen in either normal plasma or Factor XI-deficient plasma. Platelets from normal donors did not migrate towards collagen in plasma deficient in or depleted of Factor XI (Lowenhaupt 1978). Thus it may be that Factor XI in plasma or on the platelet membrane interacts with biochemically intact collagen to generate or release chemotactic factors from an exposed collagen surface. Alternatively, chemoattractants could be produced by the action of collagen on plasma.

Since the response of several other cell types to stimulation by a single chemoattractant includes phenomena other than directed movement, e.g. enzyme release (Showell et al. 1976), or increased adhesion to foreign surfaces (O'Flaherty et al. 1978b; Smith et al. 1979; Varani et al. 1981; Varani and Fantone 1982) it is interesting to speculate that in the case of platelets also, adhesion and aggregation may be under the influence of the same chemotactic factors that initiate directed movement. If so, the formation of the platelet plug could be seen as the end result of a single response with a number of components rather than a series of separately regulated responses. With reference to this concept, it has been observed that, as with chemotaxis, the ability of collagen to promote platelet adhesion or aggregation is lost after chemical or structural modification of the molecule (Brass and Bensusan 1974; Jaffe and Deykin 1974). Further examination of this speculation will require a more precise characterization of the molecular structure of the collagen-derived chemotactic factors and their interaction with the platelet. It will also be important to determine if Type IV collagen can act as a source of chemotactic activity since this is the collagen likely to be exposed as a consequence of injury to endothelial cells.

7.3.3.3. Endothelial cells and smooth muscle cells

The activation of endothelial cells during the response to tissue injury may have implications from several standpoints. First, the repair of injured tissue (either to its original state or by the formation of scar tissue) requires the formation of new blood vessels. This is accomplished by the ingrowth of new capillary sprouts from existing vessels into the injured site (Schoefl 1963; Cliff 1965). Second, injury to the luminal side of major vessels results in the denudation of the endothelial layer which is repaired by the mobilization of the endothelial cells at the periphery of the wound (Hirsch and Robertson 1977; Sholley et al. 1977). It has been shown that vascular smooth muscle cells also undergo activation after luminal injury (Poole et al. 1971). The properly controlled response of both cell types is essential for repair of the injured vessel to occur.

Studies have shown that endothelial cells are motile in vitro and are capable of demonstrating both chemokinetic and chemotactic responses. Glaser et al. (1980b) demonstrated that fetal bovine aortic endothelial cells responded in a Boyden Chamber chemotaxis assay to extracts of bovine retina as well as to extracts prepared from several other tissues. The migratory response to these factors was found to be chemotactic as indicated by the Zigmond-Hirsch checkerboard analysis but increased random motility was also stimulated by the extracts in the absence of a gradient. Since these tissues, particularly retinal tissues (Glaser et al. 1980a), are known to be potent stimulators of angiogenesis, it is tempting to suggest that directional migration of the endothelial cells toward the source of an attracting factor contribute to the angiogenic response.

In addition to the Boyden Chamber assay, endothelial cell migration has also been demonstrated with other procedures such as the wound culture and agarose assay techniques (Thorgeirsson and Robertson 1978b; Thorgeirsson et al. 1979; Wall et al. 1978). It has been shown that the repopulation of a typical, "mechanical" wound in an endothelial cell monolayer occurs as a result of both migration and proliferation (Thorgeirsson and Robertson 1978a; Thorgeirsson et al. 1979; Wall et al. 1978). The two processes can be separated since the kinetics of the two responses are different (proliferation occurs after migration has begun) and since migration will occur even when replication has been blocked by radiation. Although the formation of the wound provides the stimulus for both proliferation and migration, there is some question as to whether additional factors modulate these responses. Wall et al. (1978) showed that a heat-stable platelet factor increased the rate of endothelial cell migration in agarose. This chemokinetic effect was not observed with fibroblast growth factor, macrophage-conditioned medium or zymosan-activated fresh human serum. Using a slightly different assay, Thorgeirsson et al. (1979) also demonstrated endothelial migration in vitro and separated the effects of migration from proliferation. However, in their studies, they were not able to demonstrate chemokinetic effects with platelet-derived factors.

Like endothelial cells, smooth muscle cells also demonstrate motility in agarose (Thorgeirsson et al. 1979). However, certain differences in the pattern of migration between the two cell types are observed. For example, endothelial cells migrate as a group and nearly every cell is in contact with many other cells. Smooth muscle cells, in contrast, migrate individually. At the boundary between the seeded cells and the advancing front, the smooth muscle cells tend to be arranged in tightly packed sheets of parallel, spindle-shaped cells. When sera from platelet-rich and platelet-poor plasma were compared, the platelet-rich plasma was much more effective in supporting migration. Further studies indicated that not only was motility enhanced in the platelet-rich plasma, but proliferation was also enhanced (Thorgeirsson and Robertson, 1978a, 1978a, b).

The relationship between these in vitro observations on endothelial cell and smooth muscle cell motility and the biological behavior of the same cells in vivo can only be speculated at. In relation to atherosclerosis, it has been postulated that injury leads to platelet adherence to the subendothelial basement membrane with a resulting stimulation of smooth muscle migration and proliferation. As a result of these processes, an accumulation of smooth muscle cells occurs with a resulting intimal thickening. Simultaneous to this, endothelial cell proliferation and migration occur, leading to a restoration of the platelet-resistant lining. If a complete endothelial lining can be effected, smooth muscle activity will be limited and the lesion will not be progressive. On the other hand, if the damage to the endothelial lining is too great, a complete restoration may not be possible. As a result, smooth muscle activity continues and the progressive, atherosclerotic lesion develops.

In summary, then, stimulated migration of both endothelial cells and smooth muscle cells has been demonstrated in vitro. With endothelial cells, at least, true chemotactic migration has been shown. Whether these responses in vitro reflect behavior which is relevant in vivo is not known with certainty. However, conditions exist during the process of wound healing which should be favorable to the activation of both endothelial cells as well as smooth muscle cells. Given the fact that these conditions exist, it is not unreasonable to assume that these processes do play a role.

7.3.4. Tumor cell invasion and metastasis

Hayashi and his co-workers published a series of papers during the early 1970's in which they described chemotactic responses in several tumor cell lines (Hayashi et al. 1970; Yoshida et al. 1970; Ozaki et al. 1971; Ushijima et al. 1976). They were able to cause metastatic tumors to develop at specific skin sites injected with chemotactic factors and postulated that tumor cell metastasis may be influenced by chemotactic factors in much the same way as leukocyte localization at inflammatory sites. Following these initial observations, Ward and his colleagues (Romualdez and Ward 1975; Romualdez et al. 1976; Orr et al. 1978; Orr et al. 1979a;) and other investigators (Spiro and Mundy 1980; Mundy et al 1981; Gauss-Muller et al. 1980;

Thorgeirsson et al. 1982) described chemotactic responses in a variety of tumor cell types. Since several recent reviews have been written on various aspects of the tumor cell response to chemotactic factors (Varani 1982; Orr and Varani 1982; Varani and Ward 1982; Varani et al. 1981a) no attempt will be made here to duplicate these. We will, however, describe very recent findings from our laboratory which support a possible role for chemotactic responses in tumor cell invasion and metastasis. These findings relate to the generation of chemotactic factors for tumor cells in vivo from the fifth component of complement (C5).

Previous in vitro studies had shown that either C5 or the leukocyte chemotactic factor C5a could serve as a source from which the C5-derived tumor cell chemotactic factor could be generated (Romualdez et al 1976; Orr et al 1978). The active, tumor cell chemotactic factor was produced from either C5 or C5a by proteolytic cleavage. In addition to trypsin, the neutral proteases isolated from several tissues as well as the leukocyte lysosomal enzymes, elastase and cathepsin G

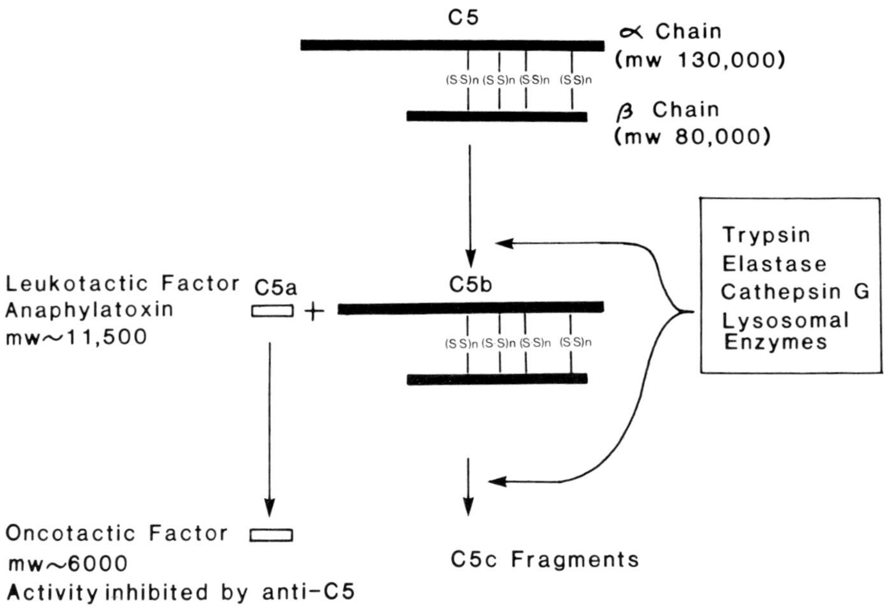

Fig. 7. Chemotactic factors from C5. The intact C5 molecule can be cleaved by a variety of proteolytic enzymes to produce a leukotactic factor (C5a) or a tumor cell chemotactic factor. The leukotactic C5a can itself be further cleaved to produce the tumor cell chemotactic factor.

were able to produce the active factor from native C5 (Romualdez et al. 1976; Orr et al. 1979c). These observations are shown schematically in Figure 7. The kinetics of leukocyte and tumor cell chemotactic activity generation from C5 are shown in Figure 8. The generation of tumor cell chemotactic activity from zymosan-activated serum is also shown in Figure 8. Since both the substrate and the lysosomal hydrolases are likely to be found at sites of acute inflammation, we predicted that inflammatory exudate fluids would provide an appropriate environment for the generation of the C5 chemotactic factor for tumor cells in vivo.

Recent experimental evidence suggests that this prediction is in fact correct. Experimentally, the factor was generated in the exudate fluid, induced in Sprague-Dawley rats by the intraperitoneal injection of glycogen. The quantity of chemotactic activity and the period of time during which it could be detected correlated with the inflammatory reaction measured by the cellular composition of the exudate and its

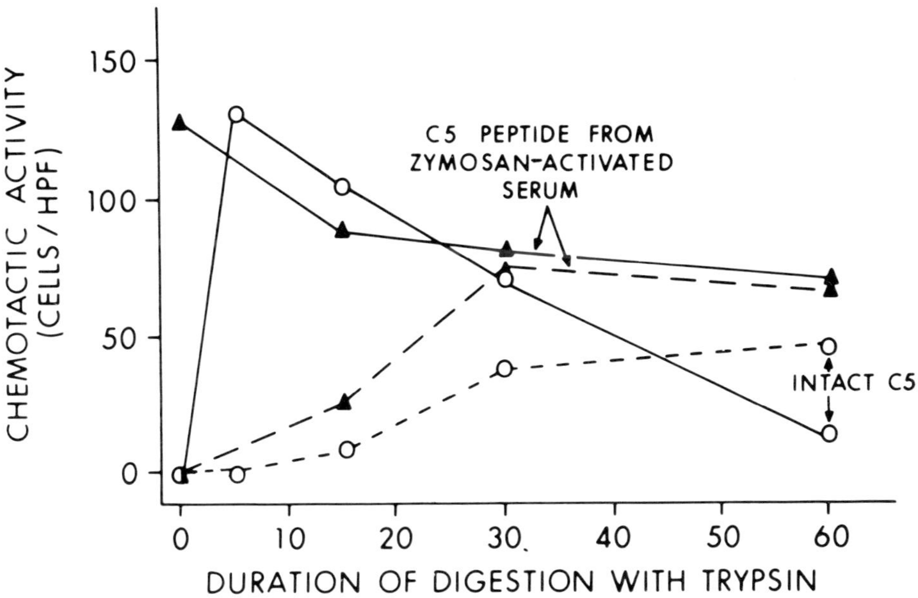

Fig. 8. Generation of chemotactic factors from C5. When intact, C5 is used as the substrate; limited proteolytic digestion produces the leukocyte chemotactic factor without generating the tumor cell chemotactic factor. With increasing digestion, chemotactic activity for leukocytes falls off and concomitantly, chemotactic activity for tumor cells is generated. When zymosan-activated serum (containing C5a) is used as the starting material, limited proteolytic cleavage produces a drop in leukocyte chemotactic activity concomitant with the generation of the chemotactic activity for tumor cells. (See Romualdez et al. 1976; Orr et al. 1978; 1979a, c.)

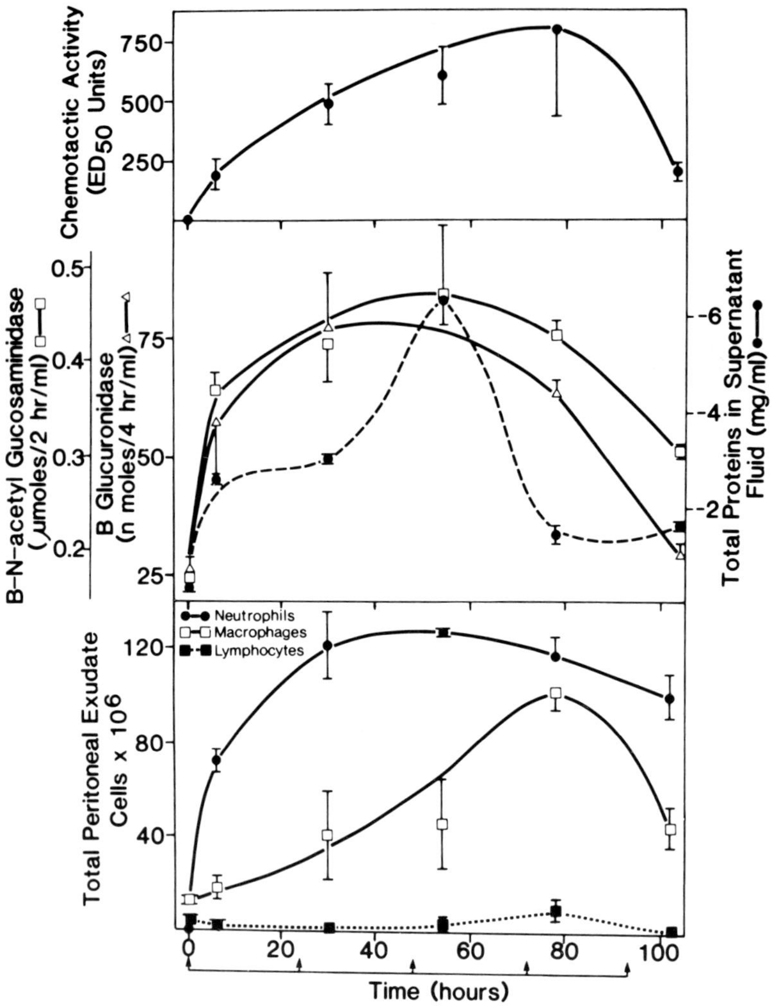

Fig. 9. Generation of chemotactic activity for tumor cells in inflammatory exudates. Sprague-Dawley rats were given an intraperitoneal injection of glycogen at time zero. At various times later, the peritoneal fluid was harvested and analyzed. The appearance of chemotactic activity for tumor cells is depicted in the top panel. The appearance of total proteins and lysosomal hydrolyases is shown in the middle panel. In the bottom panel can be seen the cellular composition of the peritoneal fluid (Orr et al. 1982a, b).

content of protein and lysosomal enzymes (Fig. 9). This factor was identified as the C5-derived chemotactic factor by its behavior in gel-filtration (estimated molecular weight ~6000 daltons) and by antibody-blocking studies (activity blocked by anti-C5 but not by anti-C3 or anti-C4). Further, the activity was not found in exudate fluids of rats depleted of serum complement by cobra venom factor.

The finding of the chemotactic activity in the exudate fluids may be significant because during the time of its presence, intravenously injected, chemotactically responsive tumor cells arrested in the mesenteries and formed metastases in much greater numbers than in normal controls: animals depleted of complement during the experimental period, or animals given intraperitoneal injections of histamine. The growth of tumor cells in vitro was not promoted by peritoneal exudate fluids nor was the size of the individual metastases greater than in control animals (Orr et al. 1982b). These findings are very similar to the finding made when preformed chemotactic factors were injected into the peritoneal cavity of animals bearing circulating tumor cells (Lam et al. 1981; Orr et al. 1982a).

These studies have been extended to human effusions. The C5-derived chemotactic factor was detected in 15 human inflammatory and neoplastic effusions including ascites, pleural effusions and cerebrospinal fluids. It was not found in normal plasma or normal CSF but could be generated from normal plasma by incubating extracts of exudate cells with normal plasma or with purified C5. Human tumor cells from one of the effusions demonstrated chemotaxis towards a factor in autologous ascites and towards the C5-derived chemotactic factor prepared in vitro (unpublished data). These studies provide evidence that the C5-derived chemotactic factor can be generated in vivo and can influence the metastatic behavior of chemotactically responsive circulating tumor cells. In our opinion, these findings offer one explanation for the observed tendency of human and experimental tumors to metastasize to sites of tissue injury.

7.4. BIOLOGICAL BASIS OF THE CHEMOTACTIC RESPONSE

It is clear from the studies described above that diverse cell types are capable of chemotactic responses. The biological basis, for the most part, of these responses has not been probed in detail. Only with leukocytes has a systematic study been made to delineate the biochemical and cell-biological basis for responsiveness. While it is not our intention to review the leukocyte studies, a brief synopsis of the major findings in leukocytes is warranted, as other cell types are invariably compared with them. A very recent review on the molecular and cellular mechanisms of leukocyte chemotaxis is available (Snyderman and Goetzl, 1981). Briefly, leukocyte chemotaxis is initiated by the binding of chemoattractants to specific plasma membrane receptors. Following binding, rapid alterations in membrane potential, cyclic nucleotide levels and ion fluxes are observed. Membrane protein and phospholipid alterations occur. Arachidonic acid is released from the membrane phospholipids and is subsequently metabolized through both the cyclo-oxygenase and lipoxygenase pathways to produce bioactive intermediates. Within minutes, microtubule structures and microfilaments undergo reorganization. Some, or all, of these changes are no doubt responsible for the morphological changes undergone by stimulated cells and for the subsequent movement of the cells toward the source of the attractant. It should be pointed out that activation of leukocytes by chemotactic factors leads to a number of physiological responses in addition to chemotactic and chemokinetic motility. These include hyperadherence to foreign surfaces (O'Flaherty et al. 1978a, b; Spagnuolo and Ellner 1980; Smith et al. 1979b), cell to cell aggregation (O'Flaherty and Ward 1978) and lysosomal enzyme release (Showell et al. 1976).

Are these biochemical and physiological responses unique to leukocytes or does chemotactic activation of other cells lead to similar changes? While only a limited amount of evidence is available at present, it does appear that the chemotactic activation pathway in non-leukocytic cells is similar to that of leukocytes.

Studies by Chiang and his colleagues with normal human fibroblasts (Chiang et al. 1978) indicated that these cells have receptors for α_1 chains of Type I collagen. ^{14}C-labeled peptide bound to the cells in a time-dependent manner which was concentration-dependent and displaceable with unlabeled peptide. Scatchard plot analysis of the binding data indicated that there are 1.6×10^6 binding sites per cell with an association constant of 1.1×10^7/M. Dose—response curves of peptide binding and chemotactic activity correlated closely.

Studies in our own laboratory with the Walker 256 rat carcinosarcoma line indicated that these cells also have specific binding sites for the synthetic chemotactic tripeptide FMLP (unpublished observation). Our studies have indicated, however, only a very small number of sites per cell (1.2×10^4 per cell). While this appears to be a very small number of specific sites per cell, it must be remembered that this is a very heterogeneous tumor and that only about 10—15% of the cells respond to the same peptide in functional assays. Studies with many other responsive cell types will have to be done before the full range of variability in chemotactic peptide binding is known. Suffice it to say that these limited studies do suggest that in non-leukocytic cells, as in leukocytes, the responses induced by chemotactic peptides follow from the initial binding of the factor at specific membrane sites.

Is the sequence of events which occurs in non-leukocytic cells after binding of the chemotactic factor similar to what occurs in leukocytes? Very few studies have been done to address this question and those which have, have used a limited number of cell types. However, in spite of the small amount of data, there are indications of similarities. In our studies with the Walker carcinosarcoma cells, we observed that chemotactic factor and phorbol ester-induced adherence were temperature-dependent events and completely inhibited by 2-deoxyglucose and iodoacetate. Similar findings had been made previously in leukocytes (Borel 1973; Carruthers 1967; O'Flaherty et al. 1977a). Likewise, we observed no inhibition of tumor cell chemotaxis or adherence in the presence of cyclohexamide and this also has been reported with leukocytes. In contrast, however, it has been reported that normal

TABLE 1.
Inhibition of chemotactic factor-induced adherence and motility in non-leukocytic cells

Agent	Finding
2-Deoxyglucose and iodoacetate	Both metabolic inhibitors completely block chemotactic factor-induced motility and adherence of Walker 256 carcinosarcoma cells (Varani et al. 1981b; Wass et al. 1980; Varani and Fantone 1982)
Cycloheximide	No effect on chemotactic factor-induced adherence and motility in Walker tumor cells (Varani and Fantone 1982; Wass et al. 1980). Dramatically inhibits chemotactic motility in normal human fibroblasts (Gauss-Müller et al. 1980)
Colchicine and vinblastine	Inhibit random and chemotactic motility in Walker tumor cells (Spiro and Mundy 1980). Inhibit chemotactic factor-induced adherence in the same cells (Varani and Fantone 1982)
Cytochalasin B	Inhibits random and chemotactic motility in Walker tumor cells (Spiro and Mundy 1980). Inhibits chemotactic factor-induced adherence in the same cells (Varani and Fantone 1982). Inhibits chemokinetic motility in endothelial cells and smooth muscle cells (Thorgeirsson et al. 1979)

fibroblast chemotaxis was inhibited by protein synthesis inhibitors (Gauss-Müller et al. 1980). Thus, there appears to be variability (not unexpectedly) among diverse population of non-leukocytic cells. Several groups of researchers have shown that chemotactic factor-induced responses (i.e. motility and adherence) are inhibited by colchicine and cytochalasin B (Gauss-Müller et al. 1980; Spiro and Mundy 1980; Varani 1982; Varani and Fantone 1982). These findings, which suggest that the responses require an intact cytoskeleton are also similar to observations made with leukocytes (Allison et al. 1971; Goldstein et al. 1973). A summary of these findings is presented in Table 1.

Several studies have indicated that, in leukocytes, arachidonic acid, which is released from membrane phospholipids during chemotactic activation, is the source of potent, internal mediators of the chemotactic response (Borgeat and Samuelsson 1979; Goetzl and Sun 1979). Using a series of inhibitors known to block phospholipase A_2 activity or metabolism of arachidonic acid through the lipoxygenase pathway we have been able to inhibit chemotactic peptide and phorbol ester-induced adherence of the Walker carcinosarcoma cells (Varani 1982; Varani and Fantone 1982). The inhibitors used include p-bromophenacyl bromide, nordihydroguaiaretic acid and 5,8,11,14-eicosatetraynoic acid. On the other hand, inhibitors of cyclo-oxygenase activity, including acetylsalicylic acid and indomethacin, were much less effective. A summary of these data is given in Table 2. The effects seen with indomethacin are particularly interesting. At high concentration (10^{-3} mol l^{-1}) we did obtain some inhibition. However, when the cells were pretreated for 12 hours with lower doses ($10^{-5}-10^{-6}$ mol l^{-1}) and then stimulated, the response was dramatically enhanced compared to non-pretreated control cells. Enhancement of responsiveness with low doses of indomethacin is thought to be nearly diagnostic of lipoxygenase involvement. The enhancing effect of low-dose indomethacin treatment may reflect the fact that cyclo-oxygenase metabolism of arachidonic acid is blocked and thereby more substrate is available for metabolism through the lipoxygenase pathway. This explanation must be considered tentative, of course, until qualitative and quantitative assessments of the arachidonic acid metabolites produced under control and stimulated conditions are made.

There is also evidence to suggest a role for cyclo-oxygenase metabolites in the

TABLE 2.
Effects of inhibitors of phospholipid and arachidonic acid metabolism on stimulated adherence of Walker cells

Agent	Finding
Bromophenacyl bromide	This inhibitor of phospholipase A_2 blocks chemotactic factor-induced adherence of Walker cells by 80% at 10^{-5} mol l^{-1}
Nordihydroguaiaretic acid	This lipoxygenase inhibitor blocks chemotactic factor-induced adherence of Walker cells by 90% at 10^{-5} mol l^{-1}
5,8,11,14-Eicosatetraynoic acid	This competitive inhibitor of arachidonic acid inhibits phorbol ester-induced adherence of Walker cells by 50% at 10^{-4} mol l^{-1}
Indomethacin	At high concentrations (10^{-3} mol l^{-1}) a 50% inhibition of chemotactic factor-induced adherence of Walker cells is seen. When the cells are treated with low concentrations ($10^{-5}-10^{-6}$ mol l^{-1}) for 12−16 hours, chemotactic factor-induced adherence is enhanced

See for details Varani and Fantone 1982 and Varani 1982.

regulation of chemotactic responses. The cyclo-oxygenase products, which include the classic prostaglandins (PGE_1, PGE_2) and prostacyclin (PGI_2) may be involved in limiting the response. We observed that pretreatment of the tumor cells with $10^{-4}-10^{-6}$ mol l^{-1} PGE_2 inhibited their chemotactic motility (Mokashi et al. 1982). In other studies, PGI_2 as well as a long-acting PGE_1 derivative (15-methyl-PGE_1) was shown to inhibit chemotactic factor-induced tumor cell adherence (Fantone et al. 1982). Prostaglandin A_1 did not produce similar inhibition of either chemotaxis or adherence. In fact, at lower concentrations (10^{-7} mol l^{-1} and 10^{-9} mol l^{-1}), a slight stimulation of the chemotactic response was observed. Associated with the inhibition of the responses was a 4–5 fold increase in the cAMP levels of the cells. These effects could be duplicated by the addition of dibutyryl cAMP or several agents known to stimulate cAMP production. These findings suggest that arachidonic acid may serve as the source for intermediary compounds which both mediate the chemotactic response and subsequently limit it.

Independent studies by others also suggests a role for phospholipid metabolism in regulating chemotactic factor-induced responses in fibroblasts. Through the use of a variety of inhibitors which are known to inhibit transmethylation reactions or to inhibit the activity of phospholipase A_2, Gauss-Müller et al. (1980) observed a dramatic inhibition of the chemotactic response of human fibroblasts. Inhibition of transmethylase reactions like blocking the phospholipase A_2 would be expected to have the same effect as far as limiting the availability of arachidonic acid for subsequent mobilization. Likewise inhibiting both would be expected to alter the dynamics of phospholipid turnover in membranes independent of arachidonic acid.

7.5. ADHERENCE, MOTILITY AND CHEMOTAXIS

The fact that, with few exceptions, eukaryotic cells move by "pulling" themselves over a substratum implies that cell–substrate adherence is an integral part of the motility process. It is not surprising that various processes involved in the regulation of cell motility (i.e. contact inhibition, contact guidance and haptotoxis) have adherence phenomena at their base (Abercrombie 1970; Vasiliev and Gelfand 1976; Carter 1965). Likewise, recent studies from several laboratories have shown a link between adherence and chemotaxis in both leukocytes (O'Flaherty et al. 1978a, b; Spagnuolo and Ellner 1980; Smith et al. 1979a, b; Keller et al. 1979) and non-leukocytic, normal (Gauss-Müller et al. 1980; Postlethwaite et al. 1980; Seppa et al. 1980) and neoplastic cells (Varani 1982 Varani and Fantone, 1982; Varani et al. 1981a, b). While a variety of methodologies have been used in these studies — making direct comparisons difficult — and while there is some disagreement among the results obtained with these disparate methodologies, the overall finding seems to be that chemotactic factors increase the cell–substrate adhesiveness in responsive cells.

O'Flaherty et al. (1978b) used the nylon fiber adherence assay to measure adherence changes in neutrophils induced by chemotactic factors. They observed a very rapid rise in adhesiveness upon addition of several active chemotactic factors. The kinetics of the adherence response paralleled closely the kinetics of cell–cell aggregation which was also induced by the same factors (O'Flaherty and Ward 1978). It was postulated that increased adhesiveness to foreign surfaces and increased cell–cell aggregation may have a common basis. However, the two responses could be at least partially separated since cell–cell aggregation was completely inhibited in Ca^{2+}-free medium while the adherence response was only partially inhibited.

It should be pointed out that certain studies have suggested that leukocyte adherence and chemotaxis can be separated (Spagnuolo and Ellner 1980). However, even in these studies, the similarities in the two responses were much more prominent than the dissimilarities. Furthermore, Keller et al. (1979) found that under conditions in which neutrophil locomotion was stimulated, the pattern of foreign surface adherence (as measured by reflection-contrast microscopy) was altered, even if the percentage of adherent cells was not. In summary, then, these studies suggest that in leukocytes, adherence and motility phenomena are closely linked. While they can be partially separated in vitro, it is very likely that the accumulation of leukocytes at sites of inflammations (Ozaki et al. 1971) and the neutropenia which accompany the systemic introduction of chemotactic agents (O'Flaherty et al. 1977b) are likely to be due at least partially, if not primarily, to altered cell–cell and cell–substrate adhesiveness induced by the stimulating agent.

Studies conducted in our own laboratory with neoplastic cells have also shown a relationship between adhesiveness and chemotactic responses. In our studies we have shown that factors which induce chemotactic motility in the Boyden Chamber assay also induce adherence to nylon fibers over the same dose range (Varani et al. 1981a, b). Likewise, factors which inhibit the chemotactic motility of the cells in the standard Boyden Chamber assay, including the classical prostaglandins (Fantone et al. 1982); the inhibitors of energy metabolism and cytoskeleton describing agents also inhibit the adherence of the cells to nylon fibers and to plastic culture dishes (Varani 1982; Varani and Fantone 1982). Findings similar to these have been made with normal fibroblasts. That is, several factors which are known to mediate the adherence of cells to foreign surfaces have also been found to be chemotactic. In addition, the two functions – adherence and chemotaxis – are often inhibited in a co-variable way by certain inhibitors (Gauss-Müller et al. 1980).

7.6. SUMMARY AND CONCLUSIONS

Several studies during the past 10–12 years have shown that a variety of non-leukocytic cells are capable of demonstrating chemotactic motility in vitro. Recent studies have shown that although the specific factors to which the cells respond vary from cell type to cell type, the underlying basis of the response may be similar in all of the cells. Comparisons with the much better studied leukocytes suggest a common basis with these cells as well.

Although polymorphonuclear leukocytes and monocytes have served as useful models for chemotactic studies, the various cell types other than the white blood cells must continue to be investigated in their own right. Not only will differences between specific cell types be found but, in addition, certain types of studies can be done using normal or neoplastic cell lines that would be very difficult or impossible to do with leukocytes. For example, since fibroblasts and tumor cells are not end-stage cells, they can be used in biological assays and then reharvested for continued culture. In this way it will be possible to look at such questions as cell cycle influences, cell population heterogeneity, response desensitization and receptor turnover. These types of studies are very difficult or impossible to do with leukocytes, which are programmed for an early death. A further advantage with the tumor cells is that they can be grown in large quantities under controlled conditions in vivo or in vitro. Such large quantities of cells would facilitate studies involving isolation and purification of short-lived agents such as the lipoxygenase intermediates of arachidonic acid. Finally, as has already been demonstrated (Orr et al. 1981), tumor cell variants with differing chemotactic responsiveness can be isolated from a common parent tumor. The availability of such variants provides invaluable tools in efforts to understand the basis of the response in any cell.

ACKNOWLEDGEMENT

This work was supported by grants CA29550 and CA29551 from the USPHS and by a grant from the National Cancer Institute of Canada. Dr. Orr is a Clinical Research Associate of the National Cancer Institute of Canada.

REFERENCES

Abercrombie, M. (1970) Contact inhibition in tissue culture. *In Vitro 6,* 128–142.

Abercrombie, M. and Heaysman, J.E.M. (1953) Observations on the social behavior of cells in tissue culture. Speed of movement of chick heart fibroblasts in relation to their mutual contacts. *Exp. Cell Res. 5,* 111–131.

Adamson, I.Y.R. (1976) Pulmonary toxicity of bleomycin. *Environ. Health Perspect. 16,* 119–126.

Adamson, I.Y.R., Bowden, D.H. and Wyatt, J.P. (1970) A pathway to pulmonary fibrosis. An ultrastructural study of mouse and rat following radiation to the whole body and hemithorax. *Am. J. Pathol. 58,* 481–498.

Allison, A.C., Davis, P. and DePetris, S. (1971) Role of contractile microfilaments in macrophage movement and endocytosis. *Nature New Biol. 232,* 153–154.

Atherton, R.W., Radnay, E.W. and Polakoski, K.L. (1978) Spectrophotometric quantitation of mammalian spermatozoan motility. *Hum. Biol. Reprod. 18,* 624–634.

Bedford, J.M. (1975) Maturation, transport and fate of spermatozoa in the epididymis. In: D.W. Hamilton and R.O. Greep (Eds), *Handbook of Physiology, Section 7: Endocrinology, Vol. 5: Male Reproductive System,* American Physiological Society, Washington DC, p. 304.

Bedford, J.M., Calvin, H.I. and Cooper, G.W. (1973) The maturation of sperm in the human epididymis. *J. Reprod. Fertil., Suppl. 18,* 199.

Blandau, R.J. and Rumery, R.E. (1964) The relationship of swimming movements of epididymal spermatozoa to their fertilizing capacity. *Fertil. Steril. 15,* 571–576.

Borel, J.F. (1973) Effect of some drugs on the chemotaxis of rabbit neutrophils in vitro. *Experientia 29,* 676–682.

Borgeat, P. and Samuelsson, B. (1979) Arachidonic acid metabolism in polymorphonuclear leukocytes: effects of ionophore A23187. *Proc. Natl Acad. Sci. USA 76,* 2148–2152.

Brass, L.F. and Bensusan, H.B. (1974) The role of collagen quaternary structure in the platelet:collagen interaction. *J. Clin. Invest. 54,* 1480–1487.

Burk, R.R. (1973) A factor from a transformed cell line that affects cell migration. *Proc. Natl Acad. Sci. USA 70,* 369–372.

Campenot, R.B. (1977) Local control of neurite development by nerve growth factor. *Proc. Natl Acad. Sci. USA 74,* 4516–4519.

Carpenter, R.R. (1963) In vitro studies of cellular hypersensitivity. I. Specific inhibition of migration of cells from adjuvant-immunized animals by purified protein derivative and other protein antigens. *J. Immunol. 91,* 803–818.

Carruthers, B.M. (1967) Leukocyte motility. II. Effect of absence of glucose in medium; effect of presence of deoxyglucose, dinitrophenol, puromycin, actinomycin D and trypsin on the response to a chemotactic substance. *Can. J. Physiol. Pharmacol. 45,* 269–278.

Carter, S.B. (1965) Principles of cell motility: the direction of cell movement and cancer invasion. *Nature (London) 206,* 1183–1187.

Casillas, E.R. and Erickson, J. (1975) The role of carnitine in spermatozoan metabolism: substrate-induced elevations in the acetylation state of carnitine and coenzyme A in bovine and monkey spermatozoa. *Biol. Reprod. 12,* 275–283.

Chamley, J.H. and Dowel, J.J. (1975) Specificity of nerve fiber attraction to autonomic effector organs in tissue culture. *Exp. Cell Res. 90,* 1–17.

Cheever, A.W. (1965) A comparative study of Schistosoma mansoni infections in mice, gerbils, multimammate rats and hamsters. II. Qualitative pathological differences. *Am. J. Trop. Med. Hyg. 14,* 227–253.

Chiang, T.M., Postlethwaite, A.E., Beachey, E.H., Seyer, J.M. and Kang, A.H. (1978) Binding of chemotactic collagen-derived peptides to fibroblasts: The relationship to fibroblast chemotaxis. *J. Clin. Invest. 62,* 916–922.

Cliff, W.J. (1965) Kinetics of wound healing in rabbit ear chambers; a time lapse cinemicroscopic study. *Quart. J. Exp. Physiol. 50,* 79–89.

Cochrane, C.G. and Janoff, A. (1974) The Arthus reaction: A model of neutrophil and complement-mediated injury. In: B.W. Zweifach, L. Grant and R.T. McCluskey (Eds), *The Inflammatory Process,* Academic Press, Inc., New York, pp. 85–162.

Dunn, G.A. (1980) Mechanisms of fibroblast locomotion. In: A.S.G. Curtis and J.D. Pitts (Eds), *Cell Adhesion and Motility,* Cambridge University Press, New York, pp. 409–424.

Ebendal, T. (1976) The relative roles of contact inhibition and contact guidance in orientation of axons extending on aligned collagen fibrils in vitro. *Exp. Cell Res. 98,* 159–169.

Ebendal, T. and Jacobson, C.O. (1977) Tissue explants affecting extension and orientation of axons in cultured chick embryo ganglia. *Exp. Cell Res. 105,* 379–387.

Fantone, J., Kunkel, S.L. and Varani, J. (1982) Inhibition of tumor cell adherence by prostaglandins. In: *Prostaglandins and Cancer: First International Conference,* Alan R. Liss, Inc., New York, pp. 673–677.

Fray, C.S., Hoffer, A.P. and Fawcett, D.W. (1972) A re-examination of motility patterns of rat epididymal spermatozoa. *Anat. Rec. 173,* 301–307.

Gauss-Müller, V., Kleinman, H.K., Martin G.R., and Schiffman, E. (1980) Role of attachment factors and attractants in fibroblast chemotaxis. *J. Lab. Clin. Med. 96,* 1071–1080.

Glaser, B.M., D'Amore, P.A., Michels, R.G., Patz, A. and Fenselau, A. (1980a) Demonstration of vasoproliferative activity from mammalian retina. *J. Cell Biol. 84,* 298–304.

Glaser, B.M., D'Amore, P.A., Seppa, H., Seppa, S. and Schiffmann, E. (1980b) Adult tissues contain chemoattractants for vascular endothelial cells. *Nature (London) 288,* 483–484.

Goetzl, E.J. and Sun, F.F. (1979) Generation of unique monohydroxy-eicosatetraenoic acids from arachidonic acid by human neutrophils. *J. Exp. Med. 150,* 406–411.

Goldstein, J., Hoffstein, S., Gallin, J. and Weissman, G. (1973) Mechanisms of lysozomal enzyme release from human leukocytes: Microtubule assembly and membrane fusion induced by a component of complement. *Proc. Natl Acad. Sci. USA 70,* 2916–2919.

Gundersen, R.W. and Barrett, J.N. (1979) Neuronal chemotaxis: Chick dorsal root axons turn towards high concentrations of nerve growth factor. *Science 206,* 1079–1080.

Gundersen, R.W. and Barrett, J.N. (1980) Characterization of the turning response of dorsal root neurities toward nerve growth factor. *J. Cell Biol. 87,* 546–554.

Haskins, D.D. and Casillas, E.R. (1975) Selective acute arterial injury repair. I. Methodology and surface characteristics. *Atherosclerosis 28,* 271–278.

Haudenschild, C.C. and Schwartz, S.M. (1979) Endothelial regeneration II. Restitution of endothelial continuity. *Lab. Invest. 41,* 407–418.

Hayashi, H., Yoshida, K., Ozaki, T. and Ushijima, K. (1970) Chemotactic factor associated with invasion of cancer. *Nature (London) 226,* 174–175.

Hirsch, E.Z. and Robertson, A.L. (1977) Selective acute arterial injury and repair. I. Methodology and surface characteristics. *Atherosclerosis 28,* 271–278.

Isenberg, G., Rathke, P.C., Hulsmann, N., Franke, W.W. and Wohlforth-Bottermann, K.E. (1976) Cytoplasmic actomyosin fibrils in tissue culture cells: Direct proof of contractility by visualization of ATP-induced contraction in fibrils isolated by laser microbeam dissection. *Cell Tissue Res. 166,* 427–443.

Jaffe, R. and Deykin, D. (1974) Evidence for a structural requirement for the aggregation of platelets by collagen. *J. Clin. Invest. 53,* 875–883.

Johnson, R.E. and Ziff, M. (1976) Lymphokine stimulation of collagen accumulation. *J. Clin. Invest. 58,* 240–252.

Katz, D.F. and Overstreet, J.W. (1979) Biophysical aspects of human sperm movement. In: D.W. Fawcett and J.M. Bedford (Eds), *The Spermatozoon. Proceedings of the Third International Symposium on the Spermatozoon, Boston and Woods Hole, 1978,* Urban and Schwarzenberg, Baltimore, p. 413.

Keller, D.W. and Polakoski, K.L. (1975) L-Arginine stimulation of hyman sperm motility in vitro. *Biol. Reprod. 13,* 154–157.

Keller, H.U., Barandun, S., Kistler, P. and Ploem, J.S. (1979) Locomotion and adhesion of neutrophil granulocytes. Effects of albumin, fibrinogen and gamma globulins studied by reflection contrast microscopy. *Exp. Cell Res. 122,* 351–362.

Kravis, T.C., Ahmed, A., Brown, T.E., Fulmer, J.D. and Crystal, R.G. (1976) Pathogenic mechanisms in pulmonary fibrosis. Collagen-induced migration inhibition factor production and cytotoxicity mediated by lymphocytes. *J. Clin. Invest. 58,* 1223–1232.

Kreutzer, D.L., O'Flaherty, J.T., Orr W., Showell, H.J., Ward, P.A. and Becker, E.L. (1978) Quantitative comparisons of various biological responses of neutrophils to different active and inactive chemotactic factors. *Immunopharmacology 1,* 39–47.

Krystosek, A. and Seeds, N.W. (1981) Plasminogen activator release at the neuronal growth cone. *Science 213,* 1532.

Lam, W.C., Delikatny, E.J., Orr, F.W., Wass, J., Varani, J. and Ward, P.A. (1981) The chemotactic response of tumor cells. A model for cancer metastasis. *Am. J. Pathol. 104,* 69–76.

Lauffenburger, D.A. and Zigmond, S.H. (1981) Chemotactic factor concentration gradients in chemotaxis assay systems. *J. Immunol. Methods 40,* 45–60.

Lazarides, E. (1975) Tropomyosin antibody: the specific localization of tropomyosin in nonmuscle cells. *J. Cell Biol. 65,* 549–561.

Lazarides, E. and Burridge, K. (1975) α-Actinin: immunofluorescent localization of a muscle structural protein in non-muscle cells. *Cell 6,* 289–298.

Lazarides, E. and Weber, K. (1974) Actin antibody. The specific visualization of actin filaments in non-muscle cells. *Proc. Natl Acad. Sci. USA 71,* 2268–2272.

Letourneau, P.C. (1975) Cell-to-substratum adhesion and guidance of axonal elongation. *Dev. Biol. 44,* 92–101.

Letourneau, P.C. (1978) Chemotactic response of nerve fiber elongation to nerve growth factor. *Dev. Biol. 66,* 183–196.

Lindemann, C.B. (1980) Requirements for motility in mammalian sperm. In: A. Steinberger and E. Steinberger (Eds), *Testicular Development, Structure and Function,* Raven Press, New York, p. 473.

Lowenhaupt, R.W. (1978) Human platelet chemotaxis: requirement for plasma factor(s) and the role of collagen. *Am. J. Physiol. Heart Circ. Physiol. 4,* 1423–1428.

Lowenhaupt, R.W., Miller, M.A. and Glueck, H.I. (1973) Platelet migration and chemotaxis demonstrated in vitro. *Thromb. Res. 3,* 477–486.

Lowenhaupt, R.W., Glueck, H.I., Miller, M.A. and Kline, D.L. (1977) Factors which influence blood platelet migration. *J. Lab. Clin. Med. 90,* 37–45.

Lqbal, M., Shivaji, S., Vijayasarathy, S. and Balarm, P. (1980) Synthetic peptides as chemoattractants for bull spermatozoa. Structure activity correlations. *Biochem. Biophys. Res. Commun. 96,* 235–242.

Malech, H.L., Root, R.K. and Gallin, J.I. (1977) Structural analysis of human neutrophil migration. Centriole, microtubule, and microfilament orientation and function during chemotaxis. *J. Cell Biol. 75,* 666–693.

Marasco, W.A., Becker, E.L. and Oliver, J.M. (1980) The ionic basis of chemotaxis. Separate cation requirements for neutrophil orientation and locomotion in a gradient of chemotactic peptide. *Am. J. Pathol. 98,* 749–768.

Marcus, A.J. and Zucker, M.B. (1965) *The Physiology of Blood Platelets: Recent Biochemical and Clinical Research,* Grune and Stratton, New York.

Mobley, W.C., Server, A.C., Ishi, D.N., Riplelle, R.J. and Shooter, E.M. (1977) Nerve growth factor. *N. Engl. J. Med. 297,* 1096.

Mokashi, S., Delikatny, J. and Orr, W. (1982) Relationship between chemotaxis, chemotactic modulators and cyclic nucleotide levels in tumor cells (Abstr.). *Fed. Proc. 41,* 334.

Mundy, G.R., DeMartino, S. and Rowe, D.W. (1981) Collagen and collagen-derived fragments are chemotactic for tumor cells. *J. Clin. Invest. 68,* 1102–1105.

Nelson, R.D., Fiegel, V.D. and Simmons, R.L. (1976) Chemotaxis of human polymorphonuclear neutrophils under agarose: morphologic changes associated with the chemotactic response. *J. Immunol. 117,* 1676–1683.

O'Flaherty, J.T. and Ward, P.A. (1978) Leukocyte aggregation induced by chemotactic factors. A review. *Inflammation 3,* 177–194.

O'Flaherty, J.T., Kreutzer, D.L., Showell, H.J. and Ward, P.A. (1977a) Influence of inhibitors of cellular function on chemotactic factor-induced neutrophil aggregation. *J. Immunol. 119,* 1751–1756.

O'Flaherty, J.T., Showell, H.J. and Ward, P.A. (1977b) Neutropenia induced by systemic infusion of chemotactic factor. *J. Immunol. 118,* 1586–1589.

O'Flaherty, J.T., Kreutzer, D.L. and Ward, P.A. (1978a) Chemotactic factor influences on the aggregation, swelling, and foreign surface adhesiveness of human leukocytes. *Am. J. Pathol. 90,* 537–550.

O'Flaherty, J.T., Kreutzer, D.L. and Ward, P.A. (1978b) The influence of chemotactic factors on neutrophil adhesiveness. *Inflammation 3,* 37–48.

Orr, F.W. and Varani, J. (1982) Chemotactic mechanisms and cancer metastasis. *Pathol. Annual,* p. 12.

Orr, W., Varani, J. and Ward, P.A. (1978) Characteristics of the chemotactic responses of neoplastic cells to a factor derived from the fifth component of complement. *Am. J. Pathol. 93,* 405–422.

Orr, W., Phan, S.H., Varani, J., Ward, P.A., Kreutzer, D.L., Webster, R.O. and Henson, P.M. (1979a) Chemotactic factor for tumor cells derived from the C5a fragment of complement component C5. *Proc. Natl Acad. Sci. USA 76,* 1986–1989.

Orr, W., Varani, J., Gondek, M.D., Ward, P.A. and Mundy, G.R. (1979b) Chemotactic responses of tumor cells to products of resorbing bone. *Science 203,* 176–179.

Orr, F.W., Varani, J., Kreutzer, D.L., Senior, R.M. and Ward, P.A. (1979c) Digestion of the fifth component of complement by leukocyte enzymes. Sequential generation of chemotactic activities for leukocytes and for tumor cells. *Am. J. Pathol. 94,* 75–84.

Orr, F.W., Varani, J., Delikatny, J., Join, N. and Ward, P.A. (1981) Comparison of the chemotactic responsiveness of two fibrosarcoma subpopulations of differing malignancy. *Am. J. Pathol. 102,* 160–167.

Orr, F.W., Lam, W.C., Delikatny, E.J., Mokashi, S. and Varani, J. (1982a) Localization of 125-iododeoxyuridine-labeled tumor cells at tissue sites injected with chemotactic stimuli: invasion and metastasis, in press.

Orr, W., Mokashi, S. and Delikatny, J. (1982b) Tumor cell chemotactic factor in inflammatory exudates and its effect on metastasis. *Am. J. Pathol. 108,* 112–118.

Ozaki, T., Yoshida, K., Ushijima, K. and Hayaski, H. (1971) Studies on the mechanisms of invasion in cancer. II. In vivo effects of a factor chemotactic for cancer cells. *Int. J. Cancer 7,* 93−100.

Poole, J.C.F. (1970) Chronic inflammation and tuberculosis. In: H.W. Florey (Ed.), *General Pathology,* W.B. Saunders Co., Philadelphia, p. 1194.

Poole, J.C.F., Cromwell, S.B. and Benditt, E.P. (1971) Behavior of smooth muscle cells and formation of extracellular structures in the reaction of the arterial wall to injury. *Am. J. Pathol. 62,* 391−414.

Postlethwaite, A.E. and Kang, A.H. (1980) Characterization of a guinea pig lymphocyte-derived chemotactic factor for fibroblasts. *J. Immunol. 124,* 1462−1466.

Postlethwaite, A.E., Snyderman, R. and Kang, A.H. (1976) The chemotactic attraction of human fibroblasts to a lymphocyte-derived factor. *J. Exp. Med 144,* 1188−1203.

Postlethwaite, A.E., Seyer, J.M. and Kang, A.H. (1978) Chemotactic attraction of human fibroblasts to type I, II, and III collagen and collagen-derived peptides. *Proc. Natl Acad. Sci. USA 75,* 871−875.

Postlethwaite, A.E., Snyderman, R. and Kang, A.H. (1979) Generation of a fibroblast chemotactic factor in serum by activation of complement. *J. Clin. Invest. 64,* 1379−1385.

Postlethwaite, A.E., Keski-Oja, J., Balian, G. and Kang, A.H. (1980) Induction of fibroblast chemotaxis by fibronectin: Localization of the chemotactic region to a 140,000-molecular weight non-gelatin-binding fragment. *J. Exp. Med. 153,* 494−499.

Romualdez, A.G. and Ward, P.A. (1975) A unique complement-derived chemotactic factor for tumor cells. *Proc. Natl Acad. Sci. USA 72,* 4128−4132.

Romualdez, A.G., Ward, P.A. and Torikata, T. (1976) Relationship between the C5 peptides chemotactic for leukocytes and tumor cells. *J. Immunol 117,* 1762−1766.

Schill, W.B. (1975) Stimulation of sperm motility by kinins in fresh and 24 hours aged human ejaculates. *Andrologia 7,* 135.

Schill, W.B., Pritsch, W. and Preissler, G. (1979) Effect of caffeine and kallikrein on cryo-preserved human spermatozoa. *Int. J. Fertil. 24,* 27−32.

Schoefl, G.L. (1963) Studies on inflammation. III. Growing capillaries: Their structure and permeability. *Virchows Arch. Pathol. Anat. 337,* 97−141.

Schoenfeld, C., Amelar, R.D. and Dubin, L. (1975) Stimulation of ejaculated human spermatozoa by caffeine. *Fertil. Steril. 26,* 158−166.

Seppa, H., Seppa, S., Yamada, K.M. and Grotendorst, G.R. (1980) The cell-binding fragment of fibronectin and platelet-derived growth factor are chemoattractants for fibroblasts (Abstract). *J. Cell Biol. 87,* 323.

Sholley, M.M., Gimbrone, M.A. and Cotran, R.S. (1977) Cellular migration and replication in endothelial regeneration; a study using irradiated endothelial cultures. *Lab. Invest. 36,* 18−25.

Showell, H.J., Freer, R.J., Zigmond, S.H., Schiffman, E., Aswanikumar, S., Corcoran, B. and Becker, E.L. (1976) The structure activity relations of synthetic peptides as chemotactic factors and inducers of lysozomal enzyme secretion for neutrophils. *J. Exp. Med. 143,* 1154−1169.

Smith, C.W., Hollers, J.C., Patrick, R.A. and Hassett, C. (1979a) Motility and adhesiveness in human neutrophils. Effects of chemotactic factors. *J. Clin. Invest. 63,* 221−229.

Smith, R.P., Lackie, J.M. and Wilkinson, P.C. (1979b) The effect of chemotactic factors on the adhesiveness of rabbit neutrophil granulocytes. *Exp. Cell Res. 122,* 169−177.

Snyderman, R. and Goetzl, E.J. (1981) Molecular and cellular mechanisms of leukocyte chemotaxis. *Science 213,* 830−836.

Spagnuolo, P.J. and Ellner, J.J. (1980) Comparative stimulation of granulocyte adherence and chemotaxis by bacterial products. *Infect. Immun. 27,* 519−524.

Spiro, T.P. and Mundy, G.R. (1980) In vitro migration of Walker 256 carcinosarcoma cells: dependence on microtubule and microfilament function. *J. Nat. Cancer Inst. 65,* 463−467.

Stossel, T.P. (1978) The mechanism of leukocyte locomotion. In: J.I. Gallin and P.G. Quie (Eds), *Leukocyte Chemotaxis: Methods, Physiology and Clinical Implications,* Raven Press, New York, pp. 143−157.

Sutter, S., Riopelle, R.J. and Harris-Warrick, R.M. (1977) Characterization of two distinct classes of high affinity binding sites for nerve growth factor on sensory ganglion cells from chick embryos. *Soc. Neurosci. 3,* 461.

Tampion, D. and Gibbons, R.A. (1963) Swimming rate of bull spermatozoa in various media and the effect of dilution. *J. Reprod. Fertil. 5,* 259−275.

Tanphaichitr, N. (1977) In vitro stimulation of human sperm motility by acetyl carnitine. *Int. J. Fertil. 22,* 85−91.

Thorgeirsson, G. and Robertson, A.L. (1978a) Platelet factor and the human vascular wall: Variation in growth response between endothelial and medial smooth muscle cells. *Atherosclerosis 30,* 67−68.

Thorgeirsson, G. and Robertson, A.L. (1978b) Platelet factors and the human vascular wall. II. Serum factors are not required for endothelial cell proliferation and migration. *Atherosclerosis 31,* 231−238.

Thorgeirsson, G., Robertson, A.L. and Cowan, D.H. (1979) Migration of human vascular endothelial and smooth muscle cells. *Lab. Invest. 41,* 51−61.

Thorgeirsson, U.P., Kalebic, T., Russo, R.G. and Liotta, L.A. (1982) Effects of chemotactic agents and protease inhibitors on tumor cell invasion of native human connective tissue barriers in vitro (Abstract). *Fed. Proc. 41,* 334.

Tremblay, R.R., Chapdelaine, P. and Mailhot, J. (1979) α-1-4-Glucosidase activity in human semen: variations with number and motility of spermatozoa. *Fertil. Steril. 31,* 592−595.

Ushijima, K., Nishi, H., Ishikura, A. and Hayashi, H. (1976) Characterization of two different factors chemotactic for cancer cells from tumor tissue. *Virchows Arch. B 21,* 119−131.

Valone, F.H., Austen, K.F. and Goetzl, E.J. (1974) Modulation of the random migration of human platelets. *J. Clin. Invest. 54,* 110−1106.

Van Winkle, W. (1967) The fibroblast in wound healing. *Surg. Gynec. Obstet. 124,* 369−386.

Varani, J. (1982) The chemotaxis of metastatic tumor cells. *Cancer Metastasis Rev., 1,* 17−28.

Varani, J. and Fantone, J.C. (1982) Phorbol myristate acetate-induced adherence of Walker 256 carcinosarcoma cells. *Cancer Res. 42,* 190−197.

Varani, J. and Ward, P.A. (1982) Tumor cell chemotaxis. In: I. Hart and L. Liotta, (Eds), *The Biological Basis of Metastasis,* Martinus Nijhoff, The Hague, pp. 99−112.

Varani, J., Orr, W. and Ward, P.A. (1978) A comparison of the migration patterns of normal and malignant cells in two assay systems. *Am. J. Pathol. 90,* 159−172.

Varani, J., Ward, P.A. and Orr, W. (1981a) Immunobiology of chemotaxis and metastasis. In: H. Waters (Ed), *The Handbook of Cancer Immunology, Vol. 7,* Garland STPM Press, New York, pp. 101−124.

Varani, J., Wass, J.A., Piontek, J.E. and Ward, P.A. (1981b) Chemotactic factor-induced adherence of tumor cells. *Cell Biol. Int. Rep. 5,* 525−530.

Vasiliev, J.M. and Gelfand, I.M. (1976) Morphogenetic reactions and locomotory behavior of transformed cells in culture. In: L. Weiss (Ed.), *Fundamental Aspects of Metastasis,* Elsevier/North-Holland Publishing Co., Inc., New York, pp. 71−98.

Vijayasarathy, S., Shivaji, S., Lqbal, M. and Balaram, P. (1980) Formyl-Met-Lew-Phe induces chemotaxis and acrosomal enzyme release in bull sperm. *FEBS Lett. 115,* 178−180.

Wahl, S.M., Wahl, L.M. and McCarthy, J.B. (1978) Lymphocyte-mediated activation of fibroblast proliferation and collagen production. *J. Immunol. 121,* 942−946.

Wall, R.T., Harker, L.A. and Striker, G.E. (1978) Human endothelial cell migration: Stimulation by a released platelet factor. *Lab. Invest. 39,* 523−529.

Ward, P.A. and Cochrane, C.G. (1965) Bound complement and immunological vasculitis. *J. Exp. Med. 121,* 215−234.

Wass, J., Varani, J., Piontek, G., Goff, D. and Ward, P.A. (1980) Characteristics of the chemotactic factor-mediated cell swelling response of tumor cells. *J. Natl Cancer Inst. 66,* 927−933.

Weber, K. and Gröschel-Stewart, U. (1974) Antibody to myosin: The specific visualization of myosin-containing filaments in nonmuscle cells. *Proc. Natl Acad. Sci. USA 71,* 4561−4564.

Yanagimachi, R. (1966) Time and process of sperm penetration into hamster ova in vivo and in vitro. *J. Reprod. Fertil. 11,* 359−370.

Yoshida, K., Ozaki, T., Ushijima, K. and Hayashi, H. (1970) Studies on the mechanisms of invasion in cancer. I. Isolation and purification of a factor chemotactic for cancer cells. *Int. J. Cancer 6,* 123−132.

Zigmond, S.H. (1977) Ability of polymorphonuclear leukocytes to orient in gradients of chemotactic factors. *J. Cell Biol. 75,* 606−616.

Zigmond, S.H. and Hirsch, J.G. (1973) Leukocyte locomotion and chemotaxis: New methods for evaluation, and demonstration of a cell-derived chemotactic factor. *J. Exp. Med. 137,* 387−410.

CHAPTER 8

Inflammatory mechanisms in the eye

STEVEN L. KUNKEL
Department of Pathology, University of Michigan Medical School, Ann Arbor, Michigan 48109

and

ALAN SUGAR
Department of Ophthalmology, University of Michigan Medical School, Ann Arbor, Michigan 48109

8.1. INTRODUCTION

The application of discoveries in the field of immunology to the visual system has historically been a slow process. Within the last two decades this trend has been reversed and many important contributions have been made by investigators dealing with the immunological aspects of ocular diseases. These studies have focused mainly on the cellular aspects of eye diseases and the cellular and humoral immune responses involved in ocular inflammation. Still, the eye remains an enigmatic organ with regard to immune/inflammatory responses because of its many unique immunologic and anatomic properties.

These unusual anatomic properties of the eye include specific barriers which control the movement of inflammatory mediators and antigens into and out of the eye. This is particularly true of the tissues that comprise the cornea and lens. These two ocular structures allow only limited access of serum components and immune cells, due to their anatomic location and lack of vascularity. The vasculature of the eye in itself is special, since the tight intercellular junctions of the retinal pigment epithelium greatly limit the ability of inflammatory mediators and antigens to cross the endothelial barrier. Also, a blood—aqueous barrier exists which controls the movement of antigens and mediators from the circulating blood to the aqueous humor. In addition to barriers which can control the movement of molecules between the blood and various eye tissues, another anatomical peculiarity is the absence of a lymphatic drainage system in the anterior chamber, cornea and lens of the eye. Thus, these structures of the eye fall into the category of immunologically privileged sites, i.e. tissue exempt from normal reactions imposed by their histo-incompatible status. A full discussion of ocular immunologically privileged sites is beyond the scope of this review, but it must be mentioned that the examination of these ocular tissues has resulted in many excellent contributions to transplantation and tumor immunology, which have been reviewed elsewhere (Barker and Billingham 1977).

Although the eye does possess unique anatomical structures which allow for relative isolation, immunocompetent cells are not entirely excluded. Mast cells are a common constituent in the iris, choroid, and conjunctiva, while lymphocytes can be found in many of the ocular tissues. Interestingly, the processing of antigens appears to occur outside the eye itself, but sensitized lymphocytes can migrate to the eye and recruit other inflammatory cells. Thus, the afferent limb of the immune process appears to take place initially outside ocular tissue, even when the antigenic challenge is given directly into the eye (Shimada and Silverstein 1975).

Although the actual antigen-processing mechanism probably occurs in extraocular areas, immunoglobulins of all the major subclasses have been found in various eye tissues. Of special interest is the high concentration of secretory immunoglobulin (IgA) in the tear film and IgG in the cornea (Chandler et al. 1975).

In addition to the presence of antibodies in various ocular tissues, another extremely important collection of proteins, the complement components, are present in the eye to defend against invasive organisms. Components involved in either the classic complement pathway or the alternate complement pathway have been detected in the eye especially the tear film, by a number of investigators (Bluestone et al. 1973; Chandler et al. 1975; Yamamoto and Allansmith 1979). In the latter study, tears from normal volunteers were found to possess complement proteins C3 through C9 each displaying hemolytic activity. Both pathways of complement activation are extremely important as defense mechanisms. The classic pathway can be activated by either immune complexes (antigen—antibody complexes) or by antibody aggregates, while the alternate pathway of complement activation is set into action by specific compounds found on the surface of bacteria (lipopolysaccharides) and fungi (zymosan). The external eye has clearly been shown to possess antibody that performs a definite protective role (Little et al. 1969). The presence of antibody, in conjunction with fully functional complement cascades, offers the ocular surface an immune defense mechanism similar to that found in other human organ systems. Although these two systems offer a very powerful and effective immunological protective mechanism, they may also participate in intense ocular inflammatory reactions resulting in tissue damage. Thus, inflammatory eye reactions resulting from activation of endogenous immune components are similar to the inflammatory reaction found in other tissues. Since immune mechanisms in the eye can potentially mediate many biological reactions (such as leukocyte chemotaxis; bacterial and viral clearance; cell membrane lysis; and the release of oxygen radicals, vasoactive mediators, lysosomal enzymes, and prostaglandins from inflammatory cells), it is appropriate to review the potential role of inflammatory mediators in the eye.

8.2. MEDIATORS DERIVED FROM INFLAMMATORY CELLS AND IMMUNE REACTIONS

8.2.1. Complement and its split products

As described above, complement components of both the classic and alternative pathways have been demonstrated to be important in the defense of the ocular surface only in the past few years. Yet in other systems the complement cascade has been recognized as an important humoral defense mechanism for decades (Muller-Eberhard 1975). The mobilization and sequential activation of the complement system has a number of biological consequences, many times independent of the tissue where the activation occurs. Not only does activation of the complement system cause irreversible structural and functional changes in target cell membranes, which can result in a cytotoxic outcome, but the activation of this system generates a number of phlogistic products that are intimately tied to the acute inflammatory system.

Activation of the complement system, whether in lacrimal fluid or serum, can occur by two separate pathways (Fig. 1). The classic pathway is composed of 11 seperate proteins, which interact in a sequential cascade when activated by antigen—antibody complexes. The activation of the classical complement pathway occurs via a recognition process, whereby the first component of complement binds to the Fc fraction of certain classes of IgG or all IgM antibody that is bound to the surface of a target cell. This initial binding sets in motion an enzymatic cascade which processes the subsequent complement components (Hyslop et al. 1970), resulting in the release of inflammatory mediators and the formation of a multimolecular membrane attack complex (Capel et al. 1978; Chenoweth and Hugli 1980; Podack and Muller-Eberhard 1980). As with the classical pathway, activation of the alternative pathway results in the sequential interaction of several discrete serum proteins (Mann et al. 1980). Although the first three classical complement components (C1, C4, and C2) are not involved in the alternative pathway activation, the end result is similar; phlogistic peptides are generated and target cell lysis occurs. Functionally the two pathways are quite similar, but the initial activation methods are very diverse. As shown in Table 1, the methods of alternative and classical complement pathway activation are dependent upon a plethora of compounds, many of which can be found associated with ocular tissue (Mondino et al. 1978; Berman 1979).

Upon activation of either the classical or alternative complement pathway in the eye, a number of potent inflammatory peptides may be produced (Table 2). Two important split products of complement activation derived from C3 and C5 are the classical anaphylatoxins, C3a and C5a (Hugli and Muller-Eberhard 1978). Although originally defined as spasmogenic factors, the anaphylatoxins are now recognized to possess additional functional characteristics (Ward and Newman 1969; Grant et al. 1975). Thus, the generation of complement-derived anaphylatoxins in ocular tissue,

A. Classic Complement Pathway

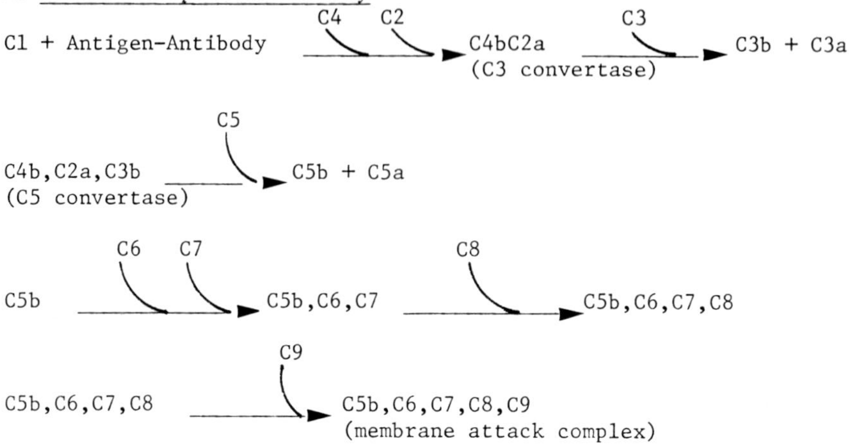

B. Alternative Complement Pathway

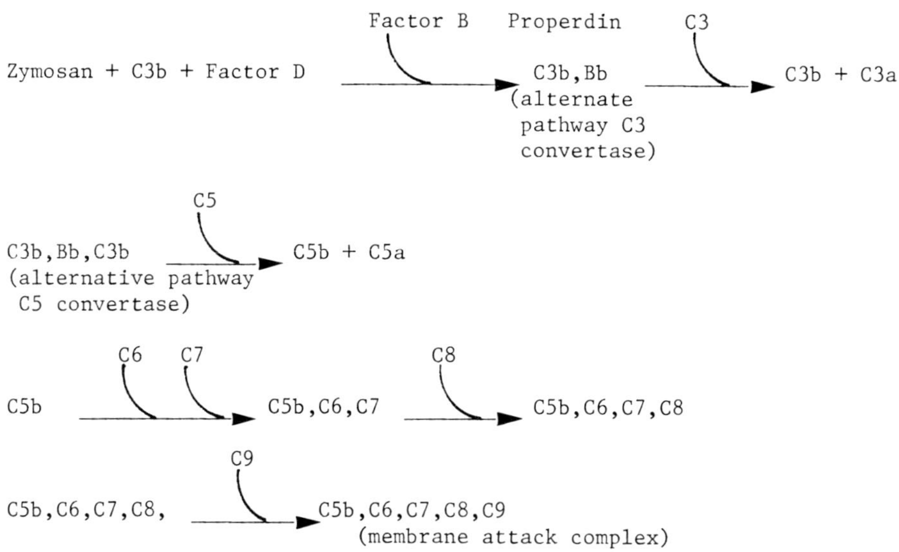

TABLE 1.
Biological complements involved in the activation of the classic or alternative complement pathway

A: Classic complement pathway activators
1. Immune complexes (antigen—antibody complexes)
   a) IgM
   b) IgG (subclasses 1—4)
2. Aggregated antibodies
3. C-reactive protein (an acute inflammatory phase protein)
4. Proteases
   a) Bacterial (bacteria origin)
   b) Host (tissue origin)

B: Alternative complement pathway activators
1. Components found in bacterial cell walls
2. Cobra venom factor (CVF)
3. Inulin
4. Components found in yeast cell walls (zymosan)
5. Lipopolysaccharides
6. C3 nephritic factor (antibody directed against C3b-dependent C3 convertase)

←

Fig. 1. Activation of the complement cascade can occur via the classic (A) or alternative (B) pathway. Antigen—antibody complexes can activate the classic pathway by binding and activating the first complement component (C1). In succession, C1 can act on C4 and C2, resulting in an enzyme complex (C3 convertase) which can cleave C3. One of the cleavage products from C3, C3b, interacts with the C3 convertase (C4b, C2a) to form the C5 convertase (C4b, C2a, C3b). This enzyme cleaves C5, generating C5b, which serves as the nidus for the binding of the terminal complement components, C6—C9, and the formation of the membrane attack complex. The alternative complement pathway is set in motion by the binding of C3b + Factor Bb in the presence of properdin to a stimulus, e.g. zymosan, forming the alternative pathway C3 convertase. This enzyme complex cleaves C3, producing more C3b, which can feed back and amplify the C3 convertase. As more C3b is bound to the alternative pathway C3 convertase, alternative pathway C5 convertase is formed which cleaves C5 and generates C5b. The C5b can now bind the terminal complement components and form the membrane attack complex as in the classic complement pathway. For a recent review on complement activation see Kunkel, S.L., Fantone, J.C. and Ward, P.A. (1981) Complement-mediated inflammatory reactions. *Pathobiology 11,* 127.

TABLE 2.
Inflammatory mediators generated by activation of either the classic or alternative complement pathway

Mediator	Parent component	Biological activity
1. Anaphylatoxins		
a) C3a	C3	-Induces smooth muscle contraction -Induces vascular permeability changes -Induces histamine release from certain inflammatory cells
b) C5a	C5	-Induces smooth muscle contraction -Induces vascular permeability changes -Induces histamine release from certain inflammatory cells -Induces polymorphonuclear leukocyte aggregation -Potent chemotactic peptide for inflammatory cells
2. C5a des arg; C5a minus C-terminal arginine	C5, C5a	-Induces release of inflammatory mediators (lysosomal enzymes) from inflammatory cells -Chemotactic for inflammatory cells in presence of serum factor
3. C3b	C3	-Both C3b and C4b can function as opsonins which can: -Promote phagocytosis
4. C4b	C4	-Solubilize immune complexes
5. Membrane attack complex	C5, C6, C7 C8, C9	-C5b−C9 are all involved in target cell membrane alterations which lead to target cell lysis

as in other organ systems, can induce the release of histamine from mast cells (Morrison et al. 1975), increase vascular permeability (Hugli and Muller-Eberhard 1978), and serve as a potent signal for the recruitment of inflammatory cells (Ward and Newman 1969). The importance of complement activation and its subsequent role in inflammatory eye disease has been extensively examined in a number of experimental eye disorders (Marak et al. 1977, 1979; Okada and Shimada 1980). In each of the above investigations the depletion of serum complement levels by cobra venom factor (C3 inactivator) resulted in the suppression of immune complex-induced, complement-dependent inflammatory processes. In the latter investigation complement depletion not only resulted in a decreased acute ocular inflammatory cell infiltrate, but permeability changes were also suppressed. The permeability changes were monitored by determining the relative amount of fluorescein-labeled serum albumin leaking into the anterior chamber during the ocular inflammation. In this study the intensity of fluorescence was continuously monitored by the use of a slit-lamp fluorophotometer (Dyster-Aas et al. 1969). The immediate permeability response in the experimental immune complex ocular model was completely suppressed in the animals given C3 inactivator. However, a slight increase in the permeability response in these animals was observed in the later phase of ocular edema.

In addition to C3 inactivator inhibiting the ocular inflammatory reactions resulting from the Arthus reaction in the eye, a number of other experimental ocular diseases are suppressed by complement depletion (Marak et al. 1977). These include experimental lens-induced endophthalmitis and experimental allergic uveitis. Although the use of C3 inactivator from cobra venom is already known to inhibit inflammation in a variety of immune complex-mediated diseases, the continued use of this protein as a probe to examine experimental inflammatory ocular diseases will be an important tool in future research.

Only recently have split products from complement activation been examined for their ability to induce ocular inflammatory reactions (Ben-Zvi et al. 1981). Upon infusion of C5a, the small molecular weight chemotactic peptide derived from C5, into the cornea, vitreous, or conjunctiva, an intense inflammatory reaction developed 2−48 hours post injection. The time course of the C5a-induced inflammatory reaction was shown to be dependent upon the ocular tissue involved. The peak inflammatory reaction occurred 2, 4, and 24 hours post infusion of C5a in the conjunctiva, cornea, and vitreous, respectively. The type of inflammatory reaction induced by C5a challenge was very similar to that induced by antigen−antibody-dependent Arthus type reactions; especially upon administration of this complement-derived fragment into the conjunctiva and cornea. The inflammatory cell infiltrates, caused by C5a, into these two ocular tissues were predominantly polymorphonuclear leukocytes. The C5a-induced inflammatory response in the vitreous was shown to be delayed, occurring 24−48 hours post infusion, and the inflammatory cell infiltrate was composed of both neutrophils and mononuclear cells. The observation that C5a can cause an infiltrate of inflammatory cells when infused into certain ocular tissues is of paramount importance. For, once the acute inflammatory cells are recruited into an area, a number of phlogistic mediators may be generated from the cells, resulting in tissue injury. Again C5a may play an important role by directing the release of superoxide anion (Becker et al. 1979), lysosomal enzyme (Henson 1980) and causing the aggregation of leukocytes (O'Flaherty and Ward 1978). Thus, the generation of a potent inflammatory mediator such as C5a in the eye can have a profound effect on the recruitment of inflammatory cells and the subsequent release

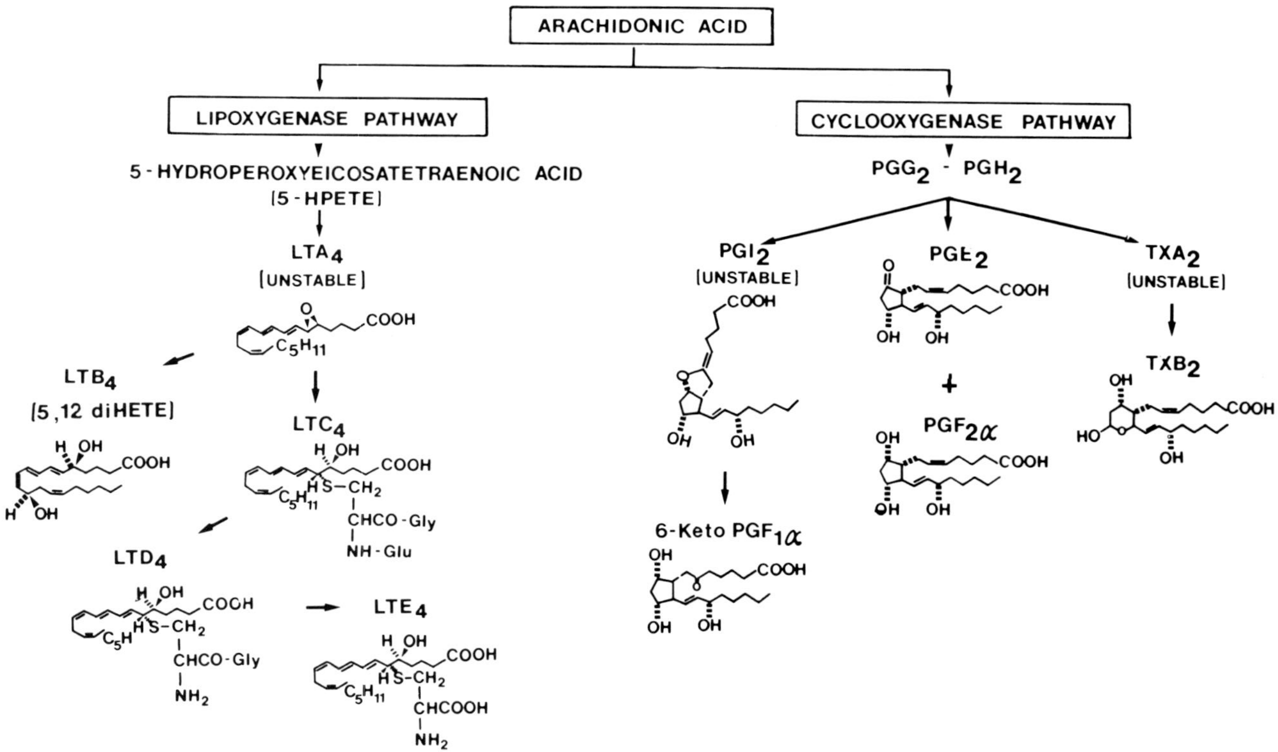

Fig. 2. Arachidonic acid metabolism can occur by two enzymatic systems; the cyclo-oxygenase pathway, which leads to the production of prostacyclin, thromboxanes and the classical prostaglandins, and the lipoxygenase pathway, whereby the various leukotrienes are synthesized.

of tissue-destructive compounds. It is interesting to note that the inflammatory reaction induced by the intra-ocular challenge with C5a could be suppressed with a number of pharmacological agents including: quinacrine, steroids, 5,8,11,14-eicosatetraynoic acid (ETYA; a non-metabolic analog of arachidonic acid), and indomethacin. Either topical application or subconjunctival injection of the above pharmacological agents was effective in reducing the inflammatory reaction, probably by virtue of suppressing the production of cyclo-oxygenase and lipoxygenase products (Hanna and Keatts 1967).

8.2.2. Cyclo-oxygenase and lipoxygenase products

As previously stated, inhibition of arachidonic acid metabolism has been demonstrated to suppress acute ocular inflammatory reactions. This is especially important since not only are prostaglandins found in normal ocular tissues, but these cyclo-oxygenase products have been found in the inflamed anterior chamber of the eye (Eakins et al. 1972c).

It has been recognized that characteristic lipid mediators are synthesized during an inflammatory reaction, independent of the organ or tissue under investigation. The major substrate for both the cyclo-oxygenase or lipoxygenase enzymes in mammalian systems is arachidonic acid. The enzymes necessary to convert arachidonic acid – in addition to other essential fatty acids – into cyclo-oxygenase products are found in most cells of the body. The synthesis of arachidonic acid by either the lipoxygenase or cyclo-oxygenase system must be initiated by the release of fatty acid (arachidonic acid) substrate from the phospholipids in cellular membrances by phospholipases. Once this occurs, arachidonic acid derivatives may be synthesized by the above enzyme systems into a number of potent biologically active lipids (Fig. 2).

It is important to recognize that many of the products produced by the metabolism of arachidonic acid are highly unstable in biological fluids and include the endoperoxides PGG_2 and PGH_2, TXA_2 and PGI_2. Even though these compounds possess half-lives measured in seconds, their activity in biological systems is extremely potent (Vane 1976; Horton 1979). The activities of these biologically active lipids produced by various inflammatory cells are outlined in Table 3. In addition to the phlogistic mediators produced by products of arachidonic acid metabolism, prostacyclin and prostaglandins of the E-series have been shown to suppress various effector systems of the inflammatory response. Investigations concerning the immunoregulatory activity of PGE compounds have shown that by virtue of increasing intracellular cyclic AMP levels lymphocyte-mediated cytotoxicity can be inhibited (Henney et al. 1971), IgE-induced release of histamine from mast cells may be suppressed (Lichtenstein and DiBernado 1971), and the release of lysosomal enzymes from polymorphonuclear leukocytes can be controlled (Zurier et al. 1975). In addition, pharmacological doses of PGE have been demonstrated to suppress acute and chronic inflammation in experimental models

TABLE 3.
Biological functions of arachidonic acids products

Cyclo-oxygenase products	Properties
Prostacyclin (PGI_2)	-Potent inhibitor of platelet aggregation -Causes vasodilatation -Can inhibit certain inflammatory cell functions -Stimulates adenylate cyclase
Prostaglandin E (PGE)	-Can inhibit platelet aggregation -Causes vasodilatation -Can inhibit the release of mediators from inflammatory cells -Stimulates adenylate cyclase -Can enhance Fc receptors on neutrophils
Thromboxane (TXA_2, TXB_2)	-Potent platelet-aggregating agent -Causes vasoconstriction
Lipoxygenase products	
Leukotriene A_4	-Unstable
Leukotriene B_4 (LTB_4)	-Potent chemotactic agent -Induces chemokinesis -Can induce the release of mediators from inflammatory cells -Can enhance C3b receptors on neutrophils -Can regulate inflammatory cell functions -Induces neutrophil aggregation -Induces vascular permeability changes
Leukotriene C_4 (LTC_4)	-Cause potent contraction of smooth muscle -Induce tracheal constriction
Leukotriene D_4 (LTD_4)	-Induce pulmonary airway constriction
Leukotriene E_4 (LTE_4)	-Increase vascular permeability

(Kunkel et al. 1979, 1981). A regulatory mechanism for prostaglandin E compounds has been demonstrated in other systems. The release of noradrenaline from the spleen in response to sympathetic nerve stimulation is inhibited by PGE, on the other hand the release of this prostaglandin occurs when the spleen contracts in response to sympathetic nerve stimulation. Therefore, by a feedback mechanism, involving prostaglandins, the contracting smooth muscle can reduce the stimulus that leads to the contraction. In a similar feedback fashion, prostaglandin release during an inflammatory response may be a defense mechanism aimed at minimizing tissue injury.

Whether prostaglandins play a dominant immunomodulatory role in ocular reactions is not clearly understood. Yet, inflammatory reactions in ocular tissue, especially the uveal tract, are definitely influenced by prostaglandins. The injection of bovine serum albumin into the vitreous of sensitized rabbits leads to an intense immunologic uveitis with the production of high PGE levels. Fluid isolated from the aqueous humor was found to contain up to 150 ng of PGE/ml, as compared to 2 ng/ml in control aqueous (Eakins et al. 1972b). In clinical cases PGE_2 levels in the aqueous humor of patients with uveitis ranged from 20−56 ng/ml compared to 2 ng/ml from specimens collected from eyes with uveitis controlled with corticosteroids (Eakins et al. 1972a). Prostaglandin E levels have also been reported to be elevated in the aqueous humor of human eyes with Behcet's disease (Masuda et al. 1973). As with other inflammatory reactions, a large number of ocular immune reactions appear to be modulated by prostaglandins. The biological role of the prostaglandins with regard to pro- or anti-inflammatory activity is still not clear, much more work needs to be done to clarify the role of prostaglandins in the eye.

8.2.3. Toxic products from oxygen metabolism

Recent experimental evidence suggests that oxygen metabolites may be responsible for tissue injury associated with inflammatory reactions (Klebanoff 1980). These toxic oxygen metabolites are generated from activated granulocytes which have been recruited into an area of inflammation (Fig. 3). The ability of these oxygen metabolic

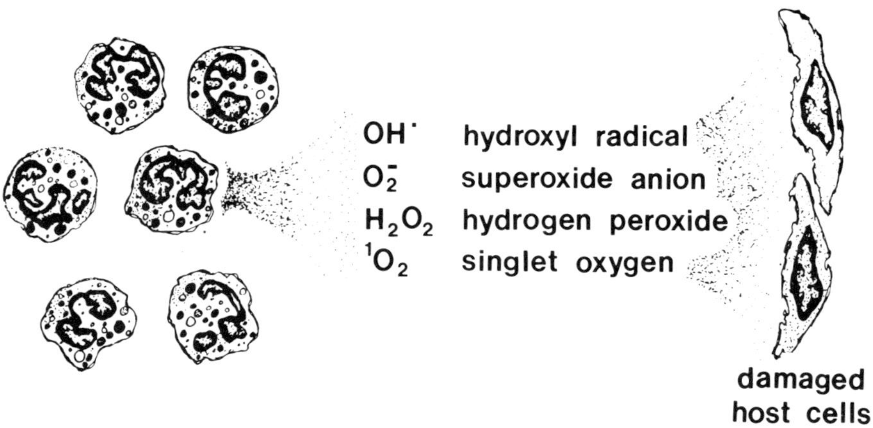

Fig. 3. Generation and release of toxic oxygen products from granulocytes recruited to an area of ocular inflammation can result in tissue destruction by polymerizing, oxidizing, or fragmenting components which make up the membrane of the host's cells.

products to cause cytotoxic damage has been clearly demonstrated in in-vitro systems whereby free radicals are enzymatically generated using xanthine oxidase and myeloperoxidase (Rosen and Klebanoff 1977; Nathan et al. 1979). Additional evidence for the role of oxygen metabolites in inducing tissue injury stems from investigations where inhibitors of specific free radicals have been shown to block the cytotoxic effects of neutrophils and activated macrophages (Weiss et al. 1978; Nathan et al. 1979). Subsequently, the suppression of immune complex-induced vasculitis has been demonstrated by systemic administration of superoxide dismutase, thus indicating that superoxide anion is involved in acute inflammation (Petrone et al. 1980). It appears that the release of these toxic oxygen products from inflammatory cells can cause tissue destruction in many organ systems, including the eye. Recent investigations have demonstrated that the generation of toxic oxygen products in ocular tissue can result in substantial damage (Goosey et al. 1981). In this specific investigation, singlet oxygen was shown to cause destruction of human lens tissue. Despite the current advances in our understanding of the role of oxygen metabolites and free radicals in initiating cytotoxic damage and tissue injury, there remains a paucity of evidence directed at understanding the role of oxygen toxic products in ocular inflammation.

8.2.4. Products of lysosomal enzyme release from inflammatory cells

The influx of neutrophils and mononuclear phagocytes into ocular tissue may be seen as the hallmark of inflammation and their presence significantly contributes to both the injury and, later, the repair seen in normal situations. The ability of these inflammatory cells to phagocytose, kill, and digest invasive organisms represents a critical factor in host defense mechanisms. The ability to intracellularly digest phagocytosed organisms or compounds is wholly or in part due to the secretion of degradative enzymes into phagocytic vacuoles. Associated with this phenomenon is the non-specific release of these enzymes into the inflammatory milieu through the process of enzyme regurgitation (Fig. 4). This results in the release of enzymes capable of degrading normal tissue at the inflammatory site. Once phagocytic cells accumulate in an area of ocular inflammation, the tissue degradation due to collagenase and other hydrolases released from these cells can be observed (Kenyon et al. 1979).

Recent investigations into the secretion of collagenase from polymorphonuclear leukocytes during corneal ulceration due to alkali burns have demonstrated the potent role of hydrolytic enzymes in ocular inflammation (Berman 1980). Experimental corneal ulcerations using a plethora of etiological agents have shown that the host's inflammatory cells are involved in the production of hydrolases which effect matrix damage leading to ocular ulceration (Meyers 1975; Kessler et al. 1977).

In addition, both bacterial and viral infections of the eye can result in recruitment

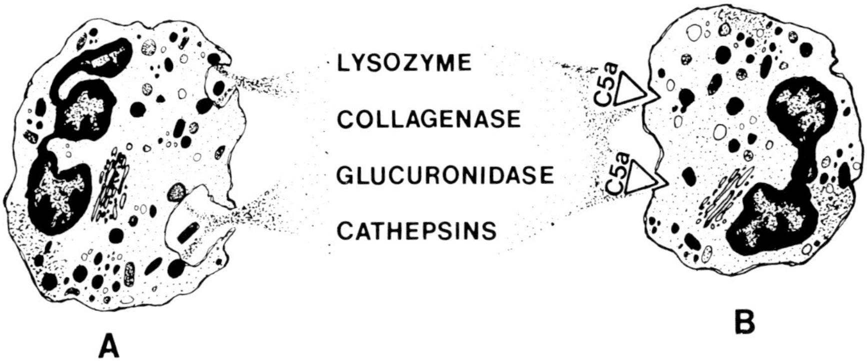

Fig. 4. The release of lysosomal enzymes from granulocytes recruited to an area of ocular inflammation can occur through distinct mechanisms including: (A) regurgitation, while phagocytizing particles, or (B) binding of components to specific membrane receptors (e.g. C5a) on the cell surface.

of polymorphonuclear leukocytes and monocyte/macrophages resulting in the release of enzymes responsible for matrix damage.

Thus, strong experimental evidence does support the role of enzyme secretion from inflammatory cells and subsequent ocular tissue damage. This is particularly true of the neutrophil-dependent ulcerations due to the degradation of stromal matrix after physical insult, alkali and thermal burns, or in response to invasion by bacterial or viral agents.

8.3. EXPERIMENTAL MODELS OF EYE DISEASE

In order to examine the role of inflammatory mediators in ocular inflammation, experimental animal models must be available in which an inflammatory response can be easily elicited. Presently a number of models exist in which ocular inflammatory mechanisms can be studied, the majority of which involve infecting the eye with a specific invasive organism (parasitic, bacterial, or viral) or inducing chemical damage to the eye (alkali burns). The intraocular challenge with a specific antigen in a sensitized host (Arthus reactions) can also result in an acute inflammatory response and provide a unique model for the investigation of antigen–antibody-dependent complement-mediated immune responses. In addition, the ocular response to intravenous administration of lipopolysaccharide (LPS) has been used as an animal model for acute iridocyclitis and as a means to examine alterations in ocular vascular permeability (Howes et al. 1971, 1979).

8.3.1. Ocular inflammation due to infectious microorganisms

The pathogenesis of ocular inflammation due to infectious diseases is determined by a number of factors including: the virulence of the agent, the host's immune response, and the anatomical site where the injection occurs. With these factors taken into consideration, a number of animal models have been developed to examine the inflammatory response due to parasitic, bacterial and viral infections. Helminthic and protozoan eye injections are known to cause blinding diseases whose immunopathological mechanisms are not entirely clear. A useful model for examining parasitic diseases of the eye involves the use of *Toxocara canis* and *Ascaris suum* infections of the guinea pig eye (Donelly et al. 1977). The experimental intravitreal infection of guinea pig eyes with *T. canis* or *A. suum* larvae (or soluble extract) resulted in an intense infiltration of eosinophils into the anterior chamber and uveal tract; followed by the development of intraocular reagin antibodies (Rockey et al. 1979). As observed with other tissues infected with helminthic parasites (Mahmoud et al. 1975), individual larvae in the eye are surrounded by granulomatous tissue composed mainly of eosinophils and it is this inflammatory cell which is probably responsible for their destruction. Experimental intravitreal infection using helminthic larvae represents a classical model to examine both the role of IgE antibody and eosinophils in intraocular diseases. Not only can one examine the beneficial role of the eosinophils by studying the intraocular cytotoxic mechanisms for parasite destruction, but the widespread release of inflammatory mediators contained within, or generated by, eosinophils can also be studied. This is important in that it allows for the investigation of eosinophil-dependent destruction of ocular components. Although the role of eosinophils in many inflammatory reactions remains enigmatic, continued investigation of this inflammatory cell in ocular disease deserves further consideration.

Infectious organisms are known to invade a number of ocular tissues, but those sites which produce the greatest morbidity upon infection are the cornea, conjunctiva, retina, and choroid (Jones 1978). Bacterial infections of the corneal stroma can lead to a keratitis and result in serious visual impairment. Thus, animal models of bacterial keratitis are extremely important in examining the host's response to ocular bacterial infections. Bacterial keratitis can be produced by a number of methods ranging from intrastromal inoculations (Van Horn et al. 1980) to topical infection after a corneal scratch (Joy 1942). Using the former challenge, Pseudomonas keratitis in guinea pigs has been assessed by a variety of methods. The following sequence of events is known to occur in response to experimental keratitis: 8 hours after infection, inflammatory cells are observed in the anterior section of the stroma; by 14−18 hours a dense accumulation of both polymorphonuclear leukocytes and monocytes is observed in the mid-stroma; 24 hours after challenge, a dense infiltrate of neutrophils extends to the limbus. At this time, neutrophils appear degranulated and contain bacteria in their phagolysosomes, as determined by electron microscopy. By 24−32 hours necrosis and connective tissue breakdown have occurred, resulting in ulceration of the epithelium. Again by the use of electron microscopy, bacteria can be found in degranulated neutrophils for up to 88 hours post inoculation. This sequestration of certain bacteria (i.e. Pseudomonas) in inflammatory cells may explain the recurrence of Pseudomonas in corneal infections despite chemotherapy (Wilson and Ahearn 1977).

Bacterial infection and its role in ocular tissue damage can occur by two general mechanisms: (a) the in-vivo production of enzymes or toxins from the bacterium itself or (b) the release of specific inflammatory mediators from phagocytic cells. Tissue damage resulting from the latter case has been described in a former section of this review. The important role of phagocytes and their inflammatory mediators in bacterial eye infections has recently been examined using experimental keratitis (Kessler et al. 1977). The intrastromal challenge with heat-killed bacteria causes an acute infiltrate of neutrophils which progresses to an extensive ulceration. Treatment with anti-inflammatory steroids significantly reduced the neutrophil infiltrate and prevented much of the ulceration. Thus, ocular inflammation due to bacterial eye infections and subsequent tissue damage may be due more to the host's response to the invasive organism than to the invasive organism itself.

In addition, experimental animals, made neutropenic by cyclophosphamide treatment (Hazzlet et al. 1977) or whole-body X-irradiation (Chusid and Davis 1979) and then challenged with an intracorneal injection of bacteria, demonstrated a rapidly progressing ocular infection. Both of the above studies demonstrate that polymorphonuclear leukocytes play a major role in the response of the cornea to bacterial infections and that neutropenia can drastically alter the outcome of ocular infections. Thus the presence of inflammatory cells in ocular diseases can be both beneficial: as phagocytic cells to remove bacteria, or harmful: as secretory cells releasing degradative lysosomal enzymes.

In Section 8.3.2., antibodies were shown to play a major role in the immunopathogenesis of ocular diseases. Although antibodies do play a major role in defending ocular structures against a number of invasive organisms, this defense does not seem to be as protective against viral infections. This is especially evident in cases where recurrent ocular herpes infections are common in the presence of antibody directed against herpes antigens. Experimental evidence now supports the role of cell-mediated immunity as the major defense mechanism in the eye to protect against viral infections (Meyers 1975). Recently many experimental models have been developed to examine ocular inflammatory mechanisms directed against viral infections, especially herpes simplex virus (HSV) (Meyers and Chitjian 1976; Meyers-Elliott and Chitjian 1980). Upon primary HSV infection of the eye, both circulating levels of IgG and tear IgA levels rise. Although IgA directed against HSV can neutralize the virus in certain cases, the presence in tears is transient and lasts approximately 90—120 days (Centifanto and Kaufman 1980). As stated above, humoral immune responses are not by themselves totally effective in preventing ocular HSV infections. More important to the host in defense against HSV infections of the eye are the cell-mediated type immune responses (Jacobs et al. 1976; Nehmias et al. 1976). This is shown by the important role of lymphokines, activated macrophages, and sensitized lymphocytes to HSV antigen in the ocular tissue during a HSV infection.

Macrophages can play an important protective role in ocular HSV infections as killer cells directed against virus particles or virus-infected cells. Macrophages have been shown to inhibit the replication of HSV and thus aid in stopping the spread of the infection (Stevens and Cook 1971). Also, a combination of antibody- and cell-mediated mechanisms is important in ocular antibody-dependent cell-mediated cytotoxicity; a key defense mechanism active during many viral infections.

8.3.2. Experimental immune complex ocular vasculitis

As stated previously, the ability of lymphocytes contained in various components of the eye to produce antibody may be of significance for antibody-mediated mechanisms in the genesis of ocular inflammation. The role of antigen–antibody reactions in ocular diseases has been extensively examined using both the passive and active Arthus reactions (Witmer 1955; Waksman and Bullington 1956; Okada and Shimada 1980). The Arthus reaction is an experimental model in which the interaction of complement, antigen, and antibody leads to a severe vasculitis that is recognizable by edema, induration, erythema, and hemorrhage. This vasculitis depends upon the interaction of four key components in the vascular bed: polymorphonuclear leukocytes, antigen, antibody, and complement. The interaction of these components usually occurs in the following manner: precipitation of the immune complexes within the walls of the blood vessels of the eye; the fixation of serum complement to these complexes with the generation of complement-derived chemotactic factors; the recruitment of neutrophils to the site of the deposited immune complexes; the phagocytosis of the complexes and degranulation of the neutrophils; and the production of toxic oxygen products and release of degradative enzymes, resulting in the destruction of host tissues. This vasculitis induced by the immune complexes is inhibitable by depleting the animal of neutrophils and/or complement (Cochrane 1965). The immunological event that leads to ocular immune complex vasculitis, i.e. the interaction of complement and immune complexes within vessel walls, is very similar to the dermal Arthus reaction (Ward and Cochrane 1965). However, a striking difference lies in the persistence of immune complexes in retinal vessels for as long as one week post challenge, whereas immune complexes in the skin are removed in hours. This difference is explained by the retention of antigen in the various tissues. The vitreous slowly releases antigen, resulting in prolonged presentation in the retinal vessel walls. This idea of continual antigen presentation is supported by a classic investigation examining the release of radioactive antigen over a number of days following intravitreal challenge (Fernando 1960). Again, it can be observed that neutrophil accumulation and subsequent mediator release can be responsible for ocular tissue damage, whether the initial insulting agent is an invasive organism or antigen–antibody complex.

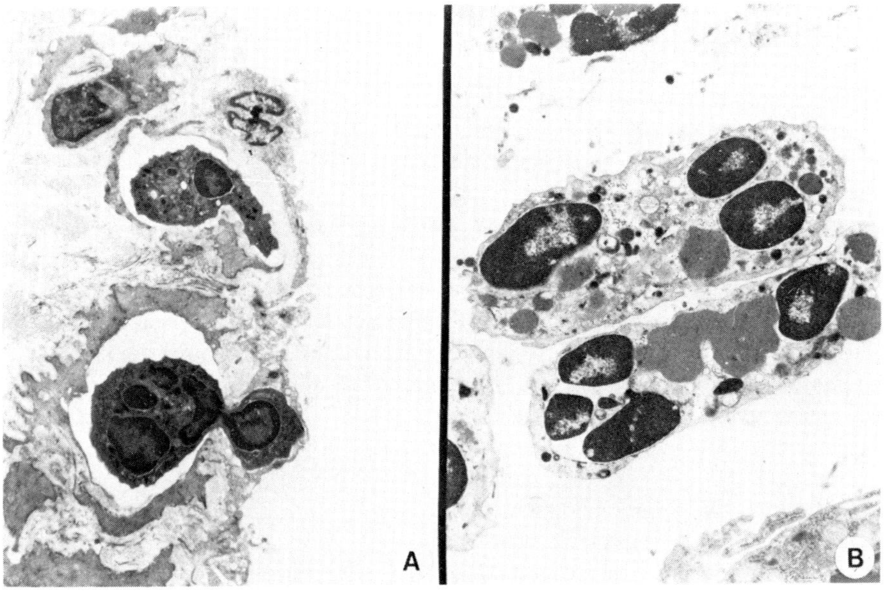

Fig. 5. Electron micrograph of neutrophils being recruited through chemotaxis to an area of inflammation (A) and neutrophils phagocytosing immune complexes (B), as demonstrated by electron dense immune complexes contained within the neutrophil's phagolysosome.

In the classical Arthus-type ocular reactions, experimental animals are actively sensitized against a particular antigen. After the animal has mounted an antibody response, the homologous antigen is given intravitreally. Within 5 hours an intense infiltrate of neutrophils occurs in the area of immune complex deposition. As shown by electron microscopy in Figure 5, the area of vascular antigen—antibody deposition contains neutrophils full of electron-dense immune complexes in their phagolysosomes.

8.3.3. Ocular inflammation due to alkali burns

Clinical cases of severe alkali burns, especially of the cornea, can be debilitating, especially when different tissues of the eye are involved (Brown et al. 1970). Recent studies have demonstrated that polymorphonuclear leukocytes do play an important role in the breakdown of the corneal matrix after alkali burns (Kenyon et al. 1979). The role of neutrophil-dependent matrix degradation in the alkali burn model is very similar to the apparent neutrophil-dependent matrix damage seen after Pseudomonas and herpes infections of the cornea. After severe alkali burns, induced by applying a filter paper disk wetted with 4-N-sodium hydroxide to the cornea, an intense accumulation of neutrophils occurred concomitant with stromal ulceration. The inflammatory cells appear extremely active, since they contain a number of phagolysosomes and an absence of lysosomal granules (indicative of degranulation). The role of neutrophil degranulation in corneal ulcerations is extremely important, since these inflammatory cells may release extracellular collagenase and cause further matrix degradation.

In addition, granulocytes may release plasminogen activator. This phenomenon is extremely important in the light of recent studies which have shown that the ulcerating stroma can release plasminogen activator and contribute to the plasmin-mediated activation of latent collagenase (Berman 1978). Latent corneal collagenase produced by fibroblasts may also be activated by neutrophil proteases released in the inflammatory area (Hook et al. 1973). Although the initial alkali insult can induce direct ocular tissue damage, neutrophils and their armament of lysosomal enzymes are clearly involved in the subsequent pathological ulceration.

8.3.4. Ocular inflammation due to endotoxemia

The ocular response to intravenous challenge with bacterial lipopolysaccharide (LPS) results in an acute iridocyclitis (Ayo 1943) in addition to alterations in ocular vascular permeability (Howes and McKay 1975). This response to LPS is known to be extremely sensitive, since previous studies have shown that quantities of LPS as small as 0.25 – 1.00 μg/kg were able to induce alterations in ocular vascular permeability (Levine and Breinen 1959). Various methods have been used in an attempt to quantitate the protein leakage; ranging from direct ocular paracentesis (Ayo 1943) to the use of photoelectric devices to assay the aqueous flare produced by the permeable vasculature (Bengtsson 1976). Interestingly, the ocular permeability change due to systemic LPS treatment is dose-dependent and appears as a bell-shaped curve; where both very low doses and doses above 200 μg/kg result in little permeability change (Howes and McKay 1975). The reason why extremely high doses of LPS are not effective may relate to feedback mechanisms between the various inflammatory mediators which are involved in both systemic and ocular responses to endotoxin.

Inhibition of prostaglandin, serotonin or histamine release can inhibit the ocular permeability response to LPS (Gilbert 1959; Howes and McKay 1975; Fletcher and Ramwell 1978). However, systemic treatment with arachidonic acid (the metabolic precursor of prostaglandin synthesis), prostaglandin of the E-series, or serotonin can also prevent the ocular leakage due to permeability changes (Gilbert 1959). Thus, ocular capillary leakage can be initiated and inhibited by the same mediators. This may explain why the higher doses of LPS, which can induce mediator release, can act to inhibit vascular permeability. Also, higher doses of LPS may increase systemic hypertension and reduce the permeability by decreasing intravascular pressure.

Since very small doses of circulating endotoxin can induce ocular capillary leakage, there is a possibility that gram-negative bacterial infections can result in an uveitis or a disorder not unlike Reiter's syndrome. This may occur by circulating LPS, released from a focal area of infection, leaking into ocular tissue and initiating an inflammatory response.

Endotoxin-induced ocular permeability primarily affects the capillaries in the iridial extension of the ciliary processes. The ease in quantitating the vascular permeability changes, plus the precise anatomical location where the LPS is active, makes this model ideal for examining vascular permeability alterations in the eye.

Basic research concerning inflammatory eye disorders continues to make significant contributions to the understanding of specific ocular diseases.

The final goal of the above research is the direct application of the knowledge to the disease state; at times a somewhat idealistic situation, especially with regard to the many enigmatic ocular inflammatory diseases discussed below.

8.4. AUTOIMMUNE PROCESSES OF THE EYE

Autoimmune processes have been presumed to occur in all ocular tissues although strict evidence for their autoimmune etiology is lacking in most (Witebsky and Milgram 1964). Examples include involvement of the lids by "collagen—vascular" disease, the conjunctiva by cicatricial pemphigoid, corneal Mooren's ulcer, lens-induced uveitis or "phacoanaphylaxis", and several forms of chorioretinitis. Several conditions with some evidence for an autoimmune basis will be discussed.

8.4.1. Sympathetic ophthalmia

Sympathetic ophthalmia is a granulomatous inflammatory disease of the uveal tract occurring in both eyes after penetrating injury to one eye. Its incidence is reported to be 1 to 2 cases per 1000 traumatic perforations of the eye and one case per 10,000 intraocular surgical procedures (Liddy and Stuart 1972; Blodi 1979). Clinically, there is usually onset of both anterior and posterior uveitis from two weeks to several years following injury, although most cases begin within 3 months. Typically subretinal exudation from choroidal infiltration leads to localized yellow subretinal nodules known as Dalen-Fuchs spots (Marak 1979). Vitritis, optic neuritis and the secondary changes of severe uveitis may follow.

Histologically, sympathetic ophthalmia is characterized by infiltration of the uveal tract with lymphocytes, epithelioid cells, and often giant cells which may contain pigment granules. Typically the choriocapillaris, the inner vascular layer of the choroid, and the retina are spared, although the retina may be elevated by uveal effusion and there may be inflammatory cells within the retina (Lubin and Albert 1979). Eosinophils may be present early in the course of the disease and plasma cell infiltration of the choroid has been shown in 60% of enucleated eyes (Lubin et al.

1980). "Phacoanaphylaxis", a neutrophilic infiltration of the lens, is seen in 23 to 46% of cases (Blodi 1959; Lubin et al. 1980).

Several etiologies have been proposed for sympathetic ophthalmia, including hypersensitivitiy to choroidal pigment and various forms of infection. Positive skin tests have been demonstrated to a uveal antigen mixture (McPherson and Woods 1948) and leukocyte migration inhibition has been stimulated by uveal pigment (Hammer 1974). Current research, however, is directed at an antigen derived from retinal rod outer segments designated "S" antigen. Injection of this antigen in complete Freunds adjuvant causes experimental autoimmune uveoretinitis in animals, a condition with features similar to sympathetic ophthalmia and Vogt-Koyanagi-Harada syndrome (Marak 1979; Faure 1980). Viral etiologies have been disputed (Lubin et al. 1980). It is possible that an as yet unidentified infectious agent plays a role as an adjuvant.

Sympathetic ophthalmia has a variable chronic course with periods of remission. It may lead to blindness, although treatment with steroids and immunosuppressive drugs has improved the prognosis. Enucleation of the injured eye within two weeks of injury prevents development of sympathetic ophthalmia, but the low incidence and possibility that the injured eye may have better vision than the "sympathizing" eye make enucleation unwise unless there is no potential for vision. Early enucleation of the injured eye after the onset of sympathetic ophthalmia may be of some small benefit (Lubin et al. 1980).

Some patients with sympathetic ophthalmia develop systemic lesions with poliosis, vitiligo, tinnitus and meningeal irritation. These symptoms and the ocular features, as well as experimental models, provide overlap with the Vogt-Koyanagi-Harada syndrome (Marak 1979; Faure 1980).

8.4.2. Vogt-Koyanagi-Harada syndrome

Vogt-Koyanagi-Harada (V-K-H) syndrome is a rare form of uveitis associated with meningeal irritation, poliosis, vitiligo, and hearing changes. The Vogt-Koyanagi syndrome may be separated by more severe anterior segment ocular inflammation and skin changes. Harada's disease is characterized by posterior uveitis with exudative retinal detachment and meningitis. As these syndromes are often made indistinguishable by their overlapping features they are usually combined as V-K-H.

The typical ocular features are bilateral anterior uveitis with iris nodules and exudative retinal detachment followed by pigmentary retinal changes. In milder cases the disease lasts several months, whereas more severe forms may last several years. Only about one-third of cases have central nervous system, ear, or skin involvement (Ohno et al. 1977). The visual prognosis is considerably poorer in those with systemic disease, although it is improved by steroid therapy (Ohno et al. 1977). The histopathology is similar to that of sympathetic ophthalmia with granulomatous choroidal infiltration (Perry and Font 1977); plasma cells are a prominent feature.

Chorioretinal scarring and pigment migration are more common and severe than is seen in sympathetic ophthalmia. Patients with Vogt-Koyanagi syndrome have granuloma formation in the uvea, while those with Harada's disease are likely to have a non-granulomatous infiltration.

Although the etiology of V-K-H is unknown, genetic factors have been considered. The disease has a predilection for pigmented individuals and is a common cause of uveitis in Japan while rare in the United States. The Japanese subtype of HLA-BW22 (HLA-BW54) has an increased prevalence in Japanese patients but not in Americans or Japanese living in the US (Ohno et al. 1976; Tagawa et al. 1976). An HLA-D antigen, LD-Wa, is also increased in affected Japanese (Tagawa and Sugiura 1979). Humoral and cellular immunity to uveal antigen or melanocytes have been demonstrated by leukocyte migration inhibition, lymphocyte-mediated cytotoxicity and antibody-dependent cell-mediated cytotoxicity tests (Hammer 1974; Tagawa and Sugiura 1979). Viral etiologies have also been suggested by the occasional finding of virus-like particles in ocular tissues (Morris and Schlaegel 1964).

8.4.3. Reiter's syndrome

Reiter's syndrome is primarily a systemic disease characterized by urethritis, conjunctivitis and arthritis. Skin lesions of keratoderma blennorrhagicum and mucosal involvement may occur. The disease occurs predominantly in young males. The most common ocular feature is a bilateral mucopurulent conjunctivitis which lasts a few months and is self-limited. Papillae form in the palpebral conjunctiva. A punctate keratitis may develop and superficial stromal corneal opacities may occur (Schachter and Dawson 1978). Anterior uveitis occurs in from 8 to 40% of patients (Friedlaender 1979).

Several etiologies have been proposed for Reiter's syndrome and it is likely that several may be factors. Associations with venereally acquired non-gonococcal urethritis and outbreaks following Shigella dysentery suggested an infectious agent. Chlamydiae have been isolated from the urethra, joints, and conjunctiva from some groups studied, but not from others (Schachter and Dawson 1978). The incidence of the HLA antigen B27 of about 80% in these patients suggests a genetic factor and possibly altered immune reactivity (Brewerton et al. 1973). The combination of documented infection, anterior uveitis and other features of Reiter's syndrome, and HLA-B27 has been documented following infection with Yersinia (Saari et al. 1980a), Salmonella (Saari et al. 1980b) and Campylobacter (Saari and Karaunen 1980). Thus, this inflammatory disease may be the result of an inherited immune responsiveness triggered by infection with any of several agents. The association between uveitis and HLA-B27 in ankylosing spondylitis and psoriatic arthritis suggests that further understanding of this system may lead to new approaches to auto-immune disease.

8.4.4. Behçet's syndrome

Behcet's syndrome may likewise have combined genetic and environmental bases. This condition is common in the Middle East and Japan but rare in the United States. The major criteria for diagnosis are buccal ulcerations (aphthae), genital ulceration, eye lesions and skin lesions. Minor criteria include arthritis, thrombophlebitis, gastrointestinal lesions, cardiovascular involvement, and central nervous system involvement (Mason and Barnes 1969). The basic pathologic process involved is an occlusive vasculitis in the affected tissues. The eye is involved in 70–85% of patients (Michelson et al. 1980). Iridocyclitis, often with hypopyon, is a frequent presenting sign. Blindness may occur from secondary cataract and glaucoma. More often, however, visual loss is the result of retinal vasculitis with periphlebitis, arteriolitis and arteriolar occlusion. Optic neuritis may occur. In one study the average time from onset of disease to loss of useful vision in both eyes was less than 3.5 years (Mamo 1970). Treatment with cytotoxic drugs, especially chlorambucil, is often effective in preventing visual loss and neurologic complications (Mamo 1976).

The etiology of the vasculitis in Behcet's disease is unknown. Circulating antibodies to oral mucosa and elevated serum complement titers have been detected (Kogure et al. 1976). It has been disputed whether the vascular lesion represents an Arthus reaction (Cooper et al. 1971). Abnormalities of cell-mediated immunity have been detected, but may be secondary. As in Reiter's syndrome an association with an HLA antigen suggests immunogenetic factors. HLA-B5 is significantly elevated in Behçet's patients (Ohno et al. 1975).

8.4.5. Cicatricial pemphigoid

Cicatricial pemphigoid is a disease of skin and mucous membranes, with chronic recurrent blister formation and progressive scarring. It occurs primarily in elderly women. Ocular involvement begins with redness, irritation and dryness, often mistaken for minor infection. As conjunctival shrinkage occurs, secondary lid changes with trichiasis develop. Finally, corneal scarring and ulceration lead to blindness. The progressive course of this bilateral condition is not significantly altered by medical therapy (Mondino and Brown 1981). In skin, subepithelial bullae are formed with inflammatory cells, lymphocytes and PMNs, along the basement membrane zone. The conjunctival epithelium is keratinized and there is loss of goblet cells.

Antinuclear antibodies have been found in patients with ocular pemphigoid (Waltman and Yarian 1974). IgG antibodies to an antigen in the basement membrane zone of skin are detectable in most patients with bullous pemphigoid, a related condition, and less frequently in cicatricial pemphigoid (Mondino et al. 1977a). Complement component C3 and IgG are bound to conjunctival basement membrane (Fernando 1960). An experimental model has been developed based on injection of IgG from bullous pemphigoid patients into rabbit cornea. Histologic and immunochemical changes of the skin in pemphigoid are reproduced in the corneal epithelium (Anhalt et al. 1981). A similar approach using antibodies from cicatricial pemphigoid is being studied. An association with HLA-B12 has been demonstrated (Mondino and Brown 1981).

8.5. ALLERGIC KERATITIS

Corneal involvement in allergic reactions is less frequent than conjunctival involvement and is often concurrent with allergic conjunctivitis.

8.5.1. Atopic keratoconjunctivitis

Atopic keratoconjunctivitis occurs in patients with atopic dermatitis. The conjunctivitis is discussed above and is characterized by itching, tearing, and redness. The keratitis causes pain, photophobia and blurred vision. Punctate epithelial keratitis, ulceration and vascularization may develop. Conjunctival scarring and lid changes can also cause secondary corneal epithelial disease and scarring.

8.5.2. Vernal catarrh

Vernal catarrh is a special form of atopic keratoconjunctivitis. The cornea is involved in several ways. Small white dots are seen in the epithelium near the limbus. Called Trantas' dots, they are made up of degenerating eosinophils and epithelial cells. Fine diffuse punctate keratitis may decrease vision significantly. Large corneal epithelial defects are occasionaly seen. In the limbal form of vernal catarrh, large papillae occur in the limbal conjunctiva and overlap the cornea. A fine pannus, vascular growth into the cornea beneath the epithelium, is frequently seen superiorly.

8.5.3. Staphylococcal marginal corneal ulceration

Staphylococcal marginal corneal ulceration is presumed to be an immunologically mediated result of staphylococcal infection of the lids and conjunctiva. An inferior punctate epithelial keratitis is frequently seen in patients with staphylococcal blepharitis. White infiltrates occur in the peripheral corneal stroma, separated from the limbus by a narrow clear zone. These catarrhal infiltrates have not been studied histologically in humans but PMNs are seen in scrapings from their surface. They have been reproduced experimentally by topical ocular application of Staphylococci in rabbits immunized to inactive organisms (Mondino et al. 1981). These experimental lesions are composed of a mixed mononuclear and PMN infiltrate in the anterior stroma. Peripheral corneal infiltrates are seen in other allergic processes such as an acute reaction to an intravenous radio-opaque dye (Baum and Bierstock

1978). They have also been seen in patients with presumably auto-immune diseases, including inflammatory bowel disease and Wegener's granulomatosis (Shulman and Sugar 1981). The location of these lesions near limbus may relate to diffusion of immune mediators from the limbal vasculature into the avascular cornea. A similar process may lead to the Wessely Ring phenomenon. These are ring-shaped corneal infiltrates concentric with the limbus. They may be present between the limbus and a central infectious corneal ulcer, particularly herpes simplex corneal stromal lesions. Neutrophils and complement products are found in experimentally produced lesions (Mondino et al. 1977b). In many instances these lesions may represent an immune complex-mediated process. Topical drugs may cause contact keratitis but the conjunctiva is much more frequently involved.

8.6. OCULAR TRANSPLANTATION IMMUNITY

Successful transplantation of the human cornea was first performed 75 years ago, long before our current understanding of transplantation immunology developed. This success was attributed in early transplantation immunologic studies to the cornea being a "privileged" site with lack of histocompatibility antigens or isolation from the immune system (Billingham et al. 1954). The avascularity of the cornea does limit access of antigens to the reticuloendothelial system, the afferent limb and sensitized cells to the cornea, the efferent limb of immunity. But it was demonstrated in 1951 that skin transplantation from the same donor stimulated corneal graft rejection in rabbits, suggesting that corneal graft failure could have an immune basis (Maumenee 1951). It has since been demonstrated in animals and humans that all layers of the cornea, the epithelium, stroma and endothelium, could be rejected separately (Khodadoust and Silverstein 1969; Allredge and Krachmer 1981). Endothelial rejection is the most common, and the most important, as both stromal keratocytes and epithelium may be replaced by host cells while the donor endothelium persists and is not replaced by host cells if damaged (Polack et al. 1964). The incidence of endothelial rejection is from 6 to 44% (Allredge and Krachmer 1981) and is lowest in avascular host corneas (Khodadoust and Silverstein 1972). Endothelial rejection typically begins at a site of vessel ingrowth to the graft with clumps of white cells, keratic precipitates, on the endothelium. These precipitates then move in a line across the graft, leaving destroyed endothelial cells and resulting corneal edema in their wake. Stromal rejection is less common and usually occurs along with endothelial rejection. It is characterized by dense stromal infiltration by white cells. Epithelial rejection is probably more frequent than is generally recognized. An elevated ridge travels across the epithelium, usually with normal-appearing epithelium before and after. It may be associated with other forms of rejection, or independent. Subepithelial infiltrates in the superficial stroma, nebulous circular white opacities, also may occur as a manifestation of rejection (Krachmer and Alldredge 1978). Rejection can usually be stopped by vigorous steroid therapy, but about 10% of grafts still fail.

Because of the high success rate of keratoplasty with unmatched donor tissue, HLA typing and cross-matching are usually not carried out. It is likely that HLA antigens are expressed on corneal cells, although the presence of Langerhans cells expressing the DR locus has been disputed (Streilein et al. 1979; Rodrigues et al. 1981). Cytotoxic antibodies can develop in patients following corneal grafting but their relationship to rejection is unclear (Stack et al. 1973). Patients having positive titers prior to grafting are more likely to suffer irreversible rejection. In poor-prognosis cases, those with a heavily vascularized recipient cornea, the degree of HLA matching correlates with graft success in several studies (Vannas 1975; Batchelor et al. 1976). An increased incidence of rejection has been found in recipients bearing antigens HLA-B27 or B12 (Vannas et al. 1977); preliminary studies in our own patients have failed to confirm this (R. Meyer and A. Sugar, unpublished data).

Transplantation of other ocular tissues has been carried out primarily for structural purposes. Sclera may be grafted and, although it is probably rejected, the acellular collagen framework persists and scars. Most conjunctival grafting has been done with autologous tissue, although cadaver conjunctival transplantation is being studied for use in severe ocular surface disease.

8.7. OTHER INFLAMMATORY EYE DISEASES

8.7.1. Infections

As in other sites, ocular infections and the resulting pathologic changes are affected by the virulence of the infecting organism, the local and systemic inflammatory—immune response of the patient, and the anatomic features of the infected tissues. Many of the anatomic features of the eye, however, make it unique as a site for infection. The ocular surface is constantly exposed to the environment and is readily accessible to organisms present on the lids and in the sinuses. The tears provide mechanical protection as well as immunoglobulins, lysozymes, and other protecting substances. The corneal epithelium acts as a mechanical barrier to penetration of most organisms with the exception of Neisseria species and *Corynebacterium diphtheriae*, which will penetrate an intact epithelium. Descemet's membrane, the basement membrane of the corneal endothelium, also acts as a mechanical barrier to intraocular penetration. The cornea, lens, and vitreous are avascular structures, limiting access of inflammatory mediators to these sites when infected. Healing as well may be delayed by avascularity. Penetration of antimicrobial agents into these tissues is limited by both the poor blood supply and the barriers to diffusion into intraocular fluids from vessels of the ciliary body; the blood—aqueous barrier, and the vitreous, the blood—retinal barrier. Because these three tissues are optically clear, an inflammatory response and subsequent healing are helpful in controlling infection and may lead to loss of transparency and, thus, loss of vision.

The conjunctiva is a mucous membrane with scanty underlying stroma. It is susceptible to bacterial infection by numerous organisms, most commonly Staphylococci, Streptococci, Haemophilus, Neisseria, and Moraxella species. A purulent or mucopurulent discharge is usually present in acute bacterial conjunctivitis, which may be self-limited or progress to involvement of the cornea. Such conjunctivitis is usually responsive to topical antibiotic therapy.

8.7.1.1. *Viral conjunctivitis*

Viral conjunctivitis is more common than the bacterial form, the most important being that caused by several types of adenovirus, particularly Types 8 and 19. Epidemic keratoconjunctivitis (EKC), caused by these viruses is characterized by rapid onset of severe conjunctival inflammation with pseudomembrane formation and formation of lymphoid follicles in the conjunctival stroma. An epithelial keratitis develops, often followed by subepithelial infiltrates in the corneal stroma, localized lymphocyte collections in response to viral antigens in the stroma. Whereas the conjunctivitis resolves within two weeks, the corneal infiltrates may last for months or years.

8.7.1.2. *Chlamydial conjunctivitis*

Chlamydial conjunctivitis is a major cause of blindness in many parts of the world. In the United States, *Chlamydia trachomatis* causes neonatal or adult inclusion conjunctivitis, a sexually transmitted disease. This is associated with mucoid discharge, conjunctival follicles, punctate keratitis, and usually mild conjunctival scarring. It may last for several months if untreated. Endemic trachoma is a chronic conjunctival infection of children with *C. trachomatis* serotypes A, B and C. Untreated it leads to severe conjunctival scarring, secondary infection and corneal opacity.

Corneal infections are usually a greater threat to vision than conjunctival infections because of the risk of permanent opacity.

8.7.1.3. *Bacterial corneal ulcers*

Bacterial corneal ulcers or abscesses can be caused by a variety of organisms. The most common are Pseudomonas, Staphylococcus and Streptococcus species. As bacterial ulcers can be rapidly destructive to the corneal stroma, they require prompt treatment based on cytologic and culture identification of the organism. Neutrophils and phagocytes enter the cornea from limbal vessels after activation of the complement system by either the classic or alternative pathway (Mondino et al. 1980). Collagenases and proteoglycanases released from leukocyte lysosomes can enhance destruction of the cornea as well as the bacteria. Pseudomonas, in addition, produces proteases which rapidly liquify the corneal stroma so that corneal perforation may follow within 48 hours of onset of infection. Treatment with antibiotics applied as drops to the cornea gives high drug levels in the corneal stroma; supplemental subconjunctival antibiotic injections may enhance these levels.

8.7.1.4. Fungal keratitis

Fungal keratitis appears frequently in the southern United States but rarely in cooler climates. It often follows injury by vegetable material or prolonged treatment with local steroids and antibiotics. The most common organisms are Aspergillus, Fusarium and Candida. Although the course of infection is less rapid than with bacterial infection, treatment is made more difficult by delay in diagnosis and inadequate antifungal agents.

8.7.1.5. Herpes simplex keratitis

Herpes simplex keratitis is the leading infectious cause of corneal blindness in the United States and the most important ocular viral infection. Ocular infection is usually a recurrent infection with Type I herpes simplex from a latent reservoir in the trigeminal ganglion, although the eye may be involved in primary disease. Usually only one eye is involved, although bilateral disease occurs, especially in immunodeficient hosts. Corneal epithelial involvement is due to actively replicating virus and often takes a branching "dendritic" pattern. These lesions respond to treatment with topical antiviral agents although they tend to recur. Deep corneal involvement may take one of several forms. Disciform keratitis is characterized by a localized, disc-shaped area of corneal edema and infiltration with keratic precipitates. Virus cannot be cultured from the cornea in this form of keratitis, although viral antigens are detectable. Deep stromal keratitis with dense cellular infiltration and necrosis may occur, leading to permanent corneal opacity and occasional perforation. Replicating virus is present in this form of the disease. When necrosis is present polymorphonuclear cells predominate but lymphocytes, plasma cells and macrophages are present in less severe forms (Metcalf et al. 1976). Both cellular and humoral immunity herpes virus have been demonstrated, although cellular immunity is thought to play the greatest role in control of infection (Meyers 1975; Nesburn 1981). Current research is aimed in part at eliminating latent viral reservoirs in ganglion cells and understanding immune modulation of recurrence.

8.7.1.6. Scleritis

Scleritis is an inflammatory cell infiltration of the sclera. It is often of unknown etiology although it may be associated with the "collagen–vascular" disease, herpes zoster infection and autoimmune processes. It is rare for the sclera to be directly involved in infectious processes. The scleral infiltration may be divided into superficial forms — episcleritis — and deep forms — true scleritis. Scleritis can be divided into diffuse, nodular, necrotizing and posterior forms (Watson and Hazleman 1976). Therapy often requires the use of systemic non-steroidal anti-inflammatory agents and/or systemic steroids. The course is chronic and painful and in the severe necrotizing forms may lead to extensive loss of scleral tissue. Little is known of the immunology of scleritis except that it relates to associated systemic disease.

We have discussed a number of entities causing ocular inflammatory disease. Because of the limited scope of this chapter, many entities have not been described in detail and many other inflammatory conditions have been ignored. The application of current immunologic knowledge and techniques to the study of ocular tissues and to these conditions affecting the eye is now only in its initial stage and is incomplete when compared to a similar application to other human tissues. Better knowledge of ocular immunology is clearly needed.

REFERENCES

Alldredge, O. and Krachmer, J. (1981) Clinical types of corneal transplant rejection. *Arch. Ophthalmol. 99,* 599.

Anhalt, G., Bahn, C., Labib, R. et al. (1981) Pathogenic effects of bullous pemphigoid autoantibodies in rabbit corneal epithelium. *J. Clin. Invest. 68,* 1097.

Ayo, C. (1943) A toxic ocular reaction. I. New properties of Schwartzmann toxins. *J. Immunol. 46,* 113.

Barker, C.F. and Billingham, R.E. (1977) Immunologically privileged sites. *Adv. Immunol. 25,* 1−54.

Batchelor, J., Casey, T., Gibbs, D. et al (1976) HLA matching and corneal grafting. *Lancet 1,* 551.

Baum, J. and Bierstock, S. (1978) Peripheral corneal infiltrates following intravenous injection of diatrizoate meglumine. *Am. J. Ophthalmol. 85,* 613.

Becker, E.L., Sigman, M. and Oliver, J.M. (1979) Superoxide production induced in rabbit leukocytes by synthetic chemotactic peptides and S23187. *Am. J. Pathol. 95,* 81.

Bengtsson, E. (1976) The effect of imidazole on the disruption of the blood−aqueous barrier in the rabbit eye. *Invest. Ophthalmol. 15,* 315.

Ben-Zvi, A., Rodrigues, M., Gery, I. and Schiffman, E. (1981) Induction of inflammation by synthetic mediators. In: A. Suran, I. Gery and R. Nussenblatt (Eds), *Proceedings, 'Immunology of the Eye' Workshop III, Immunol. Abstr. Spec. Suppl.,* p. 21.

Berman, M. (1978) Regulation of collagenase. *Trans. Ophthalmol. Soc. UK 98,* 397.

Berman, M. (1979) Regulation of collagenase in corneal ulcerations. *Trans. Ophthalmol. Soc. UK. 99,* 399.

Berman, M.B. (1980) Collagenase and corneal ulceration. In: D.E. Woolley and J.M. Evanson (Eds), *Collagenase in Normal and Pathological Connective Tissues,* John Wiley and Sons, New York, p. 141.

Billingham, R., Brent, L. and Medawar, P. (1954) Quantitative studies on tissue transplantation immunity: Origin, strength and duration of actively and adoptively acquired immunity. *Proc. R. Soc. Lond. 143,* 58.

Blodi, F. (1959) Sympathetic uveitis as an allergic phenomenon. *Trans. Am. Acad. Ophthalmol. Otolaryngol. 63,* 642−649.

Blodi, F. (1979) Sympathetic uveitis. In: Freeman H. (Ed.), *Ocular Trauma,* Appleton-Century-Crofts, New York, pp. 417−427.

Bluestone, R., Easty, D.L., Goldberg, L.S., Jones B.R. and Pettit, T.H. (1973) Lacrimal immunoglobulins and complement quantified by counter-immunoelectrophoresis. *Br. J. Ophthalmol. 59,* 279.

Brewerton, D., Caffrey, M., Nicholls, A. et al. (1973) Reiter's disease and HLA-27. *Lancet 2,* 996.

Brown, S., Weller, C. and Akiya, S. (1970) Pathogenesis of ulcers of the alkali-burned cornea. *Arch. Ophthalmol. 83,* 205.

Capel, P.J., Groeneboer, O. and Pondman, K.W. (1978) The binding of activated C3 to polysaccharide and immunoglobulins. *J. Immunol. 121,* 2566.

Centifanto, Y.M. and Kaufman, H.F. (1980) The development of tear antibodies and herpes simplex keratitis. In: D.H. Dayton et al. (Eds), *The Secretory Immunologic System,* Department of Public Health NIH Publ. No. 331.

Chandler, J.W., Leder, R., Kaufman, H.E. and Caldwell, J.R. (1975) Quantitative determination of complement components and immunoglobulins in tears and aqueous humor. *Invest. Ophthalmol. 13,* 151–153.

Chenoweth, D.E. and Hugli, T.E. (1980) Human C5a and C5a analogs as probes of the neutrophil C5a receptor. *Mol. Immunol. 17,* 151.

Chusid, M.J. and Davis, S.D. (1979) Experimental bacterial keratitis in neutropenic guinea pigs: polymorphonuclear leukocytes in corneal host defense. *Infect. Immun. 24,* 948.

Cochrane, C.G. (1965) The Arthus reaction. In: B. Zweifach and R.T. McCluskey (Eds), *The Inflammatory Process,* Academic Press, New York, p. 613.

Cooper, D., Penny, R. and Fiddes, P. (1971) Autologous plasma sensitization in Behcet's disease. *Lancet 1,* 910.

Donnelly, J.J., Rockey, J.H. and Soulsby, E.J.L. (1977) Intraocular IgE antibody induced in guinea pigs with Ascaris suum larvae. *Invest. Ophthalmol. Visual Sci. 16,* 976.

Dyster-Aas, H.K., Fritz, H. and Krakau, C.F. (1969) Quantitation of endotoxin-induced protein increase in the aqueous humor of the rabbit's eye. *Acta Pathol. Microbiol. Scand. 77,* 739.

Eakins, K.E., Whitelock, R.A.F., Bennett, A. and Martenet, A.C. (1972a) Prostaglandin-like activity in ocular inflammation. *Br. Med. J. 3,* 452.

Eakins, K.E., Whitelock, R.A.F., Perkins, K., Bennett A. and Unger, W.G. (1972b) Release of prostaglandin in ocular inflammation in the rabbit. *Nature (London) 239,* 248.

Eakins, K.E., Whitelock, R.A.F., Perkins, E.S. and Unger, W.G. (1972c) Release of prostaglandins in ocular inflammation in the rabbit. *Nature (London) 239,* 748.

Faure, J-P. (1980) Autoimmunity and the retina. *Curr. Top. Eye Res. 2,* 215–302.

Fernando, A.N. (1960) Immunologic studies with ^{131}I-labeled antigen in experimental uveitis. *Arch. Ophthalmol. 63,* 162.

Fletcher, J.R. and Ramwell, P.W. (1970) E. coli endotoxin shock in the baboon. Treatment with lidocaine or indomethacin. In: B. Samuelsson and R. Paoletti (Eds), *Prostaglandin and Thromboxane Research, Vol. 3,* Raven Press, New York, p. 183.

Friedlaender, M. (1979) *Allergy and Immunology of the Eye,* Harper and Row, Hagerstown, MD, p. 218.

Gilbert, R.P. (1959) Effects of antihistamine and antiserotonin drugs on vascular responses to E. coli endotoxin in the cat. *Proc. Exp. Biol. Med. 100,* 346.

Goosey, J.D., Zigler, J.S., Matheson, B.C. and Kinoshita, J.H. (1981) Effects of singlet oxygen on human lens crystallins in vitro. *Invest. Ophthalmol. Visual Sci. 20,* 679.

Grant, J.A., Depree, E. and Goldman, A.S. (1975) Complement-mediated release of histamine from human leukocytes. *J. Immunol. 114,* 1101.

Hammer, H. (1974) Cellular hypersensitivity to uveal pigment confirmed by leukocyte migration tests in sympathetic ophthalmitis and Vogt-Koyanagi-Harada syndrome. *Br. J. Ophthalmol. 58,* 773–776.

Hanna, C. and Keatts, H.C. (1967) Indomethacin in ocular inflammation. *Arch. Ophthalmol. 77,* 555.

Hazlett, H.D., Rosen, D.D. and Berk, R.S. (1977) Pseudomonas eye infections in cyclophosphamide treated mice. *Invest. Ophthalmol. Visual Sci. 16,* 649.

Henney, C.S., Bourne, H.R. and Lichtenstein, L.M. (1971) The role of cyclic AMP in the specific cytolytic activity of lymphocytes. *J. Immunol. 108,* 1526.

Henson, P.M. (1980) Mechanisms of exocytosis in phagocytic inflammatory cells. *Am. J. Pathol. 101,* 494.

Hook, R., Hook, C. and Brown, S. (1973) Fibroblast collagenase partial purification and characterization. *Invest. Ophthalmol. 12,* 771.

Horton, E.W. (1979) Prostanoids in health and disease; chemistry, biochemistry and pharmacological activity of prostanoids. In: S.M. Roberts and F. Scheinnmann (Eds), *Chemistry, Biochemistry and Pharmacological Activity of Prostanoids,* Pergamon Press, New York, pp. 4–12.

Howes, E.L. and McKay, D.G. (1975) Comparison of the ocular effects of circulating endotoxin and immune complexes: Role of vasoactive amines. *J. Immunol. 114,* 737.

Howes, E.L., McKay, D.G. and Aronson, S.B. (1971) An ultrastructural study of the ciliary process in the rabbit following systemic administration of bacterial endotoxin. *Lab. Invest. 24,* 217.

Howes, E.L., Aronson, S.B. and McKay, D.G. (1979) Ocular vascular permeability. The effects of systemic administration of bacterial endotoxin. *Arch. Ophthalmol. 84,* 360.

Hugli, T.E. and Muller-Eberhard, H.J. (1978) Anaphylatoxins: C3a and C5a. *Adv. Immunol. 26,* 1.

Hyslop, N.E., Dourmashkin, R.R. and Porter, R.R. (1970) The fixation of complement and the activation of complement. *J. Exp. Med. 131,* 783.

Jacobs, R.P., Aurelion, L. and Cole, G.A. (1976) Cell mediated immune response to herpes simplex virus: type-specific lymphoproliferative responses in lymph nodes draining the sites of primary infection. *J. Immunol. 116,* 1520.

Jones, D.B. (1978) Pathogenesis of bacterial and fungal keratitis. *Trans. Ophthalmol. Soc. UK 98,* 367.

Joy, N.H. (1942) Treatment of experimental Bacillus pyocyaneus ulcer of the cornea with sulfopyridine. *Arch. Ophthalmol. 27,* 1135.

Kenyon, K.R., Berman, M., Rose, J. and Gage, J. (1979) Prevention of stromal ulceration in the alkali-burned rabbit cornea by glued on contact lens. Evidence for the role of polymorphonuclear leukocytes in collagen degradation. *Invest. Ophthalmol. Visual Sci. 18,* 570.

Kessler, E., Mondino, R. and Brown, S. (1977) The corneal response to pps. aeruginosa; Histopathic and enzymatic characterization. *Invest. Ophthalmol. Visual Sci. 16,* 116.

Khodadoust, A. and Silverstein, A. (1969) Transplantation and rejection of individual layers of the cornea. *Invest. Ophthalmol. 8,* 180.

Khodadoust, A. and Silverstein, A. (1972) Studies on the nature of the privilege enjoyed by corneal allografts. *Invest. Ophthalmol. 11,* 137.

Klebanoff, S.J. (1980) Oxygen metabolism and the toxic properties of phagocytes. *Ann. Intern. Med. 93,* 480.

Kogure, M., Shimada, K. and Hara, H. (1976) Complement titer in patients with Behçet's disease. *Acta Soc. Ophthalmol. Jpn 75,* 1260.

Krachmer, J. and Alldredge, O. (1978) Subepithelial infiltrates: a probable sign of corneal graft rejection. *Arch. Ophthalmol. 96,* 2234.

Kunkel, S.L., Thrall, R.T., Kunkel, R.G., Ward, P.A. and Zurier, R.B. (1979) Suppression of immune complex vasculitis in rats by prostaglandins. *J. Clin. Invest. 64,* 1525.

Kunkel, S.L., Ogawa, H., Conran, P., Ward, P.A. and Zurier, R.B. (1981) Suppression of acute and chronic inflammation by orally administrated prostaglandins. *Arthritis Rheum. 24,* 1151.

Levine, R.Z. and Breinen, G.M. (1959) Ocular effects of endotoxin. *Arch. Ophthalmol. 61,* 568.

Lichtenstein, L.M. and DiBernado, R. (1971) The immediate allergic response; in vitro action of cyclic AMP and other drugs on the two stages of histamine release. *J. Immunol. 107,* 1131.

Liddy, M. and Stuart, J. (1972) Sympathetic ophthalmia in Canada. *Can. J. Ophthalmol. 7,* 157–159.

Little, J. M., Centifanto Y.M. and Kaufman, H.E. (1969) Immunoglobulins in human tears. *Am. J. Ophthalmol. 68,* 898.

Lubin, J. and Albert, D. (1979) Sympathetic ophthalmia, ample room for controversy. *Surv. Ophthalmol. 24,* 137–140.

Lubin, J., Albert, D. and Weinstein, M. (1980) Sixty-five years of sympathetic ophthalmia, a clinicopathologic review of 105 cases (1913–1978). *Ophthalmology 87,* 109–121.

Mahmoud, A.A.F., Warren, K. S. and Peters, P.A. (1975) A role for the eosinophil in acquired resistance to Schistosoma mansoni infections as determined by antieosinophil serum. *J. Exp. Med. 142,* 805.

Mamo, J. (1970) The rate of visual loss in Behçet's disease. *Arch. Ophthalmol. 84,* 451–452.

Mamo, J. (1976) Treatment of Behçet disease with chlorambucil. *Arch. Ophthalmol. 94,* 580–583.

Mann, J., O'Brian, R., Rosen, F.S. and Babior, B.M. (1980) Studies on binding of C3b to surfaces. *J. Immunol. 124,* 1531.

Marak, G. (1979) Recent adventures in sympathetic ophthalmia. *Surv. Ophthalmol. 24,* 141–156.

Marak, G.E., Font, R.L., Alepa, F.P. and Ward, P.A. (1977) Effects of C3 inactivator factor on the development of experimental lens-induced granulomatous endophthalmitis. *Ophthalmic Res. 9,* 416.

Marak, G.E., Wacker, W.B., Jack, R. and Ward, P.A. (1979) Effects of complement depletion and experimental allergic uveitis. *Ophthalmic Res. 11,* 97.

Mason, R. and Barnes, C. (1969) Behçet's syndrome with arthritis. *Ann. Rheum. Dis. 28,* 95–103.

Masuda, K., Izawa, Y. and Mishima, S. (1973) Prostaglandin and uveitis: a preliminary report. *Jpn J. Ophthalmol. 17,* 166.

Maumenee, A. (1951) The influence of donor–recipient sensitization on corneal grafts. *Am. J. Ophthalmol. 34,* 142.

McPherson, S. and Woods, A. (1948) The significance of the intracutaneous test for hypersensitivity to uveal pigment. *Am J. Ophthalmol. 31,* 35.

Metcalf, J., McNeill, J. and Kaufman, H. (1976) Experimental disciform edema and necrotizing keratitis in the rabbit. *Invest. Ophthalmol. 15,* 979.

Meyers, R.L. (1975) Immunology of herpes simplex virus infection. *Int. Ophthalmol. Clin. 15,* 37.

Meyers, R. and Chitjian, P. (1976) Immunology of herpes-virus infection: immunity to herpes simplex virus in eye infections. *Surv. Ophthalmol. 21,* 194.

Meyers-Elliot, R.M. and Chitjian, P. (1980) Induction of cell-mediated immunity in herpes simplex virus keratitis. *Invest. Ophthalmol. Visual Sci. 19,* 920.

Michelson, J., Michelson, P. and Chisari, F. (1980) Subretinal neovascular membrane and disciform scar in Behçet's disease. *Am. J. Ophthalmol. 90,* 182–185.

Mondino, B. and Brown, S. (1981) Ocular cicatricial pemphigoid. *Ophthalmology 88,* 95.

Mondino, B., Ross, A., Rabin, B. et al. (1977a) Autoimmune phenomena in ocular cicatricial pemphigoid. *Am. J. Ophthalmol. 83,* 443.

Mondino, B., Rabin, B., Kessler, E. et al. (1977b) Corneal rings with Gram-negative bacteria. *Arch. Ophthalmol. 95,* 2222.

Mondino, B.J., Brown, S.I., Rabin, B.S. and Bruno, J. (1978) Alternative pathway activation of complement in a Proteus mirabilis ulceration of the cornea. *Arch. Ophthalmol. 96,* 1159.

Mondino, B., Ratajczak, H., Goldberg, D. et al. (1980) Alternate and classical pathway components of complement in the normal cornea. *Arch. Ophthalmol. 98,* 346.

Mondino, B., Kowalski, R., Ratajczak, H. et al. (1981) Rabbit model of phlyctenulosis and catarrhal infiltrates. *Arch. Ophthalmol. 98,* 891–895.

Morris, R. and Schlaegel, T. (1964) Virus-like inclusion bodies in subretinal fluid in uveoencephalitis. *Am. J. Ophthalmol. 58,* 940.

Morrison, D.C., Roseer, J.F. and Henson, P.M. (1975) Two distinct mechanisms for the initiation of mast cell degranulation. *Int. Arch. Allergy. 49,* 172.

Muller-Eberhard, H.J. (1975) Complement. *Ann. Rev. Biochem. 44,* 697.

Nathan, C.F., Brukner, L., Silverstein, S.L. and Cohn, Z.A. (1979) Extracellular cytolysis by activated macrophages and granulocytes. *J. Exp. Med. 149,* 100.

Nehmias, A.J., Visintine, A.M., Caldwell, D.R. and Wilson, L.A. (1976) Eye infections with herpes simplex virus in neonates. *Surv. Ophthalmol. 21,* 100.

Nesburn, A. (1981) Immunological aspects of ocular herpes simplex disease. In: A. Suran, I. Gery and R. Nussenblatt (Eds), *Proceedings, "Immunology of the eye" Workshop III, Immunol. Abstr. Spec. Suppl.,* p. 21.

O'Flaherty, J.T. and Ward, P.A. (1978) Leukocyte aggregation induced by chemotactic factors. *Inflammation 3,* 177.

Ohno, S., Nakayama, E., Sugiura, S. et al. (1975) Specific histocompatibility antigens associated with Behçet's disease. *Am. J. Ophthalmol. 80,* 636.

Ohno, S., Char, D., Kimura, S. and O'Connor, G. (1976) HLA and Vogt-Koyanagi-Harade syndrome. *N. Engl. J. Med. 295,* 788.

Ohno, S., Char, D., Kimura, S. and O'Connor, D. (1977) Vogt-Koyanagi-Harada syndrome. *Am. J. Ophthalmol. 83,* 735–740.

Okada, M. and Shimada, K. (1980) Effects of various pharmacologic agents on allergic inflammation of the eye. *Invest. Ophthalmol. Visual Sci. 19,* 176.

Perry, H. and Font, R. (1977) Clinical and histopathologic observations in severe Vogt-Koyanagi-Harada syndrome. *Am. J. Ophthalmol. 83,* 242–254.

Petrone, W.F., English, D.K., Wong, K. and McCord, J.M. (1980) Free radicals and inflammation: The superoxide dependent activation of a neutrophil chemotactic factor in plasma. *Proc. Natl Acad. Sci. USA 77,* 1159.

Podack, E.R. and Muller-Eberhard, H.J. (1980) 5C5b-9 Complex of complement: Formation of the dimeric membrane attack complex by removal of S-protein. *J. Immunol. 124,* 1779.

Polack, F., Smelser, G. and Rose, J. (1964) Long term survival of isotopically labeled stromal and endothelial cells in corneal homografts. *Am. J. Ophthalmol. 57,* 67.

Rockey, J.H., Donnelly, J.J., Stromberg, B.E. and Soulsberg, E.J.L. (1979) Immunopathology of Toxocara canis and Ascarus suum infections of the eye: the role of the eosinophil. *Invest. Ophthalmol. Visual Sci. 18,* 1172–1184.

Rodrigues, M., Rowden, G., Hackett, J. et al. (1981) Langerhans cells in the normal conjunctive and peripherial cornea of selected species. *Invest. Ophthalmol. Visual Sci. 21,* 759.

Rosen, H. and Klebanoff, S.J. (1977) Formation of singlet oxygen by the myeloperoxidase-mediated antimicrobial system. *J. Biol. Chem. 252,* 4803.

Saari, K. and Kauranen, O. (1980) Ocular inflammation in Reiter's syndrome associated with Campylobacter jejuni enteritis. *Am. J. Ophthalmol. 90,* 572–573.

Saari, K., Laitinen, O., Leirisalo, M. et al. (1980a) Ocular inflammation associated with Yersinia infection. *Am. J. Ophthalmol. 89,* 84–95.

Saari, K., Vilppula, A., Lassus, A. et al. (1980b) Ocular inflammation in Reiter's disease after Salmonella enteritis. *Am. J. Ophthalmol. 90,* 63–68.

Schachter, J. and Dawson, R. (1978) *Human Chlamydial Infections,* PSG Publishing, Littleton, MA, pp. 141–152.

Schulman, M. and Sugar, A. (1981) Peripheral corneal infiltrates in inflammatory bowel disease. *Ann. Ophthalmol. 13,* 109.

Shimada, K. and Silverstein, M.A. (1975) Local antibody formation. *Invest. Ophthalmol. 14,* 572–583.

Stack, W., Opelz, G., Newsome, D. et al. (1973) Sensitization to human leukocyte antigen by corneal transplantation. *Invest. Ophthalmol. 12,* 639.

Stevens, J.G. and Cook, M.L. (1971) Restriction of herpes simplex virus by macrophages. An analysis of cell–virus interaction. *J. Exp. Med. 133,* 19.

Streilein, J., Toews, G. and Bergstresser, P. (1979) Corneal allografts fail to express Ia antigens. *Nature (London) 282,* 326.

Tagawa, Y. and Sugiura, S. (1979) Immunogenetical studies on Vogt-Koyanagi-Harada Disease. In: A. Silverstein and G. O'Connor (Eds), *Immunology and Immunopathology of the Eye,* Masson Publications, New York, pp. 81–89.

Tagawa, Y., Sugiura, S., Yakura, H. et al. (1976) HLA and Vogt-Koyanagi-Harada syndrome. *N. Engl. J. Med. 295,* 173.

Vane, J.R. (1976) Prostaglandins as mediators of inflammation. In: B. Samuelsson and R. Paoletti (Eds), *Advances in Prostaglandin and Thromboxane Research, Vol. 1,* Raven Press, New York, pp. 791–798.

Van Horn, D.L., Davis, S.D., Hyndiuk, R.A. and Peterson, H.J. (1980) Pathogenesis of experimental Pseudomonas keratitis in the rabbit: bacteriological, clinical, and microscopic observations. *Invest. Ophthalmol. Visual Sci. 19,* 679.

Vannas, S. (1975) Histocompatibility in corneal grafting. *Invest. Ophthalmol. 14,* 883.

Vannas, S., Vannas, A. and Tiilikainen, A. (1977) Corneal transplantation reaction in avascular keratoconus patients due to HLA-associated immune aberration against infection. *Invest. Ophthalmol 16,* 644.

Waksman, B.H. and Bullington, S.J. (1956) A quantitative study of passive Arthus reaction in the rabbit eye. *J. Immunol. 76,* 441.

Waltman, S. and Yarian, D. (1974) Circulating autoantibodies in ocular pemphigoid. *Am. J. Ophthalmol. 77,* 891.

Ward, P.A. and Cochrane, C.G. (1965) Bound complement and immunologic injury of blood vessels. *J. Exp. Med. 121,* 215.

Ward, P.A. and Newman, L.J. (1969) A neutrophil chemotactic factor from human C5. *J. Immunol. 102,* 93.

Watson, P.G. and Hazleman, B. (1976) *The Sclera and Systemic Disorders,* W.B. Saunders Co. Philadelphia.

Weiss, S.J., Ruitagi, P.K. and LoBuglio, A.F. (1978) Human granulocyte generation of hydroxyl radicals. *J. Exp. Med. 147,* 316.

Wilson, L.A. and Ahearn, D.G. (1977) Pseudomonas-induced corneal ulcers associated with contaminated eye mascaras. *Am. J. Ophthalmol. 84,* 112.

Witebsky, E. and Milgram, F. (1964) The nature of autosensitization with particular reference to the eye. In: A. Maumenee and A. Silverstein (Eds), *Immunology of Uveitis,* Williams and Wilkins, Baltimore.

Witmer, R. (1955) Antibody formation in the rabbit eye studied with fluorescein-labeled antibody. *Arch. Ophthalmol. 53,* 311.

Yamamoto, G.K. and Allansmith M.R. (1979) Complement in tears from normal humans. *Am. J. Ophthalmol. 88,* 758.

Zurier, R.B., Weissmann, G., Haffstein, S. and Tia, M.H. (1974) Mechanisms of lysosomal enzyme release from human leukocytes. II. Effects of cAMP and cGMP, autonomic agonists and agents which affect microtubular function. *J. Clin. Invest. 53,* 297.

CHAPTER 9

Inflammatory diseases of the liver

F. WILLIAM ORR
Department of Pathology, University of Manitoba, Winnipeg, Canada

and

GERALD D. ILIFFE
Department of Internal Medicine, University of Manitoba, Winnipeg, Canada

9.1. INTRODUCTION

Immunologic mechanisms are considered to be involved in the production of hepatocellular damage in many types of hepatitis. However, a detailed understanding of these processes has not been achieved. Studies to date have provided evidence that both humoral and cellular immune reactions occur in many forms of liver disease and that different mechanisms may operate together. The pathogenesis of viral hepatitis Type B is best understood mainly because of the large body of information concerning the hepatitis B virus developed since Blumberg's discovery of the "Australia antigen" (Blumberg 1964) and its association with classic long-incubation, post-transfusion viral hepatitis (Prince 1968).

In this review we have outlined the pathogenesis of several clinically important liver diseases with particular emphasis on the importance of inflammation in their genesis.

9.2. HEPATITIS B

9.2.1. Hepatitis B virus (HBV)

The complete hepatitis B virion (HBV) is represented by the 42-nm spherical Dane particle which contains an internal nucleocapsid 27 nm in diameter. The 7-nm lipoprotein envelope of the Dane particle carries the antigenic determinants originally associated with the Australia antigen (HBsAg).

The nucleocapsid core of the Dane particle is revealed after removal of the outer viral envelope by the detergent "Tween 80" (Almeida et al. 1971). The core carries antigenic determinants associated with the HBcAg and the HBeAg, circular double-stranded DNA (Hirschman et al. 1974), DNA polymerase activity (Robinson and Greenman 1974; Kaplan et al. 1973) and a protein kinase activity (Albin and Robinson 1980). The viral DNA is double-stranded for approximately 70% of its length and single-stranded for the remainder. It weighs about $1.6-2.0 \times 10^6$ daltons and has ~3200 nucleotide pairs. Dane particle DNA has been cloned in *Escherichia coli* and the production of both HBcAg and HBsAg obtained (Burrell et al. 1979; Galibert et al. 1979; Snisky et al. 1979; Valenzuela et al. 1979; Charnay et al. 1980). The DNA-dependent polymerase can use the single-stranded portion of the DNA as a template to close the ring (Summers et al. 1975).

The HBV genome has been mapped by restriction endonuclease analysis (Valenzuela et al. 1979) and differences appear to exist between various HBV subtypes. These studies have also permitted isolation and determination of the gene sequences for surface antigen and core antigen (Pasek et al. 1979). The nucleotide sequences show that HBsAg and HBcAg are encoded by HBV-DNA. Whether the coding capacity of the viral genome can account for all the known HBV polypeptides appears to be controversial. It may be that the antigenic diversity can be accounted for by polymerization of smaller peptide sub-units which are similar in size and amino acid composition. At present four distinct antigenic markers are associated with HBV.

9.2.2. Hepatitis B antigens

9.2.2.1. Hepatitis B surface antigen (HBsAg)

In addition to being detectable on the outer shell of the Dane particle, HBsAg can be expressed in the cytoplasm and plasma membrane of infected hepatocytes and in the blood of persons infected with HBV.

Initially the three morphologic forms found in serum attracted the greatest attention. These are 22-nm spheres and 22-nm filaments, varying up to several hundred nm in length (Bayer et al. 1968; Dane et al. 1970), and the Dane particle, which is occasionally present without a detectable central core (Stannard and Hodgkiss 1979). The spheres and filaments represent an incomplete viral coat, specified by the viral genome, and, like the viral envelope, contain lipid (Kim and Bissel 1971), carbohydrate (Shiraishi et al. 1980) and protein (Robinson 1977). In the circulation they have a half-life of 3.3 days (Drouet et al. 1975). Sensitive methods are now available for detection of HBsAg in serum, e.g. radioimmunoassay and ELISA (enzyme-linked immunosorbent assay).

Purified HBsAg has three major polypeptides with molecular weights of 22,000, 27,000 and 68,000. It seems likely that the largest of these peptides is composed of the smaller two and that the 27,000-dalton peptide is a glycosylated version of the smallest. All three have a similar amino acid composition (Shiraishi et al. 1980) and

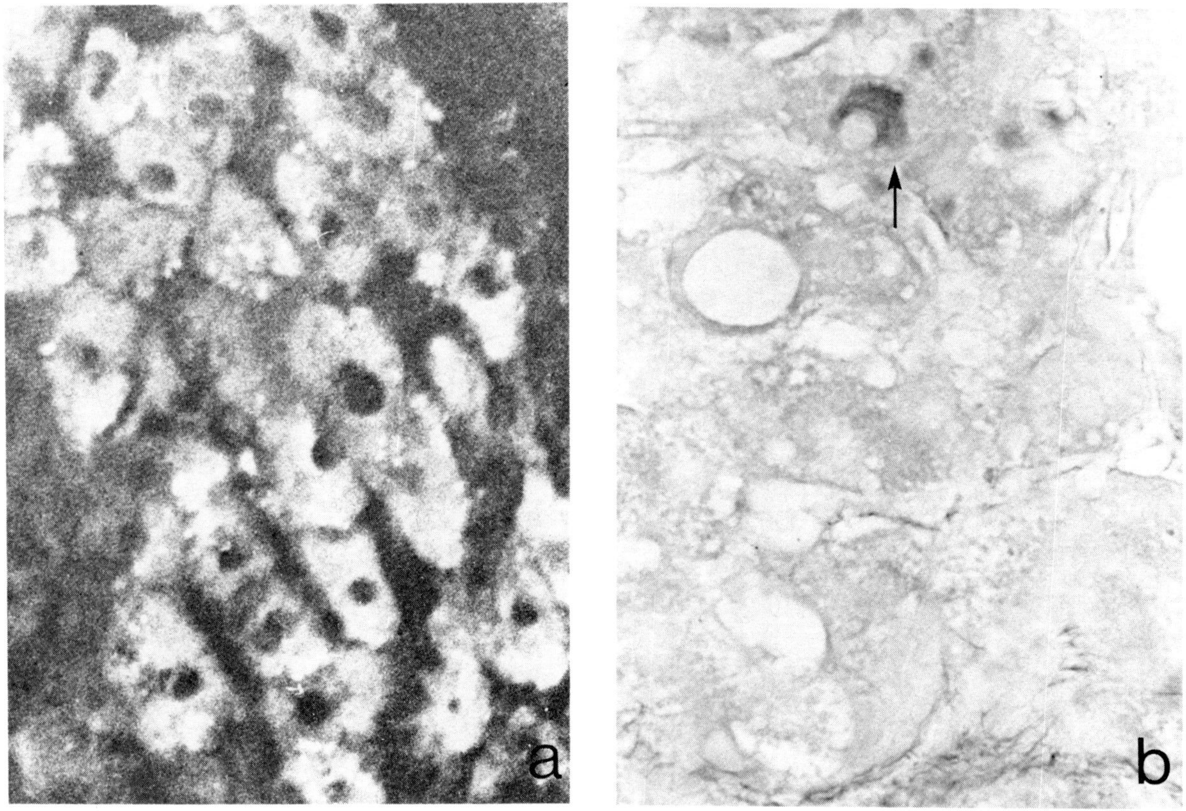

Fig. 1. HBsAg in the hepatocytes of a patient with HBV-related chronic active liver disease: (a) Cytoplasmic fluorescence is demonstrated by the indirect fluorescent antibody technique using anti-HBs. (b) Section from another specimen stained with aldehyde fuchsin. Staining of HBsAg is shown by the arrow. (originals x 440.)

are likely coded for by one nucleotide sequence in the viral genome (Tiollais et al. 1981). The formation of these peptide aggregates may be necessary for the antigenic expression of HBsAg (Mishiro et al. 1980).

In the cytoplasm of infected hepatocytes, HBsAg can be detected by a number of methods including immunofluorescence microscopy, peroxidase-antiperoxidase staining techniques, and electron and immunoelectron microscopy (Fig. 1) (Hadziyannis et al. 1972; Gerber et al. 1974; Gudat et al. 1975; Huang 1975; Huang and Neurath 1979). The presence of antigen in serum is associated with 20−30 nm filamentous material in proliferated and dilated cisternae of hepatocyte smooth endoplasmic reticulum, where synthesis seems likely to take place (Stein et al. 1972). In this location HBsAg has been associated with several morphologic forms and it seems possible that these may correspond to the filaments, spheres and Dane particles detectable in the serum (Huang and Neurath 1979), and that they may be excess coat material of the hepatitis B virus.

In "healthy" carriers of HBV, i.e. persons infected with HBV who show no signs of hepatocellular injury, the cytoplasm of injected cells may have a "ground glass" appearance on light microscopy (Hadziyannis et al. 1973). In tissue sections, cells carrying HBsAg stain with orcein aldehyde fuchsin and aldehyde thionine, possibly due to disulfide bonds in HBsAg (Shikata et al. 1974). This technique can be applied to the retrospective analysis of formalin-fixed tissue sections. In isolated hepatocytes HBsAg has been located in the plasma membrane during the early phase of acute hepatitis B in carriers (Alberti et al. 1976; Furata et al. 1975), and persons with HBV-related chronic hepatitis (Ray et al. 1976).

HBsAg appears in the sera of patients with acute hepatitis B virus hepatitis approximately 2-8 weeks before the onset of detectable clinical or biochemical disease. It persists for 1−12 weeks and disappears during convalescence, followed by the appearance of specific antibodies (Prince 1968; Hoofnagle et al. 1978). The antigen may persist in the serum of approximately 5% of patients recovering from acute hepatitis (Hoofnagle et al. 1978) or more frequently in persons with mild or subclinical infection (Barker and Murray 1971). High, persistent titers of HBsAg during the acute phase of hepatitis B may signal the development of chronic hepatitis (Deinhardt 1980).

HBsAg has a group-specific determinant "a" and two sets of mutually exclusive subtype determinants "d/y" and "w/r" (LeBouvier and Williams 1975). Subdivisions of the group-specific determinant "a" have been made and these have been useful for epidemiologic analysis.

HBsAg-associated particles from some persons carry receptors for polymerized serum albumin (O'Neill 1979; Imai et al. 1979) and the presence of the receptor may correlate with HBeAg, thus reflecting infectivity (see below).

9.2.2.2. Hepatitis B core antigen (HBcAg)

HBcAg and core antigen-associated particles have been detected in the nuclei and cytoplasm of infected hepatic parenchymal cells but, unlike HBsAg, are not found in the plasma. In the nucleus HBcAg-related particles appear as non-coated spherical 24–27-nm structures by transmission electron microscopy and these have been found to carry the antigenic determinants of HBcAg by immuno-electron microscopy (Nowoslawski et al. 1970; Gerber et al. 1974; Huang and Neurath 1979). The molecular weight of core antigen is $\sim$19,000 daltons (Pasek et al. 1979) (Fig. 2).

HBcAg has been found in close association with the hepatocyte plasma membrane by immunofluorescence and core antigen-associated particles have been found in the intracytoplasmic submembranous region by electron microscopy (Ray et al. 1976; Gudat and Bianchi 1977). There is evidence that HBcAg synthesis may take place in the endoplasmic reticulum of hepatocytes (Yamada and Nakane 1977). Large numbers of core particles can be detected occasionally in conventional tissue sections of HBcAg-positive immunosuppressed persons, where they appear as granular, eosinophilic inclusions, designated "sanded nuclei" (Bianchi and Gudat 1976).

9.2.2.3. Hepatitis B e-antigen (HBeAg)

The precise nature of HBeAg is controversial. It has been variously postulated to be a soluble, non-particulate protein with characteristics of an 11S gamma-globulin and a molecular weight of 3×10^5 daltons (Magnius and Espmark 1972; Magnius et al. 1975), part of the antigenic site of the Dane particle surface (Neurath et al. 1976; Lam et al. 1977), a complex of lactic dehydrogenase isoenzyme LDH_5 with HBs (Vyas et al. 1977), the DNA polymerase itself (Hirschman 1975) or a host-specific immunoglobulin (Neurath and Strick 1977). There are several antigenic subtypes and various molecular forms have been ascribed to the antigen (Takahashi et al. 1979a, b; Vnek et al. 1979; Blanchy et al. 1980). HBeAg correlates with the presence of the Dane particle, i.e. the infective, complete HBV. HBeAg-positive sera are highly infective (Alter et al. 1976; Okada et al. 1976), associated with DNA polymerase activity, and with acute and chronic liver disease (Takahashi et al. 1976; Hess et al. 1977). The antigen has been located in both nuclei and cytoplasm of hepatocytes in HBV-associated liver disease (Arnold et al. 1977; Trepo et al. 1972). The presence of HBeAg in the serum is generally interpreted to indicate active viral replication and persistently high titers of HBeAg in persons with HBV infection may indicate possible transition to chronic liver disease (Aldershvile et al. 1980).

9.2.2.4. Hepatitis B delta-antigen (HBδAg)

The delta antigen is the most recently described of the HBV-related antigens (Rizzetto et al. 1977). It has been found in the nuclei of HBsAg-positive patients with chronic hepatitis, and in immunosuppressed persons, but not in acute hepatitis or healthy carriers. In HBδAg-positive liver cells core particles are absent by electron microscopy, but the nuclei contain indistinct granules, 20–30 nm in diameter which bind peroxidase-labeled anti-HB (Canese et al. 1979).

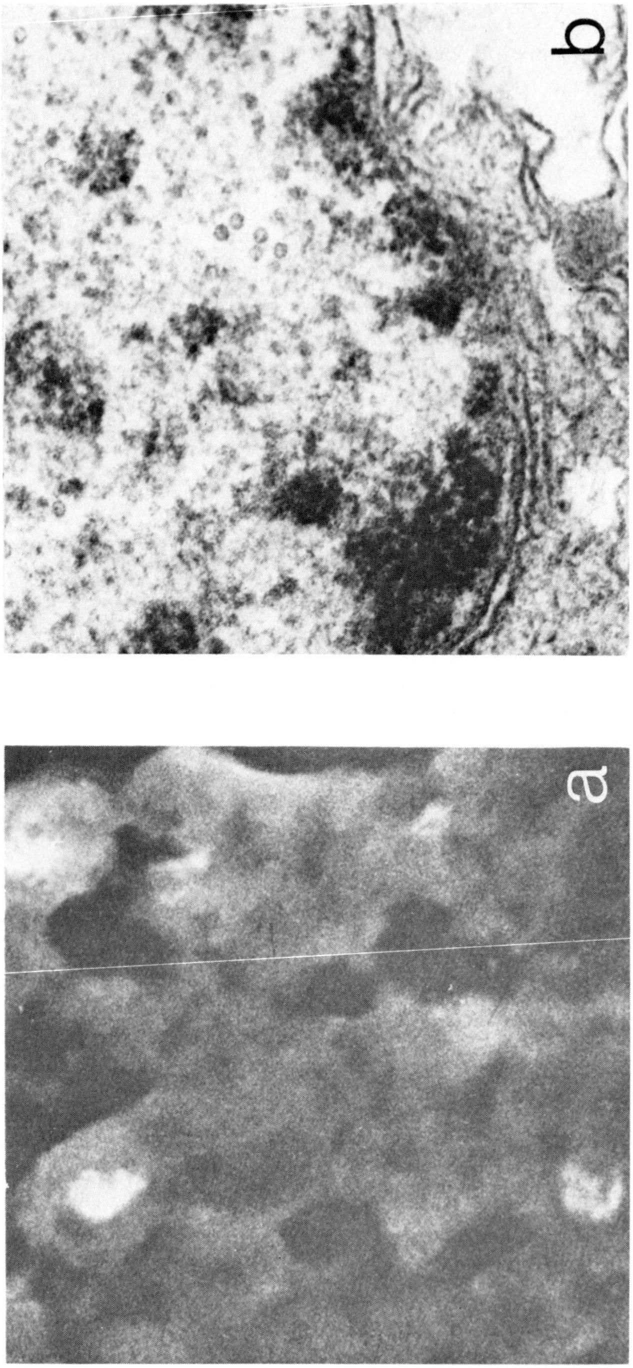

Fig. 2. HBcAg and intranuclear core particles in the liver of a patient with HBV-related chronic active liver disease. (a) Intranuclear HBcAg detected by the indirect fluorescent antibody technique (original x 500). (b) 27 nm-intranuclear core particles visualized by transmission electron microscopy (x 92,500).

9.2.3. Antibodies to hepatitis B virus-associated antigens

Humoral responses to HBsAg, HBcAg, and HBeAg have been studied and the acute-phase responses are shown in Figure 3. In the serum of patients with acute hepatitis B, disappearance of HBV-related antigens is followed by the appearance of specific antibodies, anti-HBc and anti-HBe (2−10 weeks), followed by anti-HBs during convalescence (Hoofnagle et al. 1978).

9.2.3.1. Anti-HBs

Conversion from HBsAg to anti-HBs generally correlates with elimination of virus-associated (HBsAg-positive) particles from the serum and is usually associated with resolution of the hepatic inflammatory process. A strong but incomplete cross-immunity exists for various subtypes of HBsAg.

Anti-HBs has protective properties against re-infection and this has formed the basis for production of an effective vaccine against HBV. Human serum containing HBV treated to inactivate its infectivity has been shown to act as a vaccine, protecting completely or reducing the severity of illness in susceptible persons later challenged with HBV (Krugman et al. 1971). This observation led to development of a vaccine composed of non-infective HBsAg particles isolated from the plasma of long-term carriers. This vaccine has been tested recently in a group at high risk of hepatitis B infection (homosexual men) and has been found to be a safe and effective prevention against illness in persons who received a full course of injections and developed anti-HBs (Szmuness et al. 1980). Monoclonal antibodies with high affinity for HBsAg have been produced by somatic cell hybrids and offer the possibility for development of specific immunoprophylactic agents for passive immunization (Wands and Zurawaki 1981).

9.2.3.2. Anti-HBc

Antibodies to HBc have been detected in all forms of HBV infection but especially high titers occur in chronic hepatitis B infection. In acute hepatitis B, high titers are usually measurable during the clinical manifestations of the disease and may last for many years, although in general the antibody persists up to 2 years after remission (Gerlich et al. 1980). Anti-HBc has been used as a marker for determining the prevalence of HBV infection in epidemiologic studies. Although anti-HBc is unrelated to the presence of Dane particles in the serum, anti-HBc may indicate continued HBV replication (Gerlich et al. 1980) and blood with high anti-HBc titers may be infectious (Hoofnagle et al. 1978). Because anti-HBc can be formed in HBsAg-positive HBcAg-negative carriers, it is regarded as lacking in protective effect against HBV infection.

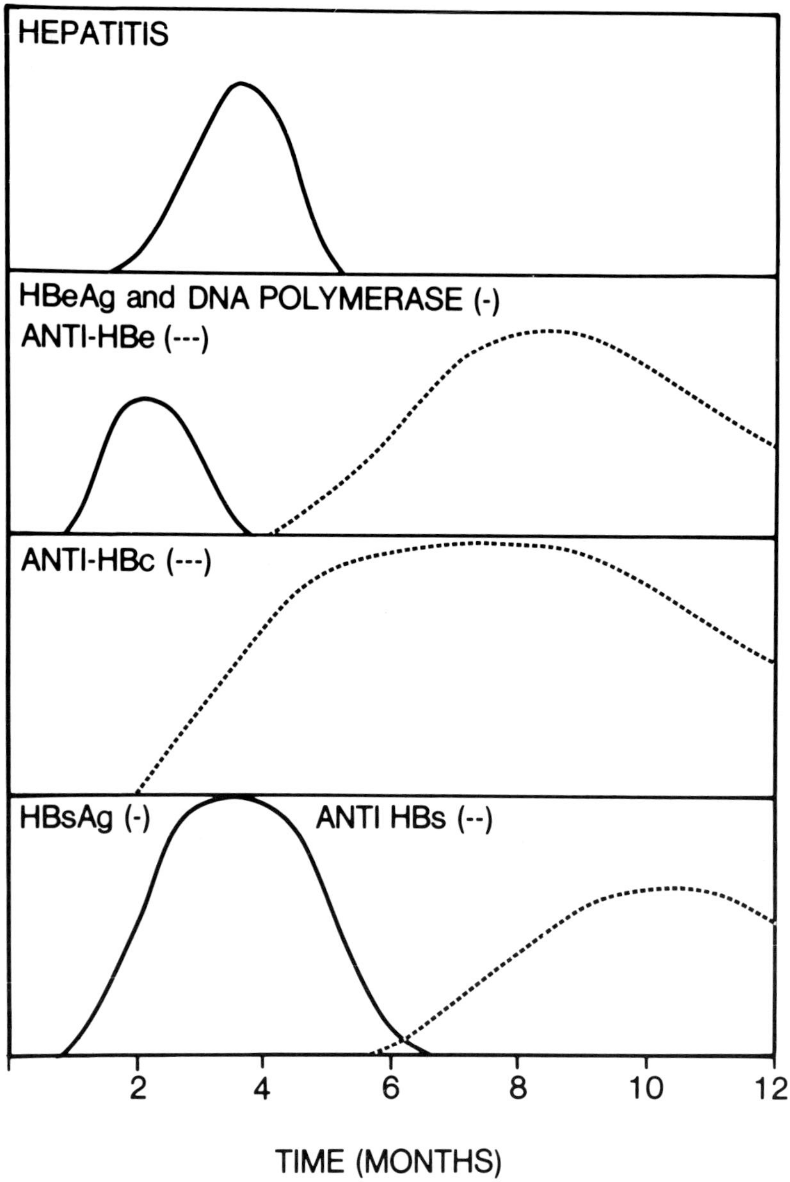

Fig. 3. Serological expression of HBV-related antigens and humoral immune responses typical of acute self-limited hepatitis B.

9.2.3.3. *Anti-HBe*

During acute hepatitis, anti-HBe can be detected by radioimmunoassay in low titers during the period between clearance of HBsAg in the serum and the appearance of anti-HBs (Aikawa et al. 1978; Frosner et al. 1978; Mushahwar et al. 1978). Its appearance seems to correlate with the suppression of active HBcAg replication, disappearance of Dane particles and HBcAg from the blood (Bianchi and Gudat 1979). While anti-HBe is usually associated with the disappearance of HBsAg, "healthy" HBsAg carriers sometimes have measurable anti-HBe with absent HBeAg, absent DNA polymerase activity, and absent Dane particles (Hess et al. 1977; Arnold et al. 1978; DeFranchis et al. 1980). These data indicate the lack of protective effect by anti-HBe.

9.2.4. *HBV-related immune complex disease*

9.2.4.1. *Hepatocellular injury*

In the normal liver Kupffer cells and possibly hepatocytes (via receptors for IgGFc and C3) clear antigens and immune complexes originating in the gastrointestinal tract (Wisse and Knook 1979). While the liver is largely resistant to damage by immune complexes, experimental liver lesions, so-called Auer hepatitis, can be caused by the administration of preformed immune complexes (Paronetto and Popper 1965) or by intravenous administration of antigen to previously sensitized animals (Fennel 1965). Repeated administration of heterologous serum or albumin to animals with toxic liver injury can potentiate hepatocellular injury, possibly due to the deposition of immune complexes on hepatocytes (Paronetto and Popper 1966).

Anti-HBs, anti-HBc and complement have been found in and eluted from hepatocytes containing hepatitis B antigens. Morphologically these immunoglobulin deposits appear as linear or lumpy deposits on the liver cell membranes (Hopf et al. 1976, 1981). HBcAg/anti-HBc complement-fixing immune complexes have been found in the nuclei of hepatocytes of some patients with HBsAg-positive chronic liver disease (Gerber et al. 1976; Arnold and Meyer zum Buschenfelde 1977) and may signal the later development of chronic active liver disease (Rizzetto et al. 1976). The significance of these findings in relationship to hepatocellular injury is not clear since they are not seen invariably and they could be explained on the basis of an epiphenomenon occurring after hepatocellular injury has taken place. In favor of this is the observation of Nowoslawski et al. (1975) that such complexes are most frequent in fulminant hepatitis. Alternatively, they might represent in-situ immune complex formation since IgG and/or IgM and IgA can be regularly found in HBcAg-containing nuclei of hepatocytes and can fix complement in vitro (Ray et al. 1979).

Isolated hepatocytes from patients with HBsAg-negative chronic active hepatitis revealed linear and granular patterns of in-vivo fixed IgG. The target antigen was not defined and one explanation of these findings is binding to Fc or C3 receptors of IgG (Hopf et al. 1976). Yet, IgG from patients with HBsAg-positive chronic hepatitis and from patients with autoimmune chronic hepatitis has been shown to bind to Chang liver cells which are deficient in Fc and C3 receptors for IgG. Absorption of the sera from HBsAg-positive patients with purified liver-specific protein (LSP) abolished IgG binding but only partial inhibition was obtained in sera from patients with autoimmune chronic active hepatitis. This finding suggested that two autoantibodies can be associated with chronic hepatitis and that HBV infection may permit expression of LSP. Recent experiments by Hopf et al. indicate that the hepatic clearance of immune complexes is a function of both hepatocytes and non-parenchymal cells (Hopf et al. 1981). It may be that some of the demonstrations of immune complex formation cited above reflect hepatocellular uptake of preformed, circulating immune complexes. The morphology of hepatocellular injury seen in HBV-related disease does not suggest immune complex mediation. The cytotoxic injuries related to immune complexes usually elicit polymorphonuclear infiltrates secondary to generation of complement-derived chemotactic factors for leukocytes, but the lymphocyte is the dominant cell in viral related hepatitis.

9.2.4.2. Circulating immune complexes

Ten to twenty percent of patients with acute HB experience symptoms of a serum sickness-like illness during the prodromal period. These symptoms include arthralgias, arthritis and urticaria (Alpert et al. 1971). There is now evidence from many workers that this transient prodromal illness, glomerulonephritis, polyarteritis nodosa, and other extrahepatic lesions can be related to the formation of immune complexes between HBV-related antigens and host-complement and immunoglobulins.

The serum from many patients with acute and chronic forms of hepatitis B is anticomplementary (Shulman and Barker 1969), reactive in the ^{125}I-C1q binding assay (Nydegger et al. 1974; Thomas et al. 1978), and positive for immune complexes in the Raji cell radioimmunoassay (Theofilopoulos et al. 1976). Electron microscopy of serum from patients with hepatitis has revealed complexes of spherical and filamentous HBsAg-associated particles with or without Dane particles (Almeida and Waterson 1969; Gocke et al. 1970; Bianchi and Gudat 1979). Antibodies capable of agglutinating Dane particles and tubules appear in chronic HB following elimination of Dane particles from the blood and elimination of HBc-producing cells from the liver (Neurath et al. 1976; Gudat and Bianchi 1977). Anti-HBe-positive sera are also capable of agglutinating Dane particles and clinically anti-HBe correlated with an absence of HBcAg and Dane particles in the serum (Bianchi and Gudat 1979). HBsAg, anti-HBs and complement components have been isolated from cryoproteins found in the sera of patients with acute and chronic HB (Wands et al. 1975a; McIntosh et al. 1976). Treatments which would be expected to cause disruption of immune complexes have caused expression of both HBsAg and anti-HBs in hepatitis sera which appeared to contain only one of these moieties (Millman et al. 1970; Madalinski et al. 1974). During the prodromal serum sickness-like illness associated with acute HB, decreased C3 and C4 levels have been found (Alpert et al. 1971) and immune complexes containing HBsAg and anti-HBs have been found by several methods (Madalinski and Bragiel 1979; Pernice et al. 1979). For example, HBsAg, C3 and IgM have been found in the walls of blood vessels of skin lesions from two patients with this prodromal illness (Dienstag et al. 1978). A finding consistent with increased utilization or consumption of complement components in patients with HBsAg-positive chronic active hepatitis is an increased fractional catabolic rate of C3 compared to albumin (Thomas et al. 1979).

Polymerases have been reported in the serum of some patients with hepatitis and it seems possible that these could be related to the formation of complexes between serum albumin and HBsAg (O'Neill 1979). The formation of such complexes may in turn lead to development of autoantibodies against polymerized albumin. It seems possible that attachment of HBV to hepatocytes could be facilitated by HBsAg-polymerized albumin complexes (Lenkei et al. 1977; Thung and Gerber 1981).

HBeAg occurs in both a free (unbound) form and bound to IgG. The ratio of these two forms has been reported to shift from the unbound to the bound form in the course of acute HB and may be related to the formation of immune complexes (Takahashi et al. 1979b).

While the evidence for immune complex formation is strong, there are other possible explanations for these findings. The hepatitis-related components of these immune complexes may be co-precipitated with antigens having other specificities. The formation of acute-phase reactants or aggregated immunoglobulins might account for some of these observations (Lawley et al. 1980).

9.2.4.3. Glomerulonephritis

Glomerulonephritis associated with granular deposits containing IgM, IgG, IgA, C3, and HBsAg has been documented by several authors (Combes et al. 1971; Brzosko et al. 1974; Kohler et al. 1974a; Knieser et al. 1974). These immune complexes are located mainly in the epimembranous and intramembranous or mesangial zones. Anti-HBs has been eluted from affected glomeruli (Ozawa et al. 1976). By electron microscopy, spherical virus-like particles, other particles of 50–100 nm, and tubular structures have been found in these deposits. The presence of HBsAg has been confirmed by immuno-electron microscopy (Knieser et al. 1974). The histologic lesions seen in association with these complexes have included membranous glomerulonephritis, membranoproliferative glomerulonephritis, mesangioproliferative glomerulonephritis and acute proliferative glomerulonephritis (Brzosko 1974; Kohler 1974; Knieser et al. 1974).

Glomerulonephritis has been seen in association with most forms of hepatitis B virus infection. In at least two studies of children with glomerulonephritis and/or nephrotic syndrome, HBV infection was linked to glomerular disease, although immune complex deposits with HBsAg were not always seen (Brzosko et al. 1974; Kleinknecht et al. 1979). HBcAg immune complexes have also been detected in children with subclinical HBV infection and membranous glomerulonephritis (Slusarczyk et al. 1980). In children with membranous glomerulonephritis complexes composed of HBeAg, IgG and C3 have also been found (Takekoshi et al. 1979; Ito et al. 1981). Glomerular deposits with immune complexes have been found by electron microscopy and by immunofluorescence microscopy in primates inoculated with HBsAg-containing plasma (Gyorkey et al. 1975).

9.2.4.4. *Polyarteritis nodosa*

Approximately 31 to 69% of patients with polyarteritis nodosa have HBs-antigenemia and/or anti-HBs (Sergent et al. 1976; Trepo et al. 1974). The serum of these patients has been shown to contain immune complexes by the Raji cell assay, C1q precipitation, electron microscopy and ultracentrifugation (Gocke et al. 1970; Trepo et al. 1974; Fye et al. 1977). By immunofluorescence microscopy granular deposits of HBsAg, immunoglobulin and C3 have been found in the vascular lesions, located along the internal elastic lamina of damaged vessels (Michalak 1978; Gocke et al. 1970). The amount of deposited immune complexes correlated with the severity of the vascular lesion, and the complexes were noted to be absent from healed lesions. In one series there was a positive correlation between the severity of liver damage and the amount of HBsAg-containing immune complexes in the vascular lesions (Nowoslawski et al. 1975). However, the liver lesions associated with HBV-related polyarteritis nodosa vary from minimal hepatitis to chronic active liver disease (Sergent et al. 1976). Apart from possible signs of liver disease, the clinical features of polyarteritis in these patients are similar to those of patients not known to have HBV infection (Sergent et al. 1976). Other evidence of immune complex disease may be found (Michalak 1978).

9.2.4.5. *Arthritis*

In the joints, arthralgia and arthritis have been described in a number of cases of acute and chronic HB (Wands et al. 1975a) in which circulating immune complexes HBsAg, IgG, IgM, IgA, C3, C4, C5 and C3 activator fragment have been described. These immune complexes were only noted in those patients with frank arthritis and were not found in patients with chronic HB without arthritis. HBsAg has been demonstrated in the inflamed joint of a patient with chronic active hepatitis and arthritis (Schumacher and Gall 1974) and particles of various sizes (20−25 nm and 40−60 nm) were seen via electron microscopy in the synovial lining cells, deep synovial cells and endothelial cells.

9.2.4.6. *Other diseases associated with HBV-related immune complexes*

HBsAg and anti-HBs were found in the cryoprecipitates of patients with essential mixed cryoglobulinemia (Levo et al. 1977). HBsAg, IgM, C3, C4 and 20-nm particles have been found in the skin lesions of a patient with cutaneous purpura and the serum cryoprecipitates contained HBsAg and IgM anti-HBs (Gower et al. 1973). HBV-related immune complexes have been related to childhood papular acrodermatitis (Gianotti 1978).

9.2.5. Anti-HBs-mediated cytotoxic reactions

There is little evidence to support a role for this mechanism in hepatocellular injury seen in HBV infections. Fluorescence microscopy has demonstrated the presence of immunoglobulins fixed to hepatocellular membranes in HBsAg-positive chronic hepatitis but not in healthy carriers (Hopf et al. 1976; Alberti et al. 1976). The corresponding target antigen has not been identified. Passive transfer of anti-HBs has not been shown to cause liver injury (Reed et al. 1973; Kohler et al. 1974b). The temporal relationship between hepatocellular injury and the appearance of anti-HBs (at the termination of HBV infection) and the fact that anti-HBs is not seen in all cases of acute HB does not support a role for anti-HBs-dependent, cell-mediated cytotoxicity in the mechanism of hepatocellular injury, although binding to cell membranes is not excluded by these observations.

9.2.6. Cell-mediated responses to HBV-related antigens

Using the leukocyte migration inhibition test, several investigators have documented the development of cell-mediated immunity against HBsAg in patients with acute limited hepatitis type B (Yeung-Laiwah et al. 1973; DeMoura et al. 1975; Meyer zum Buschenfelde et al. 1976; Aldershvile et al. 1977). Some have noted a decreased incidence of positive tests in patients after recovery (Meyer zum Buschenfelde et al. 1976; Aldersvhile et al. 1977). Patients with chronic HBsAg-positive virus infections have a lower incidence of positive tests and these may fluctuate considerably over the course of the illness (Ito et al. 1972; DeMoura et al. 1975; Meyer zum Buschenfelde et al. 1976; Aldersvhile et al. 1977). Many "healthy" chronic carriers of HBsAg have tests indicating a lack of cell-mediated immunity against HBsAg (Yeung-Laiwah et al. 1973). In general these results support the concept of a correlation between the development of cell-mediated immunity, limitation of the illness and clearance of the antigen from serum and liver tissue. These observations are in agreement with studies using lymphocyte stimulation as a marker of cell-mediated immunity (Yeung-Laiwah et al. 1973; Tong et al. 1975). They correlate with the results of one study in which the cytotoxicity of patients' lymphocytes was measured against HBsAg-coated chicken erythrocytes and in which the T-lymphocyte subpopulation was found to be cytotoxic (Alberti et al. 1977). This latter study in particular supports the concept that the hepatocellular damage in HB is mediated by T-lymphocytes reacting with hepatocytes which express the HBsAg on their plasma membranes.

Conflicting data have been obtained in a study using as a target the hepatoma cell line PLC/PRF/5, which expresses HBsAg on the plasma membrane. Dienstag and Bhan (1980) found that peripheral blood monocyte-mediated cytotoxicity was enhanced in chronic, but not acute HBV infection and that this enhanced cytotoxicity was unrelated to the expression of virus-specific antigens (HBsAg) by the target cells. The data were interpreted to indicate that there is non-specific enhancement of effector cell activity in chronic HBV infection rather than recognition of virus-specific antigens. The NK cell (natural killer cell) was identified as a possible mediator of hepatocellular injury (Dienstag and Bhan 1980). Possible mechanisms for increased NK cell activity could be interferon production or an increase in absolute numbers of NK cells. In a similar study, Chisari et al. (1981b), using the same hepatoma cell line (shown to express both HBsAg and LSP), were unable to demonstrate evidence of increased HBsAg-directed or LSP-directed cytotoxic effector cell activity of NK cells or cytotoxic T cells. On the other hand, defects in two distinct suppressor cell populations were identified during the course of acute hepatitis B (Chisari et al. 1981a). These defects tended to return to normal with recovery, but remained abnormal in patients with chronic hepatitis. In this study, as in others, the degree of immunologic dysfunction was difficult to correlate with biochemical measurement of hepatocellular injury. Chisari et al. (1981a, b) suggest that defects in suppressor cell function might permit normally suppressed, cytotoxic lymphocytes to attack host antigenic targets, e.g. LSP, to which the cells are normally tolerant. A suggested mechanism is that circulating immune complexes may interfere with "T"-suppressor cell function (Kakumu et al. 1980).

At this time there is general agreement that many of the early in-vitro studies of cell-mediated cytotoxicity have failed to evaluate the antigenic specificity of the target cells and that such in-vitro models of hepatic injury are likely to be difficult to evaluate until suitable target cells become available. Such cells will have to express the immunologically accessible antigens which are involved in HB. This problem is obviously difficult since it is quite possible that these antigens have not been completely defined.

9.2.7. Relationships between antigenic expression, immune responses, and clinical presentation of HBV infection

HBV infection is related to (Table 1) a spectrum of clinical disease including an apparently "healthy" carrier state without evidence of hepatocellular injury, acute hepatitis B, several forms of chronic infection, some leading to cirrhosis, and hepatoma.

9.2.7.1. Acute viral hepatitis

In the normergic host HBV infection results in an acute illness from which, provided it is not a fulminant hepatitis, the patient recovers without apparent sequelae (Fig. 4). HBsAg and HBcAg can be detected in only a small proportion of biopsies from patients with acute HB (Gudat et al. 1975; Ray et al. 1976). The virus is eliminated during the course of the illness, concurrent with which the patient shows sero-conversion from HBsAg to anti-HBs. Anti-HBs may remain for some months following the clinical illness, whereas anti-HBc may remain for many years (Hansson 1976). Anti-HBe may also persist for some months following clearance of the virus (Hess et al. 1977; Arnold et al. 1978). The development of cell-mediated immunity to HBsAg can be identified in most cases (Aldershvile et al. 1977).

TABLE 1.
Correlations between expression of hepatitis B viral antigens, clinical disease and immune status

Clinical disease	HBV expression		Immunologic response			
	In liver	In serum	Reaction type*	Immune status	Humoral reaction	Cellular response to HBsAg
Acute, self-limited viral hepatitis	Absent (HBsAg or HBcAg before necrosis)	HBsAg Dane particles DNA polymerase HBcAg Immune complexes	Elimination	Normal	Anti-HBc Anti-HBe Anti-HBs	Present Also against LSP
Carrier state	a) Predominant HBcAg Less HBsAg	Dane particles HBeAg	HBcAg	Immuno-suppression Tolerance Neonates	Dane particle–tubular complexes Anti-HBc	Absent or defective
Chronic persistent hepatitis	b) Predominant HBsAg Absent HBcAg	HBsAg		Unresponsive to HBsAg	Anti-HBc Anti-HBe	Absent or defective
Chronic active liver disease	c) Focal HBsAg Focal HBcAg	Dane particles HBeAg	Focal HBcAg	Variable immune insufficiency	Dane particle–tubular complexes Anti-HBc	Present, often defective Also against LSP

*Reaction patterns described by Gudat et al. 1975 and Bianchi and Gudat 1979. For details, see text.

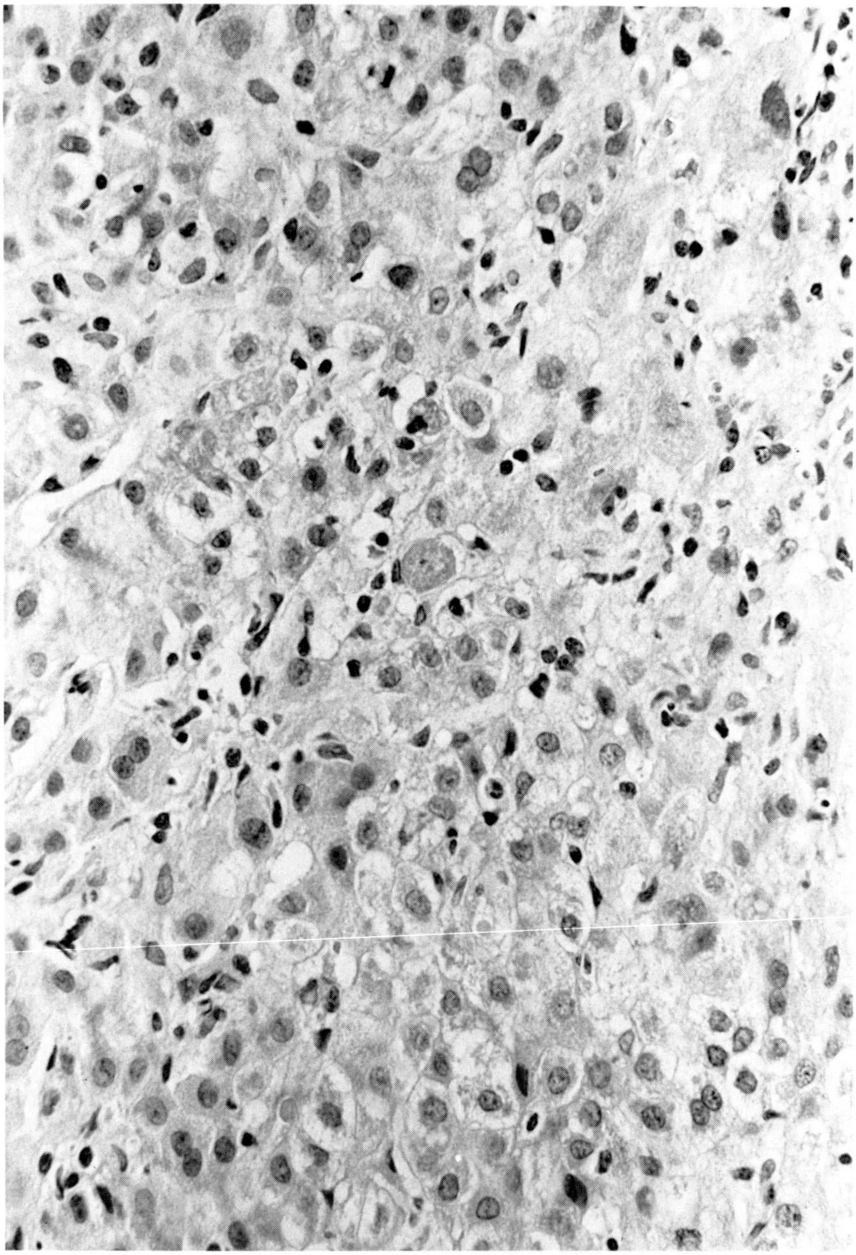

Fig. 4. Acute viral hepatitis B: Foci of parenchymal cell necrosis and lymphocytic infiltration are scattered in a patchy manner throughout the liver lobule. Some hepatocytes are swollen and hydropic; others are shrunken and have an intensely acidophilic cytoplasm, so-called acidophilic (Councilman) bodies. (H + E x 525; original x 100).

9.2.7.2. Chronic persistent hepatitis

In the majority of patients, chronic persistent hepatitis appears to be a benign disease in which infiltrates of lymphocytes and macrophages persist within the liver. These inflammatory infiltrates are classically confined to the portal tract areas and inflammation does not usually breach the limiting plate, but histological overlap can occur between chronic persistent hepatitis and chronic active liver disease. Clinically the patient feels well. There is usually an associated mild hyperbilirubinemia, and mild elevations of serum transaminases are often present. The disease may persist for one to two years, but usually runs a benign course and resolves without sequelae. Several patterns of antigenic expression and immunologic responsiveness have been identified (Gudat et al. 1975; Bianchi and Gudat 1979).

1. Immunosuppression type is characterized by abundant HBcAg in hepatocellular nuclei and cytoplasmic HBsAg in many of the liver cells. In this variant anti-HBs and anti-HBc are usually lacking, even though immune complexes can be found in approximately half of these cases. This clinical variant may occur spontaneously or in immunosuppressed patients following renal transplant or chemotherapy. It is assumed in the immunosuppressed patient that it is cellular immunity which is mainly being suppressed, resulting in incomplete elimination of the virus. In those cases occurring spontaneously, the cause is less apparent.

2. In the second group, as in the healthy carrier, there is abundant expression of HBsAg in up to 80% of the liver cells, but HBc is absent from tissue. Anti-HBs is absent in this group, but occasionally circulating immune complexes are found containing tubular HBsAg. It is felt that this group of patients lack cell-mediated immunity to HBsAg, which with the lack of anti-HBs reflects both humoral and cellular unresponsiveness to HBsAg (Yeung-Laiwah 1971; Dudley et al. 1972; Irwin et al. 1974; Schumacher et al. 1974; Lee et al. 1975). The attack of the virus, however, appears to be sufficient to effectively eliminate or suppress HBcAg-expressing cells and Dane particle-associated antigens.

3. The third group of patients with chronic persistent hepatitis have a pattern of tissue antigen expression similar to that found in chronic active liver disease, i.e. these patients show focal spotty lesions of HBcAg but little or no detectable HBs within hepatocytes. Some of these patients later develop true chronic active liver disease (Bianchi and Gudat 1979).

9.2.7.3. Healthy carrier state

This is a condition in which there is little or no evidence of liver cell damage. HBV antigens may be expressed in one of two ways. The carrier state may exist with sheets of HBcAg within the cells with only occasional cells showing evidence of HBsAg or there may be no evidence of HBcAg with abundant expression of HBsAg. Both these types of expression have been described above in chronic persistent hepatitis.

9.2.7.4. Chronic active liver disease (CALD)

In this group of patients there is evidence of an active and an aggressive inflammatory infiltrate composed of lymphocytes and plasma cells, focused at the portal tract (Fig. 5). The portal tracts of the inflammatory cells invade the parenchyma of the liver, resulting in destruction of neighboring hepatocytes (piecemeal necrosis). In these zones hepatocytes may undergo cell division (rosette formation), and the resulting destruction is accompanied by fibrosis. The fibrosis may join neighboring portal tracts (portal tract linkage), and in a small group of patients may progress to cirrhosis with generalized destruction of liver architecture, regenerative nodules and linkage to central veins, resulting in shunting of blood within the liver (MacSween 1980). The clinical expression of this disease is variable and correlates to some extent with the severity of histological damage. The patients may experience little or no symptoms in the early phases and the diagnosis is suspected on the evidence of a rising bilirubin and rising transaminase level (MacKay 1978). This pattern may be seen in recovering acute viral hepatitis and the term "chronic active liver disease" is usually reserved for patients who have shown evidence of activity for more than six months following their initial episode of acute hepatitis. However, cases of complete recovery from viral hepatitis have been noted to take as long as 12 months (Reynolds 1980). Most cases of CALD following HBV appear to settle with the passage of time. The place of steroid therapy in this group remains controversial. A few cases will progress to cirrhosis with the gradual evolution of both clinical and biochemical evidence of severe liver disease.

The antigenic expression in cases of CALD to HB shows focal spotty appearance of HBcAg within hepatocytes often with associated membrane HBsAg (Gudat et al. 1975). There appears to be an inverse relationship between the amount of HBcAg present within the liver and the degree of inflammation. When HBcAg is detected within liver cells, Dane particles, often associated with HBcAg, appear in the blood and with the more aggressive forms of CALD there appears to be a higher instance of spontaneous immune complexes composed of the Dane particles and tubules (Bianchi and Gudat 1979). Anti-HBe appears rarely, but anti-HBc is often found in high titers. As described above, the results of studies of cell-mediated immunity are more difficult to interpret. It is felt that, unlike the patient in whom there is generalized HBcAg present with liver (i.e. the picture seen in the immunosuppressed patient), the patient with CALD is able to mount an immunological assault on the virus that is sufficient to eliminate some but not all, of the viral antigens. This continued assault results in progressive destruction of the liver over a protracted period.

Therapy of this condition could be directed in two opposite directions. If the immunologic assault could be improved this might result initially in increased destruction within the liver, but might also lead to complete elimination of the virus and a resulting cure. Alternatively, suppression of the immune response might lead to a greater tolerance of virus with a lessening of hepatic destruction, but prolongation of the infection.

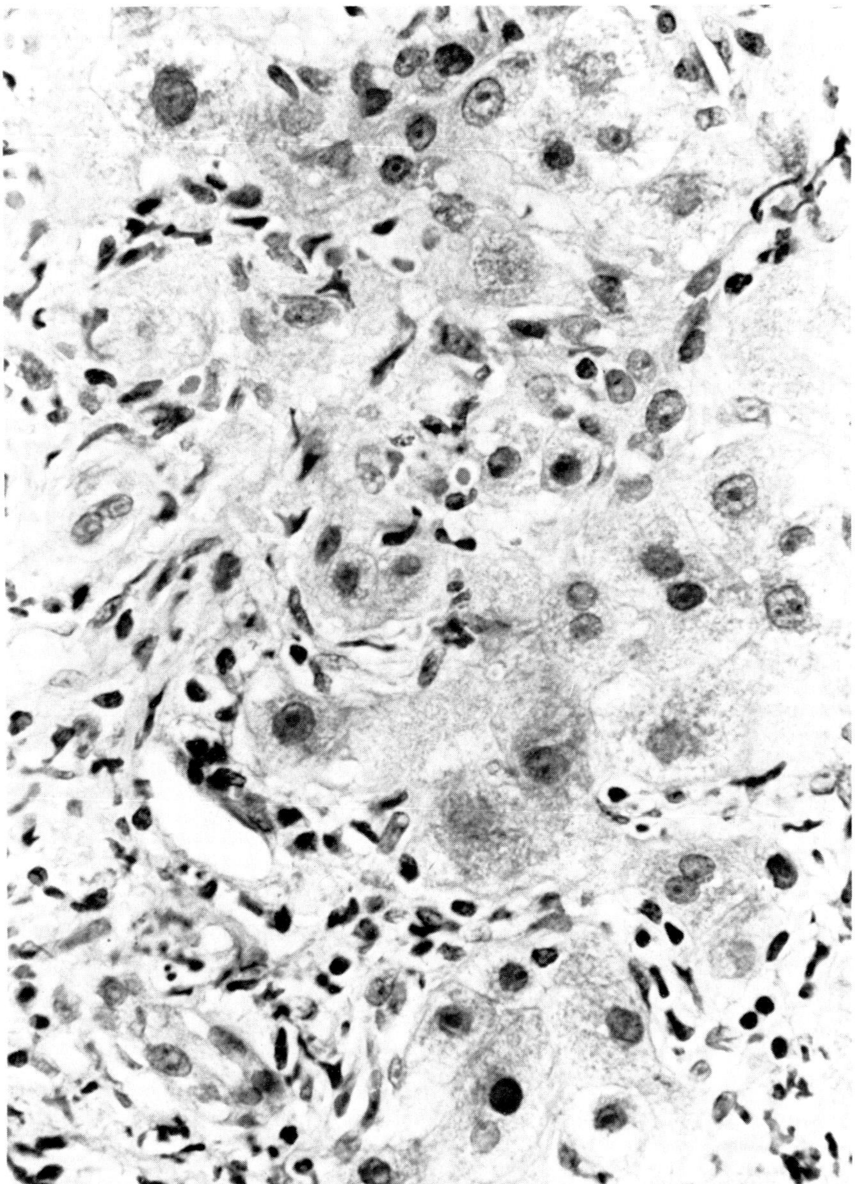

Fig. 5. Chronic active liver disease: Hepatocytes at the junction between the lobular parenchyma and the portal area are surrounded by an infiltrate of lymphocytes, macrophages, and fibroblasts (piecemeal necrosis). Small groups of cells are completely surrounded by the inflammatory process (H + E x 1300; original x 250).

9.2.7.5. Additional clinical observations
There is additional clinical evidence that hepatocellular injury in HB is mediated by inflammatory mechanisms rather than by a direct cytopathic effect.

Numerous studies have demonstrated inverse correlations between the histologic and serologic expression of HBsAg and hepatocellular injury. For example, in tissue sections, cells containing HBsAg are almost never seen in acute hepatitis and are numerous in chronic hepatitis carriers who lack significant hepatocellular injury (Gudat et al. 1975; Ray et al. 1976). Liver necrosis may be absent or of low grade in immunosuppressed renal transplant patients and in chronic carriers who lack demonstrable cell-mediated immunity to HBsAg (Gudat et al. 1975; El Sheikh et al. 1978). If immunosuppressive therapy is stopped in an HBsAg-positive person, fulminant hepatocellular necrosis may occur (Galbraith et al. 1975). A role for cellular rather than humoral mechanisms is supported by observations that chronic hepatitis can occur in patients with agammaglobulinemia (Tong et al. 1977). Further, transient increases in the severity of hepatitis follow transfusion of lymphocytes from convalescent patients, administration of transfer factor, or immunostimulatory agents, e.g. levamisole (Kohler et al. 1974b; Jain et al. 1977; DeCree et al. 1974).

9.2.7.6. Hepatocellular carcinoma (HCC)
There is now a large body of evidence that HBV infection is a major etiological factor in primary carcinoma of liver parenchyma. Epidemiologic studies have shown a higher frequency of serum markers of current HBV infection in patients with hepatocellular carcinoma than in controls (Welsh et al. 1976; Szmuness 1978; Hadziyannis 1980; Pettigrew et al. 1976).

Population studies from countries with varying incidences of HCC demonstrate positive correlations between the incidence of tumor and the prevalence of HBsAg carrier state, measured by radioimmunoassay (Hadziyannis 1980). HBV antigens, especially HBsAg, have been found in tumor tissue itself (Nazarewicz et al. 1977) in liver tissue adjacent to HBsAg- and HBcAg-negative tumor (Hadziyannis et al. 1976; Shikata 1976) and in the sera of patients with cytologically dysplastic liver cells (Anthony et al. 1973). Virus-like particles, 23 nm in diameter, have been found in the hepatocellular tissue (Campion et al. 1972). HBsAg with spherical and tubular particles has been recovered from the tissue culture medium of hepatocellular carcinoma cell lines (MacNab et al. 1976; Aden et al. 1979).

HBV-DNA has been found to be integrated in the cellular DNA of hepatoma tissue (Summers et al. 1978; Zuckerman 1978; Brechot et al. 1980) in a human hepatoma cell line (Chakraborty et al. 1980; Edman et al. 1980) and in the non-tumorous areas of liver of patients with hepatomas (Gerber et al. 1979).

Several mechanisms have been proposed for the pathogenesis of HBV-related hepatocellular carcinoma, but experimental proof of these is lacking. Minor chronic liver damage, resulting from chronic HBV infection, could lead to continuous regeneration and emergence of malignant transformed cells. Alterations in the metabolism of hepatocytes infected by HBV could facilitate the processes of chemical carcinogenesis. Incorporation of viral DNA into the liver cell genome, could result directly in malignant transformation.

It has not been resolved whether there are differences in the manner that viral DNA is incorporated in hepatitis or hepatoma or even if (as seems likely) incorporation of viral DNA into the host genome is an invariable result of HBV infection. Immunologic studies of this group are lacking.

9.3. HEPATITIS A VIRUS INFECTION

HAV infection occurs world wide, and is especially frequent in poor socioeconomic settings since the primary means of transmission is by the fecal to oral route. Other forms of transmission are possible, but are less likely to be of epidemiologic importance. Often producing subclinical illness, HAV infection is frequently undetected, but such cases may serve to maintain the existence of the virus (Dienstag 1980).

9.3.1. General characteristics of the virus

HAV, regarded as an enterovirus, was first observed by immuno-electron microscopy of fecal ultrafiltrates obtained from clinical acute phase stools of volunteers inoculated with Willowbrook MS-1 strain of hepatitis virus. Immune aggregates were formed when these ultrafiltrates were incubated with convalescent serum or pooled globulins, and revealed 27-nm virus-like particles (Feinstone et al. 1973). Unlike HBV, the virus lacks an envelope and appears to consist of a genome and surrounding virus capsid only. Two morphologic variants occur, "full" particles, containing nucleic acid and "empty" particles, devoid of nucleic acid (Dienstag 1980). The HAV genome is composed of single-stranded RNA with a mean molecular weight of 1.9×10^6 daltons (Siegl and Frosner 1978). There are three major polypeptides with molecular weights of 34,000, 25,500 and 23,000 daltons (Coulepis et al. 1978). The virus has one antigenic identity (Provost et al. 1975; Dienstag et al. 1976b) and this has been used to develop antisera specific for HAV. These antisera have made possible many of the recent basic and epidemiologic studies concerning hepatitis A.

9.3.2. Virus replication

Studies on HAV have been facilitated by susceptibility of the chimpanzee and marmoset to infection by HAV with resulting illness similar to that in man (Dienstag et al. 1976a). Following inoculation, HAV can be detected in the hepatocyte cytoplasm by immunofluorescence microscopy, the greatest amount of virus being found just before and during biochemical evidence of cell injury (Mathiesen et al. 1977). 27-nm HAV particles can be found by electron microscopy and immuno-electron microscopy in cytoplasmic vesicles of hepatocytes and Kupffer cells (Shimizu et al. 1978). In these studies the virus was not found in the hepatocyte nucleus.

Viral infection of the liver is accompanied by viremia mainly in the late incubation period, and it seems likely that this is related to entry of the virus into the blood via the hepatic sinusoids. Likewise, fecal shedding, maximal during the preclinical period, seems to be the consequence of biliary excretion of virus formed in the liver, since evidence for intestinal viral replication has not been found (Mathiesen et al. 1978; Dienstag 1980). HAV has been propagated in primary explant cultures of marmoset liver and in a rhesus monkey fetal kidney cell line. In these systems HAV has been identified in cultured cells and in culture medium but is not cytopathic (Provost and Hilleman 1979). Attempts to culture the virus in human cell lines are being made.

9.3.3. *Clinical features of human disease*

Following inoculation, a short incubation period (2–6 weeks) is followed by an illness very similar to acute HB. The liver morphology in HAV infection is similar to that in uncomplicated HB. Many cases are subclinical and unlike HBV, HAV seems not to be a cause of chronic active liver disease, nor has an association with hepatocellular carcinoma been documented.

9.3.4. *Immunologic responses*

Anti-HAV generally appears coincident with or before evidence of hepatocellular necrosis. Antibody levels peak several months after the acute illness and remain detectable for an indefinite period of time (Frosner et al. 1977). During the acute illness anti-HAV is mainly of the IgM type (Bradley et al. 1977) and is accompanied by high serum IgM levels, not all of which can be accounted for by generation of anti-HAV. The titer of anti-HAV does not regularly correlate with the severity of disease.

Circulating immune complexes may account for depressed serum complement levels (Baer et al. 1977), anticomplementary activity (Provost et al. 1975), and positive C1q binding assays (Thomas et al. 1978) in patients with proven or likely hepatitis A. Glomerular deposits of HAV have been detected in experimental hepatitis A in the marmoset (Mathiesen et al. 1978). Clinically detectable immune complex disease is uncommon, however, although a small proportion of patients may experience a prodrome with skin rashes and arthralgias. Defects in the ability of lymphocytes to form rosettes with sheep red blood cells have been found in patients with hepatitis A and the serum may contain a rosette-inhibitory factor (Chisari et al. 1977). Studies of cellular immune responsiveness to HAV infection are lacking.

9.3.5. *Pathogenesis*

The pathogenesis of hepatocellular injury in hepatitis A has not been determined. One possibility is that HAV (unlike HBV) acts as a cytopathic agent, without the requirement of immune mechanisms. In favor of this are the possibility of hepatocyte necrosis following a very short (7-day) incubation period (Provost et al. 1977) and direct correlations between hepatocellular injury and release of virus from liver cells into the stools (Frosner et al. 1977). Further, a chronic, asymptomatic carrier state is not seen. On the other hand, a cytopathic effect is not seen in cultured cells used to propagate the virus (Provost and Hilleman 1979) and, as pointed out, the histology of acute hepatitis A showing lymphocytic infiltration of the liver is in general indistinguishable from that of acute hepatitis B.

9.4. HEPATOCELLULAR ANTIGENS

Potentially antigenic components have been identified in association with hepatocyte intracytoplasmic organelles, such as mitochondria and ribosomes (Labro et al. 1978). Most recent studies on hepatocellular antigens have been directed toward understanding the antigenic nature of the plasma membrane since the introduction of foreign antigenic components into the hepatocellular plasma membrane, e.g. HBV, could theoretically generate exposed target sites for immunologic attack. It is also likely that hepatocellular membrane proteins serve as targets for autoimmune injury. At least one of the identifiable immunogenic components seems to be specific to the hepatocyte surface membrane. Other hepatocellular antigens are common to many organs and as such may be involved in multisystem disease.

9.4.1. *Liver-specific protein*

This is a high molecular weight, non-species-specific lipoprotein associated with plasma membrane fractions. It was isolated by Meyer zum Buschenfelde and Miescher from fresh human liver by homogenization, followed by ultracentrifugation and gel filtration (Meyer zum Buschenfelde and Miescher 1972). The organ-specific components of the preparation are unstable and buffer compositions are extremely important for the retention of antigenic integrity (McFarlane et al. 1977). The molecular weight, estimated by gel filtration chromatography, is likely to be between 4×10^6 daltons and 20×10^6 daltons, but this is difficult to determine with certainty because (a) preparations contain phospholipids and triglycerides and (b) there are several major and minor components when the preparations are analyzed by sodium dodecyl sulfate polyarylamide gel electrophoresis. Removal of the lipid component from liver-specific protein preparations abolishes its antigenicity (McFarlane et al. 1977).

There is controversy concerning the antigenic specifity of liver-specific proteins.

Hutteroth and Meyer zum Buschenfelde (1978a) found that it contains at least two liver-specific determinants, one being human-specific and the other cross-reactive between species (see also Manns et al. 1980b). However, Behrens and co-workers have been unable to detect organ-specific antigens (Behrens and Paronetto 1979; Behrens et al. 1979). The identification of such organ-specific components depends upon generating a specific antibody response to liver-specific protein in an immunized animal, and these antibodies must be detectable after absorption of antibodies to non-hepatocellular tissue, a process during which the organ-specific component may be lost if denatured during immunization, if weakly antigenic, or if excessively labile. Resolution of the multiple antigenic specificities of liver-specific protein preparations is likely to be achieved most easily by analysis of monoclonal antibodies which have been generated in response to immunization to crude preparations (Chisari 1980). Studies have failed to demonstrate immunologic identity between liver-specific protein and the various antigenic components associated with the hepatitis B virus (Hess et al., cited by Meyer zum Buschenfelde et al. 1979).

9.4.2. Liver membrane antigen (LMA)

This is a non-species-specific antigen, located on the hepatocyte surface, defined primarily by its reaction with an antibody which can be detected in the serum of hypergammaglobulinemic patients with HBsAg-negative chronic active hepatitis (Hopf et al. 1976). Affinity chromatography, using immunoglobulin from LMS-positive, HBsAg-negative sera, has been employed to isolate this antigen from both rabbit and human liver where it is located in the 100,000 x *g* supernatants of liver homogenates (Meyer zum Buschenfelde et al. 1979). Analysis of this preparation by crossed immuno-electrophoresis failed to demonstrate immunologic cross-reactivity with anti-liver specific protein, normal serum, or anti-human plasma protein (Meyer zum Buschenfelde et al. 1979). Immunologic identity of LMA isolated from different species has been demonstrated by tandem crossed immuno-electrophoresis (Hutteroth and Meyer zum Buschenfelde 1978b). However, there is controversy concerning the specificity of liver membrane antigen since it has been reported that the linear pattern of fluorescent staining produced by LMA-positive sera on rabbit hepatocytes can be abolished by absorbing the sera with human LSP, suggesting that the antigen against which anti-LMA is directed is a component of LSP (Hopf et al. 1976). In addition, high titers of liver-specific protein antibodies have been detected by radioimmunoassay in sera such as those used to isolate LMA (Jensen et al. 1978; Gerber et al. 1979).

9.4.3. Biliary tract antigens

Several bile-specific protein components (distinct from plasma proteins) have been identified (Englert et al. 1970; Espinosa 1976). Normal human gallbladder bile contains a protein fraction against which in-vitro cellular immune responses can be demonstrated in patients with primary biliary cirrhosis (McFarlane et al. 1979). This biliary protein has been found to contain three distinct antigens. By immunofluorescence microscopy, one of these has been associated with the canalicular portion of the hepatocyte membrane and another with the intrahepatic bile duct epithelium. However, all three antigens demonstrate cross-reactivity with other tissues (Wojcicka 1979).

9.4.4. Humoral immune responses to hepatocellular antigens

9.4.4.1. Antibodies to liver-specific protein and liver membrane antigen

Using sensitive radioimmunoassays, serum antibodies to components of human LSP preparations have been found in a majority of patients with HBsAg-positive and HBsAg-negative acute viral hepatitis, CALD, alcoholic cirrhosis and primary biliary cirrhosis. Patients with CALD had the highest titers and those with chronic persistent hepatitis had generally lower frequency and lower titers of anti-LSP, suggesting correlations between the level of antibody and the intensity of liver injury as determined by histologic or biochemical assessment (Jensen et al. 1978; Kakumu et al. 1979). In these studies the mean antibody titer tended to be higher in HBsAg-negative cases but this was not found by Manns et al. (1980a). In cases of acute hepatitis, anti-LSP decreased in titer or disappeared within several months of resolution.

Anti-LMA has been found in several inflammatory liver diseases, including HBsAg-negative chronic hepatitis and HBsAg-negative non-alcoholic cirrhosis. These antibodies are rarely found in HBsAg-positive liver disease (Tage-Jensen et al. 1977; Manns et al. 1980a).

The relevance of anti-LSP and anti-LMA to the pathogenesis of hepatocellular injury in acute or chronic hepatitis is uncertain. The relatively greater frequency of anti-LMA in HBsAg-negative liver disease has suggested that anti-LMA may be characteristic of "autoimmune hepatitis"

9.4.4.2. Non-organ-, non-species-specific antibodies

This group of antibodies has been detected in a number of liver diseases, but they are not restricted to any subgroup or even to liver disease. These antibodies include anti-mitochondrial antibody, commonly associated with primary biliary cirrhosis, antinuclear antibody and anti-smooth muscle antibodies of HBsAg-negative chronic hepatitis (Meyer zum Buschenfelde 1976). Antinuclear antibodies are usually directed against the DNA—protein complex, rarely against native DNA and then only during active disease (MacKay 1978). Anti-smooth muscle antibodies occur in many liver and non-liver diseases and have a wide spectrum of reactivity with smooth muscle and other tissues. The antigen is most likely actin but may include other cytoskeletal components such as tubulin or intermediate filaments (Toh 1979). Antimitochondrial antibodies, directed again the inner membranes of mitochondria, are discussed further in the section of this paper concerned with primary biliary cirrhosis. Other non-specific antibody responses (e.g. to measles and rubella) occur in liver disease, likely due to general stimulation of the humoral immune mechanisms. These antibodies have not been shown to have a significant pathogenic effect and are likely to be epiphenomena rather than mediators of cell injury.

9.4.5. *Cell-mediated responses to liver-specific protein*

Lymphocyte transformation (Thestrup-Pedersen et al. 1976) and leukocyte migration inhibition (Lee et al. 1977; Manns et al. 1980a) to liver-specific protein preparations have been demonstrated in patients with acute viral hepatitis, CALD and active cirrhosis in the active phase of these diseases. Such patients have been shown to have effector lymphocytes that are cytotoxic to autologous and heterologous hepatocytes and to avian red blood cells coated with human liver-specific protein preparations (Paronetto and Vernace 1975; Wands and Isselbacher 1975; Fernandez-Cruz et al. 1978; Vogten et al. 1978). The intensity of both humoral and cellular immune responses seems to correlate with the activity of the inflammatory process (measured by histologic and biochemical means). Studies using lymphocyte subpopulations suggest that the cytotoxic effector cells are present in the B-cell enriched fraction and may be K cells (Cochrane et al. 1976). Thus antibody-dependent cytotoxicity directed against a liver membrane protein may be a mechanism of hepatocyte destruction. While the in-vitro reactions can be blocked by adding human liver-specific protein to the system, identification of the target molecules has not been achieved because of the crude nature of liver-specific protein preparations.

9.4.6. *Experimental hepatitis induced by LSP*

Prolonged immunization of rabbits with preparations of crude or purified human liver-specific protein in complete Freund's adjuvant resulted in the development of histologic lesions of chronic active hepatitis, demonstration of serum antibody against liver-specific protein, deposits of hepatocyte membrane-bound immunoglobulin, and cellular immune responses (delayed hypersensitivity on skin testing) to human and rabbit liver-specific protein preparations (Meyer zum Buschenfelde et al. 1972). The cellular and humoral responses to human liver-specific protein correlated with the histologic changes. Parenterally administered rabbit liver-specific protein was able to neutralize the pathologic effects of immunization with human liver-specific protein.

9.5. CHRONIC ACTIVE LIVER DISEASE (CALD)

Chronic active hepatitis is defined by an international committee on nomenclature as a disease lasting more than six months with signs of activity characterized by increased levels of serum aminotransferase and immunoglobulins and with morphologic changes consisting of chronic inflammatory reactions in the portal tracts and in the surrounding limiting plates, i.e. periportal hepatitis (Fogarty International Proceedings 1976). The term chronic active liver disease was introduced in order to include a wider-spectrum chronic inflammatory liver disease, ranging from chronic persistent hepatitis (non-progressive hepatitis with an intact hepatic architecture) to active, advanced cirrhosis (Summerskill 1974).

The use of the term CALD implies both histological and temporal criteria, but does not imply any specific etiology. There are at least three major etiologic subgroups which are not necessarily identifiable on the basis of histologic criteria.

9.5.1. Viral-related chronic active liver disease

Hepatitis B-related chronic active liver disease has been discussed earlier. To date there is no evidence that hepatitis A virus infections produce chronic hepatitis. Together, chronic hepatitis B and hepatitis non-A,non-B are the most important etiologic agents in this group.

9.5.1.1. Chronic active liver disease related to non-A,non-B hepatitis

Non-A,non-B hepatitis has recently been implicated in the development of CALD. The histological picture is the same as for other forms of chronic active liver disease. Non-A,non-B may in fact represent more than one disease. Virus-like particles, possibly representing two distinct etiologic agents, have been found in the endoplasmic reticulum and nuclei of liver cells in chimpanzees infected with serum and blood products from carriers of non-A,non-B hepatitis (Jackson et al. 1979; Tsiquave et al. 1980). Hepatitis B-like virus particles were found in the serum and liver homogenates of patients with non-A,non-B hepatitis (Hantz et al. 1980). The existence of an antigen–antibody system, specific for non-A,non-B hepatitis has been described (Tabor et al. 1979; Vitvitski et al. 1979). Chronic liver disease due to non-A,non-B infection appears to be particularly common following blood transfusion; percentages ranging from 33 to 46 (Purcell et al. 1976; Koretz et al. 1976). It appears that chronic non-A,non-B hepatitis, while common following transfusion is also common in drug addicts (58% in a recent series) (Rakela and Redeker 1979). The pathogenesis, long-term outlook and response to steroid therapy of this subgroup of patients with virally induced CALD remains to be ascertained.

9.5.2. Autoimmune-associated chronic liver disease

This subgroup of patients with chronic active liver disease show similar histological features, but have no evidence of preceding hepatitis B infection. The picture is most commonly seen in women, often with evidence of other associated autoimmune diseases: sicca syndrome, arthralgia, hemolytic anemia, inflammatory bowel disease and renal tubular acidosis (Golding et al. 1973). This group of patients commonly show serological markers of autoimmune disease. These include non-organ-, non-species-specific antibodies to smooth muscle and occasionally to mitochondria, antinuclear antibodies, LE cells, antibodies to double-stranded DNA and hypergammaglobulinemia (MacKay 1978). The histocompatibility types HLA-B8 and HLA-DW3 are frequent (Paronetto and Sagnelli 1980). The biochemical picture is similar to that seen in chronic liver disease secondary to HBV. A good response to corticosteroid therapy may be expected in those patients who have active piecemeal necrosis and inflammation and show marked enzyme elevations (Summerskill et al. 1975). The strong markers of autoimmune disease and the good response to corticosteroids suggest that the immune processes operating in this form of CALD differ from that found in chronic liver disease secondary to hepatitis B virus. Antibodies to LSP have been described in both the autoimmune variety of CALD and that secondary to HB (Jensen et al. 1978; Kakumu et al. 1979; Manns et al. 1980a). The presence of anti-LSP does not appear to correlate well with enzymatic evidence of activity of the disease.

Liver membrane autoantibody in one study appeared to relate closely to HBsAg-negative CALD (Tage-Jensen et al. 1977).

Reduction in total circulating T cells has been reported and a defect in suppressor T-cell function has been postulated in both virus-related and virus-unrelated CALD (Williams et al. 1980). Peripheral blood lymphocytes from such patients have been shown to be cytotoxic for autologous liver cells (Wands and Isselbacher 1975; Paronetto and Vernace 1975), Chang cells (Wands and Isselbacher 1975; Jacques et al. 1976) and rabbit hepatocytes (Thomson et al. 1974; Vergani et al. 1979). In one group of patients with auto-immune CALD, lymphocytes cytotoxic to autologous hepatocytes were located in non-T-cell fractions, the cytotoxicity was blocked by the addition of excessive amounts of LSP and the cytotoxicity in vitro, although not present in all patients, showed a significant correlation with the activity of the disease assessed histologically (Vergani et al. 1979). The authors felt that the mechanism was likely to be antibody-dependent cell-mediated cytotoxicity in which K cells became attached to the hepatocyte membrane via an antibody reacting with an antigen on the liver cell. The fact that this cytotoxicity was blocked by the addition of LSP suggested that this was the target for the attack on the cell. An incidental finding was the fact that hepatocytes obtained from patients with CALD were more susceptible to damage by lymphocytes obtained from normal subjects. It was suggested that these hepatocytes might be coated in vivo with antibodies to which K cells present in the normal lymphocyte population bind in vitro.

Suppressor T-cell function defects have been noted in patients with autoimmune type CALD and in four out of five such patients tested serially the defect correlated well with indices of disease activity. Conversely, in patients who were positive for HBsAg or non-A,non-B, normal supressor T-cell function was noted (Tremolada et al. 1980). It seems possible that while liver-specific autoimmune reactions have been detected in both "auto-immune" and virus-related groups (Jensen et al. 1978), different mechanisms may be responsible for maintaining the disease process in these

TABLE 2.
Major distinctions between HBV-related and autoimmune CALD*

Clinical feature	HBV-related disease		Autoimmune
	HBs +ve	HBs −ve	
Females	26	52	80
Survival − 5 years	57	88	85
HBcAg	58	0	0
HBcAg	44	0	0
Anti-HBs	0	30	10
Anti-HBc	94	100	0
Anti-HBc	48	0	0

*Data from Paronetto et al. 1980. All values expressed as percent of total.

two groups. Indeed, as documented by Paronetto and Sagnelli (1980) the long-term prognosis of the two groups is different (Table 2).

9.5.3. Drug-induced chronic active liver disease

A number of drugs have been shown to produce the histological picture of CALD. These drugs include methyldopa, isoniazid, halothane, dantrolene and nitrofurantoin (Maddrey and Boitnott 1977; Utili and Boitnott 1977; Black et al. 1980; Sharp et al. 1980). The mechanisms by which drugs produce this lesion are unknown but it appears not to be a toxic reaction. It has been postulated that in certain susceptible individuals the drug and/or one of its metabolites is involved in the formation of a neo-antigen on the cell membrane with subsequent immune-mediated attack being directed at the altered cell with resulting hepatic necrosis. To date it has not been shown that chronic liver disease persists following the removal of the offending drug.

9.5.4. Miscellaneous group

It should be noted that the histological picture of CALD may, at times, be seen in other conditions. These include: primary biliary cirrhosis, alcoholic hepatitis, Wilson's disease and patients with liver disease associated with α_1-antitrypsin deficiency.

9.6. ALCOHOL-INDUCED LIVER DISEASE

The spectrum of histologic lesions produced by alcohol-induced injury to the liver may take three distinct histological forms (Fig. 6): (1) Steatosis of the liver in which hepatocytes become ballooned with large amounts of intracellular fat. (2) Alcoholic hepatitis in which there is hepatocellular necrosis with inflammation, both within the portal tracts and the parenchyma of the liver. (3) Cirrhosis of the liver.

These three forms are not mutually exclusive and all three may coexist within the same patient. It is felt, however, that steatosis of the liver represents the result of acute and recent ingestion of alcohol, usually disappearing if the patient stops drinking. The latter two forms, i.e. alcoholic hepatitis and cirrhosis, represent the effects of more chronic ingestion of alcohol and both forms may progress in the absence of continued drinking (Powell and Klatskin 1968; Hardison and Lee 1966). This progression of liver disease, despite the removal of the offending drug, differs from other known forms of drug-induced liver disease (see Section 9.5.3.).

Alcoholic hepatitis may show features indistinguishable from other forms of CALD. The apparent increase in susceptibility to alcohol-induced liver disease by women, and the possible HLA-B40 association with alcoholic cirrhosis, the presence of both humoral and cell-mediated immune reactions and the progression of the liver disease in many patients, despite withdrawal of the drug, suggests that autoimmune mechanisms may play an important part in its development.

9.6.1. Direct toxicity of alcohol

Alcohol-induced liver disease appears to some extent to be dose-related (Saunders et al. 1981; Pequignot 1961) and though the correlation between dose, length of history and histology is not good (Brunt et al. 1974), it appears from present data that the ingestion of more than 80 g of alcohol per day in men, and 40 g per day in women carries a marked increased risk factor for developing alcoholic liver disease. The differences in sex and dosage required for damage, and in the progression of the disease following withdrawal of alcohol suggest that other mechanisms are important (Galambos 1974).

Some of the changes in alcoholic liver disease may be secondary to failure of the microtubule-dependent secretory apparatus of the cell. It has been postulated that alcoholic hyaline accumulation is a response to the antimicrotubular action of ethanol. Acutely in rats, ethanol impedes the secretion of lipoproteins and serum proteins by hepatocytes. A similar effect is noted with other agents that interfere with the function of the microtubules, e.g. colchicine (Stein et al. 1974; LeMarchand et al. 1974; Feldman et al. 1975; Stein and Stein 1967). Alcoholic hyaline accumulation is noted in animals fed such microtubular agents (French and Davies 1975). Chronic ingestion of alcohol in rats leads to impaired export of proteins and lipids. A similar defect is noted for liver albumin and transferrin (Baroana et al. 1975; Stein et al. 1974; LeMarchand et al. 1974; Feldman et al. 1975; Stein and Stein 1967; Redman

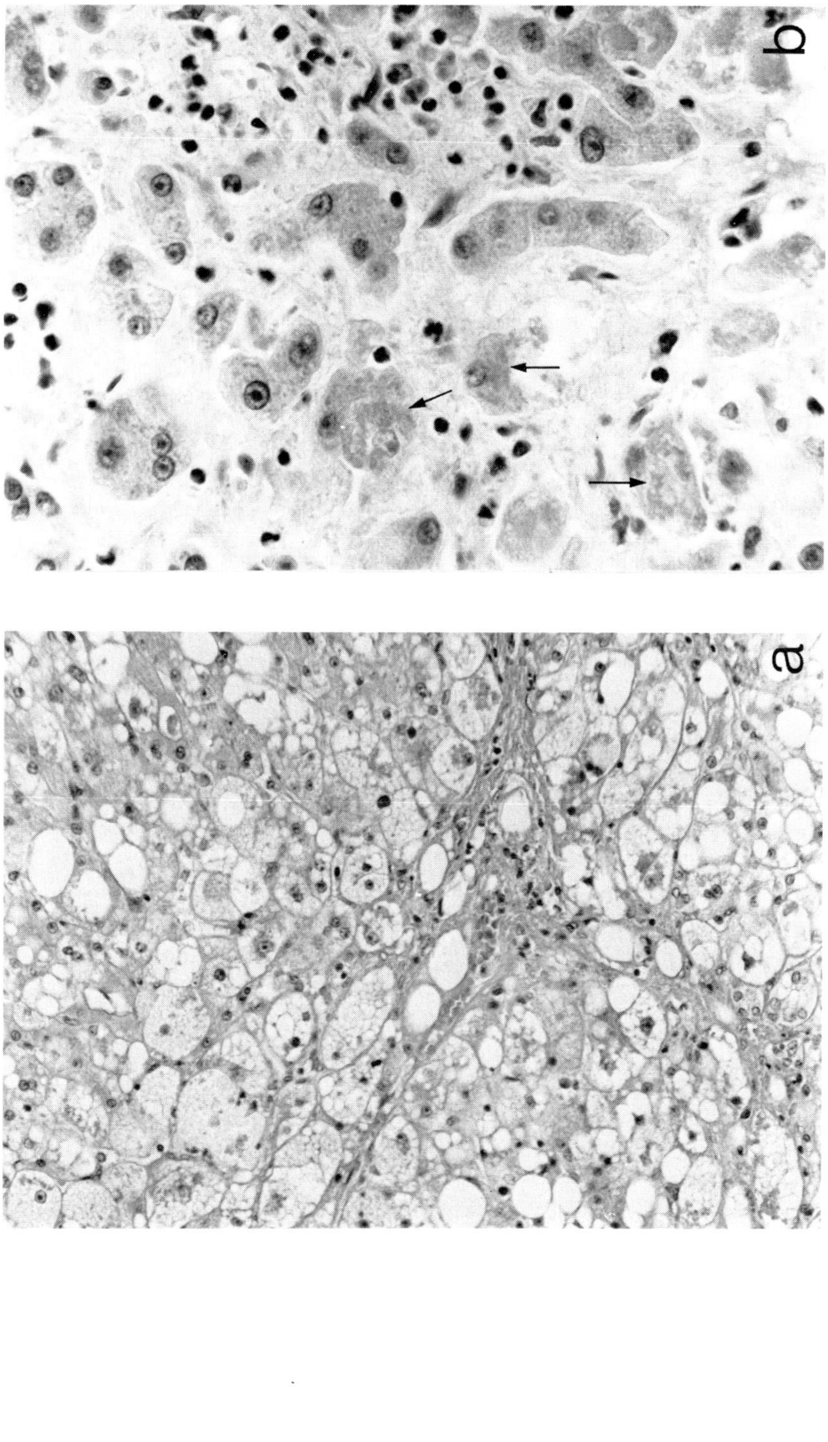

Fig. 6. Alcoholic liver disease: (a) Alcoholic fatty liver with healed alcoholic hepatitis. Many cells contain small and large droplets of intracytoplasmic fat. A thin fibrous scar radiates outward from the central vein in this photograph and is likely the sequel of previous acute alcoholic hepatitis. (b) Acute alcoholic hepatitis. Hepatocytes contain intracytoplasmic hyaline (Mallory bodies). The tissue is infiltrated by polymorphonuclear leukocytes (H + E x 525; original x 100).

et al. 1975a, b; Annable and Cooper 1974; Madsen 1969; Ehrenreich et al. 1973; Dzieniszewski et al. 1976; Prugh et al. 1976; Baroana et al. 1977). This failure of export from the cell leads to an increasing amount of intrahepatic lipid and protein. A similar effect has been noted with mice fed griseofulvin, another antimicrotubular agent, in which the cells become ballooned with the retained products and may contain alcoholic hyaline (French et al. 1977b; Denk et al. 1975, 1976). The hyaline-containing hepatocytes first appear in the centrolobular location (Denk et al. 1976) and they may progress to form Councilman bodies (Denk et al. 1976). These changes initially develop in the centrilobular area, which represents the most hypoxic zone of the liver. It is in this area that alcoholic hyaline appears first in man (Gerber and Popper 1972).

The above observations suggest that a direct toxic effect of ethanol, possibly mediated through its antimicrotubular effect, is important in initiating liver damage secondary to alcohol.

9.6.2. Humoral responses

9.6.2.1. Mallory bodies (alcoholic hyaline) and anti-Mallory-body antibodies

Mallory bodies, while not specific for alcohol-induced liver disease, are highly suggestive of the diagnosis and are felt to represent intrahepatic accumulations of alcoholic hyaline. The number of Mallory bodies found within hepatocytes may have some prognostic implications. The postoperative death rate was noted to be significantly higher if hyaline was found in more than 10% of hepatocytes in a needle biopsy obtained preoperatively in patients going for a portacaval anastomosis (Lang et al. 1978). Correlation was better with the Mallory body findings than with Child's classification. The same poor prognosis was observed in such patients who did not undergo surgery (Greenwood et al. 1972). If, as suggested above, Mallory-body filaments represent the accumulation of intermediate filaments secondary to damage to the microtubular system, do they themselves have importance in the development of alcohol-induced liver disease or, alternatively, are they simply markers of the disease process? The fact that they may be demonstrated following chronic administration of other antimicrotubular substances, such as griseofulvin and colchicine (Denk et al. 1975, 1976), and the fact that their production in tissue culture experiments within hepatocytes did not lead to cell death, suggest that they are not of primary importance. Antibodies to Mallory bodies and immune complexes have been noted in the serum and liver, respectively, of patients with alcoholic hepatitis (Kanagasundaram et al. 1977). It has been suggested that such complexes could account for the polymorphonuclear chemotaxis seen in such patients.

9.6.2.2. Other antibodies

Mallory antibodies appear to be absent in other forms of liver disease and may help in the differential diagnosis. Their importance in the pathogenesis of the disease remains uncertain. The fact that alcohol-induced liver disease appears to be more common in women, who have an increased propensity for autoimmune diseases, might suggest that immune mechanisms were more important in this subgroup. This gained support from the common finding of smooth muscle antibodies and antinuclear antibodies in women with alcohol-induced liver disease. In one series 45.4% of women with alcohol-induced liver disease, compared with 23.4% of men, had antibodies to smooth muscle. It was also noted that their mean serum IgG and IgM concentrations were higher (Krasner et al. 1977). Antibodies to liver membrane have been demonstrated in some, but not all patients with alcohol-induced liver disease. The prevalence of such antibodies appears to correlate to some extent with the severity of the histological lesion being more common in cirrhotics (MacSween et al. 1980a). HB antibodies were found in 34% of a group of 82 patients with biopsy-proven cirrhosis who were HBsAg-negative. The antibodies present were directed against core and for surface antigen, i.e. anti-HBc and anti-HBs. This suggests a higher incidence of prior infection with HB. Whether it is important in the pathogenesis of the disease, or only reflects an increased risk of alcohol-induced liver disease when ethanol is ingested by a patient with a previously damaged liver, is unclear (MacSween et al. 1980b).

9.6.3. Cell-mediated immunity

Lymphocyte-mediated cytotoxicity has been shown towards isolated hepatocytes in patients with alcoholic hepatitis (Cochrane et al. 1977). The cytotoxic effect was blocked by LSP and was present with T-cell depleted, but not B- or K-cell depleted sera. This suggests that an antibody-dependent cell-mediated response is involved (MacSween et al. 1980a). The prominent lymphocytic infiltration within the parenchyma of the liver in alcoholic hepatitis also supports the suggestion of a role for cell-mediated immunity in the pathogenesis of alcohol-induced liver disease, often with a similar picture to that seen in chronic active liver disease (Brunt et al. 1974). The lymphocytic infiltration is most frequent in the more advanced forms of disease and, in particular, in those patients with Mallory bodies (Christoffersen and Julh 1971). T lymphocytes have been shown to increase in alcoholic hepatitis in three studies (Husby et al. 1975; Sanchez-Tapias et al. 1977; French et al. 1977a), often associated with low peripheral blood levels. It has been suggested that the fall in the peripheral blood might be secondary to sequestration of T lymphocytes within the liver, perhaps resulting from antigen—antibody binding of the liver cells and lymphocyte plasma membranes. In-vitro cytotoxicity of the lymphocytes to hepatocytes has been demonstrated with blood from alcoholic hepatitis patients (Kakumu and Leevy 1977) and from baboons fed ethanol chronically (Paronetto and Lieber 1976). It has been suggested that chronic ethanol ingestion may lead to sensitization of lymphocytes to a liver cell antigen (Leevy et al. 1976; Sanchez-Tapias et al. 1977; Kanagasundaram et al. 1977; Zetterman et al. 1976) and such sensitization with resulting adherence of lymphocytes to hepatocytes leads to hepatocellular necrosis. This might be mediated either by activated T cells or antibody-associated K lymphocytes (Sanchez-Tapias et al. 1977). "T"-suppressor cells appear to be present in normal amounts in alcohol-induced liver disease (Routhier et al. 1980).

9.6.4. *Genetic factors*

The apparent susceptibility of women to the effects of alcohol suggests that genetic factors may be important. The results of studies of HLA typing have yielded conflicting data. HLA-B40 was noted to be increased in patients with alcoholic cirrhosis in one study (Bell and Nordhagen 1980), but not in two other studies (Seignalet et al. 1980; Gluud et al. 1980). HLA-B8 has been noted to be increased in patients with alcoholic liver disease (Bailey et al. 1976; Thomas et al. 1979), but not in other studies (Bell and Nordhagen 1978; Morris et al. 1977; Gluud et al. 1980).

9.7. PRIMARY BILIARY CIRRHOSIS

The diagnosis of primary biliary cirrhosis is based upon characteristic progressive histological features which have been well reviewed (Christensen et al. 1980; et al. 1978; Popper and Schaffner 1970). The resulting staging suggests a progressive assault directed at the intrahepatic biliary tree, resulting eventually in cirrhosis: Stage I, inflammatory destruction of intrahepatic bile ducts; Stage II, proliferation of ductules; Stage III, fibrosis, and Stage IV, cirrhosis. This staging has been criticized (Dickson et al. 1979), in that the staging based on liver biopsy does not always correlate well with the clinical stage of the disease, and an alternative staging has been proposed, namely: Stage I, portal stage (portal hepatitis); Stage II, periportal stage (periportal hepatitis); Stage III, septal stage (septal fibrosis or bridging necrosis or both); and Stage IV, cirrhosis (see Fig. 7).

The demonstration of a patent extrahepatic biliary tree is necessary for diagnosis, as similar histological features may develop following long-term biliary tract obstruction. The clinical pattern of primary biliary cirrhosis has been well documented (Sherlock and Scheuer 1974; Orlin et al. 1980). There is progressive cholestasis. More than 90% of the patients are female and show a positive anti-mitochondrial antibody, the titer rising with progression of the disease. Hypergammaglobulinemia is common, in particular elevation of immunoglobulin M.

Many of the features of primary biliary cirrhosis suggest that immunological mechanisms are important in the development and progression of the disease. The etiology remains unknown, but the early histological features and the development of antibodies directed against the inner membrane of mitochondria, progressing in titer in concert with the disease process, suggest that the bile duct is the prime target for attack.

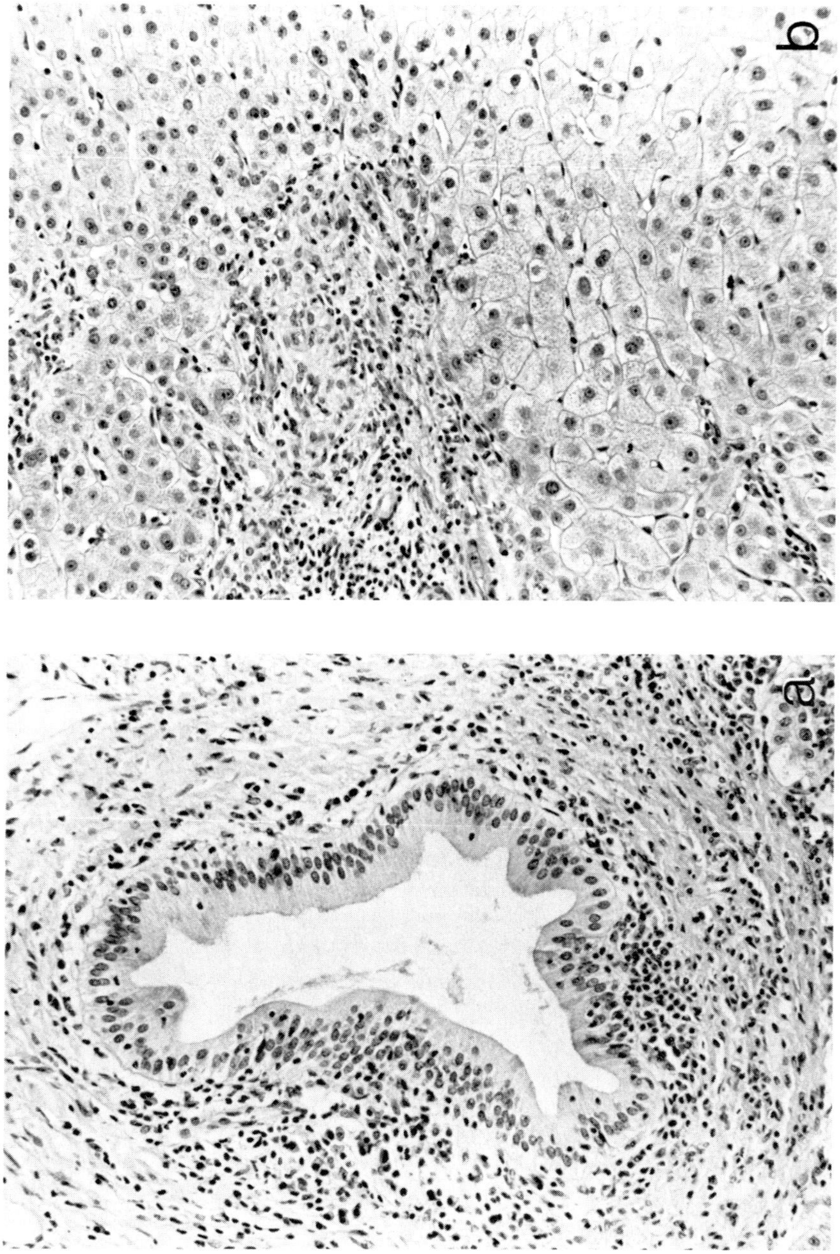

Fig. 7. Primary biliary cirrhosis: (a) First-stage lesion. A large bile duct is infiltrated by lymphocytes and plasma cells. The term "non-suppurative destructive cholangitis" is used to describe this lesion. (b) Second-stage lesion. There is piecemeal necrosis, resulting in an appearance similar to that of chronic active liver disease. (H + E x 525; original x 100).

9.7.1. *Humoral immune responses*

9.7.1.1. *Hypergammaglobulinemia*

Hypergammaglobulinemia is common in primary biliary cirrhosis, in particular elevations of immunoglobulin M. Hypergammaglobulinemia is common in all forms of chronic liver disease and two principal mechanisms have been postulated.

(1) It is a reflection of a humoral immune process directed specifically against the liver.

(2) It represents an epiphenomenon in which, as the Kupffer cell population declines or becomes impaired, more antigenic material becomes available to the reticuloendothelial system at large, resulting in increased antibody production. If the second postulate were correct one might expect a rise in immunoglobulin levels as patients reach the histological stage of cirrhosis. No such apparent change was discernible from the analysis of immunoglobulin levels in 236 patients with primary biliary cirrhosis (Christensen et al. 1980).

9.7.1.2. *Antimitochondrial antibody*

The antimitochondrial antibody is an antibody directed against the inner membrane of the mitochondria of all cells (Berg et al. 1969; Ben-Yoseph et al. 1974) which, though not specific for primary biliary cirrhosis, in high titer is highly suggestive of the diagnosis. This antibody may occasionally be present in chronic active liver disease (Berg et al. 1969), but usually in low titer. Two forms of antimitochondrial antibody have been demonstrated. The first, known as M2, is that normally occurring in primary biliary cirrhosis and consists of a trypsin-sensitive ATPase-associated antigen of the inner mitochondrial membrane. The second, known as M4, is an antibody directed against a trypsin-insensitive mitochondrial antigen which is possibly located on the outer mitochondrial membrane. This second antibody (M4) may represent a marker for a subgroup of chronic liver disease in showing features of chronic active liver disease (Berg et al. 1980). Though Type M2 antimitochondrial antibodies provide a useful marker for the disease, it is unlikely that they play a major role in its pathogenesis because: (1) Antimitochondrial antibodies occur in small numbers of apparently normal patients. (2) Antimitochondrial antibodies are present in low titer in conjunction with other forms of liver disease (chronic active hepatitis). (3) The antibody does not disappear with steroid therapy or following hepatic transplantation (Dickson et al. 1979).

9.7.1.3. *Anti-LSP*

Antibodies to human liver membrane lipoprotein have been described in some patients with primary biliary cirrhosis and a close correlation was noted between the percentage binding of ^{125}I-labeled LSP by serum and the extent of piecemeal necrosis of periportal hepatocytes on liver biospy (Tsantoulas et al. 1980). It was felt that the late appearance of antibodies to LSP made it unlikely that it was involved in the primary pathogenic process.

9.7.1.4. *Other antibody responses*

Primary biliary cirrhosis has commonly been linked with many other autoimmune diseases (Sherlock and Scheuer 1974; Bodenheimer and Schaffner 1979; Christensen et al. 1980; Fleming et al. 1978; Rai et al. 1977; Logan et al. 1978; Iliffe and Owen 1979; Hamlyn et al. 1980; Ahlqvist 1980; Akyol et al. 1980; Crowe et al. 1980). In conjunction with this, many other autoantibodies have been noted, including anti-smooth muscle antibody (Irvine, 1968), bile canalicular antibody (MacSween et al. 1973), renal tubular cell antibody (Chanarin et al. 1974), thyroid antibodies, antinuclear factor and antibodies to double-stranded DNA.

9.7.2. *Immune complexes*

Immune complexes can be demonstrated by the Raji cell radioimmunoassay in 60 to 95% of patients (Thomas et al. 1978; Gupta et al. 1978). Some correlation has been observed between elevations of immunoglobulin G and M and the severity of portal inflammation, but not with the pathological stage of the disease. The presence of immune complexes was greatest in those cases of PBC associated with other autoimmune disorders (Gupta et al. 1977).

Levels of serum complement have been variably affected in primary biliary cirrhosis. Lower levels of C3 have been found in association with circulating immune complexes (Gupta et al. 1977) and increased C3 catabolism has been noted (Potter et al. 1976), but increased catabolism did not correlate well with the histological stage of the disease. In a further study (Wands et al. 1978) the alternate complement pathway was implicated by the finding of cleavage products of factor B in 40% of the patients with PBC. In another study the importance of the classic pathway of complement in primary biliary cirrhosis was evidenced by the finding of marked increased catabolic rates of C1q in five patients with primary biliary cirrhosis (Potter et al. 1980).

9.7.3. *Cell-mediated immunity*

Alterations in cell-mediated immunity have also been implicated in the pathogenesis of primary biliary cirrhosis. The importance of cell-mediated immunity is supported by the frequent finding of granulomas within the portal areas. It has been suggested by Tsantoulas et al. that such granulomas usually contain activated T lymphocytes (Tsantoulas et al. 1980), and that these activated T lymphocytes in close contact with periportal liver cells and T cells would be able to exert their "helper" effect to stimulate anti-LSP production. This production is thought to be normally suppressed by T-suppressor cells (Allison et al. 1971), and a defect in suppressor-T-cell function has also been demonstrated in primary biliary cirrhosis (Zetterman and Woltjen 1980; Routhier et al. 1980).

TABLE 3.
Immune markers in chronic liver disease

IMMUNE MARKERS	PRIMARY BILIARY CIRRHOSIS	CHOLESTATIC C.A.L.D.	AUTO-IMMUNE C.A.L.D.	HBV-C.A.L.D.	DRUG RELATED— a) ALCOHOL	b) OTHERS
1) ANTI-L.S.P.	+ve.	+ve.	+ve.	+ve.	+ve.	e.g. DANTRILENE ISONIAZID
2) ANTI-LMA	—	+ve.	+ve.	—	—	NITROFURANTOIN METHYL DOPA OXYPHENISATIN
3) ANTI-MITOCHONDRIAL Ab						
a) M_2	+ve.	—	—	±	±	
b) M_4	+ve.	+ve.	±			
4) MALLORY BODY Ab	—	—	—	—	+	
5) NON-SPECIFIC GRP.						?
e.g. ANTI SMOOTH MUSCLE Ab A.N.F.	+ve.	+ve.	+ve.	+ve.	+ve.	ALL RECOVER IF DRUG DISCONTINUED
6) "T" CELL SUPPRESSOR DEFECT	—	+ve.	+ve.	—	—	

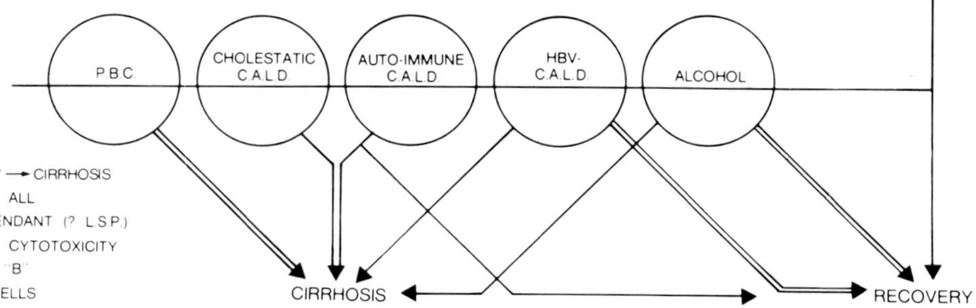

FINAL PATHWAY → CIRRHOSIS
? COMMON TO ALL
ANTIBODY DEPENDANT (? L.S.P.)
CELL MEDIATED CYTOTOXICITY
VIA SENSITIZED "B"
AND OR "NK" CELLS

The striking preponderance of women with primary biliary cirrhosis and the occasional reports of more than one case in a family suggest some genetic influence on the development of the disease. To date, however, no relationship has been found between primary biliary cirrhosis, histocompatibility antigens, ABO blood groups or rhesus blood groups (Galbraith et al. 1974; Hamlyn et al. 1974).

9.8. SUMMARY

In this article we have attempted to review the immune mechanisms operating in some commonly encountered liver diseases.

We have attempted to outline and see (Table 3) some of the more important pathways pertaining to the major subgroups of disease.

Infection of the hepatocyte by HBV is followed by proliferation of the virus and expression of viral antigens in the nucleus, cytoplasm, plasma membrane and in the serum. Expression of the viral neoantigens may be accompanied by expression of host neoantigens, LSP and LMA, and results in initiation of an immune response, without which hepatocellular injury is unlikely to occur. Humoral and cellular responses can be identified and both contribute to the immunopathology of HBV infections. There is substantial evidence that the production of antibody can be associated with the formation of immune complexes, resulting in significant extrahepatic disease, i.e. a serum sickness-like illness during the prodrome, glomerulonephritis, and arteritis. There is no strong evidence that fixation of antibody on the hepatocyte results in complement-mediated cytolysis of the hepatocyte but K-cell-mediated, antibody-dependent cytotoxicity against bound anti-LSP may contribute to the hepatocellular injury. There is strong, albeit largely indirect, information from experimental and clinical studies supporting the hypothesis that damage to hepatocytes is due, in large part, to a direct attack on infected hepatocytes by sensitized cytotoxic T cells.

Apart from HBV-related antigens, LSP is one of the best defined immunologic targets on the hepatocyte membrane. Both humoral and cellular immune responses can be demonstrated towards this antigen in many liver diseases, independent of their etiology. In experimental animals, a disease much like human chronic active hepatitis can be produced by immunization with LSP. Thus there is evidence that immune responses to LSP (and perhaps LMA) may be a final common mechanism of hepatocellular injury. It seems likely that other antigens, as yet undefined, could exist on the liver cell surface. It is not known how these antigens become expressed. Whether the expression of host antigens or even the immune responses to them are merely epiphenomena of disease, is likewise unclear.

Two markers, at present, seem to suggest that different immune mechanisms are important in the development of HB-associated chronic liver disease and autoimmune chronic active liver disease. In both, antibodies to liver-specific lipoprotein seem to be present and this liver-specific protein appears to be non-species-specific. Liver membrane autoantibodies, however, appear to be present only in the autoimmune variety of chronic active liver disease. Suppressor T-cell defects may contribute to the pathogenesis of both HBV-related and autoimmune-related chronic active liver disease.

It is likely that alcohol mediates its initial damage by a toxic effect on the microtubular system. The reasons for individual variation and, in particular, sex variation are not yet apparent, but genetic factors may be important. In the later stages of alcohol-induced liver disease its progression, despite withdrawal of alcohol, supports the hypothesis that the initiation of immunologic mechanisms contributes to its progression.

Though there is much indirect evidence to involve autoimmune processes in the development of primary biliary cirrhosis, the evidence is as yet circumstantial. This evidence includes the common findings of circulating immune complexes, antibodies directed against the inner core of mitochondria, abnormalities in immunoglobulin levels, activation of complement system, the association of other autoimmune diseases and other auto-antibodies, the presence of alterations in cell-mediated immunity and, in particular, granuloma formation. It remains to be seen which of these markers of disease are important in the pathogenesis of primary biliary cirrhosis. It may be that primary biliary cirrhosis has a multifactorial etiology, similar to chronic active liver disease, and that within different subgroups of the disease different autoimmune processes achieve varying importance.

Immunologic mechanisms contribute in a major way to the pathogenesis of several commonly encountered liver diseases. Precise delineation of these processes has not been achieved. One reason for this is that the antigenic targets or processes leading to their expression have not been defined. Another is that the effector mechanisms are likely to be multiple and interrelated. The elucidation of these pathways provides a great challenge and a better understanding will be essential for the development of rational therapies or preventive measures. One example of such success is the recent development of an effective vaccine for hepatitis B.

ACKNOWLEDGMENT

The authors gratefully acknowledge the secretarial assistance of Ms. Pat Elphick in preparing the manuscript.

REFERENCES

Aden, D.P., Fogel, A., Plotkin, S. et al. (1979) Controlled synthesis of HB_sAg in a differentiated human liver carcinoma derived cell line. *Nature (London) 282,* 615−616.

Ahlqvist, J. (1980) Primary biliary cirrhosis and graft-versus-host disease. *Lancet 2,* 207.

Aikawa, T., Sairenji, H., Furuta, S. et al. (1978) Seroconversion from hepatitis Be antigen to anti-HBe in acute hepatitis B virus infection. *N. Engl. J. Med. 298,* 439–441.

Akyol, S., Macklon, A., Griffiths, I. et al. (1980) Rheumatological and serological features of primary biliary cirrhosis. *Ann. Rheum. Dis. 39,* 186.

Alberti, A., Realdi, G., Tremolada, F. et al. (1976) Liver cell surface localization of hepatitis B antigen and of immunoglobulin in acute and chronic hepatitis and in liver cirrhosis. *Clin. Exp. Immunol. 25,* 396–402.

Alberti, A., Realdi, G., Bortolotti, F. et al. (1977) T-lymphocytes cytotoxicity to HB_sAg-coated target cells in hepatitis B virus infection. *Gut 18,* 1004–1009.

Albin, C. and Robinson, W.S. (1980) Protein kinase activity in hepatitis B virus. *J. Virol. 34,* 297–302.

Aldershvile, J., Dietrichson, O., Hardt, F. et al. (1977) Humoral and cell-mediated immunity to hepatitis B virus antigens in acute and chronic liver disease. *Scand. J. Gastroenterol. 12,* 917–922.

Aldershvile, J., Frosner, G.G., Neilsen, J.O. et al. (1980) Hepatitis Be antigen and antibody measured by radioimmunoassay in acute hepatitis B surface antigen-positive hepatitis. *J. Infect. Dis. 141,* 293–298.

Allison, A.C., Denman, A.M. and Barnes, R.D. (1971) Cooperating and controlling function of thymus derived lymphocytes in relation to autoimmunity. *Lancet 2,* 135–40.

Almeida, J.D. and Waterson, A.P. (1969) Immune complexes in hepatitis. *Lancet 2,* 983–986.

Almeida, J.D., Rubenstein, D. and Stott, E.J. (1971) New antigen-antibody system in Australia-antigen-positive hepatitis. *Lancet 2,* 1225–1228.

Alpert, E., Isselbacher, K.J. and Schur, P.H. (1971) The pathogenesis of arthritis associated with acute viral hepatitis. Complement-component studies. *N. Engl. J. Med. 285,* 185–189.

Alter, H.J., Seeff, L.B., Kaplan, P.M. et al. (1976) Type B hepatitis: the infectivity of blood positive for e antigen and DNA polymerase after accidental needlestick exposure. *N. Engl. J. Med. 295,* 909–913.

Annable, W. and Cooper, C. (1974) Inhibition of release of hepatitic triglyceride by ethanol-A reappraisal. *Biochem. Pharmacol. 23,* 2063–2068.

Anthony, P.P., Vogel, C.L. and Barker, L.F. (1973) Liver cell dysplasia: a premalignant condition. *J. Clin. Pathol. 26,* 217–223.

Arnold, W. and Meyer zum Buschenfelde, K.H. (1977) Immune complexes of HB_cAg/anti-HB_c in nuclei of HB_sAg-positive chronic liver disease. *N. Engl. J. Med. 296,* 818.

Arnold, W., Neilson, J.O., Hardt, F. et al. (1977) Localization of e-antigen in nuclei of hepatocytes in HB_sAg-positive liver diseases. *Gut 19,* 994–996.

Arnold, W., Hess, G., Purcell, RH. et al. (1978) Anti-HB_c, HB_eAg and DNA polymerase activity in healthy HB_sAg carriers and patients with inflammatory liver disease. *Klin. Wochenschr. 56,* 297–303.

Baer, G.M. Walker, J.A. and Yager, P.A. (1977) Studies of an outbreak of acute hepatitis A. I. Complement level fluctuation. *J. Med. Virol. 1,* 1–7.

Bailey, R.J., Krasner, N., Eddleston, A.L.W.F. et al. (1976) Histocompatibility antigens, autoantibodies and immunoglobulins in alcoholic liver disease. *Br. Med. J. 2,* 727–729.

Barker, L.F. and Murray, R. (1971) Acquisition of hepatitis-associated antigen. Clinical features in young adults. *J. Am. Med. Assoc. 216,* 1970–1976.

Baroana, E., Leo, M.A., Borowsky, S.A. et al. (1975) Alcoholic hepatomegaly: accumulation of protein in the liver. *Science 190,* 794−795.

Baroana, E., Leo, M.A., Borowsky, S.A. et al. (1977) Pathogenesis of alcohol-induced accumulation of protein in the liver. *J. Clin. Invest. 60,* 546−554.

Batai, G., Anbrus, M., Paal, H. et al. (1975) Hepatitis-B antigenemia associated with progressive cirrhosis and membranous glomerulonephritis. *Lancet 1,* 102−103.

Bayer, M.E., Blumberg, B.S. and Werner, B. (1968) Particles associated with Australia antigen in sera of patients with leukaemia, Down's syndrome and hepatitis. *Nature (London) 218,* 1057−1059.

Behrens, U.J. and Paronetto, F. (1979) Studies on "Liver specific" antigens. I. Evaluation of the liver specificity of "LSP" and "LP-2". *Gastroenterology 77,* 1045−1052.

Behrens, U.J., Vernace, S. and Paronetto, F. (1979) Studies on "Liver-specific" antigens. II. Detection of serum antibodies to liver and kidney cell membrane antigens in patients with chronic liver disease. *Gastroenterology 77,* 1053−1061.

Bell, H. and Nordhagen, R. (1978) Association between HLA-BW40 and alcoholic liver disease with cirrhosis. *Br. Med. J. 1,* 822.

Bell, H. and Nordhagen, R. (1980) ALA antigens in alcoholics, with special reference to alcoholic cirrhosis. *Scand. J. Gastroenterol. 15,* 453−456.

Ben-Yoseph, Y., Shapira, E. and Doniach, D. (1974) Further purification of the mitochondrial inner membrane autoantigen reacting with primary biliary cirrhosis sera. *Immunology 26,* 311−321.

Berg, P.A., Muscatello, U., Horne, R.W., Roitt, I.M. et al. (1969) Mitochondrial antibodies in primary biliary cirrhosis. II. The complement fixing antigen as a component of mitochondrial inner membranes. *Br. J. Exp. Pathol. 50,* 200−208.

Berg, P.A., Sayers, T., Wiedmann, K.H. et al. (1980) Serological classification of chronic cholestatic liver disease by the use of two different types of antimitochondrial antibodies. *Lancet 2,* 1329−1332.

Bianchi, L. and Gudat, F. (1976) Sanded nuclei in hepatitis B. *Lab. Invest. 35,* 1−5.

Bianchi, L. and Gudat, F. (1979) Immunopathology of hepatitis B. *Prog. Liver Dis. 6,* 371−391.

Black, M., Rabin, L. and Schatz, N. (1980) Nitrofurantoin-induced chronic active hepatitis. *Ann. Intern. Med. 92,* 62−64.

Blanchy, B., Hantz, O., Vitvitski, L. et al. (1980) Two low molecular weight peptides as common determinants to different molecular forms and specificities of hepatitis B_e antigen (HB_eAg). *J. Med. Virol. 5,* 39−46.

Blumberg, B.S. (1964) Polymorphisms of the serum proteins and the development of iso-precipitins in transfused patients. *Bull. N.Y. Acad. Med. 40,* 377−86.

Bodenheimer, H. and Schaffner, F. (1979) State of the Art. Primary biliary cirrhosis and the immune system. *Am. J. Gastroenterol. 72,* 285−296.

Bradley, D.W., Maynard, J.E., Hindman, S.H. et al. (1977) Serodiagnosis of viral hepatitis A: detection of acute phase immunoglobulin M anti-hepatitis A virus by radioimmunoassay. *J. Clin. Microbiol. 5,* 521−530.

Brechot, C., Pourcel, C., Louise, A. et al. (1980) Presence of integrated hepatitis B virus DNA sequences in cellular DNA of human hepatocellular carcinoma. *Nature (London) 286,* 533−535.

Brunt, P.W., Kew, M.C., Scheuer, P.J. et al. (1974) Studies in alcoholic liver disease in Britain. I. Clinical and pathological patterns related to natural history. *Gut 15,* 52–58.

Brzosko, W.J., Krawczynski, K., Nazarewicz, T. et al. (1974) Glomerulonephritis associated with hepatitis B surface antigen immune complexes in children. *Lancet 2,* 477–481.

Burrell, C.J., MacKay, P., Greenaway, P.J. et al. (1979) Expression in E. coli of hepatitis B virus DNA sequences cloned in plasmid pBR322. *Nature (London) 279,* 43–47.

Campion, E.C., Ludbrook, J., McLeod, G.M. et al. (1972) Primary hepatoma and hepatitis-associated antigen in a young white woman. *Br. Med. J. 4,* 149–152.

Canese, M.G., Rizzetto, M., Arico, S. et al. (1979) An ultrastructural and immunohistochemical study on the δ antigen associated with the hepatitis B virus. *J. Pathol. 128,* 169–176.

Chakraborty, P.R., Ruiz-Opazo, N., Shouval, D. et al. (1980) Identification of integrated hepatitis B virus DNA and expression of viral RNA in an HB_sAg-producing human hepatocellular carcinoma cell line. *Nature (London) 286,* 531–533.

Chanarin, I., Loewi, G., Tavill, A.S. et al. (1974) Defect of renal tubular acidification with antibody to loop of Henle. *Lancet 2,* 317–318.

Charnay, P., Gervais, M., Louise, A. et al. (1980) Biosynthesis of hepatitis B virus surface antigen in Escherichia coli. *Nature (London) 286,* 893–895.

Chisari, F.V. (1980) Liver-specific protein in perspective. *Gastroenterology 78,* 168–170.

Chisari, F.V., Routenberg, J.A., Fiala, M. et al. (1977) Extrinsic modulation of human T-lymphocyte E rosette function associated with prolonged hepatocellular injury after viral hepatitis. *J. Clin. Invest. 59,* 134–142.

Chisari, F.V., Castle, K.L., Xavier, C. et al. (1981a) Functional properties of lymphocyte subpopulations in hepatitis B virus infection. I. Suppressor cell control of T-lymphocyte responsiveness. *J. Immunol. 126,* 38–44.

Chisari, F.V., Bieber, M.S., Josepho, C.A. et al. (1981b) Functional properties of lymphocyte subpopulations in hepatitis B virus infection. II. Cytotoxic effector cell killing of targets that naturally express hepatitis B surface antigen and liver-specific lipoprotein. *J. Immunol. 126,* 45–49.

Christensen, E., Crowe, J., Doniach, D. et al. (1980) Clinical pattern and course of disease in primary biliary cirrhosis based on an analysis of 236 patients. *Gastroenterology 78,* 236–246.

Christoffersen, P. and Julh, E. (1971) Mallory bodies in liver biopsies with fatty changes but no cirrhosis. *Acta Pathol. Microbiol. Scand., Sect. A, 79,* 201–207.

Cochrane, A.M.G., Moussouros, A. and Thomson, A.D. (1976) Antibody-dependent, cell-mediated (K-cell) cytotoxicity against isolated rabbit hepatocytes in chronic active hepatitis. *Lancet 1,* 441–444.

Cochrane, A.M.G., Moussouros, A., Portmann, B. et al. (1977) Lymphocyte toxicity for isolated hepatocytes in alcoholic liver disease. *Gastroenterology 72,* 918–923.

Combes, B., Stasny, P., Shorey, J. et al. (1971) Glomerulonephritis with deposits of Australia antigen-antibody complexes in glomerular membrane. *Lancet 2,* 234–237.

Coulepis, A.G., Locarnini, S.A., Ferris, A.A. et al. (1978) The polypeptides of hepatitis A virus. *Intervirology 10,* 24–31.

Crowe, J., Christensen, E., Butler, J. et al. (1980) Primary biliary cirrhosis: the prevalence of hypothyroidism and its relationship to thyroid autoantibodies and sicca syndrome. *Gastroenterology 78,* 1437–1441.

Dane, D.S., Cameron, C.H. and Briggs, M. (1970) Virus-like particles in serum of patients with Australia-antigen-associated hepatitis. *Lancet 1,* 695–698.

DeCree, J., Verhaegen, H., De Cock, W. et al. (1974) The effect of levamisole on the immunologic response of HBAg positive patients. *Digestion 10,* 306.

DeFranchis, R., D'Arminio, A., Vecchi, M. et al. (1980) Chronic asymptomatic HB_sAg carriers: histological abnormalities and diagnostic and prognostic value of serologic markers of the HBV. *Gastroenterology 79,* 521–527.

Deinhardt, F. (1980) Medical perspective: predictive value of markers of hepatitis virus infection. *J. Infect. Dis. 141,* 299–305.

DeKretser, T.A., McFarlane, I.G., Eddleston, A.L.W.F. et al. (1980) A species-non-specific liver plasma-membrane antigen and its involvement in chronic active hepatitis. *Biochem. J. 186,* 679–685.

DeMoura, M.C., Vernace, S.J. and Paronetto, F. (1975) Cell-mediated immune reactivity to hepatitis B-surface antigen in liver disease. *Gastroenterology 69,* 310–317.

Denk, H. and Eckerstorfer, R. (1977) Colchicine-induced Mallory body formation in the mouse. *Lab. Invest. 36,* 563–565.

Denk, H., Gschnait, F. and Wolff, K. (1975) Hepatocellular hyaline (Mallory bodies) in longterm griseofulvin-treated mice: a new experimental model for the study of hyaline formation. *Lab. Invest. 32,* 773–776.

Denk, H., Eckerstorfer, R., Gschnait, F. et al. (1976) Experimental induction of hepatocellular hyaline (Mallory bodies) in mice with griseofulvin treatment. *Lab. Invest. 35,* 377–382.

Dickson, E.R., Fleming, C.R. and Ludwig, J. (1979) Primary biliary cirrhosis. *Prog. Liver Dis. 6,* 487–499.

Dienstag, J. (1980) Viral hepatitis type A: virology and course. *Clin. Gastroenterol. 9,* 135–154.

Dienstag, J.L., and Bhan, A.R. (1980) Enhanced in vitro cell-mediated cytotoxicity in chronic hepatitis B virus infection: absence of specificity for virus-expressed antigen on target cell membranes. *J. Immunol. 125,* 2269–2276.

Dienstag, J.L., Popper, H. and Purcell, R.H. (1976a) The pathology of viral hepatitis types A and B in chimpanzees: a comparison. *Am. J. Pathol. 85,* 131–148.

Dienstag, J.L., Schulman, A.N., Gerety, R.J. et al. (1976b) Hepatitis A antigen isolated from liver and stool: immunologic comparison of antisera prepared in guinea pigs. *J. Immunol. 117,* 876–881.

Dienstag, J.L., Rhodes, A.R., Bhan, A.K. et al. (1978) Urticaria associated with acute viral hepatitis type B. *Ann. Intern. Med. 89,* 34–40.

Drouet, J. Courouce-Pauty, A.M., Thevenaux, A.M. et al. (1975) Kinetics of HB_s antigen in man. *Biomedicine 22,* 158–166.

Dudley, F.J., Giustino, V. and Sherlock, S. (1972) Cell-mediated immunity in patients positive for hepatitis-associated antigen. *Br. Med. J. 4,* 754–756.

Dzieniszewski, J., Tiscornia, O.M., Palasciano, G. et al. (1976) The effects of acute and chronic ethanol administration on canine bile secretion. *Dig. Dis. 21,* 1037–1043.

Edman, J.C., Gray, P., Valenzuela, P. et al. (1980) Integration of hepatitis B virus sequences and their expression in a human hepatoma cell. *Nature (London) 286,* 535–538.

Ehrenreich, J.H., Bergeron, J.M., Siekevitz, P. et al. (1973) Golgi fractions prepared from rat liver. I. Isolation procedure and morphological characterization. *J. Cell Biol. 59,* 45–72.

El Sheikh, N., Osman, C.G., Cullens, H. et al. (1978) T-lymphocyte-mediated cytotoxicity in HB_sAg-positive liver disease. *Clin. Exp. Immunol. 31,*150–157.

Englert, E., Wales, E.E. and Straight, R.C. (1970) The proteins of human gallbladder bile with and without gallstones. *Clin. Chim. Acta 29,* 319–331.

Espinosa, E. (1976) Circulating tissue antigens. III. Identification and characterization of antigens of limited and of wide body distribution in human gallbladder bile. Presence in serum of patients with hepatitis. *Clin. Exp. Immunol. 25,* 410–417.

Feinstone, S.M., Kapikian, A.Z. and Purcell, R.H. (1973) Hepatitis A: detection by immune electronmicroscopy of a virus-like antigen associated with acute illness. *Science 182,* 1026–1028.

Feldman, G., Maurice, M., Sapin, C. et al. (1975) Inhibition by colchicine of fibrinogen translocation in hepatocytes. *J. Cell Biol. 67,* 237–243.

Fennel, R.H. (1965) Chronic liver disease induced in rats by repeated anaphylactic shock. *Am. J. Pathol. 47,* 173–182.

Fernandez-Cruz, E., Escartin, P., Bootello, A. et al. (1978) Hepatocyte damage induced by lymphocytes from patients with chronic liver disease, as detected by LDH release. *Clin. Exp. Immunol. 31,* 436–442.

Fleming, C.R., Ludwig, J. and Dickson, E.R. (1978) Asymptomatic primary biliary cirrhosis. Presentation, histology, and results with D-penicillamine. *Mayo Clin. Proc. 53,* 587–593.

Fogarty International Center Proceedings No. 22 (1976) *Nomenclature, Diagnostic Criteria and Diagnostic Methodology for Diseases of the Liver and Biliary Tract,* p. 9. U.S. Government Printing Office, Washington, DC.

French, S.W. and Davies, P.L. (1975) The Mallory body in the pathogenesis of alcoholic liver disease. In: J.M. Khanna, Y. Israels and H. Kalani (Eds), *Alcoholic Liver Pathology,* Addiction Research Foundation of Ontario, Toronto, pp. 113–170.

French, S.W., Burbige, E., Luehrs, D. et al. (1977a) Percent T and B cells in the liver in alcoholic hepatitis. *Am. J. Pathol. 86* 20a (Abstr.).

French, S.W., Sim, J.S., Frank, K.E. et al. (1977b) Alcoholic hepatitis. In: M.M. Fisher and J.G. Rankin (Eds), *Alcohol and the Liver,* Plenum Press, New York, pp. 349–361.

Frosner, G.G., Overby, L.R., Flehmig, B. et al. (1977) Seroepidemiological investigation of patients and family contacts in an epidemic of hepatitis A. *J. Med. Virol. 1,* 163–173.

Frosner, G.G., Brodersen, M., Papaevangelou, G. et al. (1978) Detection of HB_eAg and anti-HBe in acute hepatitis B by a sensitive radioimmunoassay. *J. Med. Virol. 3,* 67–76.

Furuta, S. Kiyosawa, K. and Nagata, A. (1975) HB_sAg on cell membrane in symptoms-free carrier. *Lancet 2,* 227.

Fye, K., Becker, M.J., Theofilopoulos, A.N. et al. (1977) Immune complexes in hepatitis B antigen-associated periarteritis nodosa. *Am. J. Med. 62,* 783–791.

Galambos, F.T. (1974) Alcoholic hepatitis. In: F. Schnaffner, S. Sherlock and C.M. Leevy (Eds), *The Liver and its Diseases,* Intercontinental Medical Book Corp., New York, pp. 225–267.

Galbraith, R.M., Eddleston, A.L.W.F., Smith, M.G.M. et al. (1974) Histocompatibility antigens in active chronic hepatitis and primary biliary cirrhosis. *Br. Med. J. 3,* 604–605.

Galbraith, R.M., Eddleston, A.L.W.F., Williams, R. et al. (1975) Fulminant hepatic failure in leukaemia and choriocarcinoma related to withdrawal of cytotoxic drug therapy. *Lancet 2,* 528–530.

Galibert, F., Mandart, E., Fitoussi, F. et al. (1979) Nucleotide sequences of the hepatitis B virus genome (subtype AYW) cloned in E. coli. *Nature (London) 281,* 646–650.

Gerber, M.A. and Popper, H. (1972) Relation between central canals and portal tracts in alcoholic hepatitis. *Hum. Pathol. 3,* 199–207.

Gerber, M.A. and Thung S.N. (1979) The localization of hepatitis viruses in tissues. *Int. Rev. Exp. Pathol. 20,* 49–71.

Gerber, M.A., Brodin, A., Steinberg, D. et al. (1972) Periarteritis nodosa, Australia antigen and lymphatic leukemia. *N. Engl. J. Med. 286,* 14–17.

Gerber, M.A., Hadziyannis, S., Vissoulis, C. et al. (1974) Electron microscopy and immunoelectron microscopy of cytoplasmic hepatitis B antigen in hepatocytes. *Am. J. Pathol. 75,* 489–502.

Gerber, M.A., Sarno, E. and Vernace, S.J. (1976) Immune complexes in hepatocytic nuclei of HB Ag-positive chronic hepatitis. *N. Engl. J. Med. 294,* 922–925.

Gerber, M.A., Lebwohl, N., Thung, S.N. et al. (1979) Antibodies to liver-specific membrane protein in liver and kidney disease. *Gastroenterology 76,* 1281.

Gerlich, W.H., Luer, W., Thomssen, R. et al. (1980) Diagnosis of acute and inapparent hepatitis B virus infections by measurement of IgM antibody to hepatitis B core antigen. *J. Infect. Dis. 142,* 95–101.

Geubel, A.P., Keller, R.H., Summerskill, W.H.J. et al. (1976) Lymphocyte cytotoxicity and inhibition studies with autologous liver cells: observations in chronic active liver disease and the primary biliary cirrhosis syndrome. *Gastroenterology 71,* 450–456.

Gianotti F. (1978) Papular acrodermatitis of childhood. *Arch. Dis. Child. 48,* 794–799.

Gluud, C., Aldershvile, J., Dietrichson, O. et al. (1980) Human leucocyte antigens in patients with alcoholic liver cirrhosis. *Scand. J. Gastroenterol. 15,* 337–341.

Gocke, D.J., Hsu, K. and Morgan, C. (1970) Association between polyarteritis and Australia antigen. *Lancet 2,* 1149–1153.

Golding, P.L., Smith, M., Williams, R. (1973) Multisystem involvement in chronic liver disease. Studies on the incidence and pathogenesis. *Am. J. Med. 55,* 772–782.

Gower, R., Sausker, W.F., Kohler, P.F. et al. (1973) Small vessel vasculitis caused by hepatitis B virus immune complexes. *J. Allergy Clin. Immunol. 62,* 222–228.

Greenwood, S.M., Leffler, C.T. and Minkowitz, S. (1972) The increased mortality rate of open liver biopsy in alcoholic hepatitis. *Surg. Gynecol. Obstet. 134,* 600–604.

Gudat, F. and Bianchi, L. (1977) HB_sAg: a target antigen on the liver cell? In: H. Popper, L. Bianchi and W. Reutter (Eds), *Membrane Alterations as Basis of Liver Injury,* MTP Press, Lancaster, pp. 171–178.

Gudat, F., Bianchi, L., Sonnabend, W. et al. (1975) Pattern of core and surface expression in liver tissue reflects state of specific immune response in hepatitis B. *Lab. Invest. 32,* 1–9.

Gupta, R.C., Dickson, E.R. and McDuffie, F.C. (1977) Circulating immune complexes and autoimmune features in primary biliary cirrhosis: implications for pathogenesis (Abstract). *Gastroenterology 73,* 1223.

Gupta, R.C., Dickson, E.R., McDuffie, F.C. et al. (1978) Circulating IgG complexes in primary biliary cirrhosis. A serial study in forty patients followed for two years. *Clin. Exp. Immunol. 34,* 19–27.

Gyorkey, F., Hollinger, F.B., Eknoyan, G. et al. (1975) Immune complex glomerulonephritis, intranuclear particles in hepatocytes, and in vivo clearance rates in subhuman primates inoculated with HB_SAg-containing plasma. *Exp. Mol. Pathol. 22,* 350–365.

Hadziyannis, S.J. (1980) Hepatocellular carcinoma and type B hepatitis. *Clin. Gastroenterol. 9,* 117–134.

Hadziyannis, S., Vissoulis, C., Moussouros, A. et al. (1972) Cytoplasmic localisation of Australia antigen in the liver. *Lancet 1,* 976–979.

Hadziyannis, S., Gerber, M.A., Vissoulis, C. et al. (1973) Cytoplasmic hepatitis B antigen in "ground glass" hepatocytes of carriers. *Arch. Pathol. 96,* 327–330.

Hadziyannis, S., Giustozi, A., Moussouros, A. et al. (1976) Hepatitis B core and surface antigen in the liver in primary liver cell carcinoma. In: C.M. Leevy (Ed.), *Diseases of the Liver and Biliary Tract,* S. Karger, Basel, pp. 174–178.

Hamlyn, A.N., Morris, J.S. and Sherlock, S. (1974) ABO blood groups, rhesus negativity, and primary biliary cirrhosis. *Gut 15,* 480–481.

Hamlyn, A., Adams, D. and Sherlock, S. (1980) Primary or secondary sicca complex? Investigation in primary biliary cirrhosis by histocompatibility testing. *Br. Med. J. 2,* 425.

Hansson, B.C. (1976) Age and sex-related distribution of antibodies to hepatitis B surface and core antigens in a Swedish population. *Acta Pathol. Microbiol. Scand., Sect. B, 84,* 342–346.

Hantz, O., Vitvitski, L. and Trepo, C. (1980) Non-A,non-B hepatitis: identification of hepatitis-B-like virus particles in serum and liver. *J. Med. Virol. 5,* 73–86.

Hardison, W.G. and Lee, F.I. (1966) Prognosis in acute liver disease of the alcoholic patient. *N. Engl. J. Med. 275,* 61–65.

Hess, G., Neilsen, O., Arnold, W. et al. (1977) E-system and intrahepatocellular HB_CAg and HB_SAg in HB_SAg positive patients with liver diseases and healthy carriers. *Scand. J. Gastroenterol. 12,* 325–330.

Hirschman, S.Z. (1975) Integrator enzyme hypothesis for replication of hepatitis-B virus. *Lancet 2,* 436–438.

Hirschman, S.Z., Gerber, M. and Garfinkel, E. (1974) DNA purified from naked intranuclear particles of human liver infected with hepatitis B virus. *Nature (London) 251,* 540–542.

Hoofnagle, J.H., Gerety, R.J. and Barker, L.F. (1975) Antibody to the hepatitis B core antigen. *Am. J. Med. Sci. 270,* 179–187.

Hoofnagle, J.H., Seeff, L.B., Bales, Z.B. et al. (1978) Type B hepatitis after transfusion with blood containing antibody to hepatitis B core antigen. *N. Engl. J. Med. 298,* 1379–1383.

Hopf, U., Meyer zum Buschenfelde, K.H. and Arnold, W. (1976) Detection of a liver membrane autoantibody in HB_SAg-negative chronic active hepatitis. *N. Engl. J. Med. 294,* 578–582.

Hopf, U., Schaefer, H.E., Hess, G. et al. (1981) In vivo uptake of immune complexes by parenchymal and non-parenchymal liver cells in mice. *Gastroenterology 80,* 250–259.

Huang, S. (1971) Hepatitis-associated antigen hepatitis: an electron microscopic study of virus-like particles in liver cells. *Am. J. Pathol. 64,* 483–500.

Huang, S.M. (1975) Immunohistochemical demonstration of hepatitis B core and surface antigens in paraffin section. *Lab. Invest. 33,* 88–95.

Huang, S.N. and Neurath, A.R. (1979) Immunohistologic demonstration of hepatitis B viral antigens in liver with reference to its significance in liver injury. *Lab. Invest. 40,* 1–17.

Husby, H., Strickland, R.G., Caldwell, J.L. et al. (1975) Localization of T and B cells and alpha fetoprotein in hepatic biopsies from patients with liver disease. *J. Clin. Invest. 56,* 1198–1209.

Hutteroth, T.H. and Meyer zum Buschenfelde, K.H. (1978a) Antigenic relationship between Chang liver cells and human hepatocytes. *Klin. Wochenschr. 56,* 525–527.

Hutteroth, T.H. and Meyer zum Buschenfelde, K.H. (1978b) Clinical relevance of the liver-specific lipoprotein (LSP). *Acta Hepato-Gastroenterol. 25,* 243–253.

Iliffe, G. and Owen, D. (1979) An association between primary biliary cirrhosis and jejunal villous atrophy resembling coeliac disease. *Dig. Dis. Sci. 24,* 802–806.

Imai, M., Yanase, Y., Nojiri, T. et al. (1979) A receptor for polymerized human and chimpanzee albumins on hepatitis B virus particles co-occurring with HB_eAg. *Gastroenterology 76,* 242–247.

Irvine, W.J. (1968) Auto-immune and hypersensitivity phenomena in alimentary diseases. In: S.C. Dyke (Ed.), *Recent Advances in Clinical Pathology, Series V,* Churchill, Edinburgh, pp. 497–519.

Irwin Jr, G.R., Hierholzer Jr, W.J., Cimis, R. et al. (1974) Delayed hypersensitivity in hepatitis B: clinical correlates of in vitro production of migration inhibition factor. *J. Infect. Dis. 130,* 580–587.

Ito, K., Nakagawa, J., Okimoto, Y. et al. (1972) Chronic hepatitis, migration inhibition of leucocytes in presence of Australia antigen. *N. Engl. J. Med. 286,* 1005.

Ito, H., Hattori, S., Matusda, I. et al. (1981) Hepatitis Be antigen-mediated membranous glomerulonephritis: correlation of ultrastructural changes with HB_eAg in the serum and glomeruli. *Lab. Invest. 44,* 214–220.

Jackson, D., Tabor, E. and Gerety, R.J. (1979) Acute non-A,non-B hepatitis: specific ultrastructural alterations in endoplasmic reticulum of infected hepatocytes. *Lancet 1,* 1249–1250.

Jacques, E.A., de Villiers, D., Crimmins, F. et al. (1976) Effect of prednisone and azathioprine on K-cell cytotoxicity in chronic active hepatitis. *Gastroenterology 71,* 913.

Jain, S., Thomas, H.C. and Sherlock, S. (1977) Transfer factor in the attempted treatment of patients with HB_sAg-positive chronic liver disease. *Clin. Exp. Immunol. 30,* 10–15.

Jensen, D.M., McFarlane, I.G., Portmann, B. et al. (1978) Detection of antibodies directed against a liver-specific membrane lipoprotein in patients with acute and chronic active hepatitis. *N. Engl. J. Med. 299,* 1–7.

Kakumu, S. and Leevy, C.M. (1977) Lymphocyte cytotoxicity in alcoholic hepatitis. *Gastroenterology 72,* 594–597.

Kakumu, S., Arakawa, Y., Goji, H. et al. (1979) Occurrence and significance of antibody to liver-specific membrane lipoprotein by double-antibody immunoprecipitation method in sera of patients with acute and chronic liver disease. *Gastroenterology 76,* 665–672.

Kakumu, S., Hotta, R., Kashio, T. et al. (1980) Circulating immune complexes against suppressor T cells in chronic active liver disease. *Gastroenterology 79,* 1111.

Kaplan, P.M., Greenman, R.L., Gerin, J.L. et al. (1973) DNA polymerase associated with human hepatitis B antigen. *J. Virol. 12,* 995–1005.

Kanagasundaram, N., Kakumu, S., Chen, T. and Leevy,C.M. (1977) Alcoholic hyaline, antigen (AHAg) and antibody (AHAb) in alcoholic hepatitis. *Gastroenterology 73,* 1368–1373.

Karasawa, T. and Shikata, T. (1977) Necrosis of the hepatocytes with hepatitis B surface antigen. *Arch. Pathol. 101,* 280–285.

Kim, C.Y. and Bissel, D.M. (1971) Stability of the lipid and protein of hepatitis-associated (Australia) antigen. *J. Infect. Dis. 123,* 470–476.

Kleinknecht, C., Levy, M., Peix, A. et al. (1979) Membranous glomerulonephritis and hepatitis B surface antigen in children. *J. Pediatr. 95,* 946–952.

Knieser, M.R., Jenis, E.H., Lowenthal, D.T. et al. (1974) Pathogenesis of renal disease associated with viral hepatitis. *Arch. Pathol. 97,* 193–200.

Kohler, P.F., Cronin, R.E., Hammond, W.S. et al. (1974a) Chronic membranous glomerulonephritis caused by hepatitis B antigen-antibody immune complexes. *Ann. Intern. Med. 81,* 448–453.

Kohler, P.F., Trembath, J., Merrill, D.A. et al. (1974b) Immunotherapy with antibody, lymphocytes and transfer factor in chronic hepatitis B. *Clin. Immunol. Immunopathol. 2,* 465–471.

Koretz, R.L., Suffin, S.G. and Gitnick, G.L. (1976) Post-transfusion chronic liver disease. *Gastroenterology 1,* 797–803.

Krasner, N., Davis, M., Portmann, B. et al. (1977) Changing pattern of alcoholic liver disease in Great Britain: relation to sex and signs of autoimmunity. *Br. Med J. 1,* 1497–1500.

Krugman, S., Giles, J.P. and Hammond, J. (1971) Viral hepatitis type B (MS-2 strain) studies on active immunization. *J. Am. Med. Assoc. 217,* 41–45.

Labro, M.T., Andrieu, M.C., Weber, M. et al. (1978) A new pattern of non-organ and non-species-specific anti-organelle antibody detected by immunofluorescence: the mitochondrial antibody number 5. *Clin. Exp. Immunol. 31,* 357–366.

Lam, K.C., Tong, M.J. and Rakela, J. (1977) Release of e antigen from a Dane particle-rich preparation of hepatitis B virus. *Infect. Immun. 16,* 403–404.

Lang, A.P., Patel, S., Langer, B. et al. (1978) Preoperative liver biopsy and the prognosis of portosystemic shunt surgery (Abstract). *Lab. Invest. 38,* 353.

Lawley, T.J., James, S.P. and Jones, E.A. (1980) Circulating immune complexes: Their detection and potential significance in some hepatobiliary and intestinal diseases. *Gastroenterology 78,* 626–641.

LeBouvier, G.L. and Williams, A. (1975) Serotypes of hepatitis B antigen (HB_SAg): the problem of "new" determinants, as exemplified by "t". *Am. J. Med. Sci. 270,* 165–171.

Lee, W.M., Reed, W.D., Mitchell, C.G. et al. (1975) Cell-mediated immunity to hepatitis B surface antigen in blood donors with persistent antigenaemia. *Gut 16,* 416–420.

Lee, W.M., Reed, W.D., Osman, C.G., et al. (1977) Immune responses to the hepatitis B surface antigen and liver-specific lipoprotein in acute type B hepatitis. *Gut 18,* 250-257.

Leevy, C.M., Chen, T., Luisada-Opper, A. et al. (1976) Liver disease of the alcoholic: role of immunologic abnormalities in pathogenesis recognition and treatment. In: H. Popper and F. Schaffner (Eds), *Progress in Liver Disease, Vol 5,* Grune and Stratton, New York, pp. 516–530.

LeMarchand, Y., Patzelt, C., Assimacopoulos-Jeannet, F. et al. (1974) Evidence of a role of the microtubular system in the secretion of newly synthesized albumin and other proteins by the liver. *J. Clin. Invest. 53,* 1512–1517.

Lenkei, R., Babes, V.T., Dan, M.E. et al. (1977) Correlation between anti-albumin antibodies and HB_sAg in hepatic patients. *J. Med. Virol. 1,* 29–34.

Levo, Y., Gorevic, P.D., Kassab, H.J. et al. (1977) Association between hepatitis B virus and essential mixed cryoglobulinemia. *N. Engl. J. Med. 296,* 1501–1504.

Logan, R.F.A., Ferguson, A., Finlayson, N.D.C. et al. (1978) Primary biliary cirrhosis and coeliac disease. *Lancet 1,* 230–233.

MacKay, I.R. (1978) Chronic active hepatitis, cirrhosis and other diseases of the liver. In: M. Samter, D.W. Talmage, B. Rose, K.F. Austen and J.H. Vaughan (Eds), *Immunological Diseases, 3rd ed.,* Chapter 83, Little, Brown and Co., Boston.

MacNab, G.M., Alexander, J.J. and Lecatsas, G. (1976) Hepatitis B surface antigen produced by a human hepatoma cell line. *Br. J. Cancer 34,* 509–515.

MacSween, R.N.M. (1980) Pathology of viral hepatitis and its sequelae. *Clin. Gastroenterol. 9,* 23–45.

MacSween, R.N.M., Armstrong, E.M., Gray, K.G. et al. (1973) Bile canalicular antibody in primary biliary cirrhosis and in other liver diseases. *Lancet 1,* 1419–1421.

MacSween, R.N.M., Burt, A., Anthony, R.S. et al. (1980a) Liver membrane antibodies in alcoholic liver disease. *Gastroenterology 79,* 1114.

MacSween, R.N.M., Mills, P.R. and Follett, E.A.C. (1980b) Hepatitis B and other viral antibodies in alcoholic cirrhosis. *Gastroenterology 79,* 1115.

Madalinski, K. and Bragiel, I. (1979) HB_sAg immune complexes in the course of infection with hepatitis B virus. *Clin. Exp. Immunol. 36,* 371–378.

Madalinski, K., Sztachelska-Budkowska, A. and Brzosko, W.J. (1974) DEAE-cellulose chromatography: a method for dissociation of soluble immune complexes of hepatitis B antigen. *J. Infect. Dis. 129,* 371–375.

Maddrey, W.C. and Boitnott, J.K. (1977) Drug-induced chronic liver disease. *Gastroenterology 72,* 1348–1353.

Madsen, N.P. (1969) Reduced serum very low density lipoprotein levels after acute ethanol administration. *Biochem. Pharmacol. 18,* 261–262.

Magnius, L.O. and Espmark. J.A. (1972) New specificities in Australia antigen positive sera distinct from the LeBouvier determinants. *J. Immunol. 109,* 1017–1021.

Magnius, L.O., Lindholm, A., Lundin, P. et al. (1975) A new antigen-antibody system. *J. Am. Med. Assoc. 231,* 356–359.

Manns, M., Meyer zum Buschenfelde, K.H. and Hess, G. (1980a) Autoantibodies against liver-specific membrane lipoprotein in acute and chronic liver diseases: studies on organ-, species-, and disease-specificity. *Gut 21,* 955–961.

Manns, M., Meyer zum Buschenfelde, K.H. and Hutteroth, T.H. (1980b) The liver-specific protein: evidence for species-specific and non-species-specific determinants. *J. Clin. Lab. Immunol. 3,* 9–13.

Mathiesen, L.R., Feinstone, S.M., Purcell, R.H. et al. (1977) Detection of hepatitis A antigen by immunofluorescence. *Infect. Immun. 18,* 524–530.

Mathiesen, L.R., Drucker, J., Lorenz, D. et al. (1978) Localization of hepatitis A antigen in marmoset organs during acute infection with hepatitis A virus. *J. Infect. Dis. 138,* 369–377.

McFarlane, G., Wojcicka, B.M., Zucker, G.M. et al. (1977) Purification and characterization of human liver-specific lipoprotein (LSP). *Clin. Exp. Immunol. 27,* 381–390.

McFarlane, J.G., Wojcicka, B.M., Tsantoulas, D.C. et al. (1979) Leucocyte migration inhibition in response to biliary antigens in primary biliary cirrhosis, sclerosing cholangitis and other chronic liver diseases. *Gastroenterology 76,* 1333–1340.

McIntosh, R.M., Koss, M.M. and Goeke, D.J. (1976) The nature and incidence of cryoproteins in hepatitis B antigen (HB_SAg) positive patients. *Q.J. Med. 45,* 23–38.

Meyer zum Buschenfelde, K.H. and Miescher, P.A. (1972) Liver-specific antigens. Purification and characterization. *Clin. Exp. Immunol. 10,* 89–102.

Meyer zum Buschenfelde, K.H., Kossling, F.K. and Miescher, P.A. (1972) Experimental chronic active hepatitis in rabbits following immunization with human liver proteins. *Clin. Exp. Immunol. 11,* 99–108.

Meyer zum Buschenfelde, K.H., Arnold, W., Knolle, J. et al. (1976) Immunreaktionen gegenüber HB_SAg und e Antigen bei akuter Virushepatitis sowie Lebergesunden und Leberkranken HB_SAg-Tragern. *Z. Gastroenterol. 4,* 365–377.

Meyer zum Buschenfelde, K.H., Manns, M. and Hutteroth, T.H. (1979) LM-Ag and LSP — two different target antigens involved in the immunopathogenesis of chronic active hepatitis? *Clin. Exp. Immunol. 37,* 205–212.

Michalak, T. (1978) Immune complexes of hepatitis B surface antigen in the pathogenesis of periarteritis nodosa. *Am. J. Pathol. 90,* 619–628.

Millman, I., Thomas, W., Sutnick, A.L. et al. (1970) Australia antigen-antibody complexes. *Nature (London) 226,* 83–84.

Mishiro, S., Imai, M., Takahashi, K. et al. (1980) A 49,000 dalton polypeptide bearing all antigenic determinants and full immunogenicity of 22-nm hepatitis B surface antigen particles. *J. Immunol. 124,* 1589–1593.

Morris, P.J., Vaughan, H., Tait, B.D. et al. (1977) Histocompatibility antigens (HLA): association with immunopathic diseases and with response to microbial antigens. *Aust. N.Z. J. Med. 7,* 616–624.

Mushahwar, I.K., Overby, L.R., Frosner, G.G. et al. (1978) Prevalence of hepatitis Be-antigen and its antibody as detected by radioimmunoassays. *J. Med. Virol. 2,* 77–87.

Nazarewicz, T., Krawczynski, K., Slusarcauk, J. et al. (1977) Cellular localization of hepatitis B virus antigen in patients with hepato-cellular carcinoma coexisting with liver cirrhosis. *J. Infect. Dis. 135,* 298–302.

Neurath, A.R. and Strick, N. (1977) Host specificity of a serum marker for hepatitis B. Evidence that "e" antigen has the properties of an immunoglobulin. *Proc. Natl Acad. Sci. USA 74,* 1702–1706.

Neurath, A.R., Trepo, C., Chen, M. et al. (1976) Identification of additional antigenic sites on Dane particles and the tubular forms of hepatitis B surface antigen. *J. Gen. Virol. 30,* 277–285.

Nowoslawski, A., Brzosko, W.J., Madalinski, K. et al. (1970) Cellular localization of Australia antigen in the liver of patients with lymphoproliferative disorders. *Lancet 1,* 494–498.

Nowoslawski, A., Krawczynski, K., Nazarewicz, T. et al. (1975) Immunopathological aspects of hepatitis type B. *Am. J. Med. Sci. 270,* 229–239.

Nydegger, U.E., Lambert, P.H., Gerber, H. et al. (1974) Circulating immune complexes in the serum in systemic lupus erythematosus and in carriers of hepatitis B antigen. *J. Clin. Invest. 54*,297–309.

Okada, K., Kamiyama, I., Inomata, M. et al. (1976) E antigen and anti-e in the serum of asymptomatic carrier mothers as indicators of positive and negative transmission of hepatitis B virus to their infants. *N. Engl. J. Med. 294,* 746–749.

O'Neill, S.P. (1979) Interaction of hepatitis B surface antigen with polymerized human serum albumin. *J. Med. Virol. 4,* 177–185.

Orlin, J.B., Berkman, E.M., Matloff, D.S. et al. (1980) Primary biliary cirrhosis and cold autoimmune hemolytic anemia: effect of partial plasma exchange. *Gastroenterology 78 (3),* 576–578.

Ozawa, T., Levisohn, P., Orsini, E. et al. (1976) Acute immune complex disease associated with hepatitis. Etiopathogenic and immunopathologic studies of the renal lesion. *Arch. Pathol. Lab. Med. 100,* 484–486.

Paronetto, F. and Lieber, C.S. (1976) Cytotoxicity of lymphocytes in experimental alcoholic liver injury in the baboon. *Proc. Soc. Exp. Biol. Med. 153,* 495–497.

Paronetto, F. and Popper, H. (1965) Aggravation of hepatic lesions in mice by an in vivo localization of immune complexes (Auer hepatitis). *Am. J. Pathol. 47,* 549–563.

Paronetto, F. and Popper, H. (1966) Chronic liver injury induced by immunologic reactions: cirrhosis following immunization with heterologous sera. *Am. J. Pathol. 49,* 1087–1101.

Paronetto, F. and Sagnelli, E. (1980) Immunologic observations in chronic active hepatitis: a disease of different etiologies. *Pathobiol. Annu. 10,* 157–181.

Paronetto, F. and Vernace, S. (1975) Immunological studies in patients with chronic active hepatitis. Cytotoxic activity of lymphocytes to autochthonous liver cells grown in tissue culture. *Clin. Exp. Immunol. 19,* 99–104.

Pasek, M., Goto, T., Gilbert, W. et al. (1979) Hepatitis B virus genes and their expression in E. coli. *Nature (London) 282,* 575–579.

Pequignot, G. (1961) The role of alcohol in the aetiology of liver cirrhosis in France; results and significance of a systematic survey. *Münch. Med. Wochenschr. 103,* 1464–1468.

Pernice, W., Sodomann, C.P., Lüben, G. et al. (1979) Antigen-specific detection of HB_sAg-containing immune complexes in the course of hepatitis B virus infection. *Clin. Exp. Immunol. 37,* 376–380.

Pettigrew, N.M., Bagshawe, A.F., Cameron, K.M. et al. (1976) Hepatitis B surface antigenaemia in Kenyans with chronic liver disease. *Trans. R. Soc. Trop. Med. Hyg. 70,* 462–465.

Popper, H. and Schaffner, F. (1970) Nonsuppurative destructive chronic cholangitis and chronic hepatitis. In: H. Popper and F. Schaffner (Eds), *Progress in Liver Disease, Vol. 3,* Grune and Stratton, New York, pp. 336–354.

Potter, B.J., Elias, E. and Jones, E.A. (1976) Hypercatabolism of the third component of complement in patients with primary biliary cirrhosis. *J. Lab. Clin. Med. 88,* 427–439.

Potter, B.J., Elias, E., Thomas, H.C. et al. (1980) Complement metabolism in chronic liver disease: catabolism of C1q in chronic active liver disease and primary biliary cirrhosis. *Gastroenterology 78,* 1034–1040.

Powell, W.J. and Klatskin, G. (1968) Survival of patients with Laennec's cirrhosis influence of alcohol withdrawal and possible effects of recent changes in general management of the disease. *Am. J. Med. 44,* 406–429.

Prince, A.M. (1968) An antigen detected in the blood during the incubation period of serum hepatitis. *Proc. Natl Acad. Sci. USA 60,* 814–821.

Provost, P.J. and Hilleman, M.R. (1979) Propagation of human hepatitis A virus in cell culture in vitro. *Proc. Soc. Exp. Biol. Med. 160,* 213–221.

Provost, P.J., Wolanski, B.S., Miller, W.J. et al. (1975) Physical, chemical and morphologic dimensions of human hepatitis A virus strain CR326. *Proc. Soc. Exp. Biol. Med. 148,* 532–539.

Provost, P.J., Villarejos, V.M. and Hilleman M.R. (1977) Suitability of the Rufiventer marmoset as a host animal for human hepatitis A virus. *Proc. Soc. Exp. Biol. Med. 155,* 283-286.

Prugh, M.F., Gregory, D.H., Vlahcevic, J.R. et al. (1976) Role of the "microtubular Golgi" network in the hepatocellular transport of biliary lipids. *Gastroenterology 70,* A–132–990.

Purcell, R.H., Alter, H.J. and Dienstag, J.L. (1976) Non-A,non-B hepatitis. *Yale J. Biol. Med. 49,* 243–250.

Rai, G.S., Hamlyn, A.N., Dahl, M.G.C. et al. (1977) Primary biliary cirrhosis, cutaneous capillaritis and IgM-associated membranous glomerulonephritis. *Br. Med. J. 1,* 817.

Rakela, J. and Redeker, A.G. (1979) Chronic liver disease after acute non-A,non-B, viral hepatitis. *Gastroenterology 77,* 1200–1202.

Ray, M.B., Desmet, V.J., Bradburne, A.F. et al. (1976) Differential distribution of hepatitis B surface antigen and hepatitis B core antigen in the liver of hepatitis B patients. *Gastroenterology 71,* 462–469.

Ray, M.B., Desmet, V.J., Bradburne, A.F. et al. (1979) Hepatitis B core antigen immune complexes in the liver of hepatitis B patients. *Clin. Exp. Immunol. 37,* 15–24.

Redman, C.M., Banerjee, D., Howell, K. et al. (1975a) Colchicine inhibition of plasma protein release from rat hepatocytes. *J. Cell Biol. 66,* 42–59.

Redman, C.M., Banerjee, D., Howell, K. et al. (1975b) The step at which colchicine blocks the secretion of plasma protein by rat liver. *Ann. NY Acad. Sci. 253,* 780–788.

Reed, W.D., Eddleston, A.L.W.F., Cullens, H. et al. (1973) Infusion of hepatitis B antibody in antigen positive active chronic hepatitis. *Lancet 2,* 1347–1351.

Reynolds, T.B. (1980) Chronic hepatitis: current dilemmas. *Am. J Med. 69,* 485–487.

Rizzetto, M., Bonino, F., Crevelli, O. et al. (1976) Complement fixing hepatitis B core antigen immune complexes in the liver of patients with HBs antigen positive chronic disease. *Gut 17,* 837–843.

Rizzetto, M., Canese, M.G., Arico, S. et al. (1977) Immunfluorescence detection of a new antigen-antibody system (δ/anti-δ) associated to hepatitis B virus in liver and in serum of HBsAg carriers. *Gut 18,* 997–1003.

Rizzetto, M., Shih, J.W.K. and Gerlin, J.L. (1980) The hepatitis B virus-associated antigen: isolation from liver, development of solid-phase radioimmunoassay for antigen and anti-δ and partial characterization of δ antigen. *J.Immunol. 125,* 318–324.

Robinson, W.S. (1977) The genome of hepatitis B virus. *Annu. Rev. Microbiol. 31,* 357–377.

Robinson, W.S. and Greenman, R.L. (1974) DNA polymerase in the core of the human hepatitis B virus candidate. *J. Virol. 13,* 1231–1236.

Routhier, G., Goldstein, G, Tidman, N. et al. (1980) T-lymphocyte subpopulation (identified by monoclonal antibodies) in chronic liver disease. *Gastroenterology 79(5), part 2,* p. 1122.

Sanchez-Tapias, J., Thomas, H.C. and Sherlock, S. (1977) Lymphocyte population in liver biopsy specimens from patients with chronic liver disease. *Gut 18,* 472–475.

Saunders, J.B., Davis, M. and Williams, R. (1981) Do women develop alcholic liver disease more readily than men? *Br. Med. J. 282,* 1140–1143.

Schumacher, H.R. and Gall, E.P. (1974) Arthritis in acute hepatitis and chronic active hepatitis: pathology of the synovial membrane with evidence for the presence of Australia antigen in synovial membranes. *Am. J. Med. 57,* 655–664.

Schumacher, K., Maerker-Alzer, G. and Wehmer, U. (1974) A lymphocyte-inhibiting factor isolated from normal human liver. *Nature (London) 251,* 655–656.

Scott, B.B., Rajah, S.M. and Losowsky, M.S. (1977) Dantrolene-associated hepatic injury. *Gastroenterology 72,* 122–125.

Seignalet, J., Blanc, F. and Lapinski, H. (1980) Groupes HLA des cirrhotiques alcooliques. *Nouv. Presse Med. 9,* 712.

Sergent, J.S., Lockshin, M.D., Christian, C.L. et al. (1976) Vasculitis with hepatitis B antigenemia: long-term observations in nine patients. *Medicine (Baltimore) 55,* 1–18.

Sharp, J.R., Ishak, K.G. and Zimmerman, H.F. (1980) Chronic active hepatitis and severe hepatic necrosis associated with nitrofurantoin. *Ann. Intern. Med. 92,* 14–19.

Sherlock, S. and Scheuer, P.J. (1974) The presentation and diagnosis of 100 patients with primary biliary cirrhosis. In: F. Schaffner, S. Sherlock and C.M. Leevy (Eds), *The Liver and its Diseases,* Intercontinental Medical Book Corp., New York, pp. 227–235.

Shikata, T. (1976) Primary liver carcinoma and liver cirrhosis. In: K. Okuda and R.L. Peters (Eds), *Hepatocellular Carcinoma,* J. Wiley, New York, pp. 53–71.

Shikata, T., Uzawa, T., Yoshiwara, N. et al. (1974) Staining methods of Australia antigen in paraffin section. Detection of cytoplasmic inclusion bodies. *Jpn J. Exp. Med. 44,* 25–36.

Shimizu, Y.K., Mathiesen, L.R., Lorenz, D. et al. (1978) Localization of hepatitis A antigen in liver tissue by peroxidase-conjugated antibody method. Light and electron microscopic studies. *J. Immunol. 121,* 1671–1679.

Shiraishi, H., Shirachi, R., Akiyama, K. et al. (1980) Glycopeptide composition of hepatitis B surface antigen. *J. Gen. Virol. 48,* 31–38.

Shulman, N.R. and Barker, L.F. (1969) Virus like antigen, antibody, and antigen-antibody complexes in hepatitis as measured by complement fixation. *Science 165,* 304–306.

Siegl, G. and Frosner, G.G. (1978) Characterization and classification of virus particles associated with hepatitis A. II. Type and configuration of nucleic acid. *J. Virol. 26,* 48–53.

Slusarczyk, J., Michalak, T., Nazarewicz-De Mezer, T. et al. (1980) Membranous glomerulopathy associated with hepatitis B core antigen immune complexes in children. *Am. J. Pathol. 98,* 29–44.

Snisky, J.J., Siddiqui, A., Robinson, W.S. et al. (1979) Cloning and endonuclease mapping of the hepatitis B viral genome. *Nature (London) 279,* 346–348.

Stannard, L.M. and Hodgkiss, M. (1979) Morphological irregularities in Dane particle cores. *J. Gen. Virol. 45,* 509–514.

Stein, O. and Stein, Y. (1967) Lipid synthesis, intracellular transport, storage, and secretion. I. Electron microscopic radioautographic study of the liver after injection of tritiated palmitate or glycerol in fasted and ethanol-treated rats. *J. Cell Biol. 33,* 319–339.

Stein, O., Fainaru, M. and Stein, Y. (1972) Visualization of virus-like particles in endoplasmic reticulum of hepatocytes of Australia antigen carriers. *Lab. Invest. 26,* 262–269.

Stein, O., Sanger, L. and Stein, Y. (1974) Colchicine-induced inhibition of lipoprotein and protein secretion into the serum and lack of interference with secretion of biliary phospholipids and cholesterol by rat liver in vivo. *J. Cell Biol. 62,* 90–103.

Summers, J., O'Connell, A. and Millman, I. (1975) Genome of hepatitis B virus: restriction enzyme cleavage and structure of DNA extracted from Dane particles. *Proc. Natl Acad. Sci. USA 72,* 4597–4601.

Summers, J., O'Connell, A., Manpas, P. et al. (1978) Hepatitis B virus DNA in primary hepatocellular carcinoma tissue. *J. Med. Virol. 2,* 207–214.

Summerskill, W.H.J. (1974) Chronic active liver disease re-examined: prognosis hopeful. *Gastroenterology 66,* 450–464.

Summerskill, W.H.J., Korman, M.G., Ammon, H.V. et al. (1975) Prednisone for chronic active liver disease: dose titration, standard dose and combination with azathioprine compared. *Gut 16,* 876–883.

Szmuness, W. (1978) Hepatocellular carcinoma and the hepatitis B virus: evidence for a causal association. *Prog. Med. Virol. 24,* 40–69.

Szmuness, W., Stevens, C.E., Harley, E.J. et al. (1980) Hepatitis B vaccine. Demonstration of efficacy in a controlled clinical trial in a high risk population in the United States. *N. Engl. J. Med. 303,* 833–841.

Tabor, E., Mitchell, F.D., Goudeau, A.M. et al. (1979) Detection of an antigen-antibody system in serum associated with human non-A,non-B hepatitis. *J. Med. Virol. 4,* 161–169.

Tage-Jensen, U., Arnold, W., Dietrichson, O. et al. (1977) Liver-cell-membrane autoantibody specific for inflammatory liver disease. *Br. Med. J. 1,* 206–208.

Takahashi, K., Imai, M., Tsuda, F. et al. (1976) Association of Dane particles with "e" antigen in the serum of asymptomatic carriers of hepatitis B surface antigen. *J. Immunol. 117,* 102–105.

Takahashi, K., Akagane, Y. Gotanda, T. et al. (1979a) Demonstration of hepatitis Be antigen in the core of Dane particles. *J. Immunol. 122,* 275–279.

Takahashi, K., Miyakawa, Y., Gotanda, T. et al. (1979b) Shift from free "small" hepatitis Be antigen to IgG-bound "large" form in the circulation of human beings and a chimpanzee acutely infected with hepatitis B virus. *Gastroenterology 77,* 1193–1199.

Takekoshi, Y., Tanaka, M., Miyakawa, Y. et al. (1979) Free "small" and IgG-associated "large" hepatitis Be antigen in the serum and glomerular capillary walls of two patients with membranous glomerulonephritis. *N. Engl. J. Med. 300,* 814–819.

Theofilopoulos, A.N., Wilson, C.B. and Dixon, F.J. (1976) The Raji cell radioimmune assay for detecting immune complexes in human sera. *J. Clin. Invest. 57,* 169–182.

Thestrup-Pederson, K., Ladefoged, K. and Anderson, P. (1976) Lymphocyte transformation test with liver-specific protein and phytohemagglutinin in patients with liver disease. *Clin. Exp. Immunol. 24,* 1–8.

Thomas, F.B. (1974) Chronic aggressive hepatitis induced by halothane. *Ann. Intern. Med. 81,* 487–489.

Thomas, H. (1978) In: A.L.W.F. Eddleston, J.C.P. Weber and R. Williams (Eds), *Immune Reactions in Liver Disease,* Pitman Medical, Tunbridge Wells, pp. 226–228.

Thomas, H.C., DeVillers, D., Potter, B. et al. (1978) Immune complexes in acute and chronic liver disease. *Clin. Exp. Immunol. 31,* 150–157.

Thomas, H.C., Potter, B.J., Elias, E. et al. (1979) Metabolism of the third component of complement in acute type B hepatitis, HBs antigen positive glomerulonephritis, polyarteritis nodosa and HBs antigen positive and negative chronic active liver disease. *Gastroenterology 76,* 673–679.

Thomson, A.D., Cochrane, A.M.G., McFarlane, I.G. et al. (1974) Lymphocyte cytotoxicity to isolated hepatocytes in chronic active hepatitis. *Nature (London) 252,* 721–722.

Thung, S.N. and Gerber, M.A. (1981) HB_sAg-associated albumin receptors and anti-albumin antibodies in sera of patients with liver disease. *Gastroenterology 80,* 260–264.

Tiollais, P., Charnay, P. and Girish, N.V. (1981) Biology of hepatitis B virus. *Science 213,* 406–411.

Toh, B.H. (1979) Smooth muscle autoantibodies and auto-antigens. *Clin. Exp. Immunol. 38,* 621–628.

Tong, W.J., Wallace, A.M., Robert, D. et al. (1975) Lymphocyte stimulation in hepatitis B infections. *N. Engl. J. Med. 293,* 318–322.

Tong, M.J., Nies, K.M. and Redeker, A.G. (1977) Rapid progression of chronic active type B hepatitis in a patient with hypogammaglobulinemia. *Gastroenterology 73,* 1418–1421.

Tremolada, F., Fattovich, G., Panebianco, G. et al. (1980) Suppressor cell activity in viral and non-viral chronic active hepatitis. *Clin. Exp. Immunol. 40,* 89–95.

Trepo, C., Vitvitski, L. and Neurath, R. (1972) Detection of e antigen by immunofluorescence in cytoplasm of hepatocytes of HBs carriers. *Lancet 1,* 486.

Trepo, C.G., Zuckerman, A.J., Bird R.C. et al. (1974) The role of circulating hepatitis B antigen/antibody immune complexes in the pathogenesis of vascular and hepatic manifestations in polyarteritis nodosa. *J. Clin. Pathol. 27,* 863–868.

Tsantoulas, D., Perperas, A., Portmann, B. et al. (1980) Antibodies to a human liver membrane lipoprotein (LSP) in primary biliary cirrhosis. *Gut 21,* 557–560.

Tsiquave, K.N., Bird, R.G., Tovey, G. et al. (1980) Further evidence of cellular changes associated with non-A,non-B hepatitis. *J. Med. Virol. 5,* 63–71.

Utili, R., Boitnott, J.K. and Zimmerman, H.J. (1977) Dantrolene-associated hepatic injury: incidence and character. *Gastroenterology 72,* 610–616.

Valenzuela, P., Gray, P., Quiroga, M. et al. (1979) Nucleotide sequences of the gene coding for the major protein of hepatitis B virus surface antigen. *Nature (London) 280,* 815–819.

Vergani, M.G., Vergani, D., Jenkins, P.F. et al. (1979) Lymphocyte cytotoxicity to autologous hepatocytes in HB_sAg-negative chronic active hepatitis. *Clin. Exp. Immunol. 38,* 16–21.

Vitvitski, L., Prince, A.M., Trepo, C. et al. (1979) Detection of virus-associated antigen in serum and liver of patients with non-A,non-B hepatitis. *Lancet 2,* 1263–1367.

Vnek, J., Prince, A.M., Trepo, C. et al. (1979) Cryptic association of e antigen with different morphologic forms of hepatitis B surface antigen. *J. Med. Virol. 4,* 187–199.

Vogten, A.J.M., Hadzic, N., Shorter, R.G. et al. (1978) Cell-mediated cytotoxicity in chronic active liver disease: a new test system. *Gastroenterology 74,* 883–889.

Vyas, G.N., Peterson, D.L. and Townsend, R.M. (1977) Hepatitis B "e" antigen: an apparent association with lactate dehydrogenase isozyme-5. *Science 198,* 1068–1070.

Wands, J.R. and Isselbacher, K.J. (1975) Lymphocyte cytotoxicity to autologous liver cells in chronic hepatitis. *Proc. Natl Acad. Sci. USA 72,* 1301–1303.

Wands, J.R., Alpert, E. and Isselbacher, K.J. (1975a) Arthritis associated with chronic active hepatitis: complement activation and characterization of circulating immune complexes. *Gastroenterology 69,* 1286–1291.

Wands, J.R., Perrotto, J.L., Alpert, E. et al. (1975b) Cell-mediated immunity in acute and chronic hepatitis. *J. Clin. Invest. 55,* 921–929.

Wands, J.R., Dienstag, J.L., Bhan, A.K. et al. (1978) Circulating immune complexes and complement activation in primary biliary cirrhosis. *N. Engl. J. Med. 298,* 233–237.

Wands, J.R., Zurawaki Jr, V.R. (1981) High affinity monoclonal antibodies to hepatitis B surface antigen (HB_SAg) produced by somatic cell hybrids. *Gastroenterology 80,* 225–232.

Welsh, J.D., Brown, J.D., Arnold, K. et al. (1976) Hepatitis B_SAg, malaria titers and primary liver cancer in South Vietnam. *Gastroenterology 70,* 392–396.

Williams Jr, R.C., Strickland, R.G. and Montano, J.D. (1980) Subpopulations of T cells ($T\gamma$ and $T\mu$) in patients with chronic liver disease. *Clin. Immunol. Immunopathol. 15,* 616–621.

Wisse, E. and Knook, D.L. (1979) The investigation of sinusoidal cells: a new approach to the study of liver function. *Prog. Liver Dis. 6,* 153–171.

Wojcicka, B. (1979) Separation and characterization of bile antigens. In: A.L.W.F. Eddleston, J.C.P. Weber and R. Williams (Eds), *Immune Reactions in Liver Disease,* Pitman Medical, Tunbridge Wells, p. 154.

Wojciech, K.P. (1976) Cytodestructive mechanisms provoked by lymphocytes. *Am. J. Med. 61,* 1–8.

Yamada, G. and Nakane, P.K. (1977) Hepatitis B core and surface antigens in liver tissue. Light and electron microscopic localization by the peroxidase-labeled antibody method. *Lab. Invest. 36,* 649–659.

Yeung-Laiwah, A.A.C. (1971) Lymphocyte transformation by Australia antigen. *Lancet 2,* 470–471.

Yeung-Laiwah, A.A.C., Chaudhuri, A.K.R. and Anderson, J.R. (1973) Lymphocyte transformation and leukocyte migration-inhibition by Australia antigen. *Clin. Exp. Immunol. 15,* 27–34.

Zetterman, R.K. and Woltjen, J.A. (1980) Suppressor cell activity in primary biliary cirrhosis. *Dig. Dis. Sci. 25,* 104–107.

Zetterman, R.K., Luisada-Opper, A. and Leevy, C.M. (1976) Alcoholic hepatitis cell-mediated immunological response to alcoholic hyaline. *Gastroenterology 70,* 382–384.

Zuckerman, A. (1978) Hepatitis B virus and primary liver cancer. In: H. Remmer, H.M. Bolt, P. Bonnasch and H.Popper (Eds), *Primary Liver Tumors,* MTP Press, Lancaster, pp. 425–429.

CHAPTER 10

Mechanisms of immunologic injury in inflammatory bowel injury: ulcerative colitis and Crohn's disease

DAVID F. KEREN

Department of Pathology, University of Michigan Medical School, Ann Arbor, Michigan 48109

10.1. ETIOLOGY OF INFLAMMATORY BOWEL DISEASE (IBD)

The idea that a transmissible agent is responsible for chronic idiopathic inflammatory bowel disease (IBD) (ulcerative colitis and Crohn's disease) dates back at least as far as Crohn's original suggestion that a variant of *Mycobacterium tuberculosis* was responsible for the pathologic features which he described (Crohn et al. 1932).

Although numerous micro-organisms have been cultured from tissue specimens of patients with IBD, no single organism has been consistently found, and until recently it has been difficult to transfer the disease to experimental animals. The literature on the subject is detailed in an excellent recent review by Beeken (1980).

It is generally accepted that the fecal flora of the intestine is increased in patients with IBD, especially those with Crohn's disease (Cooke 1967; Van der Wiel-Korstanje and Winkler 1975; Keighley et al. 1978). This likely accounts for the many serologic studies that have demonstrated relatively high antibody titers to the common *Escherichia coli* and other micro-organisms which are less frequently found in normal individuals, some of which, such as rotavirus, are associated with gastroenteritis (DeGroote et al. 1977; Burnham et al. 1978; Tabagchali et al. 1978; Greenberg et al. 1979; Helphingstine et al. 1979; Schuller et al. 1979). Many of these serum antibodies also may relate to increased permeability of the gut epithelium by luminal antigens, as high titers of antibody to food products such as maize have also been demonstrated in patients with IBD (Davidson et al. 1979).

Whereas it appears that the more commonplace microbiologic and serologic studies have failed to yield an acceptable etiologic agent, some unconventional approaches have resulted in several plausible candidate etiologic agents for IBD.

Three groups have reported success in producing granulomas in experimental animals after injecting them with crude and then bacteria-free filtrates of intestine and involved lymph nodes from patients with IBD (Mitchell and Rees 1970; Cave et al. 1973, 1976; Taub et al. 1976, 1978; Cohen et al. 1980). Unfortunately, several careful studies by other workers have not been able to reproduce these phenomena (Bolton et al. 1973; Heatley et al. 1975; Simonowitz et al. 1977). Lastly, independent study by an authoritative gastrointestinal pathologist of some of the actual tissue sections which purported to display granulomas disclosed that some lesions were not granulomas at all (one being lymphosarcoma of aged mice and another being a leiomyosarcoma of the uterus) (Cave et al. 1979). Some of the tissue sections did contain granulomata but many of these were of the classic foreign-body type, some of which contained polarizable material (consistent with fibers of filters used to exclude bacteria) and these containing ". . . bits of hair, bone, etc. . . ." (Thayer, 1979). These findings, together with the studies that have found granulomata in animals given extracts of tissues from individuals lacking IBD, raise serious doubts over some of the original observations (Taub et al. 1976; Donnelly et al. 1977). Lastly preliminary data from a large cooperative study have been unable to reproduce the granulomas (Cave et al. 1980).

Several workers have demonstrated viral inclusions or have been able to show in-vitro cytopathic effect in tissue culture cell lines treated with extracts of tissues from patients with IBD (Aronson et al. 1975; Gitnick et al. 1979; Cave et al. 1980). Whereas there is some evidence that this may be a rheovirus-like agent (Whorwell et al. 1977; Gitnick et al. 1979; Strickland et al. 1979), other groups have not been able to confirm rheovirus as the agent causing the cytopathic effect (Kapikian et al. 1979; Phillpotts et al. 1979). Also, cytopathic effects have been produced, albeit less frequently, after inoculation of tissue cultures with homogenates of biopsy material from healthy controls (Aronson et al. 1975). This latter finding does not exclude the possibility that, although the virus-like agent is present in controls, patients with IBD may have a unique genetic susceptibility – perhaps due to receptor sites on epithelial cells which they alone possess, or perhaps due to altered immune reactivity to antigens on that viral agent – which would cause only them to express the disease.

Cytomegalovirus (CMV) has also been demonstrated in patients with IBD (Monis and Mendeloff 1961; Keren et al. 1975; Cooper et al. 1977) and its possible role as an etiologic agent in IBD has been suggested (Cooper et al. 1977). However, DNA hybridization studies found no evidence of CMV in any patients with Crohn's disease and in only 1 of 8 patients with ulcerative colitis (Roche and Huang 1977).

Attempts at using special bacterial isolation techniques have demonstrated the presence of cell-wall defective micro-organisms in tissues from patients with IBD, but not in control tissues (Burnham et al. 1978; Parent and Mitchell 1978; Belsheim et al. 1980). These isolates have not been able to reproduce lesions of IBD when injected into experimental animals (Parent et al. 1980).

Lastly, Das et al. (1980) injected homogenized tissues from patients with Crohn's disease into female nude mice, which subsequently developed lymphomas and plasma cell hyperplasia. Although production of such lymphomas is not unusual in mice as they age, Das et al. (1980) also found that sera from patients with Crohn's disease would react with the cytoplasm of these cells. Their studies suggest that a transmissible agent may produce lymphoproliferative disorders in nude mice but results in an IBD in humans.

Clearly, the final identification of the etiologic agent in IBD is not yet available. Further exploration of the CPE phenomenon, cell-wall defective bacteria and transmissible agents in experimental models may yield a definable infectious agent responsible for IBD. However, there is strong evidence that there exists an altered immune state in patients with IBD, with regard to autoimmune phenomena, altered plasma cell populations in the gut mucosa, increased killer lymphocytes and decreased suppressor T-cells. These latter, in addition to any specific inciting agent (or agents), may be responsible for the histopathologic features of IBD.

10.2. HUMORAL IMMUNITY IN IBD

10.2.1. Local antibody production

There are increased numbers of plasma cells in the lamina propria of biopsies from patients with IBD (Figs. 1 and 2). Using either immunofluorescence or immunoperoxidase, several groups have demonstrated increased numbers of immunoglobulin-containing cells in colon mucosal samples from patients with IBD (Fig. 3) as compared to colon mucosal samples from control individuals (Fig. 4) (Skinner and Whitehead 1974).

There has been some controversy, however, about the type of immunoglobulin present in these cells and its potential significance (Table 1). Early observations from several groups indicated that IgG-containing plasma cells were increased in colon biopsies from patients with IBD (Soltoft et al. 1973; Brandtzaeg et al. 1974; Skinner and Whitehead 1974; Baklien and Brandtzaeg 1975). Furthermore, Soltoft et al. (1973) noted that the increased numbers of IgG-containing cells were present both during the active and inactive stages of the disease. Conversely, Green and Fox (1975) and more recently O'Donoghue and Kumar (1979) found no difference in the numbers of IgA-, IgM-, and IgG-containing cells in the colon from patients with IBD as compared to control material.

Further, controversy exists about the content of IgE-containing plasma cells in the lamina propria of patients with IBD. Increased numbers of IgE-containing plasma cells have been found in the bronchial mucosa of asthmatics and in the small-bowel mucosa of children with milk allergy (Gerber et al. 1971; Shiner et al. 1975); therefore, the markedly increased number of IgE-containing plasma cells in rectal biopsy specimens recently reported by O'Donoghue and Kumar (1979) could indicate that an allergic mechanism is involved in IBD. However, Lloyd et al. (1975) actually found a slight decrease in IgE-containing cells in the colon of patients with

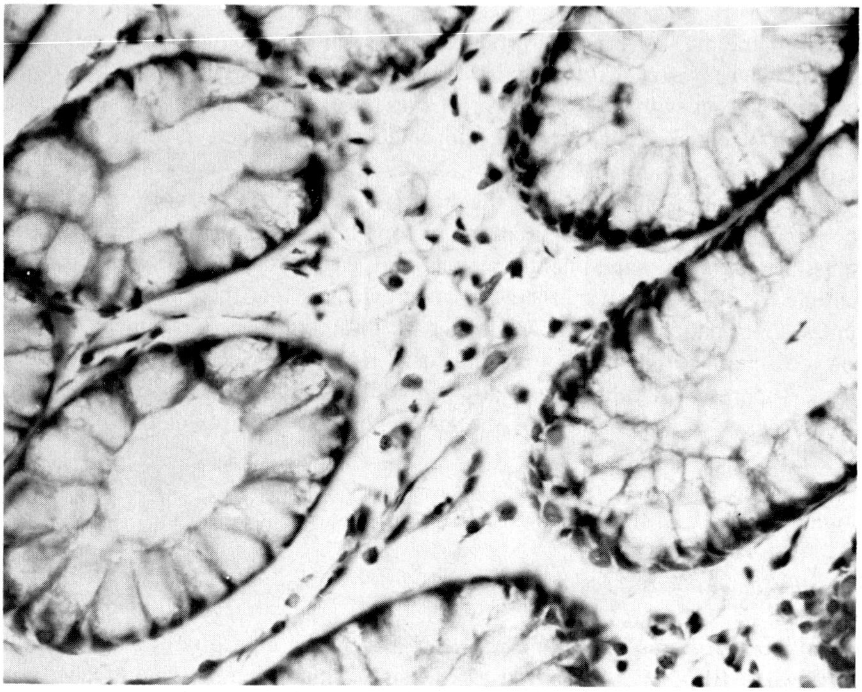

1

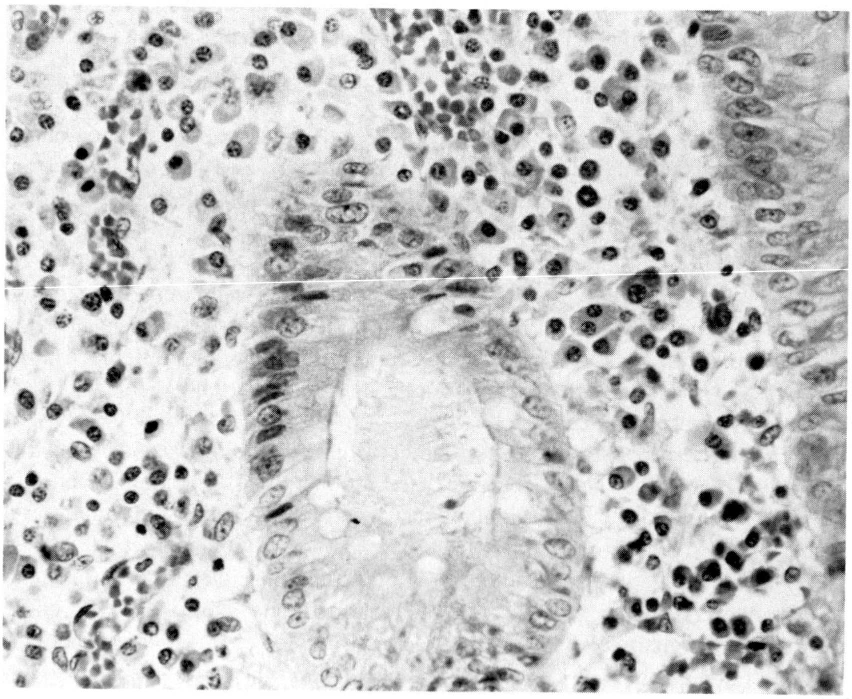

2

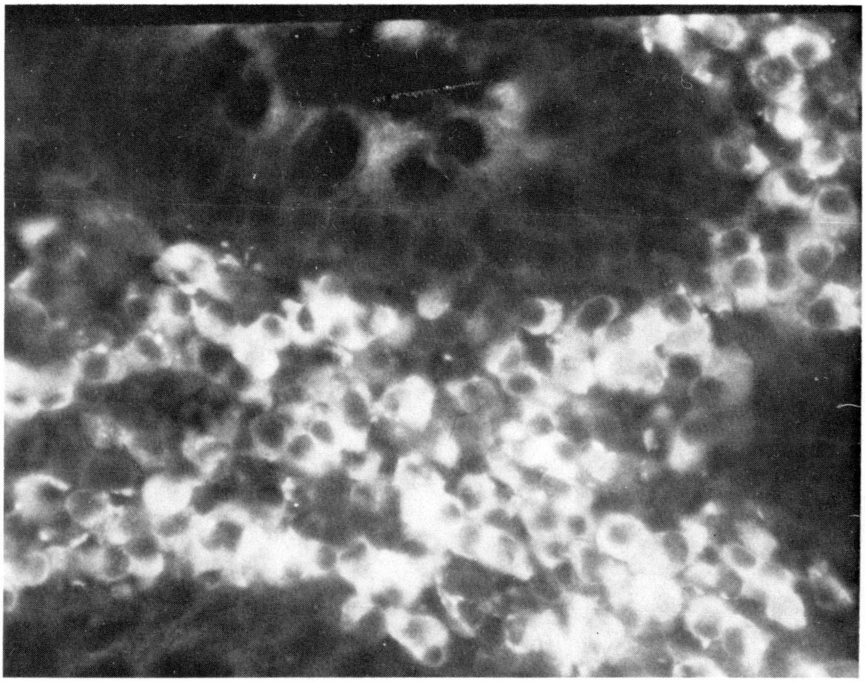

Fig. 3. Dark-field photomicrograph showing vast numbers of IgA-containing plasma cells in colon from patient with active inflammatory bowel disease. Fluorescein and anti-human IgA; x 350.

Crohn's colitis and normal numbers of these cells in patients with ulcerative colitis. Similarly, Green and Fox (1975) found normal numbers of IgE-containing cells in colons from patients with Crohn's colitis.

Indeed, this latter controversy may relate to the definition of ulcerative versus allergic proctitis. Some cases of ulcerative proctitis will eventually develop full-blown ulcerative colitis; consequently, ulcerative proctitis can be viewed as a variant in the spectrum of ulcerative colitis (Lennard-Jones et al. 1962). Alternatively, some have

←

Fig. 1. Normal colon lamina propria. H and E; x 350.

Fig. 2. Lamina propria from patient with active inflammatory bowel disease. Note a relative prominence of plasma cells. H and E; x 350.

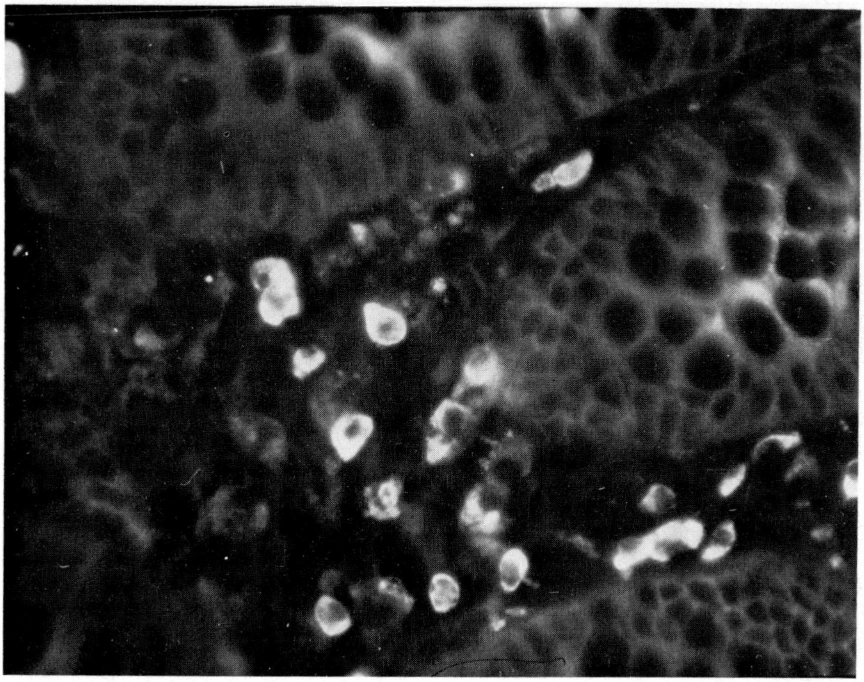

Fig. 4. Dark-field photomicrograph showing normal IgA-containing plasma cell content of control colon.

considered that ulcerative proctitis may have an allergic basis, which is consistent with the favorable response of individuals with this condition to disodium cromoglycate (Heatley et al. 1975; Heatley and James 1978). Others have noted that patients with ulcerative colitis do not generally respond well to treatment with disodium cromoglycate (Willoughby et al. 1979). Heatley et al. (1975) and, most recently, Rosekrans et al. (1980b) have presented convincing evidence that this results from the fact that allergic proctitis is a distinct clinical and pathologic entity.

In the study of Rosekrans et al. a markedly increased number of IgE-containing cells were detected in the lamina propria of rectal biopsies in 8 of 12 patients (Fig. 5) but not in patients with ulcerative colitis or Crohn's disease. All 12 of these subjects responded to therapy with disodium cromoglycate. These results (Rosekrans et al. 1980b) resolve the disparity between O'Donoghue and Kumar (1979), whose marked increase in IgE-containing cells likely reflected allergic proctitis, and (Green and Fox 1975) whose normal numbers of IgE-containing cells reflected the lack of allergic proctitis in their population.

In the case of allergic proctitis, immunohistology as used by Rosekrans et al.

TABLE 1.
Immunoglobulin-containing cells in inflammatory bowel disease

Study	IgA	IgM	IgG	IgE
Soltoft et al. (1973)	sl↑[1)]	Normal	↑[2)]	ND[3)]
Brandtzaeg et al. (1974)	sl↑	↑	↑↑↑	ND
Skinner and Whitehead (1974)	↑↑	↑↑	↑↑	ND
Baklien and Brandtzaeg (1975)	sl↑	↑	↑↑↑	ND
Green and Fox (1975)	Normal	sl↑	Normal	Normal
Lloyd et al. (1975)	ND	ND	ND	sl↓/normal[5)]
O'Donoghue and Kumar (1979)	Normal	Normal	Normal	↑↑
Rosekrans et al. (1980a)	sl↑	↑↑/sl↑[5)]	↑Active/↑[2)]	NR[4)]

1) Graded from slightly decreased (sl↓) to marked increase (↑↑↑).
2) Increased in both active and inactive disease.
3) ND = Not done.
4) NR = Data not reported.
5) Crohn/ulcerative colitis.

(1980b) has provided extremely useful information. By correlating the histopathology and clinical response to therapy with the immunohistology, Rosekrans et al. (1980b) separated out those cases with isolated proctitis and increased numbers of IgE-containing cells as allergic proctitis. Further, their results help to explain studies which hypothesized that ulcerative colitis may be related to allergy (Wright and Truelove 1965; Mee et al. 1979a).

Information about IgD-containing cells is available only in the work of Green and Fox (1975), who found normal numbers of these cells in biopsies from patients with IBD.

Some of the conflicting data with regard to IgG, IgA and IgM content in IBD tissue relate to: (1) relatively small numbers of specimens examined by each study, (2) the population selected — many studies looked only at resection specimens and hence only at the extreme cases of IBD — and (3) the relatively meager correlation with the clinical and histopathologic activity of the disease.

In order to look at larger populations and a broader spectrum of IBD, our recent studies have taken advantage of techniques which allow immunohistology to be performed on formalin-fixed, paraffin-embedded tissue (Huang et al. 1976; Qualman and Keren 1979; Clark and Keren 1982). By examining in a prospective fashion all biopsy and excision material from patients who were histopathologically classified as having IBD by the Department of Pathology at The University of Michigan over a one-year period, we have obtained a broad and in-depth view of immunoglobulin-containing cells in IBD. The results of the 115 specimens from 58 patients examined over this period were correlated with the histopathologic degree of activity. Some of our data, summarized in Table 2, demonstrate that the IgG-containing plasma cells are increased when there is histologic evidence of active IBD but not in inactive disease or in reactive mucosa (Keren et al. 1982). Similar findings were reported in a

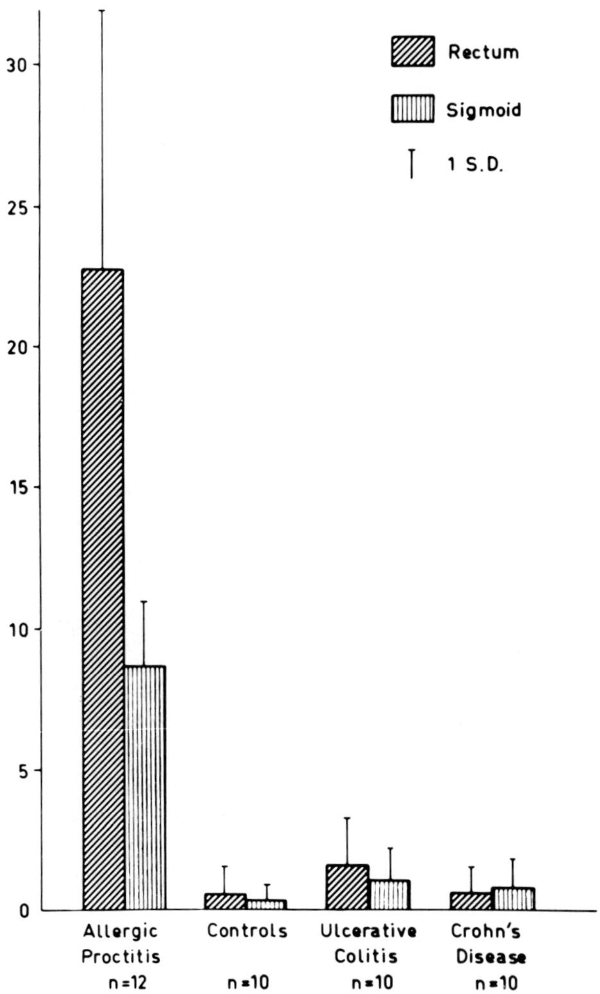

Fig. 5. Number of IgE-containing cells per mm of mucosal length. Note large numbers of IgE-containing cells in both rectum and sigmoid from patients with allergic proctitis as opposed to controls or patients with inflammatory bowel disease. (Data from Rosekrans et al. 1980b. Used with permission.)

TABLE 2.
Immunoglobulin-containing cells in colon

Histopathology	No. of specimens	IgA*	IgM	IgG
Control	11	68.6	5.4	2.5
Active IBD	23	114.8	33.9	45.3
Inactive IBD	40	80.9	12.3	9.1
Reactive mucosa	39	88.7	18.9	3.9

* Mean number of cells per high-power field.
(Data from Keren et al. 1982).

recent study by Rosekrans et al. (1980a), which used an immunoperoxidase technique on formalin-fixed, paraffin-embedded tissues and found an increase in IgG-containing cells in 10 patients with ulcerative colitis (regardless of disease activity), but in Crohn's disease, only such an increase was found in those with active disease.

10.2.2. Serum antibody levels

In serum of patients with ulcerative colitis the mean IgG, IgA and IgM concentrations are greater than those of control individuals or those of patients with Crohn's disease. However, the mean IgM level in patients with Crohn's disease is greater than that of control subjects (Hodgson and Jewell 1978); this was true even in patients receiving corticosteroid therapy.

Recently, using a sensitive radioimmunoassay technique, Delacroix and Vaerman (1981) reported that serum levels of secretory IgA (IgA coupled to secretory component) were significantly elevated in patients with Crohn's disease. These studies confirm earlier reports by Thompson et al. (1969) and Iscaki and Buffet (1978) which used less sensitive double diffusion techniques. The increased serum immunoglobulins likely reflect increased antigen load resulting from the damaged intestinal epithelium in IBD patients.

10.3. ROLE OF INFLAMMATORY MEDIATORS: COMPLEMENT AND PROSTAGLANDINS

Since the histopathology of IBD presents a classic picture of acute and, later, chronic inflammation, several studies have been performed to determine whether complement activation or prostaglandins (mediators of inflammation) are altered in patients with IBD.

It is clear that C3 is catabolized and synthesized at an increased rate in patients with IBD (Hodgson et al. 1977b; Lake et al. 1979). Lake et al. (1979) also showed that in these patients there were significant abnormalities of the alternative pathway with decreased levels of serum properdin and properdin convertase. While Lake and colleagues admit that the significance of these changes in the alternative pathway in patients with acute IBD is unclear, they suggest that their findings support an immune complex activation of complement or an activation of alternative pathway, perhaps by endotoxin. Alternatively, they suggest that C3b activation may enhance lymphocyte-mediated cytotoxicity, as has been shown in vitro by Stobo et al. (1976) with lymphocytes from IBD patients and colon cells.

Potter and colleagues (1979) found that the catabolic and synthetic rates of C1q were increased in patients with IBD. Because of this, they suggested that the classic pathway of complement activation may be important in the pathogenesis of IBD. Lake et al. (1979), however, were unable to demonstrate abnormalities of the classic complement pathway. Their findings are consistent with normal levels of the second component of complement C2 in active disease (Ward and Eastwood 1975). Additional evidence of complement activation has been provided by the recent investigations of Potter et al. (1980) in which increased serum concentrations of C1-INH (C1 esterase inhibitor) and C3b-INA (C3b inactivator) were found to be elevated in patients with active ulcerative colitis and Crohn's disease. Overall, the above studies indicate that there is activation of complement that will be consistently

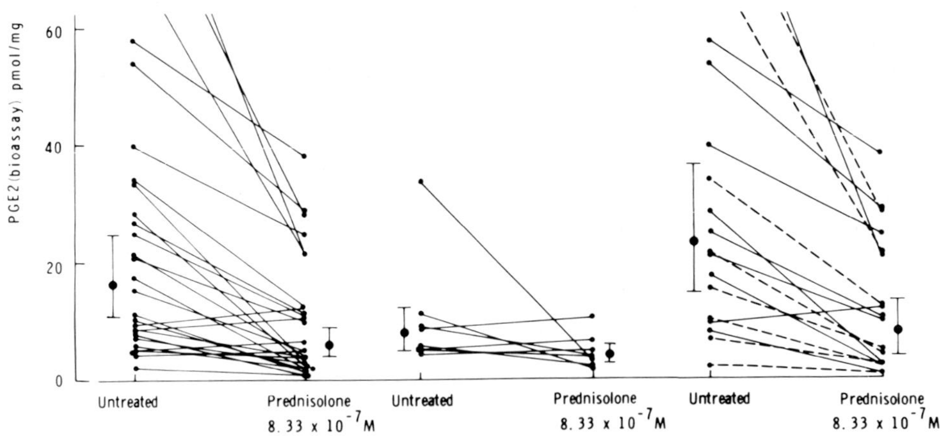

Fig. 6. Measurement of prostaglandin PGE_2 synthesized in vitro by uninflamed or inflamed biopsies. Note decrease in PGE_2 levels in tissues treated with 8.33 x 10^{-7} mol l^{-1} prednisolone. (Data from Hawkey and Truelove 1981. Used with permission.)

seen in patients with active IBD. The mechanism(s) for initiation of such complement activation is, however, unclear at the present time.

Prostaglandins have been shown to be of importance in both acute and chronic inflammatory reactions. In patients with ulcerative colitis, high levels of prostaglandins have been reported in the serum (Gould et al. 1977). This increase has been shown by Sharon et al. (1978) to be due to a rate of synthesis of prostaglandin E_2 that is twice normal in patients with ulcerative colitis. This increased synthesis of prostaglandin E_2 could be inhibited in vitro by sulfasalazine. The serum studies of Sharon et al. (1978) have been extended recently by Rampton et al. (1980), who demonstrated that the prostaglandin E_2-like material obtained by in-vivo rectal dialysis was increased over the levels found in control individuals: 3-fold in patients with ulcerative colitis in remission and 13-fold in patients with ulcerative colitis in relapse. Hawkey and Truelove (1981), using in-vitro organ culture found that the mean synthesis of prostaglandin E_2 by inflamed tissues was significantly greater than that of non-inflamed tissues (Fig. 6). This increased synthesis could be decreased by incubating the tissues with a prednisolone concentration of 8.33×10^{-7} mol l^{-1} (Fig. 6). These studies, which indicate that prednisolone and sulfasalazine can effectively modify synthesis of prostaglandin E_2, bring hope that the inflammation in inflammatory bowel disease may be ameliorated by inhibiting prostaglandin synthesis.

10.4. IMMUNE COMPLEXES AND INFLAMMATORY BOWEL DISEASE

There is good evidence from experimental models that immune complexes can produce a histopathologic picture like that seen in IBD. Hodgson et al. (1978a) and Mee et al. (1979b) showed that if preformed complexes were injected intravenously into rabbits and a non-specific acute inflammation was created simultaneously by dilute formalin enemas, a severe colitis histologically similar to ulcerative colitis would result. Formalin enemas alone did not produce this histologic picture.

Circulating immune complexes have been found in the sera of some patients with IBD (Jewell and MacLennan 1973; Hodgson et al. 1977a). However, a recent study by Kemler and Alpert (1980) using a sensitive Raji cell assay found that most patients with IBD do not have circulating immune complexes. Further, the presence of circulating immune complexes and their level did not correlate with disease severity, type, or location of disease (Fig. 7). This discrepancy may be explained in the report by Soltis et al. (1979) that aggregated immunoglobulins, rather than immune complexes, have erroneously been interpreted as immune complexes in patients with IBD. Their data using C1q precipitation demonstrated no significant difference between IBD patients and controls (Fig. 8). Furthermore, most workers, including the present author, have not been able to consistently demonstrate immunoglobulin or complement immune complex deposition in the involved tissues of patients with IBD.

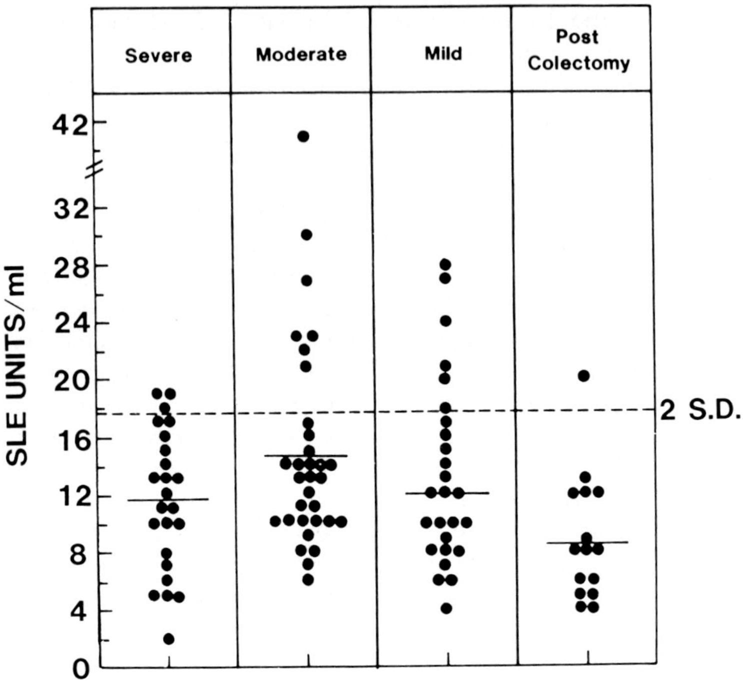

Fig. 7. Circulating immune complex levels in serum of patients with varying degrees of severity of colitis. Note lack of correlation between severity of disease and immune complex levels. (Data from Kember and Alpert 1980. Used with permission.)

Leroux-Roels et al. (1981) have pointed out the existence of circulating complexes of alkaline phosphatase and immunoglobulin in serum samples of patients with IBD. In 20 patients with IBD, alkaline phosphatase–immunoglobulin complexes were found in three and LDH (lactatic dehydrogenase) complexes in two others. Formation of complexes between immunoglobulins and enzymes has been described for several enzymes (Winship 1981). This, however, is only the second instance of association of enzyme–immunoglobulin complex with a particular disease. However, the relationship of these enzyme–immunoglobulin complexes to the inflammatory process in the bowel is not clear at present.

10.5. ANTIBODY-DEPENDENT CELL-MEDIATED CYTOTOXICITY (ADCC)

Mechanisms other than complement-dependent cytotoxicity and cell-mediated cytotoxicity by T-lymphocytes can be involved in tissue injury. ADCC was first

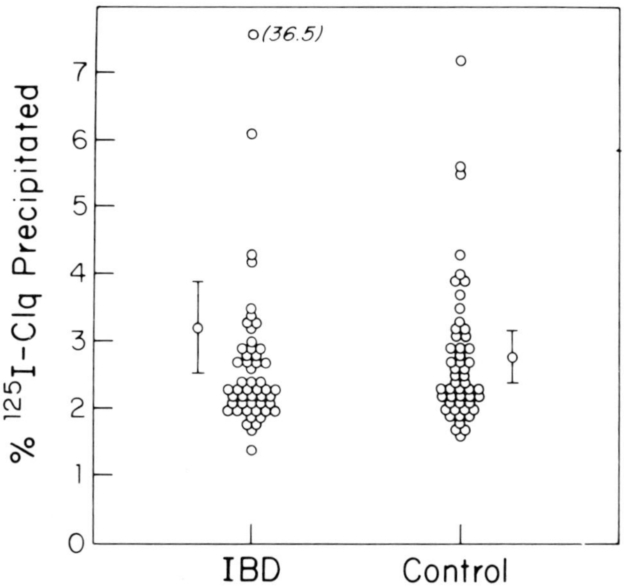

Fig. 8. Circulating immune complex levels demonstrated by ^{125}I-C1q precipitation in sera of controls and patients with IBD. There was no significant difference between the two groups. (Data from Soltis et al. 1979. Used with permission.)

described as cell damage from the collaboration of specific IgG and null-lymphocytes. Although null-lymphocytes lack surface immunoglobulin or T-cell markers when studied by conventional techniques, this cell has a receptor for the Fc portion of IgG. When ^{51}Cr-labeled target cells are reacted with specific antibody and then mixed with null-lymphocytes, membrane damage with release of ^{51}Cr results. The specific antibody alone (in the absence of complement), or null-lymphocytes alone, will not damage the cell membrane. The specificity of ADCC, therefore, is due to the antibody while the cytotoxic damage is mediated by the lymphocyte. Neutrophils, monocytes, eosinophils can mediate ADCC as well as lymphocytes.

Studies by Fanger et al. (1980) indicate that peripheral blood phagocytes have surface receptors for IgA. IgA-mediated ADCC has been demonstrated with peripheral blood effector cells but has been a relatively weak effect (Lowell et al. 1979, 1980; Keren et al. 1980; Smith et al. 1981). Shen and Fanger (1981) also have shown that specific IgA can act in synergy with IgG in mediating ADCC by neutrophils and monocytes.

Relative to the bowel epithelium, these findings may have considerable importance when viewed in context of the demonstration by Arnaud-Battandier et al. (1978) that intraepithelial lymphocytes in the guinea pig gut are enriched in killer cells that can effect ADCC. Others have found lamina propria-derived lymphocytes to be ineffective in mediating ADCC with cell-line targets although they could mediate ADCC with erythrocytes (MacDermott et al. 1980). Thus, the particular compartment (intraepithelial, lamina propria, peripheral blood, etc.) from which the effector cells were derived and target cells may have considerable influence on the results and conclusions obtained.

Eosinophils are of particular interest in this process for the gastrointestinal tract. Capron and co-workers demonstrated that eosinophils can destroy *Schistosoma mansoni* schistosomula coated with schistosomula-specific IgG 2A (Capron et al. 1978). Eosinophils bound to the antibody-coated schistosomula and damaged the surface membrane (Fig. 9). Further, factors released from mast cells enhanced eosinophil-mediated killing of schistosomula.

All the above mentioned studies provide evidence that ADCC-like phenomena exist in the bowel. That such mechanisms are operating in patients with IBD was suggested several years ago when Shorter et al. (1969) demonstrated that peripheral blood mononuclear cells from these patients were able to kill colonic epithelial cells in vitro. A non-T-, non-B-cell population was subsequently found to be responsible for mediating this damage (Stobo et al. 1976). Further, it has been shown that killer lymphocytes and monocytes are prevalent in mesenteric lymph nodes of patients with Crohn's disease but not in mesenteric nodes of control individuals (Britton et al. 1978).

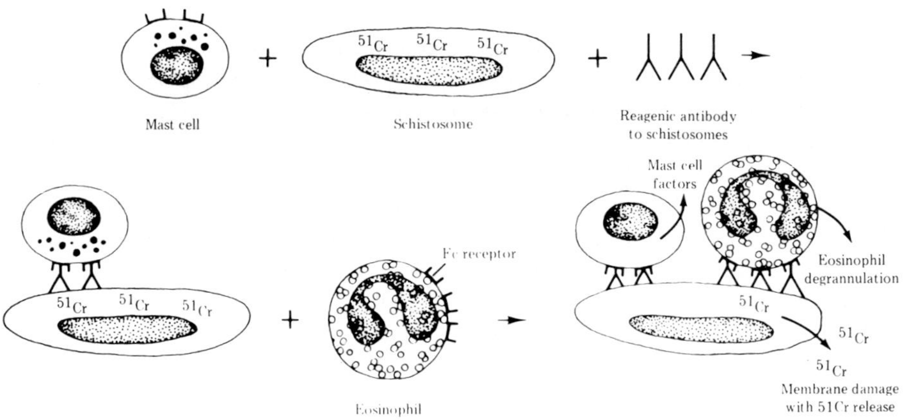

Fig. 9. Schematic representation showing damage to schistosome membranes by antibody-dependent cell-mediated cytotoxicity. Most cells seem to enhance the killing by eosinophils. (Reprinted from Keren, D.F.: *Immunology and Immunopathology of the Gastrointestinal Tract,* ASCP, 1980, with permission.)

However, for the ADCC mechanism to have meaning, specific antibodies need to be demonstrated. Such antibodies with reactivity against colonic mucosa were identified first in patients with ulcerative colitis over two decades ago (Broberger and Perlmann 1959). However, such studies were difficult to perform, technically. More recently, Carlsson et al. (1977) were able to demonstrate anti-colon antibodies in patients with inflammatory bowel disease. They found a significantly increased anti-colon antibody titer in 60% of the 148 patients examined who had Crohn's disease. Only 13% of control patients (280 individuals) had elevated titers. However, individuals with other unrelated diseases, such as urinary tract infections or cirrhosis, also had significantly increased titers in 69 and 62% respectively, of the individuals studied.

These studies indicate that a cytotoxic mechanism mediated by specific antibodies and carried out by local granulocytes, monocytes, or lymphocytes is a potential explanation for the mucosal damage in patients with inflammatory bowel disease. The specifics and their exact relationship to the disease have not yet been worked out to satisfaction. One possible problem in obtaining clear-cut information is that most studies have not looked at the specific antibodies being produced locally in the bowel (where the damage occurs!) and most studies have not used lamina propria or intraepithelial lymphocytes to look for cytotoxic damage. By using more specific, relevant, and sensitive techniques, it should be possible to sort out whether the above described phenomena are indeed related to IBD.

10.6. CELL-MEDIATED IMMUNITY IN INFLAMMATORY BOWEL DISEASE

The cell-mediated immunity of patients with IBD is impaired. In addition to poor responses against tuberculin skin tests, cutaneous anergy to dinitrochlorobenzene (DNCB; a compound that reacts with normal tissue components and which is highly immunogenic for T-cell-mediated responses) has been found in patients with IBD (Meyers et al. 1976). As an in-vitro corollary of poor cell-mediated immune function, Fiske and Falchuck (1980) have shown poor mixed-lymphocyte culture reaction of lymphocytes from the peripheral blood of patients with IBD.

Enumeration of the overall T-lymphocytes in peripheral blood has provided relatively little useful information. In recent years, it has become clear that many subpopulations of T-lymphocytes exist in broad categories such as T-killer cells, T-helper cells and T-suppressor cells. With the availability of monoclonal antibodies, a finer dissection of T-lymphocyte subpopulations is possible. Besides the use of monoclonal antibodies it has been shown that T-cells can be subclassified on the basis of their surface receptors for IgG, IgA and IgM (Pichler et al. 1978; Lum et al. 1979). These receptors are inducible by elevated serum antibody concentrations of homologous isotype (Hoover et al. 1981).

A considerable reduction in the proportion of T-cells with surface receptors for

IgM ($T\mu$) has been found in IBD patients, whether the disease was in an active phase or in remission. No difference was found in the number of $T\gamma$-cells between patients with inflammatory bowel disease and control individuals (Victorino and Hodgson 1980). In general, $T\mu$-cells are thought to be associated with helper T-cell populations and $T\gamma$-cells are enriched in suppressor T-cell populations. The number of $T\mu$-cells present correlated with the ability to mediate T-cell help with the T-cell mitogens PHA and con-A and the T- and B-cell mitogen PWM.

The decrease in $T\mu$-cells could relate to their loss into the gut lumen or to sequestration into the lamina propria of the gut. However, this would not completely satisfy the observation that $T\mu$-cells are decreased both in active and in inactive disease (in inactive disease only trivial increase in lamina propria lymphocytes would be expected). Another possibility is that lymphocytotoxic antibody which is found in most patients with IBD (Korsmeyer et al. 1975) may have selective activity for the $T\mu$-subset. Such subset lymphocytic antibody activity has already been demonstrated by Sakane et al. (1979) in patients with systemic lupus erythematosis.

In addition to decreased $T\mu$-cells, Auer et al. (1980) have reported a decrease in natural killer cell activity in patients with Crohn's disease. Natural killer cells are lymphocytes that can destroy target cells in vitro without known prior sensitization and without the aid of specific antibody. Decreased natural killer cell activity may reflect active sequestration of these cells into the gut to effect damage on gut epithelial cells.

Hodgson et al. (1978b) found that suppressor cell activity was decreased in 7 of 11 patients with IBD. Since decreased suppressor T-cells are thought to be a factor in autoimmune-disease systemic lupus erythematosis (Sakane et al. 1979), this observation is relevant to development of autoreactive phenomena such as anti-colon antibodies and lymphocytotoxic antibodies. However, more recent studies by Elson et al. (1981) indicate that suppressor T-cell activity is not impaired when one makes a detailed study by separating the suppressor T-cell population in vitro.

10.7. MUCOSAL IMMUNOCYTES AND INFLAMMATORY BOWEL DISEASE

Whereas most studies of cell-mediated immunity have looked at populations of peripheral blood lymphocytes, the lymphocyte subpopulations of key importance to study are those in the epithelium and the lamina propria of the gut. Techniques are now available which allow isolation and study of the functional capabilities of mucosal lymphocytes from patients with inflammatory bowel disease.

Most lymphocytes isolated from the gut lamina propria are T-cells with B-lymphocytes being increased in inflamed tissues (Eade et al. 1980). Likewise, studies of intraepithelial lymphocytes have found about 90% T-cells (Selby et al. 1981). This may be of great importance since intraepithelial lymphocytes were the cells that Arnaud-Battandier et al. (1978) showed to be involved in antibody-dependent cell-mediated cytotoxicity in guinea pig intestine. Both B-lymphocytes with surface IgG and IgG-synthesizing plasma cells are increased in the lamina propria of patients with IBD (Bookman and Bull 1979). This may have significance as the studies by Shen and Fanger (1981) indicate that IgG may act synergistically with IgA in mediating ADCC.

That gut lymphocytes may play a role in IBD is further suggested by a cell-mediated hypersensitivity model by Rabin and Rogers (1978), in which rabbits were sensitized with DNCB and then challenged with an intracolonic dose of DNCB. This resulted in crypt abscesses, superficial ulceration and mucous depletion resembling acute IBD. The lesions regressed, but would reappear when DNCB was reapplied to the colon. This reproduces the remissions and exacerbations seen in IBD. Also, after numerous intracolonic doses of DNCB, the animals demonstrated cutaneous hypersensitivity to colon antigens. This demonstration that T-cell hypersensitivity can produce an IBD picture is an impetus to further functional studies of mucosal lymphocytes in IBD. Glick and Falchuck (1981) reproduced the DNCB colitis model in guinea pigs and showed that their experimental animals had lamina propria lymphocytes with a greater percentage of T-cells and a greater capacity to mediate mitogen-induced cellular cytotoxicity than mucosal lymphocytes from control animals. Their data imply that the cytotoxic capability of lamina propria lymphocytes is an important determinant for production of epithelial injury in the DNCB model.

Lastly, most workers have found no significant association of HLA antigens with ulcerative colitis or Crohn's disease (Vachon et al. 1976). However, Delpre et al. (1980) found that 60 European-born Jews with ulcerative colitis had a significant association of HLA-BW35 and with HLA-AW24; there was an association with early onset of severe disease. The meaning of such HLA association is unclear but possible interpretations include: (1) HLA-BW35 may be linked to genes regulating the immune response. (2) The HLA-BW35 antigen may be a cell surface receptor for a micro-organism that is involved in initiating ulcerative colitis. (3) The "causative" micro-organism(s) contains HLA-BW35 surface antigen and a poor immune response may form to it, allowing it to dwell in the infected tissues or initiating an autoimmune type response.

The immunologic mechanisms of tissue injury to gut epithelium are beginning to be defined. By applying techniques which look directly at the local humoral and cellular immune mechanisms in the gastrointestinal tract it may soon be possible to delineate the pathogenic role of the immune system in IBD.

ACKNOWLEDGEMENT

The author thanks Mrs. MaryAnn Byrnes for her excellent assistance in preparing the manuscript. Some of Dr. Keren's data and figures used in this chapter were from work supported by The National Foundation for Ileitis and Colitis (No. 341667).

REFERENCES

Auer, I.O., Ziemer, E. and Sommer, H. (1980) Immune status in Crohn's disease. V. Decreased in vitro natural killer cell activity in peripheral blood. *Clin. Exp. Immunol. 42,* 41-49.

Arnaud-Battandier, F., Bundy, B.M., O'Neill, M., Bienenstock, J. and Nelson, D.L. (1978) Cytotoxic activities of gut mucosal lymphoid cells in guinea pigs. *J. Immunol. 121,* 1059-1063.

Aronson, M.D., Phillips, C.A., Becken, W.L. and Forsyth, B.R. (1975) Isolation and characterization of a viral agent from intestinal tissue of patients with Crohn's disease and other intestinal disorders. *Prog. Med. Virol. 21,* 165-176.

Baklien, K. and Brandtzaeg, P. (1975) Comparative mapping of the local distribution of immunoglobulin-containing cells in ulcerative colitis and Crohn's disease of the colon. *Clin. Exp. Immunol. 22,* 197-209.

Beeken, W.L. (1980) Transmissible agents in inflammatory bowel disease: 1980. *Med. Clin. North Am. 64,* 1021-1035.

Belsheim, M.R., Darwish, R., Watson, W.C. and Sullivan, S.N. (1980) Bacterial L forms in inflammatory bowel disease (Abstract). *Gastroenterology 78,* 1139.

Bolton, P.M., Owen, E., Heatley, R.V., Williams, W.J. and Hughes, L.E. (1973) Negative findings in laboratory animals for a transmissible agent in Crohn's disease. *Lancet 2,* 1122-1124.

Bookman, M.A. and Bull, D.M. (1979) Characteristics of isolated intestinal mucosal lymphoid cells in inflammatory bowel disease. *Gastroenterology 77,* 503-510.

Brandtzaeg, P., Baklien, K., Fausa, O. and Hoel, P.S. (1974) Immunohistochemical characterization of local immunoglobulin formation in ulcerative colitis. *Gastroenterology 66,* 1123-1136.

Britton, S., Eklund, A.E. and Bird, A.G. (1978) Appearance of killer (K) cells in the mesenteric lymph nodes in Crohn's disease. *Gastroenterology 75,* 218-227.

Broberger, O. and Perlmann, P. (1959) Autoantibodies in human ulcerative colitis. *J. Exp. Med. 110,* 657-674.

Burnham, W.R., Lennard-Jones, J.E., Stanford, J.L. and Bird, R.G. (1978) Mycobacteria as a possible cause of inflammatory bowel disease. *Lancet 2,* 693-696.

Capron, M., Rousseaux, J., Mazingue, C., Bazin, H. and Capron, A. (1978) Rat mast cell-eosinophil interaction in antibody-dependent eosinophil cytotoxicity to Schistosoma mansoni schistosomula. *J. Immunol. 121,* 2518-2525.

Carlsson, H.E., Lagercrantz, R. and Perlmann, P. (1977) Immunological studies in ulcerative colitis. VIII. Antibodies to colon antigen in patients with ulcerative colitis, Crohn's disease, and other diseases. *Scand. J. Gastroenterol. 12,* 707-714.

Cave, D.R., Mitchell, D.N., Kane, S.P. and Brooke, B.N. (1973) Further animal evidence of a transmissible agent in Crohn's disease. *Lancet 2,* 1120-1122.

Cave, D.R., Mitchell, D.N. and Brooke, B.N. (1976) Evidence of an agent transmissible from ulcerative colitis tissue. *Lancet 1,* 1311-1314.

Cave, D.R., Mitchell, D.N. and Brooke, B.N. (1978) Induction of granulomas in mice by Crohn's disease tissues. *Gastroenterology 75,* 632-637.

Cave, D.R., Mitchell, D.N. and Brooke, B.N. (1979) Correspondence: Induction of granulomas in mice by Crohn's disease tissues. *Gastroenterology 77,* 202-203.

Cave, D.R., Kirsner, J., McLaren, L., Strickland, R., Phillips, A., Auslander, M., Sachar, D., Janowitz, H., Shorter, R., Bartlett, J., Pitt, H., Ferin, B., Jones, M. and Gitnick, G. (1980) Infectious agents in inflammatory bowel disease (IBD): A status report (Abstract). *Gastroenterology 78,* 1185.

Clark, K.A. and Keren, D.F. (1982) Demonstration of monoclonal lymphoplasmacytic proliferations by immunofluorescence on routine formalin-fixed, paraffin-embedded tissue. *Cancer, 49,* 2376-2382.

Cohen, Z., Jirsch, D., Archibald, S., Leung, M.K. and Gardner, J. (1980) The production of granulomas in rabbit bowel (Abstract). *Gastroenterology 78,* 1152.

Cooke, E.M. (1967) A quantitative comparison of the fecal flora of patients with ulcerative colitis and that of normal persons. *J. Pathol. Bacteriol. 94,* 439-444.

Cooper, H.S., Raffensberger, E.L., Jonas, L. and Fitts Jr, W.T. (1977) Cytomegalovirus inclusions in patients with ulcerative colitis and toxic dilation requiring colonic resection. *Gastroenterology 72,* 1253-1256.

Crohn, B.B., Ginzburg, L. and Oppenheimer, G.D. (1932) Regional ileitis; a pathological and clinical entity. *J. Am. Med. Assoc. 99,* 1323-1329.

Das, K.M., Valenzuela, I. and Morecki, R. (1980) Crohn's disease lymph node homogenates produce murine lymphoma in athymic mice. *Proc. Natl Acad. Sci. USA 77,* 588-592.

Davidson, I.W., Lloyd, R.S., Whorwell, P.J. and Wright, R. (1979) Antibodies to maize in patients with Crohn's disease, ulcerative colitis and coeliac disease. *Clin. Exp. Immunol. 35,* 147-148.

DeGroote, G., Desmyter, J., Vantrappen, C. and Phillips, C.A. (1977) Rotavirus antibodies in Crohn's disease and ulcerative colitis. *Lancet 2,* 1263-1264.

Delacroix, D. and Vaerman, J.P. (1981) Reassessment of levels of secretory IgA in pathological sera using a quantitative radioimmunoassay. *Clin. Exp. Immunol. 43,* 633-640.

Delpre, G., Kadish, U., Gazet, E., Joshua, H. and Zamir, R. (1980) HLA antigens in ulcerative colitis and Crohn's disease in Israel. *Gastroenterology 78,* 1452-1457.

Donnelly, B.J., Delaney, P.V. and Healy, T.M. (1977) Evidence for a transmissible factor in Crohn's disease. *Gut 18,* 360-363.

Eade, O.E., Andre-Ukena, S., St. Moulton, C., MacPherson, B. and Beeken, W.L. (1980) Lymphocyte subpopulations of intestinal mucosa in inflammatory bowel disease. *Gut 21,* 675-682.

Elson, C.O., Graeff, A.S., James, S.P. and Strober, W. (1981) Covert suppressor T-cells in Crohn's disease. *Gastroenterology 80,* 1513-1521.

Fanger, M.W., Shen, L., Pugh, J. and Bernier, G.M. (1980) Subpopulations of human peripheral granulocytes and monocytes express receptors for IgA. *Proc. Natl Acad. Sci. USA 77,* 3640-3642.

Fiske, S.C. and Falchuk, Z.M. (1980) Impaired mixed-lymphocyte culture reactions in patients with inflammatory bowel disease. *Gastroenterology 79,* 682-686.

Gerber, M.A., Paronetto, F. and Kockwa, S. (1971) Immunohistochemical localization of IgE in asthmatic lungs. *Am. J. Pathol. 62,* 339-343.

Gitnick, G.L., Rosen, V.J., Arthur, M.H. and Hertweck, S.A. (1979) Evidence for the isolation of a new virus from ulcerative colitis patients. Comparison with virus derived from Crohn's disease. *Dig. Dis. Sci. 24,* 609-619.

Glick, M.E. and Falchuk, Z.M. (1981) Dinitrochlorobenzene-induced colitis in the guinea pig: studies of colonic lamina propria lymphocytes. *Gut 22,* 120-125.

Gould, S.R., Brash, A.R. and Conolly, M.E. (1977) Increased prostaglandin production in ulcerative colitis. *Lancet 2,* 98-99.

Green, F.H.Y. and Fox, H. (1975) The distribution of mucosal antibodies in the bowel of patients with Crohn's disease. *Gut 16,* 125-131.

Greenberg, H.B., Gebhard, R.L., McClain, C.J., Soltis, R.D and Kapikian, A.Z. (1979) Antibodies to viral gastroenteritis virus in Crohn's disease. *Gastroenterology 76,* 349-350.

Hawkey, C.J. and Truelove, S.C. (1981) Effect of prednisolone on prostaglandin synthesis by rectal mucosa in ulcerative colitis: investigation by laminar flow bioassay and radioimmunoassay. *Gut 22,* 190-193.

Heatley, R.V. and James, P.D. (1978) Eosinophils in rectal mucosa. *Gut 20,* 787-791.

Heatley, R.V., Bolton, P.M., Owen, E., Williams, W.J. and Hughes, L.E. (1975) A search for a transmissible agent in Crohn's disease. *Gut 16,* 528-532.

Heatley, R.V., Calcraft, B.J., Rhodes, J., Owen, E. and Evans, B.K. (1975) Disodium cromoglycate in the treatment of chronic proctitis. *Gut 16,* 559-563.

Helphingstine, C.J., Hentges, D.J., Campbell, B.J., Butt, J. and Barrett, J.T. (1979) Antibodies detectable by counter immunoelectrophoresis against Bacteroides antigens in serum of patients with inflammatory bowel disease. *J. Clin. Microbiol. 9,* 373-378.

Hodgson, H.J.F. and Jewell, D.P. (1978) The humoral immune system in inflammatory bowel disease. II. Immunoglobulin levels. *Am. J. Dig. Dis. 23,* 123-129.

Hodgson, H.J.F., Potter, B.J. and Jewell, D.P. (1977a) Immune complexes in ulcerative colitis and Crohn's disease. *Clin. Exp. Immunol. 29,* 187-196.

Hodgson, H.J.F., Potter, B.J. and Jewell, D.P. (1977b) C3 metabolism in ulcerative colitis and Crohn's disease. *Clin. Exp. Immunol. 29,* 490-495.

Hodgson, H.J.F., Potter, B.J., Skinner, J. and Jewell, D.P. (1978a) Immune complex-mediated colitis in rabbits. An experimental model. *Gut 19,* 225-232.

Hodgson, H.J.F., Wands, J.R. and Isselbacher, K.J. (1978b) Decreased suppressor cell activity in inflammatory bowel disease. *Clin. Exp. Immunol. 32,* 451-458.

Hoover, R.G., Dieckgralfe, B.K. and Lynch, R.G. (1981) T cells with Fc receptors for IgA: induction of T cells in vivo and in vitro by purified IgA. *J. Immunol. 127,* 1560-1563.

Huang, S., Minassian, H. and More, J.D. (1976) Application of immunofluorescent staining on paraffin sections improved by trypsin digestion. *Lab. Invest. 35,* 383-390.

Iscaki, S. and Buffet, C. (1978) Secretory IgA increase in sera of patients with liver disease. *Ric. Clin. Lab. 8 (Suppl. 1),* 287-293.

Jewell, D.P. and MacLennan, I.C.M. (1973) Circulating immune complexes in inflammatory bowel disease. *Clin. Exp. Immunol. 14,* 219-226.

Kapikian, A.Z., Barile, M.F., Wyati, R.G., Yolken, R.H., Tully, J.G., Greenberg, H.B., Kalica, A.R. and Chenock, R.M. (1979) Mycoplasma contamination in cell culture of Crohn's disease material. *Lancet 2,* 466-467.

Keighley, M.R.B., Arabi, Y., Dimock, F., Burdon, D.W., Allan, R.N. and Alexander-Williams, J. (1978) Influence of inflammatory bowel disease on intestinal microflora. *Gut 19,* 1099-1104.

Kember, B.J. and Alpert, E. (1980) Inflammatory bowel disease associated circulating immune complexes. *Gut 21,* 195-201.

Keren, D.F., Milligan, F.D., Strandberg, J.D. and Yardley, J.H. (1975) Intercurrent cytomegalovirus colitis in a patient with ulcerative colitis. *Johns Hopkins Med. J. 136,* 178-182.

Keren, D.F., Nair, M., Rosillo, M. and Schwartz, S.A. (1980) Antigen-specific secretory IgA can mediate antibody-dependent cell-mediated cytotoxicity against eukaryotic target cells (Abstract). *Gastroenterology 78,* 1194.

Keren, D.F., Appelman, H.D., Geisinger, K.R. and Foley, J.L. (1982) Immunoglobulin-containing cells in inflammatory bowel disease: correlation of immunofluorescence findings with histopathology (Abstract). *Lab. Invest., 46,* 45A.

Korsmeyer, S.J., Williams, R.C., Wilson, I.D. and Strickland, R.G. (1975) Lymphocytotoxic antibody in inflammatory bowel disease. A family study. *N. Engl. J. Med. 293,* 1117-1120.

Lake, A.J., Stitzel, A.E., Urmson, J.R., Walker, W.A. and Spitzer, R.E. (1979) Complement alterations in inflammatory bowel disease. *Gastroenterology 76,* 1374-1379.

Lennard-Jones, J.E., Cooper, G.W., Newell, A.C., Wilson, C.W.E. and Avery Jones, F. (1962) Observations on idiopathic proctitis. *Gut 3,* 201-206.

Leroux-Roels, G.G., Wieme, R.J. and DeBroe, M.E. (1981) Occurrence of enzyme-immunoglobulin complexes in chronic inflammatory bowel disease. *J. Lab. Clin. Med. 97,* 316-321.

Lloyd, G., Green, F.H.Y., Fox, H., Mani, V. and Turnberg, L.A. (1975) Mast cells and immunoglobulin E in inflammatory bowel disease. *Gut 16,* 861-886.

Lowell, G.H., Smith, L.F., Griffiss, J.M. and Brandt, B.L. (1979) Antibody-dependent monocyte-mediated antibacterial activity. *J. Exp. Med. 150,* 127-134.

Lowell, G.H., Smith, L.F., Griffiss, J.M., Brandt, B.L. and MacDermott, R.P. (1980) Antibody-dependent mononuclear cell-mediated anti-meningococcal activity. *J. Clin. Invest. 66,* 260-264.

Lum, L.G., Muchmore, A.V., Keren, D.F., Decker, J., Koski, I., Strober, W. and Blaese, R.M. (1979) A receptor for IgA on human T lymphocytes. *J. Immunol. 122,* 65-69.

MacDermott, R.P., Franklin, G.O., Jenkins, K.M., Kodner, I.J., Nash, G.S. and Weinrieb, I.J. (1980) Human intestinal mononuclear cells. I. Investigation of antibody-dependent, lectin-induced, and spontaneous cell-mediated cytotoxic capabilities. *Gastroenterology 78,* 47-56.

Mee, A.S., Brown, D. and Jewell, D.P. (1979a) Atopy in inflammatory bowel disease. *Scand. J. Gastroenterol. 14,* 743-6.

Mee, A.S., McLaughlin, J.E., Hodgson, H.J.F. and Jewell, D.P. (1979b) Chronic immune colitis in rabbits. *Gut 20,* 1-8.

Meyers, S., Sachar, D.B., Taub, R.N. and Janowitz, H.D. (1976) Anergy to dinitrochlorobenzene and depression of T-lymphocytes in Crohn's disease and ulcerative colitis. *Gut 17,* 911-920.

Mitchell, D.N. and Rees, R.J.W. (1970) Agent transmissible from Crohn's disease tissue. *Lancet 2,* 168-171.

Monis, B. and Mendeloff, A.L. (1961) Observations on inclusion bodies in normal and pathologic mucosa of the colon in man. *J. Natl Cancer Inst. 26,* 1429-1444.

O'Donoghue, D.P. and Kumar, P. (1979) Rectal IgE cells in inflammatory bowel disease. *Gut 20,* 149-153.

Parent, K. and Mitchell, P. (1978) Cell wall defective variants of Pseudomonas-like (Group Va) bacteria in Crohn's disease. *Gastroenterology 75,* 368-372.

Parent, K., Mitchell, P. and Beltros, E. (1980) Pilot animal pathogenicity studies with cell-wall defective Pseudomonas-like bacteria isolated from Crohn's disease patients (Abstract). *Gastroenterology 78,* 1233.

Phillpotts, R.J., Hermon-Taylor, J. and Brooke, B.N. (1979) Virus isolation studies in Crohn's disease. A negative report. *Gut 20,* 1057-1062.

Pichler, W.J., Lum, L. and Broder, S. (1978) Fc-receptors on human T-lymphocytes. I. Transition of Tγ to Tμ cells. *J. Immunol. 121,* 1540-1548.

Potter, B.J., Hodgson, H.J.F., Mee, A.S. and Jewell, D.P. (1979) C1q metabolism in ulcerative colitis and Crohn's disease. *Gut 20,* 1012-1019.

Potter, B.J., Brown, D.J.C., Watson, A. and Jewell, D.P. (1980) Complement inhibitors and immunoconglutinins in ulcerative colitis and Crohn's disease. *Gut 21,* 1030-1034.

Qualman, S.J. and Keren, D.F. (1979) Immunofluorescence of deparaffinized, trypsin-treated renal tissues. Preservation of antigens as adjunct to diagnosis of disease. *Lab. Invest. 41,* 483-489.

Rampton, D.S., Sladen, G.E. and Youlten, L.J.F. (1980) Rectal mucosla prostaglandin E_2 release and its relationship to disease activity, electrical potential differences, and treatment in ulcerative colitis. *Gut 22,* 591-596.

Rabin, B.S. and Rogers, S.J. (1978) A cell-mediated immune model of inflammatory bowel disease in the rabbit. *Gastroenterology 75,* 29-33.

Roche, J.K. and Huang, E.S. (1977) Viral DNA in inflammatory bowel disease: CMV-bearing cells as a target for immune-mediated enterocytolysis. *Gastroenterology 72,* 228-233.

Rosekrans, P.C.M., Meijer, C.J.L.M., Van der Wal, A.M., Cornelisse, C.J. and Lindeman, J. (1980a) Immunoglobulin containing cells in inflammatory bowel disease of the colon: a morphometric and immunohistochemical study. *Gut 21,* 941-947.

Rosekrans, P.C.M., Meyer, C.J.L.M., Van der Wal, A.M. and Lindeman, J. (1980b) Allergic proctitis, a clinical and immunopathological entity. *Gut 21,* 1017-1023.

Sakane, T., Steinberg, A.D., Reeves, J.P. and Creen, I. (1979) Studies of immune functions of patients with systemic lupus erythematosus. Complement-dependent immunoglobulin M anti-thymus derived cell antibodies preferentially inactivate suppressor cells. *J. Clin. Invest. 63,* 954-958.

Schuller, J.L., Piket-van Ulsen, J., Veeken, I.V.D., Michel, M.F. and Stolz, E. (1979) Antibodies against Chlamydin of lymphogranuloma venereum type in Crohn's disease. *Lancet 1,* 19-20.

Selby, W.S., Janossy, G. and Jewell, D.P. (1981) Immunohistological characterization of intraepithelial lymphocytes of the human gastrointestinal tract. *Gut 22,* 169-175.

Sharon, P., Ligumsky, M., Rachmilewitz, D. and Zor, U. (1978) Role of prostaglandins in ulcerative colitis. Enhanced production during active disease and inhibition by sulfasalazine. *Gastroenterology 75,* 638-640.

Shen, L. and Fanger, M.W. (1981) Secretory IgA antibodies synergize with IgG in promoting ADCC by human polymorphonuclear cells, monocytes, and lymphocytes. *Cell. Immunol. 59,* 75-81.

Shiner, M., Ballard, J. and Smith, M.E. (1975) The small intestinal mucosa in cow's milk allergy. *Lancet 1,* 136-137.

Shorter, R.G., Cardoza, M., Spencer, R.J. and Huizenga, K.A. (1969) Further studies of in vitro cytotoxicity of lymphocytes from patients with ulcerative and granulomatous colitis for allogeneic colonic epithelial cells including the effects of colectomy. *Gastroenterology 56,* 304-314.

Simonowitz, D., Block, G.E., Riddell, R.H., Kraft, S.C. and Kirsner, J.B. (1977) The production of an unusual tissue reaction in rabbit bowel injected with Crohn's disease homogenates. *Surgery 82,* 211-218.

Skinner, J.M. and Whitehead, R. (1974) The plasma cells in inflammatory disease of the colon: a quantitative study. *J. Clin. Pathol. 27,* 643-646.

Smith, L.F., Collins, H.H., Wilson, S.R., Formal, S.B., Keren, D.F. and Lowell, G.H. (1981) Secretory IgA-dependent mononuclear cell-mediated antibacterial activity (Abstract). *Fed. Proc. 40,* 1974.

Soltis, R.D., Hasz, D., Morris, M.J. and Wilson, I.D. (1979) Evidence against the presence of circulating immune complexes in chronic inflammatory bowel disease. *Gastroenterology 76,* 1380-1385.

Soltoft, J., Binder, V. and Gudmand-Hoyer, E. (1973) Intestinal immunoglobulins in ulcerative colitis. *Scand. J. Gastroenterol. 8,* 293-300.

Stobo, J.D., Tomasi, T.B., Huizenga, K.A., Spencer, R.J. and Shorter, R.G. (1976) In vitro studies of inflammatory bowel disease. Surface receptors of the mononuclear cell required to lyse allogeneic colonic epithelial cells. *Gastroenterology 70,* 171-176.

Strickland, R.G., Volpicelli, N.A., Robinson, J.M., Greenlee, L.S. and McLaren, L.C. (1979) Isolation of infectious agents from patients with inflammatory bowel disease (Abstract). *Clin. Res. 27,* 29A.

Tabagchali, S., O'Donoghue, D.P. and Bettelheim, D.A. (1978) Escherichia coli antibodies in patients with inflammatory bowel disease. *Gut 19,* 108-113.

Taub, R.N., Sachar, D., Janowitz, H. and Slitzbach, L.E. (1976) Induction of granulomas in mice by inoculation of tissue homogenates from patients with inflammatory bowel disease and sarcoidosis. *Ann. NY Acad. Sci. 278,* 560-564.

Thayer, W.R., Jr (1979) Executive summary of the AGA-NFIC sponsored workshop on infectious agents in inflammatory bowel disease. *Dig. Dis. Sci. 24,* 781-784.

Thompson, R.A., Asquith, P. and Cooke, W.T. (1969) Secretory IgA in serum. *Lancet 2,* 517-519.

Vachon, A., Gebuhrer, L. and Betuel, H. (1976) HL-A antigens in ulcerative colitis and Crohn's disease. Abstract V-18 In: J. Dansset (Ed.), *First International Symposium on HL-A and Diseases, Paris, 23-25 June, 1976,* Editions INSERM, Paris, p. 170.

Van der Wiel-Korstanje, J.A.A. and Winkler, K.C. (1975) The fecal flora in ulcerative colitis. *J. Med. Microbiol. 8,* 491-501.

Victorino, R.M.M. and Hodgson, H.J.F. (1980) Alteration in T lymphocyte subpopulations in inflammatory bowel disease. *Clin. Exp. Immunol. 41,* 156-165.

Ward, M. and Eastwood, A.S. (1975) Serum complement components C2 and C4 in inflammatory bowel disease. *Digestion 13,* 100-103.

Whorwell, P.J., Phillips, C.A., Beeken, W.L., Little, P.K. and Roessner, K.D. (1977) Isolation of reovirus-like agents from patients with Crohn's disease. *Lancet 1,* 1169-1171.

Willoughby, C.P., Heyworth, M.F., Piris, J. and Truelove, S.C. (1979) Comparison of D.S.C.G. and sulphasalazine as maintenance therapy for ulcerative colitis. *Lancet 1,* 119-122.

Winship, D.H. (1981) Immune complexes in inflammatory bowel disease: cause or coincidence? *J. Lab. Clin. Med. 97,* 313-315.

Wright, R. and Truelove, S.C. (1965) Circulating antibodies to dietary proteins in ulcerative colitis. *Br. Med. J. 2,* 142-144.

CHAPTER 11

The contact system of plasma in inflammation

CHARLES G. COCHRANE

Department of Immunopathology, Scripps Clinic and Research Foundation, La Jolla, California 92037

11.1. INTRODUCTION

In the development of inflammation, considerable activity results from the interaction between cells and activated humoral constituents of the plasma. Four principal systems in plasma are involved: the complement, contact (Hageman factor), clotting and fibrinolytic systems. These four systems have the capacity to act in concert and cross-activate one another. Components of these systems also are known to interact with cells, leading to stimulation of their function, and various cells are known to release activators of the components of these protein systems of plasma.

We will concentrate on one of these systems, the contact or Hageman factor pathway, describing its biochemistry and interactions with cells and cellular constituents that may be important in the development of inflammation.

The components of the HF system are presented in Figure 1. The physical characteristics and biochemistry of activation of the components in solution and on a negatively charged surface are the subject of a recent review from this laboratory (Cochrane and Griffin 1982). In brief, when plasma contacts a negatively charged surface, a group of proteins interacts on the surface to produce a sequence of conversions of proenzymes to enzymes. This occurs as a burst of activity in a period of seconds. Hageman factor, prekallikrein, high molecular weight (high-MW) kininogen and clotting Factor XI are the principal molecules that undergo initial proteolytic cleavage as activation occurs. This cleavage appears to be essential for the rapid activation of each component. Hageman factor binds rapidly to the surface in whole plasma and the peptide chain is cleaved so as to produce chains of 28,000 and 52,000 MW which are held together by a small disulfide bridge. Cleavage then occurs at the N-terminal site of the disulfide bridge, allowing the smaller chain, which bears the enzymatic site of Hageman factor, to dissociate into the fluid phase (Revak and Cochrane 1976). The larger fragment remains surface-bound.

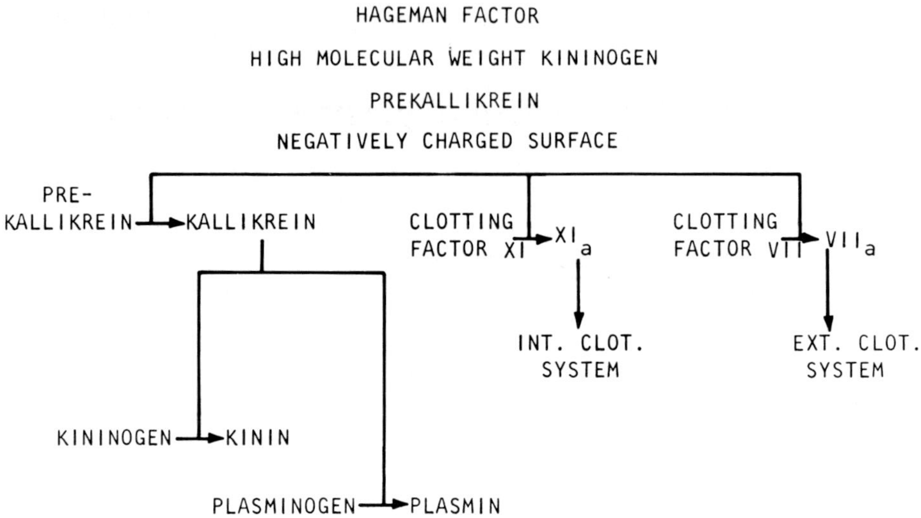

Fig. 1. Diagram of the sequences of activation of components of the Hageman factor system.

The enzyme in plasma responsible for the rapid cleavage of Hageman factor is kallikrein. Its precursor, prekallikrein, is itself cleaved into heavy and light chains and activated by Hageman factor. Thus a reciprocal activation by these two molecules has been proposed as a mechanism of activation of the contact system (Cochrane et al. 1973). The reciprocal enzymatic cleavage and activation of HF and prekallikrein is augmented by the fact that, when bound to the surface, Hageman factor is over 100-fold more susceptible to enzymatic cleavage (Griffin 1978). In the absence of prekallikrein, Hageman factor is cleaved and activated slowly, suggesting that other enzymes may play a secondary role. However, in the absence of prekallikrein, the clotting and kinin-generating activities are markedly retarded (Wuepper 1973).

Prekallikrein and Factor XI exist in plasma as a complex with high-MW kininogen (Mandle et al. 1976; Thompson and Kaplan 1977). The high-MW kininogen, acting stoichiometrically with Hageman factor (Griffin and Cochrane 1976), brings prekallikrein and Factor XI to the surface, where they are able to interact with Hageman factor (Wiggins et al. 1977). The light chain of high-MW kininogen bears a domain extremely rich in histidine residues, which apparently is responsible for the adherence of the molecule to negatively charged surfaces (Han et al. 1975). A portion of the light chain is also responsible for the complexing of high-MW kininogen with prekallikrein and Factor XI (Waldman et al. 1977; Thompson et al. 1978). Thus, high-MW kininogen acts as a cofactor, in a stoichiometric relation with Hageman factor, to promote the reciprocal activation of prekallikrein and

Hageman factor (Griffin and Cochrane 1976; Meier et al. 1977) and the cleavage and activation of Factor XI by Hageman factor.

Kallikrein rapidly dissociates from high-MW kininogen on the surface and cleaves and activates other surface-bound Hageman factor molecules (Cochrane and Revak 1980). The dissociating kallikrein also rapidly cleaves high-MW kininogen both on the surface and in fluid phase.

The initial event that triggers the activation of Hageman factor and prekallikrein is not precisely understood. While it has been thought for years that Hageman factor is activated upon binding to a surface, this has been questioned. In the absence of prekallikrein or high-MW kininogen, Hageman factor still becomes surface-bound, but does not activate and does not undergo cleavage for several minutes (well after the burst of activity that is seen in normal plasma) (Revak et al. 1977). Single-chain, zymogen Hageman factor binds ^{3}H-DFP extremely slowly, and this is not influenced by contact with a surface (Griffin 1977; Fujikawa et al. 1977). Data supporting surface activation have been presented in which zymogen or activated Hageman factor were found to activate prekallikrein at the same rate (Heimark et al. 1980). The prekallikrein was present in great excess (more that 60-fold higher concentration than that of normal plasma relative to the amount of Hageman factor used) and the possibility remained that rapid reciprocal cleavage and activation of the two molecules took place. This is especially true in view of the speed of reciprocal activation by kallikrein (Cochrane and Revak 1980). The possibility exists that an undetected exogenous enzyme could activate either prekallikrein or Hageman factor, although unequivocal evidence for this has not been obtained. And finally, the possibility that Hageman factor and prekallikrein are "active zymogens" has been raised (Cochrane and Griffin 1982). In support of this theory are the findings that both Hageman factor and prekallikrein slowly take up ^{3}H-DFP in a manner similar to that of trypsinogen. Surface binding of the Hageman factor does not alter the slow rate of uptake of the ^{3}H-DFP. In addition, zymogen HF, when brought onto a negatively charged surface in apposition with other zymogen HF molecules, leads to cleavage and "autoactivation" of the population of surface-bound HF. This latter event fails to occur when the HF molecules are less densely dispersed on the surface. We have proposed that HF and prekallikrein, when brought into contact with each other, can induce a triggering event leading to proteolytic cleavage and activation. The kallikrein binds to high-MW kininogen with relatively low affinity and rapidly dissociates, leading to cleavage of HF molecules bound elsewhere on the surface. This movement of kallikrein in fluid phase probably accounts for a great majority of activation of the HF. The kallikrein at the same time cleaves high-MW kininogen both in fluid phase and on the surface.

A summary of the molecular assembly leading to the activation of HF is given in Figure 2. At the upper left portion of the figure, HF and the complex of PK and high-MW kininogen (HMWK) are depicted in the plasma. It should be noted that Factor XI and HMWK also exist in plasma as a complex. When presented with a negatively charged surface (right side of the figure), HF and the complex of PK and HMWK

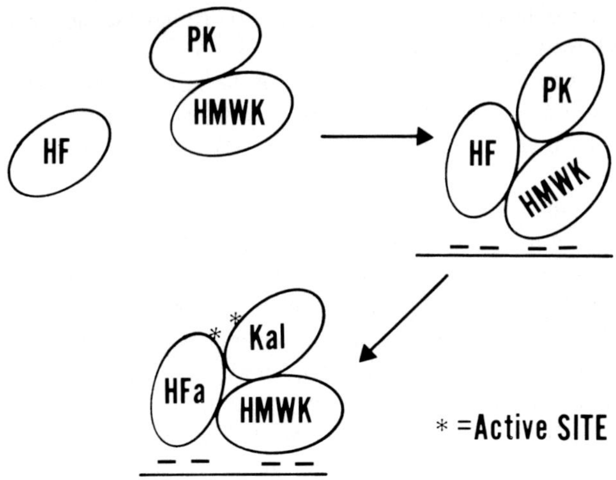

Fig. 2. Proposed mechanism of activation of Hageman factor (HF) and prekallikrein (PK), the cofactor, high-MW kininogen (HMWK). The proteins are seen in solution in the upper left. Upon contact with a negatively charged surface (right), the proteins are assembled, leading to activation of HF and PK. HMWK is cleaved in the process. See text for details.

become bound to the surface. This occurs by virtue of positively charged residues on the heavy chain of HF and a histidine-rich portion (termed Fragment 1-2) of the light chain of HMWK. The HF and PK are thus brought into apposition and activation of each takes place. This is aided by apparent conformational changes occurring in the HF upon surface contact in that the surface-bound molecule is approximately 500-fold more sensitive to enzymatic cleavage than the unbound HF.

11.2. ACTIVATION OF PROTEINS OF THE CONTACT SYSTEM BY CELLULAR ENZYMES

Several cells are now known to contain enzymes capable of cleaving and activating components of the HF system. Endothelial cells contain an enzyme(s) capable of cleaving HF into 52,000 and 28,000 MW fragments. When assessed for activity, the cleaved HF was found, in turn, to cleave and activate both prekallikrein and Factor XI, when bound to a negatively charged surface (Wiggins et al. 1980). The presence of the cofactor, high-MW kininogen, greatly enhanced the reaction with Factor XI, presumably by bringing the Factor XI to the surface where it encountered the cell enzyme-activated HF. The endothelial cell enzyme was associated with the 100,000 x *g* pellet of the cell, containing cytoplasmic and microsomal membranes, and was inhibited by diisopropylphosphofluoridate (DFP) (2 mmol/l) but not soybean trypsin inhibitor (50 g/ml), hirudin (8 mg/ml) or purified antibodies to prekallikrein or plasmin. Thus, this cell, which is located at the focal point of the initial inflammatory damage, contains an activator of the HF system.

Recent studies have revealed another pathway by which cellular constituents react with components of the HF system. In collaboration with Drs Newball, Meier, Lichtenstein and Kaplan, washed fragments of normal human lung were submitted to anaphylactic challenge and the supernatant fluid examined for the presence of histamine and enzymes capable of cleaving and activating components of the HF system. Following such challenge it was possible to isolate enzymes that cleaved HF, prekallikrein, Factor XI and high-MW kininogen, but not components of the complement system (C3, C5, C4, Factor B) or plasminogen (Newball et al. 1980). The high-MW kininogen released kinin during the interaction with enzyme, as revealed by contraction of the estrous rat uterus. The HF was cleaved in disulfide-linked fragments of 52,000 and approximately 28,000 MW, which cleaved the HF substrate D-Pro-Phe-Arg-p-nitroanalide. Prekallikrein was cleaved by an enzyme separable from the above enzymes on SP-Sephadex and DEAE-Sephacel, and was found in turn to cleave its peptide substrate Bz-Pro-Phe-Arg-p-nitroanalide (which is not cleaved by activated HF). Other assays on prekallikrein activity have not been performed. Thus, during the anaphylactic response, enzymes are released that generate activity of the HF system and release kinin. The role played by these components in anaphylaxis or similar IgE-initiated reactions remains to be determined.

Another interaction was proposed by Kaplan and Austen (1972), namely that kallikrein induces chemotaxis of neutrophils, but not eosinophils, while prekallikrein or DFP-inactivated kallikrein did not possess activity. We have attempted to repeat these observations several times using peripheral blood neutrophils and kallikrein from both rabbit and human origin without success. A wide dosage range of kallikrein was employed, and kallikrein neither augmented nor inhibited chemotaxis induced by zymosan-treated serum (unpublished observations). Recently, Dr R.C. Wiggins in our laboratory, together with Dr P. Giclas found that an intermediate component of plasma was essential for the chemotactic stimulation of rabbit neutrophils by rabbit kallikrein (Wiggins et al. 1981). Kallikrein, HF and HMWK, either alone or in combination over a wide dose range failed to stimulate chemotactic movement of neutrophils. However, in the presence of C5, kallikrein induced chemotaxis and release of β-glucuronidase. An anodally migrating species of C5 was generated by the interaction of kallikrein and C5. Thus, a novel activity of kallikrein on C5 was observed which generated a factor capable of stimulating both chemotaxis and exocytosis of neutrophils. Its relationship with C5a is not clear at present. In addition, a relationship of the C5-related chemotactic factor to the factor generated in the studies of Kaplan is uncertain.

Studies have also indicated a reaction between the contact system and platelets.

As platelets aggregate to form a hemostatic plug, they provide an activating surface for assembling coagulation factors that initiate and propagate the intrinsic coagulation pathway. Walsh (1972a) showed that ADP-stimulated platelets could shorten the clotting time of platelet-rich plasma in a HF-dependent reaction. Furthermore, he showed that collagen-stimulated platelets accelerate blood coagulation reactions that occur prior to the activation of Factor X (Walsh 1972b). In this latter case of collagen-induced coagulant activity involving platelets, it was shown that coagulant activity requiring Factor XI was generated in reactions that were partially dependent on and partially independent of HF. Recent studies employing washed human platelets and purified radiolabeled HF and Factor XI confirmed and extended these concepts (Walsh and Griffin 1980). It was demonstrated that platelets can promote the proteolytic activation of HF by kallikrein as well as the activation of Factor XI by both HF-dependent and HF-independent mechanisms.

11.3. PATHOPHYSIOLOGIC ACTIONS OF THE COMPONENTS OF THE CONTACT SYSTEM

11.3.1. Hageman factor and PF/dil

Hageman factor and PF/dil induce an increase in vascular permeability in their active form. Ratnoff and Miles (1964) employed partially activated HF to induce an increase in vascular permeability of guinea pigs. They found that a minimal dose of 2 μg in 0.1 ml volume induced increased permeability in the skin. Since the HF was only partially active and partially purified, it was uncertain whether this represented a true minimal dose.

When the HF was added to dilute plasma, the permeability effect was enhanced, leading the investigators to suspect that the HF had activated a second factor, thought to be the permeability factor of dilution (PF/dil). PF/dil, which was generated in plasma, diluted in the presence of glass (Miles and Wilhelm 1955; Wilhelm et al. 1958; Spector 1957; Kagan et al. 1963), was thought to act as a substrate for the activated HF. It was later found that PF/dil and active HF are the same (Johnston et al. 1974; Oh-Ishi and Webster 1975).

More recently, fully activated, purified guinea pig HF has been assessed for its permeability activity, and found to be active in this regard when as little as 1 ng HFa (at a concentration of 3×10^{-10} mol/l in 0.1 ml) was used. The active HF was about 10-100 times more active than bradykinin in this assay (Yamamoto and Cochrane 1981).

Following earlier reports of *hypotensive responses* in humans to infusions of albumin (Bland et al. 1973; Harrison et al. 1971a, b), a study was made of the nature of the hypotensive agent in commercial albumin preparations. β-HFa (prekallikrein activator) was found in the albumin preparations as determined by physical properties, its ability to activate prekallikrein and by its inhibition with specific antibodies to HF (Alving et al. 1978). The activity was reportedly not related to bradykinin or kallikrein in the preparation.

11.4. LEUKOCYTE ACCUMULATION IN BLOOD VESSELS AND TISSUES

Leukocyte accumulation in blood vessels and tissues occurred when HF was exposed to ellagic acid and placed in a vascular bed of rabbit ear chambers (Graham et al. 1965). The reaction reached a maximum after about 90 minutes as opposed to a more transient effect of bradykinin.

11.5. HIGH-MW KININOGEN

Aside from being the parent molecule of bradykinin generated by the hydrolytic action of plasma kallikrein, high-MW kininogen also contains the histidine-rich residue, Fragment 1-2. In the case of bovine high-MV kininogen, Fragment 1-2 and its cleavage products, Fragment 1 and Fragment 2, are released by the action of plasma kallikrein, a property not demonstrated with the human proteins. The bovine Fragment 1-2 and Fragment 2, but not Fragment 1, produce an increase in vascular permeability when administered intradermally. Matheson et al. (1976) observed a permeability reaction with 10^{-8} to 10^{-9} mol/l of Fragment 1-2, about 10^{-2} less potent than the reaction to bradykinin. An additive effect between Fragment 1-2 and bradykinin was measured. Oh-Ishi et al. (1977b) have noted in independent studies that Fragment 1-2 and Fragment 2, but not Fragment 1, induce vascular permeability to an extent of 1/100th that of bradykinin in rabbit skin. PGE_2, but not bradykinin, was found to enhance the permeability activity. It should be kept in mind that rabbits respond poorly to bradykinin or HFa in comparison to guinea pigs and primates.

Fragment 1-2 and Fragment 2 were also found to have less than 10^{-4} the activity of bradykinin in the contraction of rat uterine and guinea-pig ilial smooth muscle and 10^{-2} to 10^{-3} of the activity of bradykinin in the hypotensive response in rats (Oh-Ishi et al. 1977a).

11.6. BRADYKININ

The physiologic and pathologic effects of bradykinin are of extreme diversity and have received intensive study over the past 3-4 decades. Both in vitro and in many species of animals in vivo, the pharmacologic effects of this nonapeptide are now well recognized. Increase in vascular permeability, smooth muscle contraction, diminished arterial resistance and hypotension, vascular margination and infiltration of leukocytes into tissues, and pain are among the commonly studied responses to bradykinin. The actions have been subject to review and will not be specifically discussed here. Comparisons with active components of the contact system have been given above in this section. Bradykinin has been found in fluid such as plasma and joint fluid in numerous forms of experimental and clinical inflammatory disease. The reader is referred to recent compilations of studies of kinins (*Chemistry and Biology of the Kallikrein-Kinin System in Health and Disease,* John J. Pisano and K. Frank Austen (Eds), DHEW Publication No. (NIH) 76-791, 1976; *Kinins II,* S. Fujii, H. Moriya and T. Suzuki (Eds), Plenum Press, New York, 1979; *Bradykinin, Kallidin, and Kallikrein (Supplement),* E. Erdos (Ed), *Handbook of Experimental Pharmacology, Vol. 25 (Supplement),* Springer-Verlag, New York, 1979).

11.7. CONTACT ACTIVATION SYSTEM AND THE PLASMA RENIN—ANGIOTENSIN SYSTEM

The plasma kallikrein—kinin system and the renin—angiotensin system exhibit a number of interesting relationships. Bradykinin is hypotensive whereas angiotensin II is hypertensive. The dipeptidase converting enzyme, found principally in pulmonary endothelium, generates angiotensin II from a less active peptide, angiotensin I, by cleaving off a dipeptide (Erdos 1979). The same proteolytic enzyme destroys bradykinin by eliminating its C-terminal dipeptide, Phe-Arg (Erdos, 1979). Recently it has been shown that in-vitro activation of plasma prorenin can be effected via Factor XIIa and kallikrein.

Plasma renin liberates angiotensin I from angiotensinogen. In plasma, most renin (80-90%) circulates in zymogen form as prorenin (Derkx et al. 1976), which can be activated by trypsin, plasmin, urinary kallikrein or plasma kallikrein (Cooper et al. 1977; Sealey et al. 1978; Osmond and Loh 1978; Osmond et al. 1978; Derkx et al. 1979b). Cryoactivation of plasma or acidification followed by neutralization of plasma also results in activation of prorenin (Sealey et al. 1978; Derkx et al. 1978; Atlas et al. 1978; Osmond and Loh 1978). Experiments employing plasmas deficient in HF or prekallikrein indicated that these proteins were essential for these in-vitro activations of prorenin (Osmond et al. 1978; Millar et al. 1978; Derkx et al. 1979a; Sealey et al. 1979). Normal prorenin activation is restored by addition of kallikrein to HF-deficient plasma, but not by addition of β-HFa to prekallikrein-deficient plasma (Derkx et al. 1979a; Sealey et al. 1979). This shows that kallikrein is more directly required for prorenin activation than is HFa, although HF is presumably required for activation of prekallikrein.

The pathophysiologic significance of the activation of the renin—angiotensin system by HF- or prekallikrein-dependent pathways is not at all clear. Nor is apparent the significance of the observation that 10-20% of plasma renin exists as renin versus 80-90% present as prorenin. However, it appears that prekallikrein influences the physiologic percentage of renin versus prorenin since the level of prorenin is abnormally high and renin is abnormally low in plasma from patients with prekallikrein deficiency (Derkx et al. 1979a). In this context, one recent report that activation of the plasma kallikrein–kinin system appears unlikely to result in activation of prorenin in vivo based on their observations that kaolin-induced generation of plasma arginine esterase, presumably kallikrein, does not necessarily lead to prorenin activation (Blumberg et al. 1981). Further work will be necessary to define the potential significance of these recent in-vitro observations.

11.8. SUMMARY

The biochemistry of the components of the contact (Hageman factor) system of plasma and its activation upon surface contact are presented (Figs. 1 and 2). In addition, data are presented showing that components of the HF system may interact with enzymes of endothelial cells, enzymes derived from the anaphylactic challenge of human lung, and that kallikrein may act on C5 of the complement system to induce directional movement of neutrophils. Many studies now indicate that activated components of the contact system are capable of inducing increased vascular permeability, leukocyte accumulation, hypotension, and smooth muscle contraction. Their participation in inflammatory disease states of experimental animals and man have been recently reviewed (Cochrane and Griffin 1982).

ACKNOWLEDGEMENT

This is publication number 2640 from the Department of Immunopathology, Scripps Clinic and Research Foundation, La Jolla, CA. This work was supported in part by National Institutes of Health grants AI-17354, HL-16411, Office of Naval Research Contract N00014, and the Council for Tobacco Research.

REFERENCES

Alving, B.M., Hojima, Y., Pisano, J.J., Mason, B.M., Buckingham, R.E., Mozen, M.M. and Finlayson, J.S. (1978) *New Eng. J. Med. 229,* 66.

Atlas, S.A., Sealy, J.E. and Lavagh, J.H. (1978) *Circ. Res. 42 (Suppl. 1),* 128.

Bland, J.H.L., Laver, M.B. and Lowenstein, E. (1973) *J. Am. Med. Assoc. 224,* 1721.

Blumberg, A.L., Sealy, J.E., Atlas, S.A., Lavagh, J.H., Dharingrongartama, B. and Kaplan, A.P. (1981) *J. Lab. Clin. Med. 97,* 771.

Cochrane, C.G. and Griffin, J.H. (1982) In: F.J. Dixon and H.G. Kunkel (Eds), *Advances in Immunology, Vol. 33,* pp. 242–307. Academic Press, New York.

Cochrane, C.G. and Revak, S.D. (1980) *J. Exp. Med. 152,* 608.

Cochrane, C.G., Revak, S.D. and Wuepper, K.D. (1973) *J. Exp. Med. 138,* 1564.

Cooper, R.M., Murray, G.E. and Osmond, D.H. (1977) *Circ. Res. 40 (Suppl.1),* 171.

Derkx, F.H.M., Wenting, G.J., Man in 't Veld, A.J., Van Gool, J.M.G., Verhoeven, R.P. and Schalekamp, M.A.D.H. (1976) *Lancet 2,* 496.
Derkx, F.H.M., Tan-Tjiong, H.L. and Schalekamp, M.A.D.H. (1978) *Lancet 2,* 218.
Derkx, F.H.M., Bouma, B.N., Schalekamp, M.P.A. and Schalekamp, M.A.D.H. (1979a) *Nature (London) 280,* 315.
Derkx, F.H.M., Tan-Tjiong, H.L., Man in 't Veld, A.J., Schalekamp, M.P.A. and Schalekamp, M.A.D.H. (1979b) *Clin. Sci. 57,* 351.
Erdos, E. (Ed.) (1979) *Handbook of Experimental Pharmacology, Vol. 25 (Supplement),* Springer-Verlag, Berlin.
Fujikawa, K., Walsh, K.A. and Davie, E.W. (1977) *Biochemistry 16,* 2270.
Graham, R., Ebert, R.H., Ratnoff, O.D. and Moses, J.M. (1965) *J. Exp. Med. 121,* 807.
Griffin, J.H. (1977) *Fed. Proc. 36,* 324.
Griffin, J.H. (1978) *Proc. Natl Acad. Sci. USA 75,* 1998.
Griffin, J.H. and Cochrane, C.G. (1976) *Proc. Natl Acad. Sci. USA 73,* 2554.
Han, Y.N., Komiya, M., Iwanaga, S. and Suzuki, T. (1975) *J. Biochem. 77,* 55.
Harrison, G.A., Torda, J.A. and Schiff, P. (1971a) *Med. J. Aust. 2,* 1040.
Harrison, G.A., Torda, J.A. and Schiff, P. (1971b) *Med. J. Aust. 2,* 1308.
Heimark, R.L., Kurachi, K., Fujikawa, K. and Davie, E.W. (1980) *Nature (London) 208,* 456.
Johnston, A.R., Cochrane, C.G. and Revak, S.D. (1974) *J. Immunol. 113,* 103.
Kagan, J.L., Leddy, J.P. and Becker, E.L. (1963) *J. Clin. Invest. 42,* 1353.
Kaplan, A.P. and Austen, K.F. (1972) *J. Exp. Med. 135,* 81.
Mandle, R., Colman, R.W. and Kaplan, A.P. (1976) *Proc. Natl Acad. Sci. USA 11,* 4179.
Matheson, R.T., Miller, D.R., Lacombe, M.J., Han, Y.N., Iwanaga, S., Kato, H. and Wuepper, K.D. (1976) *J. Clin. Invest. 58,* 1395.
McGuire, W.W., Spragg, R.G., Cohen, A. and Cochrane, C.G. (1982) *J. Clin. Invest., 69,* 543.
Meier, H.K., Webster, M.E., Mandle, R., Colman, R.W. and Kaplan, A.P. (1977) *J. Clin. Invest. 60,* 18.
Miles, A.A. and Wilhelm, D.L. (1955) *Br. J. Exp. Pathol. 36,* 71.
Millar, J.A., Clappison, B.H. and Johnston, C.I. (1978) *Lancet 2,* 1376.
Newball, H.H., Meier, H.L., Kaplan, A.P., Revak, S.D., Cochrane, C.G. and Lichtenstein, L.M. (1980) *Fed. Proc. 39,* 906.
Oh-Ishi, S., Katori, M., Han, Y.N., Kanagawa, S., Kato, H. and Suzuki, T. (1977a) *Biochem. Pharmacol. 26,* 115.
Oh-Ishi, S., Tanaka, K., Katori, M., Han, Y.M., Kato, H. and Iwanaga, S. (1977b) *Life Sci. 20,* 695.
Oh-Ishi, S. and Webster, M.E. (1975) *Biochem. Pharmacol. 24,* 591.
Osmond, D.H. and Loh, A.Y. (1978) *Lancet 1,* 102.
Osmond, D.H., Lo, E.K., Loh, A.Y., Zingg, E.A. and Hedlin, A.H. (1978) *Lancet 2,* 1375.
Ratnoff, O.D. and Miles, A.A. (1964) *Br. J. Exp. Pathol. 45,* 328.
Revak, S.D. and Cochrane, C.G. (1976) *J. Clin. Invest. 57,* 852.
Revak, S.D., Cochrane, C.G. and Griffin, J.H. (1977) *J. Clin. Invest. 59,* 1167.
Sealey, J., Atlas, S.A., Laragh, J.H., Oza, N.B. and Ryan, J.W. (1978) *Nature (London) 275,* 144.

Sealey, J., Atlas, S.A., Laragh, J.H., Silverberg, M.J. and Kaplan, A.P. (1979) *Proc. Natl Acad. Sci. USA 76,* 5914.
Spector, W.G. (1957) *J. Pathol. Bacteriol. 74,* 67.
Thompson, E., Mandle, R. and Kaplan, A.P. (1977) *J. Clin. Invest. 60,* 1376.
Thompson, R.E., Mandle, R. and Kaplan, A.P. (1978) *J. Exp. Med. 147,* 488.
Waldman, R., Scicli, A.G., Scicli, G.M., Guimaraes, J.A., Carretero, O.A., Kato, H., Han, Y.N. and Iwanaga, S. (1977) *Thromb. Haemostasis 38,* 14.
Walsh, P.N. (1972a) *Br. J. Haematol. 22,* 237.
Walsh, P.N. (1972b) *Br. J. Haematol. 22,* 393.
Walsh, P.N. and Griffin, J.H. (1980) *Blood 57,* 106.
Wiggins, R.C., Bouma, B.N., Cochrane, C.G. and Griffin, J.H. (1977) *Proc. Natl Acad. Sci. USA 74,* 4636.
Wiggins, R.C., Loskutoff, D.J., Cochrane, C.G., Griffin, J.H. and Edgington, T.S. (1980) *J. Clin. Invest. 65,* 197.
Wiggins, R.C., Giclas, P.C. and Henson, P.M. (1981) *J. Exp. Med. 153,* 1391-1404.
Wilhelm, D.L., Mill, P.J., Sparrow, E.M., Mackey, M.E. and Miles, A.A. (1958) *Br. J. Exp. Pathol. 39,* 228.
Wuepper, K.D. (1973) *J. Exp. Med. 138,* 1345.
Yamamoto, T. and Cochrane, C.G. (1981) *Am. J. Pathol. 105,* 164.

CHAPTER 12

Altered inflammatory mechanisms in thermal injury

GERD O. TILL

and

PETER A. WARD

Department of Pathology, University of Michigan Medical School, Ann Arbor, Michigan 48109

12.1. INTRODUCTION

Inflammation, as a standard response to infection and trauma, usually results in a combined interaction of different humoral and cellular systems. The purpose of these cascading events is to protect the individual from dissemination of pathogens and to bring about restoration of the affected tissue and organs. In the early phases of an acute inflammatory response, the most prominent products of mediator system activation are biologically active proteins/peptides of the complement, coagulation, fibrinolytic, kinin-generating systems and lipids from arachidonate metabolism. Cells such as neutrophils and platelets also play key roles. As the inflammatory reactions progress, macrophages, lymphocytes and lymphocyte products such as lymphokines and antibodies complete the arsenal that permits the individual to survive a hazardous environment. Alterations in inflammatory mechanisms due to genetically determined or acquired deficiencies of humoral or cellular components of the inflammatory system may lead to compromises in host defenses resulting in a life-threatening situation.

A characteristic and critical feature of patients with thermal injuries is increased susceptibility to microbial infections accompanied by depression of both humoral and cellular defenses. In spite of substantial improvements in modern burn care, bacterial infections remain the leading cause of death following severe thermal injury. It seems increasingly likely that disturbances in complement and in leukocytes contribute to the pathogenesis of complications developing in burn patients. In this chapter, rather than presenting a comprehensive review of the literature, we have chosen to discuss altered inflammatory mechanisms occurring in the course of thermal injury. We will cover changes in the complement system, defects in phagocytic cells and their regulatory factors, and immunoregulatory aberrations.

12.2. SERUM COMPLEMENT IN THERMAL INJURY

It is now well recognized that activation products of the complement system contribute to the inflammatory response and to host defenses against invasion by pathogenic organisms. In an acute inflammatory reaction to local trauma and bacterial infection, complement activation products can bring about changes in vascular permeability and local blood flow, attract and activate phagocytic leukocytes, and enhance phagocytosis and intracellular killing of microbial pathogens. To demonstrate activation of complement, functional assays of individual complement components and total hemolytic complement activity as well as demonstration of complement-derived biological activities, are essential. Reduction in titers of total hemolytic complement activity alone or decrease in protein concentrations of individual complement components may be due to consumptive depletion, to increase in levels of inhibitors of the complement system, or to loss of plasma proteins due to "leaky vessels". The majority of data on complement changes in thermal injury are based on protein determinations of individual complement components, whereas the number of functional complement assays performed in burned patients is very small. Therefore, the evidence for complement activation in thermally injured patients is still weak. Data published so far are rather conflicting and, to date, neither the pathway(s) nor the mechanism of complement activation following thermal injury is totally clear.

A marked reduction in hemolytic complement activity (CH_{50} units) has been observed in patients with burns greater than 25% of total body surface (Bjornson and Alexander 1974). However, normal or elevated protein concentrations of C3 have been found. Functional assays of C3 have revealed decreases in C3 activity (Bjornson and Alexander 1974). This underlines the importance of functional hemolytic assays as opposed to immunochemical tests. Using a kinetic method of immune hemolysis, Dhennin et al. (1978) also observed a decrease in hemolytic complement activity immediately after burn. Maximum depression of complement activity occurred during the first 48 hours post-burn and was related to the size of the burn. After 48 hours complement activity rose to normal values. In patients with extensive burns, however, complement levels remained low. In patients with burn size involving less than 30% of total body surface, complement levels rose above the normal range reaching peak values at 10 days post-burn. Occurrence of infection seemed to interfere with the restoration of complement levels; very low levels of complement seem to reflect a potential risk of sepsis (Dhennin et al. 1978).

In patients suffering from major thermal injuries, Zuckerman et al. (1978) have observed depressed CH_{50} levels which quickly returned to normal or supernormal levels by the end of the first post-burn week. The highest CH_{50} levels were seen in patients with minor burns or in those who survived. In this study, significant decreases in C4 and C3 levels, as measured immunochemically, were found early after thermal injury. Depressed C4 and C3 values seemed to return to normal or supernormal levels in surviving patients. In fatally burned individuals, complement values remained suppressed until death (Zuckerman et al. 1978). These data support the observations by others (Fjellström and Arturson 1963; Dhennin et al. 1978).

Whether total hemolytic complement activity is, in fact, decreased in the early phase of thermal injury has, however, been questioned by several recent reports. In severely burned patients, Erbs et al. (1980) failed to observe decreased CH_{50} levels during the first week post-burn. On the contrary, CH_{50} titers as well as levels of C4, C2 and C3 were found to be increased during the first week post-burn and remained elevated throughout the 3-week period after thermal injury. Similar observations have been reported by Holder and Ablin (1980). Others observed a reduction of CH_{50} titers during the initial post-burn period only in septic patients (Bjornson et al. 1980). In this case, however, it should be noted that the studies had been conducted in patients who had already received infusions of fresh plasma.

12.2.1. Activity of individual complement components

Fjellström and Arturson (1963) were the first to show changes in individual complement components following thermal injury. In four cases of fatal burns, they observed a pronounced drop in the activity of C1, C4, C2 and C3 from the first day after trauma, reaching values as low as 10% of normal serum on the third day and remaining low until death. In patients with minor burn injuries, these authors failed to observe significant decreases in the four complement components. On the contrary, complement titers started to increase by the end of the first week and reached levels two to three times above those of non-burned individuals. Erbs et al. (1980) also observed a decrease in C1 activity in 20 cases studied. This drop was independent of the severity and the extent of burn injury and remained low for several weeks. When immunochemical determinations were performed, a significant decrease of the serum concentration of C1q protein was observed immediately after burn injury (Sharma et al. 1980; Bjornson et al. 1980). C1q levels returned to normal values within 10 days (Bjornson et al. 1980) or remained low even over a time period of 28 days post-burn (Sharma et al. 1980). The latter finding appears to be in accordance with the observation of prolonged low titers of C1 activity as reported by Erbs et al. (1980). The decrease in C1 activity was paralleled by a prolonged and striking increase in the serum protein concentration of the C1 esterase inhibitor (Daniels et al. 1974; Erbs et al. 1980). Immunochemical determinations of the fifth component of complement in sera of burned patients have revealed conflicting results. A decrease in serum concentration of C5 immediately after thermal injury has been reported by one group (Sharma et al. 1980) but others have not observed any changes of C5 (Bjornson et al. 1980).

12.2.2. Alternative pathway of complement activation

An inhibition of the alternative pathway of complement activation was observed when post-burn sera were incubated with inulin or cobra venom factor, both of which substances are known to activate the alternative complement pathway. As determined by C3 conversion, the activity of the alternative complement pathway has been found to be persistently decreased during a prolonged period of time following thermal injury (Bjornson et al. 1976, 1977, 1980). This has been observed in both bacteremic and non-septic burned patients (Bjornson et al. 1980). Interestingly, the concentration of properdin was also found to be decreased over the entire post-burn time (8 weeks) (Bjornson et al. 1977, 1980). Reduction in amounts of C3 conversion as well as levels of properdin correlated with increasing burn size (Bjornson et al. 1977).

In order to evaluate further the nature of the reduction in C3 conversion in sera from severely burned patients, equal parts of pooled normal serum and sera known to have abnormal C3 conversion were mixed together (Bjornson et al. 1976). This manipulation interfered with conversion of C3 following addition of inulin, as determined by radial immunodiffusion employing antisera against the B-antigen of C3. When serum depleted of properdin or C3 proactivator was mixed with an equal amount of pooled normal serum, conversion of C3 by inulin was fully restored, suggesting that decrease or depletion of essential components of the alternative pathway of complement activation is not the cause of the observed abnormality of C3 conversion related to serum from burn patients. On the basis of these observations the authors suggested that reduction in C3 conversion in burn sera results from the presence of an inhibitor (Bjornson et al. 1976). Similar observations have been reported by others. When serum from thermally injured patients was incubated, two abnormalities could be observed. Some of the sera exhibited 100% consumption of CH_{50} activity (contrasted to 57% in normal human serum) whereas in other sera CH_{50} was only partially reduced, with complement consumption being significantly less than that observed in normal serum (Holder and Ablin 1980). The authors suggested that an inhibitor of the C3 proactivator might have been produced or released as a consequence of thermal injury. The observed increase in the consumption of complement by zymosan in certain sera has been explained by increased levels of C3 proactivator (Holder and Ablin 1980).

Recently, Bjornson et al. (1980a) presented further evidence that an inhibitor of C3 conversion is present in burn sera. The authors were able to show that dialysis of burn sera partially or fully corrected the reduction in C3 conversion by inulin. Further experiments indicated that this was related to the removal of inhibitory factor following absorption to cellulose membranes of dialysis tubing and/or due to inactivation by the same material. As assessed immunochemically, the dialysis procedure did not alter concentrations of C3, C3 proactivator, C3b inactivator, properdin and other complement components, nor did it change the total hemolytic complement activity of normal as well as burn sera (Bjornson et al. 1981a).

When other components of the alternative pathway were examined in sera from burn patients, both the serum concentration of the C3 proactivator as well as the concentration of the C3b inactivator were found to be elevated within one week post-burn and remained increased during the entire study period of 8 weeks (Bjornson et al. 1977). In three patients with 42 to 70% third-degree burns involving 60 to 75% total body surface the concentration of C3 proactivator and C3b inactivator remained within normal values or showed a borderline depression (Bjornson et al. 1977).

12.2.3. Experimental studies on complement changes

With regard to clinical studies of thermal injury, limiting factors include lack of baseline values, inability to initiate investigations within a few minutes after burn injury, variation in and extent of injury and other variables such as age, treatment, and nutrition. Many of these difficulties are avoided using experimental animals.

Farrell et al. (1973) produced full-thickness burn injuries involving 25% of total body surface in anesthetized rats after exposure of the shaved backs to 99°C hot water for 20 seconds. The authors observed a rapid fall (by 35%) of total hemolytic complement activity at 6 hours (when the first post-burn blood samples were obtained). These changes in CH_{50} levels were paralleled by decreases in functional levels of C1, C3, C5 and C8. Complement activity continued to remain decreased over the first 20 hours. Thereafter, CH_{50} values increased and reached normal or supernormal levels 60 to 100 hours after burn injury. A decrease in complement activity following thermal injury of experimental animals has also been reported by others (Heideman 1979a; Till et al. 1983). After submerging 50% of the body surface of dogs under water at 80°C for 45 seconds, total hemolytic complement activity decreased to 60% within 2 hours after injury and remained low for 6 hours post-burn when the dogs were sacrificed (Heideman 1979a). In rats, a 30% decrease in total hemolytic complement activity was seen following exposure of flank skin (28% total body surface) to water of 70°C for 30 seconds (Till et al. 1983). Within 2 to 3 hours following thermal injury a drop in the levels of C4, C3 and C6 was also observed, paralleling the decrease in total complement activity.

Farrell et al. (1973) observed a simultaneous decline in serum complement activity and in the concentration of total serum protein. The authors suggested that loss of complement proteins into the burn site could account for the observed decrease in serum complement activity. On the other hand, the same authors found the activity of C9 to be increased above normal values at 6 hours post-burn. Others have observed that, in severe thermal injury, albumin is the chief protein leaking into the burn site (Fjellström and Arturson 1963).

Although some loss of complement proteins into the burn site cannot be excluded, recently published data indicate that thermal injury of skin can activate the complement system. In thermally injured rats Till et al. (1983) observed conversion of serum C3 to C3b, an indication of complement activation in vivo. Furthermore,

TABLE 1.
Humoral alterations in thermal injury

Decreased serum immunoglobulin levels
Serum inhibitory activity for neutrophil migration
Serum inhibitory activity for neutrophil phagocytosis
Inhibitory activity of the alternative pathway of complement activation
Immunosuppressive activities in serum
Activation of plasma complement, kinin-forming system, arachidonate metabolites and fibrinolytic system

when chemotaxis assays were performed employing rat peritoneal neutrophils, C5-related chemotactic activity could be detected in rat serum as early as 30 minutes post-burn. The appearance of complement-derived chemotactic activity was accompanied by a transient neutropenia which is known to occur during intravascular complement activation (Craddock et al. 1977; O'Flaherty et al. 1978). These experimental data provide strong evidence that thermal injury can induce systemic complement activation. It seems likely that depression of serum complement activity found in burned humans is due to in-vivo activation of the complement system. Recently, Nelson et al. (1983) reported that C3a and C5a anaphylatoxin (activation products of the complement system), are detectable in the serum of thermally injured patients.

12.2.4. Overview of clinical and experimental studies

Why decreases in total hemolytic complement activity have been observed inconsistently in patients with thermal injury may be explained by several reasons. The experimental data show that complement activation following thermal injury is a very early event which may be missed if early studies (3 to 6 hours post-burn) are not undertaken. Intravascular complement activation seems to be followed by an "acute-phase"-like reaction with elevation of complement levels above normal values. The severity and extent of thermal injuries may also have an effect on complement activation. It should also be mentioned that some authors conducted studies in burned patients who had already received infusions of fresh plasma, which could easily mask complement activation. As far as changes of individual complement components in sera of burned patients are concerned, similar, inconsistent data have been published and may be due to the technical problems (in analytical procedures) described above.

Another important question remains to be answered. In experimental thermal injury, the activation mechanism of the complement system is not currently known. Heideman (1979b) reported that heat-precipitated rat plasma as well as thermally injured rat tissue is able to activate complement in vitro, probably via the alternative activation pathway. This hypothesis seems to be supported by clinical observations of decreased properdin levels (Bjornson et al. 1977, 1980) and increased concentrations of C3 proactivator and C3b inhibitor (Bjornson et al. 1977, 1980, 1981a) in sera of burn patients. However, the discovery of a serum inhibitor of the alternative complement pathway in thermally injured patients (Bjornson et al. 1981b) is another possible explanation for reductions in complement levels. Experimental data demonstrating activation of complement components C1 through C8 (Farrell et al. 1973; Till et al. 1983) suggest that activation via the classic complement pathway may be occurring in thermally injured animals. However, these data do not exclude simultaneous activation of the alternative pathway.

12.3. ALTERED NEUTROPHIL FUNCTIONS IN THERMAL INJURY

Neutrophils comprise an important group of phagocytic cells involved in defense against bacterial infections. Neutrophils are produced from a common hematopoietic stem cell in the bone marrow by a process of maturation and division. Within 9–10 days the cells enter the peripheral blood, remain there for only 6–10 hours and migrate into tissues or are removed, presumably by the reticuloendothelial system. Thus, the total life time of neutrophils is only 13–15 days. The mature neutrophil is highly specialized to respond to microbial invasion by means of chemotaxis, phagocytosis, intracellular killing, digestion, and extracellular release of leukocytic products.

In spite of significant improvements in therapeutic measures, bacterial infections are still the leading cause of death in thermally injured patients. A number of conditions, such as disruption of the integrity of the skin and contamination of the wound, increased metabolic requirements in the presence of decreased nutritional intake, loss of plasma proteins, fluid and electrolytes into the burned area, and suppression of the patient's defense mechanisms all contribute to increased susceptibility to infection. Neutrophils from some patients with extensive burns have been reported to show reduced chemotactic responses and decreased intracellular microbicidal capacity.

12.3.1. Chemotactic response

In a group of 46 burned patients, Warden et al. (1974) conducted studies of neutrophil chemotaxis in vitro. The test was carried out by means of a filter technique employing blood leukocytes from thermally injured patients or from healthy volunteers as test cells and a mixture of casein and normal human serum as chemoattractant. Within the first 72 hours after injury, the chemotactic responses of the patient leukocytes correlated inversely with the burn size. For instance, involvement of 40 to 60% of total body surface area was associated in most instances with a reduction in neutrophil chemotactic responses (approximately 65 or 45% of normal values, respectively). No patient whose neutrophils showed 60% reduction in chemotactic function survived beyond 72 hours. In general, non-survivors had larger burns and significantly lower chemotactic responses (averaging 40% of normal), while survivors had smaller burns and chemotactic responses that averaged 98% of the normal response. Infection was the major cause of death, but diminished chemotactic leukocyte function was observed before clinical evidence of infection.

Studies by Warden et al. (1975) showed that in vitro incubation of a leukocyte-rich suspension from thermally injured patients with normal serum restored the depressed chemotactic response. Heat-labile serum factors were thought to be responsible for the restoration of chemotactic function. On the other hand, the same authors could show that sera obtained from thermally injured patients who had been treated with mafenide acetate or silver sulfadiazine suppressed the migration of neutrophils from normal donors, whereas sera from patients treated with silver nitrate had no inhibitory effect. Dialysis of burn sera removed the chemotaxis-suppressing factor(s), presumably related to the topical therapeutic agents. These studies demonstrate depression of normal leukocyte chemotaxis by two commonly used chemotherapeutic agents and, in addition, suggest the presence of a reversible chemotaxis defect related to a deficiency of a heat-labile factor in sera from burn patients.

Decreases in chemotactic responses of neutrophils of thermally injured patients have also been observed by other investigators (Grogan 1976a; Fikrig et al. 1977; Altman et al. 1977; Nathenson et al. 1978; Heck et al. 1980; Davis et al. 1980). In contrast to the studies of Warden et al. (1974, 1975) the defect in neutrophil chemotaxis was neither corrected by addition of normal serum (Grogan 1976) nor could an inhibitor or inactivator be demonstrated in the serum of thermally injured patients (Grogan 1976; Fikrig et al. 1977). However, in patients with burns involving 40% total surface area, serum from these patients contained a cell-directed inhibitor of neutrophil chemotaxis (Altman et al. 1977). The inhibitor was heat-stable (56°C, 30 min), non-dialyzable, and not related to topical therapeutic agents used in these patients. The important question, whether the defect in neutrophil chemotaxis is related to deficiency of a heat-labile factor or is due to the presence of a heat-stable cell-directed inhibitor requires further investigations. The observation of decreased neutrophil lysozyme levels accompanied by elevated levels in serum of lysozyme following thermal injury (Alexander 1967), together with the development of decreased chemotactic responses in neutrophils after degranulation in vitro (Gallin et al. 1978) suggest a relationship between lysosomal enzyme levels and chemotactic responsiveness of neutrophils in burn patients. Davis et al. (1980) studied 15 patients with a mean burn area of 35% of total body surface area. Blood neutrophils from these patients exhibited significantly decreased chemotaxis between the 5th and the 15th day post-burn. The depression of chemotaxis corresponded closely with the onset of septic complications and was paralleled by significantly lowered levels of lysozyme in the patients' neutrophils. These data suggest that secretion of neutrophilic specific granule contents in vivo may result in impaired neutrophil chemotaxis in thermally injured patients. The nature of this degranulative process remains to be elucidated, although complement activation with release of C5a is a likely explanation. Whether release of lysosomal enzymes is the proximate cause of depressed neutrophil chemotaxis remains to be determined. Based on recent studies by Nelson et al. (1983), who found increased levels of C5a in the serum of thermally injured patients, chemotactic deactivation (Ward and Becker 1968) of neutrophils by C5a should also be considered as a possible cause of impaired neutrophil chemotaxis in burned patients.

With regard to defects in neutrophil chemotaxis in burned patients some caution in interpretation of published data seems to be advisable. Neutrophils from thermally injured patients show significantly depressed random migration (Davis et al. 1980). Considering the fact that in most instances chemotaxis of neutrophils from burned patients has been assessed by counting the number of cells which have migrated through a micropore filter toward a chemoattractant in a given time period, it appears conceivable that less neutrophils will appear on the lower surface of test filters when the migrational capacity of these cells is impaired. To answer the question of whether the basis of the migrational defect involves random or chemotactic motility, further studies such as visual assessment of cell orientation upon contact with chemotactic factors, checkerboard analyses, and evaluation of chemoattractant-induced release of lysosomal enzymes are indicated. Recently, Davies et al. (1981) have demonstrated that neutrophils from burn patients showing depressed migrational response in the filter assay possess the same number of receptor sites for the chemotactic tripeptide F-Met-Leu-Phe when compared to cells from normal controls. Furthermore, recently published data also suggest the possibility of iatrogenically induced dysfunctions of white blood cells (see also p. 392). For example, povidone-iodine, a strong germicidal agent which is frequently used in burn wound treatment, has been shown to induce strong suppression of neutrophil migration in vitro (Connolly, Gilmore 1979). This inhibition may be related to iodine content. Since patients treated with povidone-iodine showed high levels of iodine in their serum (Ninnemann and Stein 1981), possibility of iatrogenically induced alterations of neutrophil migration in burn patients is a real possibility.

Leukocyte defects occur in a variety of different clinical states. They have been observed not only in patients with severe trauma or sepsis but have also been identified in patients with malnutrition (Edelman et al. 1973; Douglas and Schopfer 1974; Kulapongs et al. 1977). Clinical observations suggest that protein malnutrition plays an important role (Alexander et al. 1980, 1981) and it is believed that these defects can be corrected or prevented by proper dietary management.

Whether all the defects can be related to acute nutritional changes is not yet known. Some investigators have observed disturbances in leukocyte chemotaxis that seemed to be related to abnormal serum levels of either chemotactic factor inactivators and/or cell-directed inhibitors. In a patient with Listeria meningitis a chemotactic and phagocytic defect of both neutrophils and monocytes was observed (Maderazo et al. 1977). The defect could be related to the presence of a cell-directed inhibitor present in the patient's serum. The inhibitor was termed CDI (cell-directed inhibitor of leukocyte chemotaxis) and could also be demonstrated in a high percentage of sera from patients with cancer or advanced hepatic cirrhosis (Maderazo et al. 1978). CDI appears to be a natural regulator of the inflammatory response, since it is also present in normal human serum, although in very low levels. CDI is heat stable (56°C) and has an estimated molecular weight of 160,000 daltons. The inhibitor chromatographically isolates with the IgG fraction of normal or abnormal serum, but is not an autoantibody to leukocytic antigens, since CDI activity appears to be related to the Fc but not to the $F(ab)_2$ portion of the IgG molecule. The nature of the inhibition and the mechanism that governs the levels of CDI in human serum are not understood.

Another regulator of the inflammatory response that directly and irreversibly interacts with chemotactic factors such as C5a is also present in normal human serum and has been termed CFI (Berenberg and Ward 1973). CFI is an alpha globulin (Till and Ward 1975) present in very low serum concentrations (less than 10 g/ml) and has an estimated molecular weight of 140,000 daltons (Kreutzer et al. 1979). Very high levels of CFI have been observed in the sera of patients with Hodgkin's disease (Ward and Berenberg 1974), hepatic cirrhosis (Maderazo et al. 1975), sarcoidosis (Maderazo et al. 1976) and lepromatous leprosy (Ward et al. 1976). Patients with high serum levels of CDI or CFI show a picture of cutaneous anergy. In leprosy patients only half the number of leukocytes found in control patients accumulated in Rebuck skin windows (Ward et al. 1976). This suggests that high levels of CFI reduce the influx and accumulation of leukocytes at inflammatory sites. This assumption has been supported by experimental data. CFI purified from human serum, blocks a variety of immune complex-induced inflammatory reactions in the rat (Johnson et al. 1977). It seems likely that CFI inactivates the C5 chemotactic peptide C5a in statu nascendi, before its biological effects (such as neutrophil margination, aggregation and movement) are fully developed. The source of CFI is not known. Neutrophils contain chemotactic factor inactivating activities that can be ascribed to elastase and cathepsin G activities. Antiproteases, present in serum, rapidly inactivate these neutrophilic proteinases but the inhibitors have no effect on the CFI activity indicating that CFI activity in the serum is not due to the presence of leukocytic protease-like material. Recent evidence suggests that serum levels of CFI can fluctuate rapidly in response to acute inflammatory reactions. In the course of immune complex-induced vasculitis (reversed passive Arthus reactions) in rats, complement activation with release of C5-related chemotactic activity into the circulation occurs 4 to 8 hours after intradermal injection of antibody. The appearance of chemotactic activity in serum is followed by an abrupt rise of CFI levels (in serum), reaching peak values at 12 hours and declining thereafter (Till et al. 1980). Interestingly, in the same experimental animals, high levels of CDI activity also appeared in the serum. The cell-directed inhibitor of chemotaxis could be detected at 24 hours after antibody injection. CDI reached peak values at 48 hours and then gradually declined over the next 2 days.

In thermally injured rats, Till et al. (1983) observed that peak values of C5-related chemotactic activity in the serum were followed by a rapid drop of leukotactic activity below baseline values. Depression of "baseline" chemotactic activity continued for several hours. It is not known at present whether this abrupt fall in serum chemotactic activity is due to the appearance of CFI activity. In severely burned patients, states of cutaneous anergy or a delay in the rejection of skin transplants have been frequently observed (Kay 1957; Alexander and Moncrief 1966; Chambler and Batchelor 1969; Ninnemann et al. 1978). It seems likely that high serum levels of inhibitors such as CFI and CDI represent an explanation for these observations.

12.3.2. Chemotactic activity

A neutrophil chemotactic factor termed "burn leucoegresin" has been found in the pseudoglobulin fraction of extracts from rabbit skin exposed to heated (56°C) metal discs for 20 seconds (Maeda et al. 1975). The highly purified factor has a molecular weight of approximately 140,000 daltons, is relatively heat-stable and shares at least some antigenic determinants with rabbit IgG. Injection of burn leucoegresin into rabbit skin induces a pronounced emigration and accumulation of blood neutrophils at the injection site. Burn leucoegresin appears to be identical to leucoegresin extracted from skin Arthus lesions (see review by Hayashi et al. 1974).

Four hours after exposure of skin of anesthetized rats to heated metal discs (56°C, 30 s), extracts have been obtained by homogenization in phosphate-buffered saline of thermally injured and non-injured skin. In eight different animals tested there was as much as a 10-fold increase in the amount of chemotactic activity in the injured areas versus noninjured areas (Ward 1981). It is not yet known if this activity is identical to the "burn leucoegresin" described by Maeda et al. (1975) or whether the leukotactic activity is complement-derived. Normal tissue has the ability to generate chemotactic activity in the presence of complement. The ability of tissue to generate chemotactic activity resides in the soluble fraction of the tissue and is associated with fragmentation of the C3 molecule into chemotactically active peptides (Ward et al., unpublished). Earlier studies demonstrated that C3 or C5 derived chemotactic peptides are produced when tissue is injured by anoxic changes, leading to release of neutral proteases that will cleave C3 and/or C5 (Hill and Ward 1969; Ward and Hill 1970). It remains to be seen if in thermally injured tissue similar mechanisms are responsible for locally generated chemotactic activity. It is also not known whether the C5 related chemotactic activity observed in the serum of thermally injured rats (Till et al. 1983) or the C5a protein demonstrated in the serum of burned patients (Nelson et al. 1983) is generated locally (in the burned tissue) or whether a systemic intravascular complement activation is responsible for the appearance of C5 related chemotactic activity in the serum following thermal injury.

12.3.3. Opsonization and phagocytosis

In severely burned patients, a reduction in serum opsonic activity for *Pseudomonas aeruginosa* and *Escherichia coli* has been found to occur during the early acute burn phase (Bjornson and Alexander 1974). The opsonic defect disappears by the end of the third week. Since addition of normal human serum to burn serum fully restores opsonic activity, it has been suggested that the opsonic defect is due to deficiency of a serum factor(s) (Bjornson et al. 1976). Nathenson et al. (1978) observed a depression of yeast opsonic activity in sera of burned patients; this defect was accompanied by depressed chemotactic activity and decreased properdin levels. The opsonic defect could be restored by the addition of purified properdin. During the first 10 days post-burn, levels of IgG and IgA are reduced in noninfected patients (Bjornson et al. 1977). This is followed by decreased concentrations of IgM and properdin. Decreased serum levels of C3 are seen from 10 days to six weeks post-burn. However, significantly decreased opsonic activity has been observed only during sepsis (Bjornson et al. 1977), suggesting that opsonic defects occur in burned patients as a result rather than a cause of infection. Further studies by Bjornson et al. (1979, 1980) have revealed that in burned patients the activity of heat-stable opsonins (antibodies) to their infecting bacterial strains is not significantly altered, and it has been found that complement abnormalities frequently seen in these patients do not seem to predispose them to bacterial infections. An opsonic factor that perhaps could account for these unexplained observations is plasma fibronectin. Opsonic plasma fibronectin or so-called cold-insoluble globulin is an α_2-globulin with a molecular weight of approximately 450,000 daltons (Blumenstock et al. 1976, 1978; Saba et al. 1978). The opsonin stimulates macrophage phagocytosis of nonbacterial particulates (Blumenstock et al. 1976; Saba et al. 1978) and also seems to augment neutrophil phagocytosis (Lanser et al. 1980). In thermally injured patients, plasma fibronectin levels have been found to be decreased within hours after burn (Lanser et al. 1980). The opsonin concentration then increases to normal levels within 1–3 days. A second depression in circulating opsonic fibronectin can be seen in septic patients. Resolution of the septic episode is followed by complete recovery of plasma fibronectin levels (Lanser et al. 1980). The pathophysiologic role of fibronectin (opsonic and cell surface fibronectin) in burn disease warrants further experimental and clinical investigations.

The phagocytic activity of neutrophils from thermally injured patients is generally found to be normal or increased (Alexander et al. 1968a; Alexander and Wixson

1970; Grogan and Miller 1973; Curreri et al. 1973), although a decrease in ingestion of *Pseudomonas aeruginosa* by neutrophils from severely burned patients has been observed by Grogan (1976b). In patients with burns up to 30% of total body surface area, 9% of the neutrophil assays for phagocytosis reveal lower than normal results. This figure increases to 19% in patients with larger burns and is most often associated with patients who are severely ill. The phagocytic depression is usually not seen until 5 days post-burn, which suggests that the decreased ingestion is probably secondary to the burn trauma. An inhibitory effect of sera from bacteriemic burned patients on the phagocytic uptake of *Staphylococcus aureus* and *Escherichia coli* by normal neutrophils has been demonstrated by Bjornson et al. (1981b). Depressed phagocytosis was observed in 3 of 12 patients during 8 to 56 days after burn and was neither due to defective opsonization nor to cytotoxic effects (on neutrophils) of the burn sera. Further studies have revealed that the serum-mediated inhibition results from a direct interaction of the burn sera with the neutrophils. Washing of the leukocytes did not reverse the phagocytic depression. The inhibitor was non-dialyzable, suggesting a molecular weight of more than 12,000 (Bjornson et al. 1981b) and may likely be responsible for the decreased chemotactic responsiveness of neutrophils from thermally injured patients as well.

12.3.4. Bactericidal activity

The function of neutrophils in thermal injury has been extensively studied by Alexander and co-workers, who provided strong evidence of a bactericidal defect in the neutrophils of severely burned patients (Alexander et al. 1968a, b; Alexander and Wixson 1970; Alexander and Fisher 1970; Alexander et al. 1971; Alexander and Meakins 1972). Most importantly, the bactericidal abnormalities, as expressed by a neutrophil bactericidal index, are associated with an increasing incidence of bacteriemia (Alexander and Meakins 1972; Alexander et al. 1979). The neutrophil bactericidal index is calculated (following a 4-hour incubation) by dividing the number of bacteria which survive incubation with normal neutrophils into the number of bacteria surviving following incubation with neutrophils from test subjects. A neutrophil bactericidal index of 10 would mean that 10 times as many bacteria survived when incubated with patient's cells than with control neutrophils. A bactericidal index of 8 and higher is considered to be severely abnormal. Bacteria (*Staphylococcus aureus*) are counted as colonies on plates following incubation for 48 hours. Phagocytic defects can be separated from intracellular killing defects by adding streptomycin and penicillin at the beginning of incubation to kill extracellular bacteria which were not rapidly internalized. The number of surviving intracellular bacteria which are protected from these antibodies is determined following a 4-hour incubation and the phagocytosis—intracellular killing index calculated in a manner similar to the neutrophil bactericidal index.

By the use of these techniques it was found that the bactericidal defect was most apparent in patients with large burn injuries. The defect was not seen earlier than 3 to

7 days after thermal injury (Alexander et al. 1968a). The intracellular killing defect was usually associated with a significant increase in the rate of phagocytosis. These observations seem to indicate that the abnormality in intracellular killing is not directly caused by the burn injury, but due to an as yet unknown secondary event gradually evolving with time. Alexander et al. (1968a) have not observed bactericidal defects that could be ascribed to a diminished rate of phagocytosis. However, when normal neutrophils were incubated with *S. aureus* and undiluted sera from bacteriemic burn patients, Bjornson et al. (1981b) observed diminished intracellular killing which could be related to an inhibitory effect of the burn sera on the phagocytic process. The non-cytotoxic and long-lasting effect of the phagocytosis inhibitor on neutrophils was demonstrated in 3 of 12 burn patients 8 to 56 days post-burn. The isolation and characterization of this cell-directed inhibitor is of considerable importance and may help to provide an explanation for the curious defects of leukocyte function found in thermally injured patients.

In severely burned patients whose convalescence is complicated by septicemia, or in victims of trauma with a complicated clinical course, a pronounced depression of neutrophil bactericidal activity has been detected (Grogan and Miller 1973). Neutrophils from 5 and 13 out of 16 patients with trauma, complicated by infection, demonstrated significantly depressed phagocytosis and intracellular killing, respectively. In contrast, none of the traumatized patients free of complications exhibited alterations of phagocytosis or intracellular killing of *Pseudomonas aeruginosa.* These observations suggest that the leukocyte dysfunctions correlate with the presence of sepsis rather than the injury per se. Whether the reduction in intracellular killing is related to decreased bacterial uptake (eventually caused by the inhibitor described by Bjornson et al. (1981), see above) is not known.

The basis for the neutrophil bactericidal defect has not been established. Lowered levels in neutrophils of lysozyme in burned patients have been correlated with significantly decreased chemotactic activity and random migration of neutrophils between the 5th and 15th day post-injury (Davis et al. 1980). Defective mobilization of lysosomal enzymes has been suggested by Bröte and Stendahl (1975), who found

TABLE 2.
Cellular alterations in thermal injury

Decreased neutrophil and macrophage migration
Decreased neutrophil phagocytosis
Decreased neutrophil bactericidal activity
Decreased lysozyme levels in neutrophils
Decreased numbers of lymphocytes
Increased numbers of immunosuppressive mononuclear cells

normal hexose monophosphate shunt activity but impaired myeloperoxidase-mediated iodination during phagocytosis in neutrophils from thermally injured patients.

Alexander (1967) suggested that decreased concentrations of neutrophil lysosomal enzyme are a contributing factor to diminished resistance to bacterial infections in thermally injured patients. Others have related a serum inhibitor of phagocytosis to decreased intracellular killing in septic burn patients (Bjornson et al. 1981b). Curreri et al. (1973) noted a significant reduction in neutrophil bactericidal function in patients with greater than 30% total body surface burns. The functional cell defect was measured by the in vitro stimulated reduction of nitroblue tetrazolium. A fall in NBT reduction by phagocytosing neutrophils from burned patients was almost uniformly seen with the development of burn wound sepsis. The authors suggested this technique as a means of monitoring wound colonization in thermally injured patients. Significantly decreased oxygen consumption in resting and stimulated neutrophils from burned patients when compared to unburned individuals had been observed by Heck et al. (1975). However, altered cellular oxygen consumption did not correlate with stimulated NBT test, wound sepsis or burn size. Subsequent studies revealed a defect in NADH and NADP oxidase levels in the subcellular fraction of leukocytes from burned patients which was suggested to be of relevance to the reduced neutrophil bactericidal activity in thermally injured patients (Heck et al. 1979).

A marginal improvement of neutrophil bactericidal capacity was observed in thermally injured dogs treated with *Corynebacterium parvum* vaccine (Stinnett et al. 1981). The survival rate of these animals was significantly improved as compared to untreated burned dogs. It should also be mentioned that high protein diet significantly improved neutrophil bactericidal activity as well as other humoral and cellular defects in thermally injured patients (for review see Alexander et al. 1981).

12.4. LUNG INJURY SUBSEQUENT TO THERMAL TRAUMA

Pulmonary complications constitute a major threat to the burned patient even though in most cases there is not direct injury to the lung, either direct thermal injury or related to smoke/vapor inhalation. Acute respiratory distress can be observed in some patients within minutes to hours after thermal injury. Other patients develop progressive respiratory failure 1 to 5 days after being burned, and a third group of patients may develop pneumonia several weeks after thermal injury (Achauer et al. 1973). The lung appears to respond to a variety of injuries such as surgical trauma or body surface burns with damage to lung vascular endothelium and/or alveolar epithelial lining cells, resulting in interstitial and alveolar edema. In autopsies of burned patients, pulmonary edema and/or bronchopneumonia are almost always found (Achauer et al. 1973).

The pathogenesis of the acute and the progressive form of lung injury in burned

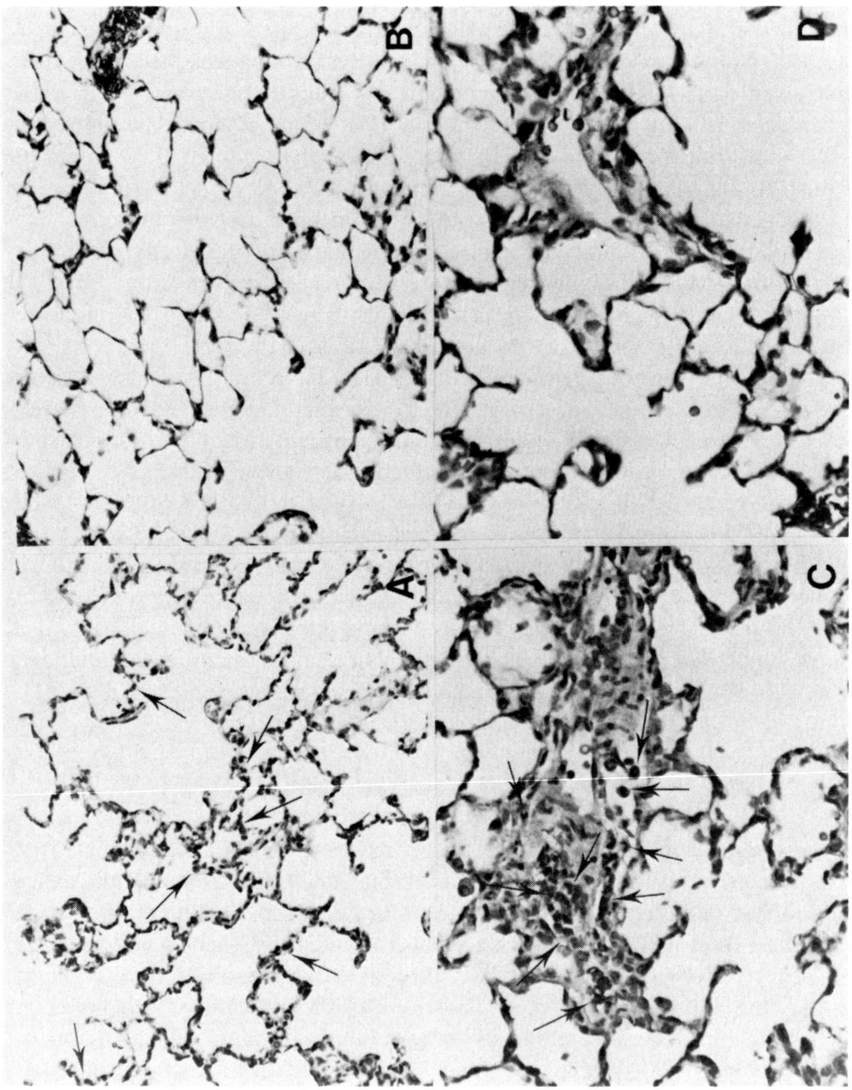

Fig 1. Fixed reactions of lungs from thermally injured (A, C) and normal (B, D) rats. While pulmonary capillary lumens in sections from the normal animals are relatively devoid of leukocytes (B, D), leuko-aggregates can be seen in the interstitial vessels of thermally injured rats (arrows, A, C). (H and E, x 180).

patients is not known, although, in some cases, smoke inhalation, direct heat or carbon monoxide poisoning may contribute to acute respiratory distress. A loss of surfactant (Matsuura 1966) or platelet-fibrin microemboli in the pulmonary vasculature (Rapaport et al. 1973) has been reported as a consequence of thermal injury. Some authors suggested that sepsis is the primary cause of increased vascular permeability with resulting pulmonary edema in burned patients (Tranbaugh et al. 1980). Vasoactive or related substances, released in response to thermal injury, have also been suggested to play a role in vascular permeability changes (Carvajal et al. 1975; Arturson and Jonsson 1979). For example, Anggard and Jonsson (1971) found prostaglandin E_1 to be increased in lymph from burned tissue. Others observed increased levels of prostacyclin (PGI_2) in lung lymph of sheep following body surface burns (Harms et al. 1981). The increase in PGI_2 has been found to correspond with microvascular changes in the lung.

Recent findings in experimental studies of thermal injury suggest that toxic oxygen species released from activated neutrophils seem to play an important role as well. Acute thermal injury (70°C, 30 s) to rat skin (28% total body surface area) resulted in intravascular complement activation and generation of C5-derived chemotactic activity which was followed by increases in lung vascular permeability (Till et al. 1983). Lung injury developed progressively during the first six hours post-burn and was paralleled by changes in complement levels. Leukoaggregates within pulmonary capillaries and the presence of intra-alveolar hemorrhage were the most prominent morphologic features (Fig. 1). In order to evaluate the pathogenic basis for the observed lung injury, rats were depleted of serum complement or neutrophils by pretreatment with cobra venom factor or antiserum against rat neutrophils prior to thermal injury. In both instances, increased vascular permeability in the lung was almost completely prevented, providing evidence of complement activation products and neutrophils as important pathogenic factors. The requirement for complement did not seem to depend on anaphylatoxin-mediated release of histamine since antihistamine treatment of animals prior to thermal injury did not alter lung vascular permeability. However, treatment of rats with a combination of catalase and superoxide dismutase almost totally protected the thermally injured animals from acute lung injury (Till et al. 1983). These findings are in agreement with observations by Hilton (1980), who showed that in thermally injured dogs treatment with superoxide dismutase reduced early plasma volume loss, and catalase reduced both early and continuing plasma volume losses. From the data by Till et al. (1983) it seems likely that the most important effect of intravascular complement activation following thermal injury is the generation of chemotactic peptide (C5a) and the subsequent activation of neutrophils with subsequent production and release of oxygen metabolites including hydrogen peroxide and superoxide anion. The ability of catalase and superoxide dismutase to protect the thermally injured animal from acute lung injury provides strong evidence that release of toxic oxygen species from neutrophils is the most significant patho-physiologic event leading to vascular injury.

Following thermal injury, various toxic factors have been described and have been associated with organ tissue damage (Allgöwer et al. 1968; Helmkamp et al. 1973; Loebl et al. 1973). In this regard, studies by Nishigaki et al. (1980), who suspected that "burn toxin" might be similar to lipid peroxides, seem to be of considerable interest. In the burned skin of rats the authors observed a sixfold increase in the concentration of lipid peroxide 3 hours post-burn. The lipid peroxide level remained high for 24 hours, then decreased, reaching control values on Day 7 post-burn. These changes in the burned skin were paralleled by changes of lipid peroxide in the serum. High serum levels of lipid peroxide were followed by increased concentrations of lipid peroxide in various organ tissues, resulting in tissue damage as measured by the release of tissue enzymes (Nishigaki et al. 1980). Since the formation of lipid peroxide in the burned skin followed by release of lipid peroxide into the blood stream resulted in damage of cells of certain organs, the authors assigned lipid peroxide as "burn toxin". These few examples of recently published data on toxic oxygen species and lipid peroxide in experimental burns seem to open a promising new avenue of clinical research to further evaluate the pathogenesis of acute and progressive lung damage in thermally injured patients.

12.5. IMMUNOLOGICAL ABERRATIONS

The observation of prolonged survival of skin allografts on severely burned patients (Branch et al. 1946; Dempster and Lennox 1951; Kay 1957; Alexander and Moncrief 1966; Chambler and Batchelor 1969; Ninnemann et al. 1978) had led to the recognition of altered cellular immunity following thermal injury. The delay in rejection time appears to be proportional to burn size (Rapaport et al. 1964; Chambler and Batchelor 1969) but is unrelated to the number of lymphocytes in the blood and is not accompanied by decreased serum levels of immunoglobulin (Ninnemann et al. 1978). Experiments in guinea pigs further supported the evidence of T-cell abnormality in thermal injury (Rapaport and Converse 1966; Solowey and Rapaport 1967). The authors have shown that tuberculin-sensitive animals have a marked depression of skin reactivity to intradermal tuberculin tests following full-thickness skin burns of 20-40% total body surface area. It is now well recognized that burn patients and animals become anergic to certain tests of delayed cutaneous hypersensitivity (Casson et al. 1966; Rapaport et al. 1968). However, the burn size appears to be critical. In patients as well as in experimental animals it has been noticed that immunological responses remain normal in burns smaller than 20% body surface area (Munster et al. 1973). In contrast to skin allografts, survival of internal organ transplants has not been found to be prolonged in burned animals (Munster et al. 1973).

Further evidence of T-cell abnormality in thermally injured patients has been provided by in vitro assays employing T-cell mitogens such as Candida antigen, phytohemagglutinin and concanavalin A. In most instances, decreased mitogen responses of peripheral blood lymphocytes from severely burned patients have been observed (Munster et al. 1973; Ishizawa et al. 1978; Miller and Baker 1979; Constantian 1979). Similar results have been obtained by the use of mixed lymphocyte culture assays showing depression of both the response as well as the stimulatory capacity of burn lymphocytes (Sakai et al. 1974). Studies of cell-mediated immunity in burned patients have also shown decreased T-cell counts (Neilan et al. 1977; Volenec et al. 1977a, b; Ishizawa et al. 1978; Sukhtankar and Sengupta 1981) and depressed lymphokine production in lymphocytes stimulated in vitro (Solowey and Rapaport 1967; Sukhtankar and Sengupta 1981). Whereas the T-cell count has been found to be depressed in patients regardless of burn size, depression of blastoid transformation and lymphokine generation has been observed only in patients with burns involving more than 25% of total body surface area (Sukhtankar and Sengupta 1981). The most pronounced depression of these parameters of cell-mediated immunity was seen 1−2 days post-burn in large-sized burns involving approximately 65% of total body surface areas. T-cell functions then recovered completely, reaching normal values on the 12th day post-burn (Sukhtankar and Sengupta 1981). The same authors also observed a strong correlation between decreased lymphokine activity and depressed bactericidal activity. This is in accordance with previous observations by Baker et al. (1979a), who noticed decreased mitogen responses in burned patients 4 to 7 days post-burn which predated clinical evidence of sepsis by 2 to 4 days. On the other hand, burn patients with only mild infections have been found to demonstrate, not a depressed, but rather an augmented mitogen response (Baker et al. 1979a). It is assumed that depressed cell-mediated immunity greatly increased the threat of sepsis in thermally injured patients. Additional experiments revealed that addition of mononuclear cells from immunosuppressed burn patients to an ongoing normal mixed leukocyte reaction significantly depressed leukocyte proliferation (Miller and Baker 1979). Addition of cells from patients with normal or increased cellular immune responses had no such effect. The results of these experiments suggest that mononuclear suppressor cells are generated as a result of thermal injury. Subsequent experiments suggested that suppressor T-lymphocytes are associated with the depressed cell-mediated immunity in thermally injured patients (Constantian 1979; Baker et al. 1979b; Wolfe et al. 1981). T-suppressor cells have also been demonstrated in thermally injured mice (Miller and Claudy 1979). The function of B-lymphocytes from burned patients appears unaffected (Rapaport and Bachvaroff 1976; Miller and Trunkey 1977; Bjornson et al. 1977).

There is increasing evidence that serum factors may be related to the generation of suppressor cell activity in thermally injured patients. For example, a factor or factors present in serum of burn patients have been shown to suppress the reactivity of normal human leukocytes to the T-lymphocyte mitogens Candida or phytohemagglutinin (Munster et al. 1973; Constantian 1978; Ninnemann et al. 1978, 1979; Wolfe et al. 1981). Constantian (1978) reported that depressive serum factors are present in a low molecular weight (10,000 daltons) polypeptide subfraction and that the activity of these factors is directly related to the severity of burn injury.

Prolonged allograft survival in thermally injured patients was found to be related to an immunosuppressive effect of post-burn serum (Ninnemann et al. 1978). This effect was found to be dependent on the presence of B-lymphocytes which participate in the generation of suppressor T-cells (Ninnemann 1979, 1980). The same author was able to demonstrate that bacterial endotoxin can initiate this suppressive effect both in vivo and in vitro (Ninnemann and Stein 1980). Ninnemann et al. (1979) also noticed that addition of post-recovery serum from burn patients to cultures of normal lymphocytes reduced the effect of autologous suppressive serum. Further studies revealed that the blocking effect of post-recovery serum was due to the presence of IgG with anti-suppressor cell activity (Ninnemann et al. 1979).

Recently published data suggest the possibility that the occurrence of suppressor lymphocytes and serum immunosuppressive factors in thermally injured patients can be iatrogenically induced. A complex of polyvinylpyrrolidone and iodine (povidone-iodine: Betadine) with strong germicidal activity, which is frequently used in the daily burn wound management, has been found to profoundly suppress phytohemagglutinin stimulation of normal lymphocytes and the reaction of normal lymphocytes in the mixed leukocyte culture (Ninnemann and Stein 1981). Incubation of normal lymphocytes in the presence of povidone-iodine for only 24 hours was enough to induce strong suppression. The iodine content of this drug was found to be responsible for this induction. This suppression has been found to be mediated by the induction of a suppressor cell population. Patients treated with povidone-iodine showed high levels of iodine in their serum. Ninnemann and Stein (1981) observed that sera with iodine concentrations of more than 70 μg per 100 ml expressed significant suppression of blastogenesis of normal lymphocytes in vitro. The suppressive effect was found to reside in the albumin fraction which contained the iodine. Since not all suppressive sera, as tested by Ninnemann and Stein (1981), displayed high iodine levels it is suggested that immunosuppression in thermally injured patients may have a multiplicity of causes. Based on clinical observations of greatly increased susceptiblity to bacterial infections and prolonged allograft survival as well as the experimental observations of suppressed lymphocyte responses, there is substantial evidence that in thermally injured patients cellular immunity is impaired due to an increase in suppressor T-cell activity.

12.6. CONCLUDING REMARKS

From the diverse observations cited above, it is clear that thermal injury ultimately produces defects in host defenses, the result of which leads to life-threatening microbial infections. Based on the known facts, no simple outline can currently explain the many defects that occur subsequent to thermal injury. Some of the outcomes, such as the state of immunosuppression, may, for instance, be secondary to abnormal production of cyclo-oxygenase products of the prostaglandin system. The question then becomes: What led to stimulation of arachidonate metabolism?

The defect in phagocytic cell function (phagocytosis, bactericidal activity, chemotactic migration) could be the result of excessive production of prostaglandin E, or cell contact with complement activation products. It is difficult to determine what is primary and what is secondary in the intertwining and reverberating circuits of the inflammatory system. To compound the confusion, we now see evidence that some of the alterations of host defenses in thermal injury may be related to therapeutic intervention. What is needed is a more thorough exploration of mediator systems both in thermally injured humans and in experimental models. It is only through a concerted effort that the tangled web of facts will become comprehensible.

REFERENCES

Achauer, B.M., Allyn, P.A., Furnas, D.W. and Bartlett, R.H. (1973) Pulmonary complications of burns: the major threat to the burn patient. *Ann. Surg. 177,* 311–319.

Alexander, J.W. (1967) Serum and leukocyte lysosomal enzymes. Derangements following severe thermal injury. *Arch. Surg. 95,* 482–490.

Alexander, J.W. and Fisher, M.W. (1970) Immunological determinants of pseudomonas infections of man accompanying severe burn injury. *J. Trauma 10,* 565–574.

Alexander, J.W. and Meakins, J.L. (1972) A physiological basis for the development of opportunistic infections in man. *Ann. Surg. 176,* 273–287.

Alexander, J.W. and Moncrief, J.A. (1966) Alterations of the immune response following severe thermal injury. *Arch. Surg. 93,* 75–83.

Alexander, J.W. and Wixson, D. (1970) Neutrophil dysfunction and sepsis in burn injury. *Surg. Gynecol. Obstet. 130,* 431–438.

Alexander, J.W., Hegg, M. and Altemeier, W.A. (1968a) Neutrophil function in selected surgical disorders. *Ann. Surg. 168,* 447–458.

Alexander, J.W., Windhorst, D.B. and Good, R.A. (1968b) Improved tests for the evaluation of neutrophil function in human disease. *J. Lab. Clin. Med. 72,* 136–148.

Alexander, J.W., Dionigi, R. and Meakins, J.L. (1971) Periodic variation in the antibacterial function of human neutrophils and its relationship to sepsis. *Ann. Surg. 173,* 206–213.

Alexander, J.W., Stinnett, J.D., Ogle, C.K., Ogle, J.D. and Morris, M.J. (1979) A comparison of immunologic profiles and their influence on bacteriemia in surgical patients with a high risk of infection. *Surgery 86,* 94–103.

Alexander, J.W., McMillan, B.G., Stinnett, J.D., Ogle, C.K., Bozian, R.C., Fisher, J.E., Oakes, J.B., Morris, M.J. and Krummel, R. (1980) Beneficial effects of aggressive protein feeding in severely burned children. *Ann. Surg. 192,* 505–516.

Alexander, J.W., Stinnett, J.D. and Ogle, C.K. (1981) Alterations in neutrophil function. In: J.L. Ninnemann (Ed.), *The Immune Consequences of Thermal Injury,* Williams and Wilkins, Baltimore, pp. 21–35.

Altman, L.C., Turukawa, C.T. and Klebanoff, S.J. (1977) Defective polymorphonuclear leukocyte function in thermally injured patients (Abstract). *Clin. Res. 25,* 117.

Allgöwer, M., Burri, C., Cueni, L., Engley, F., Fleisch, H., Gruber, U.F, Harder, F. and Russell, R.G.G. (1968) Study of burn toxins. *Ann. NY Acad. Sci. 150,* 807–815.

Anggard, E. and Jonsson, C.E. (1971) Efflux of prostaglandins in lymph from scalded tissue. *Acta Physiol. Scand. 81,* 440–447.

Arturson, G. and Jonsson, C.E. (1979) Transcapillary transport after thermal injury. *Scand. J. Plast. Reconstr. Surg. 13,* 29–38.

Baker, C.C., Miller, C.L. and Trunkey, D.D. (1979a) Predicting fatal sepsis in burn patients. *J. Trauma 19,* 641–647.

Baker, C.C., Miller, C.L., Trunkey, D.D. and Lim, R.C. (1979b) Identity of mononuclear cells which compromise the resistance of trauma patients. *J. Surg. Res. 26,* 478–487.

Berenberg, J.L. and Ward, P.A. (1973) The chemotactic factor inactivator in normal human serum. *J. Clin. Invest. 52,* 1200–1206.

Bjornson, A.B. and Alexander, J.W. (1974) Alterations of serum opsonins in patients with severe thermal injury. *J. Lab. Clin. Med. 83,* 372–382.

Bjornson, A.B., Altemeier, W.A. and Bjornson, H.S. (1976) Reduction in C3 conversion in patients with severe thermal injury. *J. Trauma 16,* 905–911.

Bjornson, A.B., Altemeier, W.A. and Bjornson, H.S. (1977) Changes in humoral components of host defense following burn trauma. *Ann. Surg. 186,* 88–96.

Bjornson, A.B., Altemeier, W.A. and Bjornson, H.S. (1979) The septic burned patient. A model for studying the role of complement and immunoglobulins in opsonization of opportunistic micro-organisms. *Ann. Surg. 189,* 515–527.

Bjornson, A.B., Altemeier, W.A. and Bjornson, H.S. (1980) Complement, opsonins, and the immune response to bacterial infection in burned patients. *Ann. Surg. 191,* 323–329.

Bjornson, A.B., Bjornson, H.S. and Altemeier, W.A. (1981a) Reduction in alternative complement pathway mediated C3 conversion following burn injury. *Ann. Surg. 194,* 224–231.

Bjornson, A.B., Bjornson, H.S. and Altemeier, W.A. (1981b) Serum-mediated inhibition of polymorphonuclear leukocyte function following burn injury. *Ann. Surg. 194,* 568–575.

Blumenstock, F.A., Saba, T.M., Weber, P. and Cho, E. (1976) Purification and biochemical characterization of a macrophage stimulating alpha 2-globulin opsonic protein. *J. Reticuloendothel. Soc. 19,* 157–172.

Blumenstock, F.A., Saba, T.M., Weber, P. and Laffin, R. (1978) Biochemical and immunological characterization of human opsonic alpha 2 SB glycoprotein: its identity with cold-insoluble globulin. *J. Biol. Chem. 253,* 4287–4291.

Branch, C.D., Wilkins, C.F. and Ross, F.P. (1946) The coagulum contact method of skin grafting in the treatment of burns and wounds. *Surgery 19,* 460–465.

Bröte, L. and Stendahl, O. (1975) The function of polymorphonuclear leukocytes after surgical trauma. *Acta Clin. Scand. 141,* 565–570.

Carvajal, H.F., Brouhard, B.H. and Linares, H.A. (1975) Effect of antihistamine-antiserotonin and ganglionic blocking agents upon increased capillary permeability following burn trauma. *J. Trauma 15,* 969–975.

Casson, P.R., Solowey, H.C. and Converse, J.M. (1966) Delayed hypersensitivity status of burned patients. *Surg. Forum 17,* 268–273.

Chambler, K. and Batchelor, J.R. (1969) Influence of defined incompatibilities and area of burn on skin-homograft survival in burned subjects. *Lancet 1,* 16–18.

Craddock, P.R., Fehr, J., Dalmasso, A.P., Brigham, K.L. and Jacob, H.S. (1977)

Hemodialysis leukopenia: pulmonary vascular leukostasis resulting from complement activation by dialyzer cellophane membranes. *J. Clin. Invest. 59,* 879–888.

Connolly, J.C. and Gilmore, O.J.A. (1979) A study of the effect of povidone-iodine on polymorphonuclear leukocytes chemotaxis. *Br. J. Exp. Pathol. 60,* 662–666.

Constantian, M.B. (1978) Association of sepsis with an immunosuppressive polypeptide in the serum of burn patients. *Ann. Surg. 188,* 209–215.

Constantian, M.B. (1979) Impaired reactivity of burn patient lymphocytes to phytohemagglutinin in autologous serum: Failure to improve responsiveness by washing in vitro. *J. Surg. Res. 27,* 84–92.

Curreri, P.W., Heck, E.L., Browne, L. and Baxter, C.R. (1973) Stimulated nitroblue tetrazolium test to assess neutrophil antibacterial function: Prediction of wound sepsis in burned patients. *Surgery 74,* 6–13.

Daniels, J.C., Larson, D.L., Abston, S. and Ritzmann, S.E. (1974) Serum protein profiles in thermal burns. II. Protease inhibitors, complement factors, and C-reactive protein. *J. Trauma 14,* 153–162.

Davis, J.M., Dineen, P. and Gallin, J.I. (1980) Neutrophil degranulation and abnormal chemotaxis after thermal injury. *J. Immunol. 124,* 1467–1471.

Davis, J.H., Illner, H., Stevens, J.M. and Dinenn, P.A.P. (1981): FMLP receptor availability in burn patients with impaired chemotaxis. *Surg. Forum 32,* 35–36.

Dempster, W.J. and Lennox, B. (1951) Experimental approach to homotransplant problem in plastic surgery: use of multiple donors. *Br. J. Plast. Surg. 4,* 81–84.

Dhennin, C., Pinon, G. and Greco, J.M. (1978) Alterations of complement system following thermal injury: use in estimation of vital prognosis. *J. Trauma 18,* 129–133.

Douglas, S.D. and Schopfer, K. (1974) Phagocyte function in protein-calorie malnutrition. *Clin. Exp. Immunol. 17,* 121–128.

Edelman, R., Suskind, R.N., Olson, R.E. and Sirisinha, S. (1973) Mechanisms of defective delayed cutaneous hypersensitivity in children with protein-calorie malnutrition. *Lancet 1,* 506–508.

Erbs, F., Müller and Opferfuch, W. (1980) Der Einfluss der Verbrennungskrankheit auf das Komplement-System. *Fortschr. Med. 98,* 397–399.

Farrell, M.F., Day, N.K., Tsakraklides, V., Good, R.A. and Day, S.B. (1973) Study of lymphocyte depletion and serum complement perturbation following acute burn trauma. *Surgery 73,* 697–705.

Fikrig, S.M., Karl, S.C. and Suntharalingam, K. (1977) Neutrophil chemotaxis in patients with burns. *Ann. Surg. 186,* 746–748.

Fjellström, K.-E. and Arturson, G. (1963) Changes in the human complement system following burn trauma. *Acta Pathol. Microbiol. Scand. 59,* 257–270.

Gallin, J.I., Wright, D.C. and Schiffmann, E. (1978) Role of secretory events in modulating human neutrophil chemotaxis. *J. Clin. Invest. 62,* 1364–1374.

Grogan, J.B. (1976a) Suppressed in vitro chemotaxis of burn neutrophils. *J. Trauma 16,* 985–988.

Grogan, J.B. (1976b) Altered neutrophil phagocytic function in burn patients. *J. Trauma 16,* 734–738.

Grogan, J.B. and Miller, R.C. (1973) Impaired function of polymorphonuclear leukocytes in patients with burns and other trauma. *Surg. Gynecol. Obstet. 137,* 784–788.

Harms, B.A., Bodai, B.I., Smith, M., Gunther, R., Flynn, J, and Demling, R.H. (1981) Prostaglandin release and altered microvascular integrity after burn injury. *J. Surg. Res. 31,* 274–280.

Hayashi, H., Yoshinaga, M. and Yamamoto, S. (1974) The nature of a mediator of leukocyte chemotaxis in inflammation. In: H. Schönfeld, R.W. Brockman and F.E. Hahn (Eds), *Antibiotics and Chemotherapy, Vol. 19: Chemotaxis: Its Biology and Biochemistry,* S. Karger, Basel, pp. 296–332.

Heck, E.L., Browne, L., Curreri, P.W. and Baxter, C.R. (1975) Evaluation of leukocyte function in burned individuals by in vitro oxygen consumption. *J. Trauma 15,* 486–489.

Heck, E.L., Edgar, M.A., Masters, B.S. and Baxter, C.R. (1979) The role of NADH-HADPH oxidase activity in the leukocyte function of burned patients. *J. Trauma 19,* 49–51.

Heck, E., Edgar, M.A., Hunt, J.L. and Baxter, C.R. (1980) A comparison of leukocyte function and burn mortality. *J. Trauma 20,* 75–77.

Heideman, M. (1979a) The effect of thermal injury on hemodynamic, respiratory and hematologic variables in relation to complement activation. *J. Trauma 19,* 239–243.

Heideman, M. (1979b) Complement activation in vitro induced by endotoxin and injured tissue. *J. Surg. Res. 26,* 670–673.

Helmkamp, G.M., Wilmore, D.W, Johnson, A.A. and Pruitt, B.A. (1973) Essential fatty acid deficiency in red cells after thermal injury: correction with intravenous fat therapy. *Am. J. Clin. Nutr. 26,* 1331–1338.

Hill, J.H. and Ward, P.A. (1969) C3 leukotactic factors produced by a tissue protease. *J. Exp. Med. 130,* 505–518.

Hilton, J.G. (1980) Effects of alterations of polyunsaturated fatty acid metabolism upon plasma volume loss induced by thermal trauma. *J. Trauma 20,* 663–668.

Holder, I.A. and Ablin, R.J. (1980) Alterations in complement in burn patients. In: J.L. Ninnemann (Ed.), *The Immune Consequences of Thermal Injury.* Williams and Wilkins, Baltimore, pp. 134–149.

Ishizawa, S., Sakai, H., Sarles, H.E., Larson, D.L. and Daniels, J.C. (1978) Effect of thymosin on T-lymphocyte functions in patients with acute thermal burns. *J. Trauma 18,* 48–52.

Johnson, K.J., Anderson, T.P. and Ward, P.A. (1977) Suppression of immune complex-induced inflammation by the chemotactic factor inactivator. *J. Clin. Invest. 59,* 951–958.

Kay, G.D. (1957) Prolonged survivial of a skin homograft in a patient with very extensive burns. *Ann. NY Acad. Sci. 64,* 767–774.

Kreutzer, D.L., Claypool, W.D. and Ward, P.A. (1979) Isolation by hydrophobic chromatography of the chemotactic factor inactivators from human serum. *Clin. Immunol. Immunopathol. 12,* 162–176.

Kulapongs, P., Edelman, R., Suskind, R. and Olsen, R.E. (1977) Defective local leukocyte mobilization in children with kvashiorkor. *Am. J. Clin. Nutr. 30,* 367–370.

Lanser, M.E., Saba, T.M. and Scovill, W.A. (1980) Opsonic glycoprotein (plasma fibronectin) levels after burn. *Ann. Surg. 192,* 776–782.

Loebl, E.C., Baxter, C.R. and Currerl, P.W. (1973) The mechanism of erythrocyte destruction in the early post-burn period. *Ann. Surg. 178,* 681–686.

Maderazo, E.G., Ward, P.A. and Quintilliani, R. (1975) Defective regulation of chemotaxis in cirrhosis. *J. Lab. Clin. Med. 85,* 621–630.

Maderazo, E.G., Ward, P.A., Woronick, C.L., Kubik, J. and DeGraff, A.C. (1976) Leukotactic dysfunction in sarcoidosis. *Ann. Intern. Med. 84,* 414–419.

Maderazo, E.G., Ward, P.A., Woronick, C.L. and Quintilliani, R. (1977) Partial characterization of a cell directed inhibitor of leukotaxis in human serum. *J. Lab. Clin. Med. 89,* 190–199.

Maderazo, E.G., Anton, T.F. and Ward, P.A. (1978) Serum-associated inhibition of leukotaxis in humans with cancer. *Clin. Immunol. Immunopathol. 9,* 166–176.

Maeda, S., Yoshinagoa, M. and Hayashi, H. (1975) Characterization of a chemotactic factor (leucoegresin) for polymorphonuclear leukocytes from thermal skin site. *Virchows Arch. B. 19,* 37–49.

Matsuura, Y., Najib, A. and Lee, W.H. (1966) Pulmonary compliance and surfactant activity in thermal burn. *Surg. Forum 17,* 86–88.

Miller, C.L. and Baker, C.C. (1979) Changes in lymphocyte activity after thermal injury. The role of suppressor cells. *J. Clin. Invest. 63,* 202–210.

Miller, C.L. and Trunkey, D.D. (1977) Thermal injury: Defects in immune response induction. *J. Surg. Res. 22,* 621–625.

Miller, C.L. and Claudy, B.J. (1979) Suppressor T-cell activity induced as a result of thermal injury. *Cell. Immunol. 44,* 201–208.

Munster, A.M., Eurenius, K., Katz, R.M., Canales, L., Foley, F.D. and Mortensen, R.F. (1973) Cell-mediated immunity after thermal injury. *Ann. Surg. 177,* 139–143.

Nathenson, G., Miller, M.E., Myers, K.A., Stitzel, A. and Spitzer, R.E. (1978) Depressed opsonic and chemotactic activities in sera of postburn patients and partial opsonic restauration with properdin and properdin convertase. *Clin. Immunol. Immunopathol. 9,* 269–276.

Neilan, B.A., Taddeini, L. and Strate, R.G. (1977) T-lymphocyte rosette formation after major burns. *J. Am. Med. Assoc. 238,* 493–296.

Nelson, R.D., Chenoweth, D.E., Solomkin, J.S. and Solem, L.D. (1983) Cytotaxin receptors on human neutrophils: modulation of C5a and peptide receptor number. In: H.U. Keller and G.O. Till (Eds), *Agents and Actions, Suppl., Vol. 12: Leukocyte Locomotion and Chemotaxis*. Birkhäuser Verlag, Basel, pp. 274–289.

Ninnemann, J.L. (1979) Activation of suppressor T-cells following thermal injury is B-cell and not accessory cell/macrophage-mediated. *Immunol. Lett. 1,* 97–99.

Ninnemann, J.L. (1980) Immunosuppression following thermal injury through B cell activation of suppressor T cells. *J. Trauma 20,* 206–213.

Ninnemann, J.I. and Stein, M.D. (1980) Bacterial endotoxin and the generation of suppressor T cells following thermal injury. *J. Trauma 20,* 959–966.

Ninnemann, J.L. and Stein, M.D. (1981) Suppressor cell induction by povidone-iodine: in vitro demonstration of a consequence of clinical burn treatment with Betadine. *J. Immunol. 126,* 1905–1908.

Ninnemann, J.L., Fisher, J.C. and Frank, H.A. (1978) Prolonged survival of human skin allografts following thermal injury. *Transplantation 25,* 69–72.

Ninnemann, J.L., Fisher, J.C. and Wachtel, T.L. (1979) Thermal injury-associated immunosuppression: occurrence and in vitro blocking effect of post recovery serum. *J. Trauma 122,* 1736–1741.

Nishigaki, I., Hagihara, M., Hiramatsu, M., Izawa, Y. and Yaki, K. (1980) Effect of thermal injury on lipid peroxide levels of rat. *Biochem. Med. 24,* 185–189.

O'Flaherty, J.T., Craddock, P.R. and Jacob, H.S. (1978) Effect of intravascular complement activation on granulocyte adhesiveness and distribution. *Blood 51,* 731–739.

Rapaport, F.T. and Bachvaroff, R.J. (1976) Kinetics of humoral responsiveness in severe thermal injury. *Ann. Surg. 184,* 51–57.

Rapaport, F.T. and Converse, J.M. (1966) Inhibition of tuberculin sensitivity by thermal injury (Abstract). *Fed. Proc. 25,* 549.

Rapaport, F.T., Converse, J.M., Horn, L., Ballantyne, D.L. and Mulholland, J.M. (1964) Altered reactivity of skin homografts in severe thermal injury. *Ann. Surg. 159,* 390–395.

Rapaport, F.T., Milgrom, F., Kano, K., Gesner, B., Solowey, A.C., Casson, P., Silverman, H.I. and Converse, J.M. (1968) Immunologic sequelae of thermal injury. *Ann. NY Acad. Sci. 150,* 1004–1008.

Rapaport, F.T., Nemirovsky, M.S., Bachvaroff, R. and Ball, S.K. (1973) Mechanisms of pulmonary damage in severe burns. *Ann. Surg. 177,* 472–477.

Saba, T.M., Blumenstock, F.A., Weber, P. and Kaplan, J.E. (1978) Physiologic role for cold-insoluble globulin in systemic host defense. Implications of its characterization as the opsonic alpha 2 SB glycoprotein. *Ann. NY Acad. Sci. 312,* 43–55.

Sakai, H., Daniels, J.C., Beathard, G.A., Lewis, S.R., Lynch, J.B. and Ritzmann, S.E. (1974) Mixed lymphocyte culture reaction in patients with acute thermal burns. *J. Trauma 14,* 53–57.

Sharma, V.K., Agarwal, D.S., Satyanand and Saha, K. (1980) Profile of complement components in patients with severe burns. *J. Trauma 20,* 976–978.

Solowey, A.C. and Rapaport, F.T. (1967) Mechanisms of tuberculin unresponsiveness in burned animals. *Surg. Forum 18,* 522–524.

Stinnett, J.D., Alexander, J.W., Morris, M.J., Dreffer, R.L., Craycraft, T.K., Anderson, P.E., Ogle, C.K. and Macmillan, B.G. (1981) Improved survival in severely burned animals using intravenous Corynebacterium parvum vaccine post injury. *Surgery 89,* 237–242.

Sukhtankar, A.Y. and Sengupta, S.R. (1981) Cellular immunity in burns. *Burns 8,* 168–171.

Till, G. and Ward, P.A. (1975) Two distinct chemotactic factor inactivators in human serum. *J. Immunol. 114,* 843–847.

Till, G., Debatin, M. and Gemsa, D. (1980) Regulatory mediators in Arthus reactions: demonstration of chemotactic factor inactivator and cell directed inhibitor activity. In: D.A. Willoughby and J.P. Giroud (Eds), *Inflammation: Mechanisms and Treatment,* MTP Press, Lancaster, England, pp. 639–645.

Till, G.O., Beauchamp, C., Menapace, D., Tourtellotte, W., Kunkel, R., Johnson, K.J. and Ward, P.A. (1983) Oxygen radical dependent lung damage following thermal injury of rat skin. *J. Trauma 23,* 269–277.

Tranbaugh, R.F., Lewis, F.R., Christensen, J.M. and Elings, V.B. (1980) Lung water changes after thermal injury. The effects of cristalloid resuscitation and sepsis. *Ann. Surg. 192,* 479–488.

Volenec, F.J., Mani, M.M., Clark, G.M., Robinson, D.W. and Humphrey, L.J. (1979a) Peripheral blood T and B lymphocytes in patients with burns. I. Test parameters and clinical evaluation of the rosette assays. *Burns 4,* 1–6.

Volenec, F.J., Mani, M.M., Clark, G.M., Robinson, D.W. and Humphrey, L.J. (1977b) Peripheral blood T and B lymphocytes in patients with burns. II. Sequential rosette analysis considering burn severity and pseudomonas sepsis. *Burns 4,* 7–13.

Ward, P.A. (1981) Chemotactic mechanisms in thermal injury. In: J.L. Ninnemann (Ed.), *The Immune Consequences of Thermal Injury,* Williams and Wilkins, Baltimore, pp. 119–126.

Ward, P.A. and Becker, E.L. (1968) The deactivation of rabbit neutrophils by chemotactic factor and the nature of the activatable esterase. *J. Exp. Med. 127,* 693–709.

Ward, P.A. and Berenberg, J.L. (1974) Defective regulation of inflammatory mediators in Hodgkin's disease. Supernormal levels of chemotactic factor inactivator. *N. Engl. J. Med. 290,* 76–80.

Ward, P.A. and Hill, J.H. (1970) C5 chemotactic fragments produced by an enzyme in lysosomal granules of neutrophils. *J. Immunol. 104,* 535–543.

Ward, P.A., Goralnick, S. and Bullock, W.E. (1976) Defective leukotaxis in patients with lepromatous leprosy. *J. Lab. Clin. Med. 87,* 1025–1032.

Warden, G.D., Mason, A.D. and Pruitt, B.A. Jr. (1974) Evaluation of leukocyte chemotaxis in vitro in thermally injured patients. *J. Clin. Invest. 54,* 1001–1004.

Warden, G.D., Mason, A.D. and Pruitt, B.A. (1975) Suppression of leukocyte chemotaxis in vitro by chemotherapeutic agents used in the management of thermal injuries. *Ann. Surg. 181,* 363–369.

Wolfe, J.H.N., Saporoschetz, I., Young, A.E., O'Connor, N.E. and Mannick, J.A. (1981) Suppressive serum, suppressor lymphocytes, and death from burns. *Ann. Surg. 193,* 513–520.

Zuckerman, L., Caprini, J.A., Lipp, V. and Vagher, J.P. (1978) Disseminated intravascular multiple systems activation (DIMSA) following thermal injury. *J. Trauma 18,* 432–439.

Subject Index

Acute Bacterial Pneumonias, 109
Acute Respiratory Failure, 134, 139
Adherence, 235
Adult Respiratory Distress Syndrome, 109
Alcohol, 308–312
Alkali Burns, 261
Allergic Proctitis, 342
Alternative Complement Pathway, 247–248
Alveolar Macrophages, 100
Alveolitis, 122
Anaphylatoxin(s), 94, 247
Anaphylaxis, 163, 165, 169, 171–174, 180, 365
  slow reacting substance (SRS-A), 163, 165, 169, 171–174, 180
Animal Models, 258
Antibasement-Membrane-Induced Nephritis, 2
Anticolon Antibodies, 351
Antibody
  antimitochondrial, 314
  dependent cell-mediated cytotoxicity (ADCC), 64–70, 348
  non-organ specific, 303
Antigens
  HLA, 353
  HLA-AW24, 353
  HLA-BW35, 353
  HLA-DrWZ, 144
Anti-Inflammatory Therapies, 137
Antineoplastic Drugs, 96
α_1-Antiprotease, 97
α_1-Antitrypsin Deficiency, 100
Arachidonic Acid, 163–175, 178–181, 194, 253
Arthritis, 290
Arthus Reaction, 257
Atopic Keratoconjunctivitis, 267
Axon, 219

B-Lymphocytes, 353
Basement Membrane, 127, 142
Basophils, 163, 169, 171, 172
Behçet's Syndrome, 266
Beryllium, 122, 123, 145
Bleomycin, 122, 134, 136, 141, 142, 144
Boyden Chamber, 212
Bradykinin, 367
Burn
  leucoegresin, 383
  toxin, 390

Carboxypeptidase-N (SCPN), 93, 94
Catalase, 47, 52, 109, 139, 140
Cell(s)
  cell-directed inhibitor of leukocyte chemotaxis, 382
  cell-mediated immunity, 291, 304, 311, 315, 318, 351
  cell-wall defective micro-organisms, 338
  endothelial cells, 226, 364
  IgA-, IgM-, and IgG-containing cells, 339
  IgA-mediated ADCC, 349
  IgD-containing cells, 343
  IgE-containing plasma cells, 339
  IgG-containing plasma cells, 339
  motility, 211
  secretory IgA, 345
  smooth muscle cells, 226
  suppressor T-cells, 352
  T-cell mediated responses, 351
  tumor cell, 227
Charge, 12

Chemotactic, 97
derived from alveolar macrophages, 98
factor(s), 164, 167, 168, 175–178, 180, 195
factor inactivator (CFI), 94, 382
Chemotaxis, 90, 211, 246
Chlamydial Conjunctivitis, 270
Cholera Toxin, 193
Chronic Active Liver Disease, 296, 304, 306
alcohol-induced, 308, 311
autoimmune, 305–307
drug-induced, 307
Chronic Granulomatous Disease, 45–46
Cicatricial Pemphigoid, 266
Circulating Immune Complexes, 347
Classical Complement Pathway, 247–248
Clotting Factor XI, 361
Cobra Venom Factor, 251
Collagen, 95, 122, 124, 125–128, 132–137, 147
metabolism, 141
synthesis, 141, 145
Type I, 125, 126, 127, 133, 134, 138, 139, 140, 141
Type II, 125, 126, 127
Type III, 125, 126, 127, 133, 134, 138, 139, 140, 141
Type IV, 125, 126, 127
Type V, AB, 125, 126, 127
Collagenase, 123, 127, 128, 130, 137, 145, 146, 147
Complement, 16, 23, 93, 123, 146, 247
C1 esterase inhibitor (C1-INH), 346
C1q, 346
C2, 346
C3, 346
C3a, 93
C3b activation, 346
C3b inactivator (C3b-INA), 346
C5a, 93, 97, 98, 103, 105
C5a-des-Arg, 94
Connective Tissue, 121, 124, 125, 131, 137–139, 145, 146
Corneal Ulceration, 267
Crohn's Disease, 337
Cryoglobulinemia, 290
Cutaneous Inflammation, 193
Cyclic AMP, 190
Cyclic GMP, 191
Cyclo-Oxygenase, 253
Cyclo-Oxygenase Pathway, 163–166, 169–172, 174, 179, 180
Cytomegalovirus, 338
Cytotoxic, 101
Cytotoxicity
antibody-dependent cellular cytotoxicity (ADCC), 64–70
and hydrogen peroxide, 51–59
and superoxide, 49–51

Degranulation, 91
Diffuse Alveolar Damage, 101
Dorsal Root Ganglia, 219

5,8,11,14-Eicosatetraynoic Acid (ETYA), 253
Elastase, 100, 129, 130
Elastin, 96, 124, 128–130, 134, 135, 138
Endothelial Cells, 226, 364
Endotoxemia, 262
Endotoxin, 105
Enzyme-Immunoglobulin Complex, 348
Eosinophil, 164, 171, 175–178, 180
chemotactic factor of anaphylaxis (ECF-A), 99
peroxidase, 41, 61, 62
Eosinophilic, 110
Epidermal Cell Mitogen, 193
Episcleritis, 271
Essential Fatty Acids, 253

F-Met-Leu-Phe, 71
Fertilization, 218
Fibrinogen, 384
Fibroblast, 134, 138, 139, 140, 141, 145, 147, 222
activating factors, 123, 145, 146, 147
chemotactic factors, 145, 146
inhibitory factors, 145
Fibronectin, 146
Formylated Peptides, 99
Formylated Signal Peptides, 99
Fungal Keratitis, 271

Glomerulonephritis, 1, 289
Glutathione, 57–58
peroxidase, 47, 52, 57
Glycosaminoglycans, 124, 130, 131, 135, 136, 138, 141
Granuloma(s), 110, 338

H-2 Haplotype, 144
Haber-Weiss (Fenton) Reaction, 43, 92, 96
Hageman Factor, 361
Hepatitis
A, 299–301
acute viral, 292
alcoholic, 308, 311
B, 279–299
B antigens, 280–283
cell mediated responses, 291
B virus, 279
antibodies to, 285–287
carrier state, 295
chronic persistent, 295
experimental, 304
non-A,non-B, 305
Hepatocellular Antigens, 301

antibodies to, 303
cell-mediated responses, 304
Hepatocellular Carcinoma, 298
Herpes Simplex Keratitis, 271
High Molecular Weight (high-MW), 361
HLA Antigens, 353
HLA-AW24, 353
HLA-BW35, 353
HLA-DrWZ, 144
Hydrogen Peroxide (H_2O_2), 40, 47, 51–59, 92, 96
and endothelial cells, 55–56
and erythrocytes, 52–54
and leukocytes, 54–55
and platelets, 54
and tumor cells, 56–58
generation, 99
Hydroperoxyeicosatetraenoic Acid (OOHETE), 164, 165, 170–172, 177–178, 180
Hydroxyeicosatetraenoic Acid (HETE), 98, 163–165, 169–171, 175–180
12-L-HETE, 198
Hydroxyl Radical, 42, 48–49, 63–64, 92, 96
Hydroxylysine, 125
Hydroxyproline, 125
Hyperoxia, 96, 138, 141, 142, 147
Hyperplastic Epidermis, 190
Hypersensitivity, 163–165, 171, 174, 180, 181
Hypersensitivity Pneumonitis, 110
Hypobromous Acid, 42
Hypochlorous Acid, 41, 62–63, 74
Hypoiodous Acid, 42
Hypotensive Responses, 366

Idiopathic Pulmonary Fibrosis, 121, 122, 131, 132, 134, 144, 146
IgA-, IgM, and IgG-containing Cells, 339
IgA-mediated ADCC, 349
IgD-containing Cells, 343
IgE-containing Plasma Cells, 339
IgG-containing Plasma Cells, 339
Immune Complex(es), 106, 107, 108, 109, 110, 111, 122, 123, 143, 144, 146, 246–248, 287–291, 300, 315, 317
Immunosuppressive, 137, 144, 146
Infections, 269
Inflammation, 163, 164, 166, 174, 175, 178–180, 361
Inflammatory Bowel Disease (IBD), 337
Intraepithelial Lymphocytes, 351
Invasion, 227
Iridocyclitis, 257

Keratoconjunctivitis, 270
Kininogen, 361, 362

Large-latticed Complexes, 11

Leukocytes, 163–173, 175–180
mononuclear, 163, 164, 168, 171–173, 175
polymorphonuclear (PMN), 163–171, 175–178, 180
Leukostasis, 105
Leukotrienes, 163–165, 169–180
LTA_4, 164, 172, 177
LTB_4, 98, 164–165, 169–170, 172–180, 195, 254
LTC_4, 165, 171–175, 180, 254
LTD_4, 171–175, 180, 254
LTE_4, 165, 171–174, 180, 254
Lipomodulin, 167, 169, 170
Lipopolysaccharide, 262
Lipoxygenase, 253
pathway, 163–166, 168–172, 175, 177–180
Liver
membrane antigen, 302, 306, 311, 317
specific protein, 301, 306, 311, 314, 317
Lung Injury Following Thermal Trauma, 387
increased vascular permeability, 388
leukoaggregates in, 388
toxic oxygen species in, 388
Lymphocyte, 98, 144, 145, 146, 147, 260
derived chemotactic factor for fibroblasts (LDCF-F), 145
intraepithelial lymphocytes, 351
null-lymphocytes, 349
Lymphokines, 98
Lysosomal Enzymes, 256

Macrophage(s), 25, 142, 144, 145, 146, 147, 165, 169, 170, 175, 180
Mallory Bodies, 308–310
Mast Cells, 164, 166–168, 171, 174
peroxidase, 41, 61, 62
Metastasis, 227
Methionine Sulfoxide, 71–74
Micropore Filter Assay, 212
Myeloperoxidase, 40–42, 43–44, 47, 59–63, 71–74, 92, 96, 97, 101, 103
deficiency, 48

NADPH Oxidase, 38, 91
Natural Killer Cell Activity, 352
Nephritis
anti-basement-membrane-induced, 2
Neutropenia, 259
Neutrophil(s), 23, 127, 146, 147, 164, 169, 176, 178, 180
Null-Lymphocytes, 349

Opsonins, 250
Oxygen-derived Free Radicals, 25
Oxygen Metabolites, 96, 100, 101, 124, 141, 255
and arachidonic acid, 70–71
and chemotactic factors, 71

and lysosomal enzymes, 59–60
and prostanoids, 73
and α_1-proteinase inhibitor, 71–73
Ozone, 138

Paraquat, 96, 124, 134, 138, 140, 141, 142
Peroxidase
glutathione, 47, 52, 57
mast cell, 41, 61, 62
PF/dil, 366
PGE, 154
PGE_2, 199, 347
$PGF_{2\alpha}$, 199
Phorbol Myristate Acetate (PMA), 45, 50, 53, 55–57, 62
Phospholipase A_2, 198
Phospholipid, 163, 166–169, 177
metabolism, 163, 166–168
methylation, 166, 168
Plasmin, 95
Plasminogen, 95
activator, 262
Platelet(s), 17, 142, 165, 166, 168–171, 175, 224
Pneumocyte
Type I, 142
Type II, 142
Pneumonitis, 122, 124, 136, 142, 143, 147
Polyarteritis Nodosa, 290
Polymorphonuclear (PMN) Leukocyte, 194, 259
Prekallikrein, 361, 362
Primary Biliary Cirrhosis, 312–317
Procollagen, 125, 126
Proline, 125
Prolyl Hydroxylase, 125, 140, 141
Properdin, 346
convertase, 346
Prostacyclin, 254
Prostaglandin(s), 163–165, 169, 171–175, 178–180, 347
PGE, 154
PGE_2, 347
$PGF_{2\alpha}$, 199
Proteases, 97, 100
Protein Kinase, 190
Pseudomonas Keratitis, 258
Psoriasis, 189
Pulmonary Edema, 105
Pulmonary Fibrosis, 103, 110, 121, 123, 124, 128, 131, 135, 138, 139, 140, 142, 143

Radiation, 122, 123, 134, 135, 142
Random Migration, 215
Reiter's Syndrome, 265
Respiratory Burst, 91, 99
Rheumatoid Arthritis, 110, 169, 179–181

Scleritis, 271
Secretory IgA, 345
Serum Sickness, 2, 106
Silica, 122, 123, 134, 142, 146
Singlet Oxygen ($^1O_2$), 42, 48, 96
Smooth Muscle Cells, 226
Smooth Muscle Contraction, 163, 165, 171, 173
Spermatozoa, 218
Steroid, 122, 135, 136, 143, 146
Stromal Keratitis, 271
Superoxide, 38–40, 46, 49–51
anion, 91, 96
dismutase (SOD), 39, 46, 101, 108, 139, 140, 256
Suppressor T-Cells, 352
Sympathetic Ophthalmia, 263
Systemic Lupus Erythematosus (SLE), 110

T-Cell Mediated Responses, 351
T-Lymphocytes, 165, 171, 177
Thermal Injury, 373
bactericidal activity of neutrophils in, 385
cellular immunity in, 390
chemotactic activity in, 384
complement activation, alternative pathway, 376
complement activity in, 374
complement components in, 375
depressive serum factors in, 391
mononuclear suppressor cells in, 391
neutrophil chemotaxis in, 379
opsonic serum activity in, 384
phagocytic activity of neutrophils in, 384
T-cell abnormality in, 390
Thermal Injury, Experimental, 377
C-5 related chemotactic activity in, 378, 384
complement activity in, 377, 378
lung injury following, 387
neutropenia in, 378
Tissue Repair, 221
Thromboxane, 254
Transplantation, 268
Tropocollagen, 125
Tumor Cell, 227

Ulcerative Colitis, 337

Vascular Permeability, 163, 171–175, 178–180, 198, 366
Vasculitis, 260
Vasodilation, 199
Vernal Catarrh, 267
Viral Conjunctivitis, 270
Viruses, 99
Vogt-Koyanagi-Harada Syndrome, 264

Wound Healing, 121, 134, 140, 146

Zymosan, 249